Book of Abstracts of the

16th World Congress of the IACAPAP

Book of Abstracts
of the
16th World Congress
of the
International Association
for Child and Adolescent Psychiatry
and Allied Professions
(IACAPAP)

22–26 August 2004, Berlin, Germany

Edited by

Helmut Remschmidt, MD, PhD, Congress President
Myron Belfer, MD, MPA, Chair Program Committee

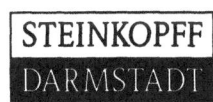
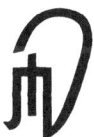

Prof. Helmut Remschmidt, MD, PhD
Department of Child and Adolescent Psychiatry
Philipps University
Hans-Sachs-Str. 6
35033 Marburg, Germany
E-Mail: remschm@med.uni-marburg.de

Prof. Myron L. Belfer, MD, MPH
Harvard Medical School
Department of Social Medicine
541 Huntington Avenue
Boston, MA 02115, USA
E-Mail: MYRON_BELFER@hms.harvard.edu

ISBN 978-3-7985-1472-0   ISBN 978-3-662-21595-1 (eBook)
DOI 10.1007/978-3-662-21595-1

Bibliographic information published by Die Deutsche Bibliothek
Die Deutsche Bibliothek lists this publication in the Deutsche Nationalbibliografie; detailed bibliographic data is available in the Internet at <http://dnb.ddb.de>.

www.steinkopff.springer.de

© Springer-Verlag Berlin Heidelberg 2004
Originally published by Steinkopff Verlag Darmstadt in 2004

Production: Heinz J. Schäfer
Typesetter: K+V Fotosatz GmbH, Beerfelden

SPIN 11014416   85/7231 – Printed on acid-free paper

Foreword

This book contains all of the abstracts of the 16th World Congress of the International Association for Child and Adolescent Psychiatry and Allied Professions (IACAPAP) held in Berlin, Aug 22–26, 2004.

The abstracts are arranged according to the type of session (main lecture, state of the art lecture, symposium, workshop, course, or poster exhibition) and the day of the conference. The abstracts of the industry-sponsored sessions are also included. A subject index is provided to help track themes of special interest. The author index allows you to find the abstract authors and the address of the first author for direct contact.

The general theme of the congress *"Facilitating Pathways: Care, Treatment and Prevention in Child and Adolescent Mental Health"* is quite inclusive and the contributions to the Congress, as reflected in the abstracts, cover the whole range of child and adolescent mental health endeavour, including all modern methods and trends in research and clinical application. The ways we understand and treat our patients are changing rapidly, and this too is reflected in the contributions to this volume, which give state-of-the-art information that should allow us to provide better care, treatment and prevention to children, adolescents and their care-givers everywhere in the world.

In spite of remarkable progress during recent years, there are still areas of major concern such as:
- magnitude of the burden of child and adolescent mental disorders
- advances made in treatment and diagnosis
- barriers to treatment
- trends in care for children and adolescents with mental disorders.

The Congress has recognized these areas of concern and given them special attention where possible.

The concern for international issues, the uniquely important role of IACAPAP, is expressed by the breadth of the contributions coming from more than 70 countries. The cultural dimension is often emphasized both in terms of differences, but importantly in an understanding of commonalities across cultures.

The editors of this volume wish to thank the members of the IACAPAP Executive Committee for continuous help and support. They thank all the authors for their valuable contributions and their excellent cooperation. They express their thanks and appreciation to the German Society for Child and Adolescent Psychiatry, Psychosomatics and Psychotherapy for the invitation to Germany and for substantial support. Further, they would like to offer their most sincere thanks to the program committee and especially to the reviewers who did an excellent job in reviewing more than 1200 submissions with remarkable results. Some compromises regarding format and the language of abstracts had to be made in order to maintain and promote a degree of uniformity and the international character of this Congress.

Finally, we thank very cordially the team of the congress organizing company CPO-Hanser and the members of the publishing company Steinkopff. Last, but not least, we wish to thank the staff members of the Marburg Department for Child and Adolescent Psychiatry for their immense engagement, untiring effort, and highly competent work.

Helmut Remschmidt, MD, PhD (Marburg/Germany)
Congress President

Myron L. Belfer, MD, MPA (Boston/USA)
Chair, Program Committee

Committees

Congress President
Professor Helmut Remschmidt, Marburg

National Scientific Committee
(Directors and professors of child and adolescent
departments at German universities)

Chairman:	Martin H. Schmidt, Mannheim
Vice-Chairmen:	Bernd Blanz, Jena
	Andreas Warnke, Würzburg
Members:	Christine Ettrich, Leipzig
	Jörg M. Fegert, Ulm
	Tilman Fürniss, Münster
	Alexander von Gontard, Homburg
	Frank Hässler, Rostock
	Johannes Hebebrand, Essen
	Beate Herpertz-Dahlmann, Aachen
	Emil Kammerer, Münster
	Günther Klosinski, Tübingen
	Ulrich Knölker, Lübeck
	Ulrike Lehmkuhl, Berlin
	Gerd Lehmkuhl, Köln
	Joest Martinius, München
	Gunther Moll, Erlangen
	Klaus-Jürgen Neumärker, Berlin
	Fritz Poustka, Frankfurt
	Franz Resch, Heidelberg
	Peter Riedesser, Hamburg
	Aribert Rothenberger, Göttingen
	Michael Scholz, Dresden
	Eberhard Schulz, Freiburg
	Michael Schulte-Markwort, Hamburg
	Gerd Schütze, Kiel

Scientific Secretaries

Gerd Schulte-Körne, Marburg
Johannes Hebebrand, Essen
Klaus Hennighausen, Freiburg
Fritz Mattejat, Marburg

Local Organizing Committee

Chairperson:	Ulrike Lehmkuhl, Berlin
Members:	Michael Huss, Berlin
	Ernst Pfeiffer, Berlin
	Harriet Salbach, Berlin

International Advisory Board

IACAPAP Executive Committee (1998–2004)

The IACAPAP Executive Committee has served as the International Advisory Board.

President:	Helmut Remschmidt, Germany
Secretary-General:	Ian M. Goodyer, UK
Treasurer:	Myron L. Belfer, USA
Honorary Presidents:	James E. Anthony, USA
	Gerald Caplan, Israel
	Colette Chiland, France
Vice-Presidents:	Ernesto Caffo, Italy
	Miguel Cherro-Aguerre, Uruguay
	Pierre Ferrari, France
	Per-Anders Rydelius, Sweden
	Herman van Engeland, Netherlands
	Kosuke Yamazaki, Japan
Assistant Secretaries:	Peter Jensen, USA
General:	Savita Malhotra, India
	Samuel Tyano, Israel
Adjunct Secretaries:	Amira Seif El Din, Egypt
	Bernard Golse, France
	Michael Hong, Korea
	Patricia Howlin, UK
	Barry Nurcombe, Australia
	John Sikorski, USA
	Andreas Warnke, Germany
Counselors:	Salvador Celia, Brazil
	Ronald Feldman, USA
	Philippe Jeammet, France
	Kari Schleimer, Sweden
	Martin H. Schmidt, Germany
Monograph Editors:	J. Gerald Young, USA
	Pierre Ferrari, France
Newsletter Editors:	Cynthia Pfeffer, USA
	Jocelyn Hattab, Israel
Editor Emeritus:	Colette Chiland, France

IACAPAP Nominating Committee

Chairperson:	Kari Schleimer, Malmö/Sweden
Members:	Salvador Celia, Porto Alegre/Brazil
	Barry Nurcombe, Brisbane/Australia

Program Committee

Chairman:	Myron L. Belfer, USA
Members:	Boris Birmaher, USA
	Ernesto Caffo, Italy
	John Fayyad, Lebanon
	Martine Flament, Canada
	Ian M. Goodyer, UK
	Philip Graham, UK
	Arturo Grau, Chile
	Late Richard Harrington, UK
	Luis Diego Herrera, Costa Rica
Members:	Michael Hong, Korea
	Shuji Honjo, Nagoya/Japan
	Philippe Jeammet, France
	Barry Nurcombe, Australia
	Brian Robertson, South Africa
	Luis Rohde, Brazil
	Per-Anders Rydelius, Sweden
	Martin H. Schmidt, Germany
	Fred Volkmar, USA
	Andreas Warnke, Germany
	Kosuke Yamazaki, Japan

Host Organization

GERMAN SOCIETY FOR CHILD AND ADOLESCENT
PSYCHIATRY, PSYCHOSOMATICS, AND PSYCHOTHERAPY

President:	Beate Herpertz-Dahlmann, Aachen
Vice Presidents:	Franz Resch, Heidelberg
	Peter Riedesser, Hamburg
Secretary-General:	Alexander von Gontard, Homburg
Treasurer:	Ulrike Lehmkuhl, Berlin
Members:	Fritz Mattejat, Marburg
	Helmut Remschmidt, Marburg (Honorary President)
	Martin H. Schmidt, Mannheim (Honorary President)
	Renate Schepker, Hamm (Chairperson of the Board of Directors of Child and Adolescent Psychiatric Hospitals in Germany)
	Christa Schaff, Weil der Stadt (Chairperson of the professional organization of German Child and Adolescent Psychiatrists)

Format Descriptions of the Scientific Program

Main Lectures
will be held every day by leading child psychiatrists and other mental health professionals and will cover major topics of the program.

State of the art Lectures
will present the recent development in a certain area with special focus on the congress theme.

Symposia
Symposia sessions last 120 minutes and focus on a specific topic, representing several points of view. There are Invited Symposia and Proposed Symposia. The organizer of the symposium chairs the session, which includes a maximum of six papers and time for discussion.

Workshops
Workshop sessions last 120 minutes. They deal with topics of special interest to child and adolescent mental health, using multiple, brief presentations of not more than 60 minutes, followed by approximately 60 minutes of discussion.

IACAPAP Courses
devoted to topics of practical relevance and given by distinguished experts are part of the educational program and will give an excellent opportunity for learning new facts and treatment procedures. Fees are charged separately for the courses: EUR 50.00 per course. Five courses are scheduled for Sunday, Aug 22, from 9 AM to 1 PM, five on Thursday, Aug 26, from 2 PM to 6 PM. This offers the opportunity to participate in two courses.

Poster Exhibition
The Poster Exhibition will be open from Monday, Aug 23, 11 AM – Thursday, Aug 26, 4 PM. The posters can stay for the whole time of the congress. Each poster author is requested to be at his or her poster from Monday – Thursday, between 1.30 and 2.30 PM. As the posters will be displayed for the whole time of the congress, this gives ample opportunities to repeatedly visit the posters and to discuss with the poster authors.

Student Tutorship Program

IACAPAP appreciates young academic colleagues in child and adolescent psychiatry. A novelty of this congress is the student tutorship program. Interested students of medicine and psychology, especially those who are currently working on their doctoral or master's theses, are especially welcome to attend the congress. They will have the opportunity to discuss their results with experienced experts.

(please see Workshop 204 on Tuesday, 24 August 2004, 17.00–19.00 h, room 43)

Free Communications

There was the possibility for a limited number of free communications. The scientific committee took the liberty to either integrate them into symposia or to accept them as posters.

Congress Monograph

A monograph devoted to and entitled with the main theme of the congress was produced for the congress. Leading child and adolescent mental health professionals from all continents reviewed and analyzed systems of care as well as innovations in the field of treatment and prevention in a transcultural perspective. The monograph is part of the congress documents.

Symposia Organized by the Industry

Satellite Symposia and Luncheon Satellite Symposia are organized by pharmaceutical companies in consultation with the Scientific Program Committee and presented during the congress.

How to Use this Book

The content of this book is divided into 8 chapters, each representing a type of session as listed in the table of contents (p. XVII). Within the chapters there are two types of entries as shown in the examples below:

- For the whole session, consisting of the session number from the program (e.g. S-002), the session topics (according to the topic list on the next page), the session title, the chairpersons and as a rule for symposia and workshops the session abstract.
- For a single presentation in a session, consisting of the contribution number from the program (e.g. S-002-010), the contribution topics, the contribution title, the author with address, the co-authors and the abstract.

Example for the whole session:

Example for a single presentation:

S-002 Topic: 23
Treatment evaluation under realistic clinical conditions
Track: Therapy and intervention
Chairperson: Helmut Remschmidt, Universität Marburg Kinder- und Jugendpsychiatrie, Marburg, Germany, remschm@med.uni-marburg.de

Treatment evaluation under realistic clinical conditions
Helmut Remschmidt, Universität Marburg, Kinder- und Jugendpsychiatrie, Marburg, Germany, remschm@med.uni-marburg.de

There are remarkable differences with regard to treatment success between experimental/controlled treatment studies and treatment studies under realistic clinical conditions. It is essential to find out which treatment matters are effective in which patients and under which conditions. Recent studies investigating this question have focused on empirical supported psychotherapeutic and combined treatment methods carried out in efficiency and effectiveness studies.

S-002-010 Topic: 6, 70
Cognitive-behavioral therapy for youth depression in community mental health clinics
John Weisz, University of California, Dept. of Psychology, Los Angeles, CA, USA, weisz@psych.ucla.edu

Objective: To describe an effectiveness test of cognitive-behavioral therapy (CBT) for youth depression in community mental health clinic settings. **Methods:** Depressed youths aged 8-15 who were referred to community mental health clinic were randomly assigned to receive either CBT or the usual care (UC) provided by the clinic. Therapists in each clinic had also been randomly assigned to learn and use CBT or to continue providing their own form of UC. Pre-treatment, post-treatment, and follow-up assessments provide evidence on the outcomes experienced by youths in the two treatment conditions. **Results:** At this time, not all youths have completed treatment in the UC condition; its duration is free to vary, and some youths have been in UC treatment for more than a year. Because this means that final outcome data are not available yet, the presentation

An author index and a topic index at the end of this book will help you to search for specific contributions.

The author index lists authors, co-authors, and chairpersons with the pagenumber of their appearance.

The topic index provides an alphabetical list of authors for each topic. Appended to the name of the author is the contribution number and the pagenumber, so that one is able to find either the session in the final program or the abstract in this book.

Topic List

1. Defining the needs for mental health services
2. Systems of care in a world wide perspective
3. Models of treatment and prevention
4. Treatment settings (day care treatment, home treatment, inpatient treatment, outpatient treatment, others)
5. Rehabilitation
6. Behavioural and cognitive therapies
7. Psychoanalytic/psychodynamic treatment
8. Interpersonal therapy
9. Group therapy and psychodrama
10. Parent training, family therapy and systemic approaches
11. Other psychotherapeutic approaches
12. Typical and atypical antipsychotics
13. Antidepressants
14. Mood stabilizers
15. Stimulants
16. Other medications
17. Pharmacotherapy in combination with other treatment methods
18. Other interventions
19. Multimodal and disorder-specific approaches to treatment and prevention
20. Internet and computer-based programs
21. School-based interventions
22. Consultation and liaison child psychiatry
23. Treatment evaluation and quality assurance
24. Developmental psychopathology
25. Child and mental health issues in the community
26. Epidemiology
27. Classification
28. Genetics
29. Neurology
30. Neuropsychology
31. Neurochemistry
32. Endocrinology
33. Immunology
34. Psychopharmacology
35. Neuroimaging techniques
36. Electrophysiology
37. Methods of clinical investigation (interviews, tests)
38. Research methods and strategies
39. Infant psychiatry
40. Child psychiatry
41. Adolescent psychiatry
42. Longitudinal studies/longterm course/follow up
43. Risk studies
44. Social psychiatry

45. Transcultural child and adolescent psychiatry/ethnic issues
46. Historical aspects
47. The child and his family
48. Attachment and interaction
49. Separation/divorce/bereavement
50. Adoption/foster care/custody
51. Child abuse and neglect
52. Violence
53. Children and war/disaster
54. Refugee children
55. Children of sick parents
56. Quality of life issues
57. Forensic child and adolescent psychiatry
58. School-based issues
59. Media
60. Self-help groups
61. Stigma and discrimination
62. Socioeconomic burden of disease
63. Training and professional issues
64. Financial issues/funding
65. Ethical issues
66. Children's rights
67. Organic and symptomatic mental disorders
68. Substance related disorders
69. Schizophrenia and other psychotic disorders
70. Mood disorders/Affective disorders
71. Anxiety and phobic disorders
72. Obsessive-compulsive disorder
73. Posttraumatic stress disorders
74. Dissociative disorders
75. Somatoform disorders
76. Sexual and gender identity disorders
77. Sleep disorders
78. Eating and feeding disorders/obesity
79. Behavioural syndromes and mental disorders associated
    with physiological dysfunction
80. Personality disorders
81. Mental retardation
82. Learning disorders, motor function disorders, speech and language disorders
83. Pervasive developmental disorders
84. Attention-deficit/hyperactivity disorders
85. Oppositional defiant and conduct disorders
86. Emotional disorders
87. Tic disorders
88. Elimination disorders (enuresis/encopresis)
89. Attachment disorders
90. Other disorders with onset usually occurring in childhood and adolescence
91. Epilepsy
92. Other somatic diseases
93. Suicide and self injurious behaviour
94. School refusal
95. Comorbidity in child psychiatry
96. Other disorders/conditions

Contents

Main Lectures

ML-001   Topic: 31, 29
Architecture of the cerebral cortex
and transmitter receptors
Chairperson: Paul Lombroso, Yale University Child Study
Center, New Haven, CT, USA, paul.lombroso@yale.edu

ML-001-001   Topic: 31, 29
Architecture of the cerebral cortex
and transmitter receptors
Karl Zilles, Forschungszentrum Jülich, Inst. für Medizin,
Germany, k.zilles@fz-juelich.de

The structural and functional heterogeneity of the human cerebral cortex was demonstrated at the beginning of the last century. The cortex was parcellated into numerous cortical areas (Brodmann, 1909; Vogt and Vogt, 1919; von Economo and Koskinas, 1925). The resulting cortical maps are based on local differences in the regional and laminar distribution of cell bodies (i.e., cytoarchitecture) or myelinated fibers (i.e., myeloarchitecture). The pioneering map of Brodmann (1909) is the reference system, if a precise anatomical localization has to be assigned to functional imaging data (e.g., functional magnetic resonance imaging (fMRI)). Such attempts, however, reveal a mismatch between the Brodmann map and the functional imaging data. The reason for this mismatch is manifold. Beside technical and methodological problems of classical cytoarchitectonic approaches, the restriction to cell bodies or myelinated nerve fibers as markers of cortical organization is apparently not sufficient to analyze the enormous functional and structural complexity of the cerebral cortex. Since transmitter receptors play a key role in neurotransmission, and are molecular markers of the cortical organization, we explored the regional and laminar distributions of receptors by using quantitative in vitro receptor autoradiography and image analysis procedures. The regional and laminar distribution patterns of 15 different receptor types and subtypes representing all classical transmitter systems (glutamate, GABA, acetylcholine, dopamine, noradrenaline, serotonin) were analyzed by labelling the receptors with highly specific, tritiated ligands in 20 micrometer thin, serial cryostat sections through complete human hemispheres. These distribution patterns were correlated with cyto- and myeloarchitectonic data in immediately adjacent sections. In some cases, a perfect match between the cyto- or myeloarchitectonic definition of cortical borders on one hand and local changes in receptor patterns on the other hand were found. However, the receptor-based parcellation of the cerebral cortex leads in many cases to more detailed cortical maps than previously described indicating the segregation of the cortex into molecular-based units. E.g., the muscarinic M2, serotoninergic 5-HT2, and noradrenergic alpha2 as well as to some degree also the GABAergic GABAA receptors show exceptionally high densities in the primary sensory areas as opposed to other cortical areas. This clearly demonstrates a molecular diversity of the cortex, and suggests that, e.g., pharmacotherapy with receptor ligands may cause different effects in the different cortical regions. Since receptors interact with each other, the balance between different receptors in each cortical region seems to be even more important than the local density of a single receptor type. To visualize this complex multimodal aspect, the "receptor fingerprint" was recently introduced as a molecular marker of cortical organization. In the present talk, a receptor fingerprint is the polar coordinate plot of the mean (averaged over all cortical layers) receptor densities of 15 receptor types and subtypes in each of the different cortical fields. The fingerprint is a graphical representation of a multidimensional feature vector representing the contribution of each receptor to the balance between all receptors in a cortical area. The analysis of the fingerprints using multidimensional scaling and cluster algorithms reveals a novel and highly segregated regional and laminar organization of the human cerebral cortex, which is the molecular basis of its diverse functions. Supported by DFG, EU, and NIH.

ML-002   Topic: 24
Gerald Caplan Lecture: What about girls?
Sex differences in psychopathology
Chairperson: Myron Belfer, Harvard Medical School
Dept. of Social Medicine, Boston, MA, USA,
myron-belfer@hms.harvard.edu

ML-002-002   Topic: 24
What about girls? Sex differences in psychopathology
Colette Chiland, Université René Descartes, Paris, France,
cchiland@wanadoo.fr

Methods: Often boys are chosen as the paradigmatic cases. But the picture is not the same for boys and girls, mutatis mutandis. Female were said to be the feeble sex; but considering psychobiological development, male are the feeble sex. We have to consider the overall psychopathology and the specific conditions. There are data scattered throughout the literature about specific conditions. But there was no consideration paid to the sex differences in psychopathology as a whole until recently. Throughout the world, and throughout childhood, there are more males than females seen in clinics, and still more treated in institutions. The sex ratio Male to Female varies with symptoms: for an example, around 6 for encopresis, 4 for autism, stammering, around 2.5 for enuresis. The reason of these various levels is unknown. We will try to discuss various hypotheses. Here is a field open for further researches.

ML-003   Topic: 83
Autism spectrum disorders
Track: Pervasive developmental disorders (PDD)
Chairperson: Herman van Engeland, University Medical
Center Child & Adolescent Psychiatry, Utrecht, Netherlands,
h.vanengeland@azu.nl

ML-003-003   Topic: 83
Autism spectrum disorders
Christopher Gillberg, University of Göteborg, Göteborg,
Sweden, christopher.gillberg@pediat.gu.se

Autistic disorder/childhood autism is now conceptualized as one of the conditions in the so called autism spectrum, which also includes Asperger syndrome, atypical autism and childhood disintegrative disorder. The autism spectrum disorders are also, controversially, referred to as pervasive developmental disorders. Both autistic disorder and the other disorders in the spectrum are much more common than previously believed. Together they affect 1 in 200 to 1 in 100 children of young school age. Symptoms are present from early childhood and the diagnosis can be made with good precision in typical cases of autistic disorder around 3 years of age and in more high-functioning individuals around 5-8 years of age. Learning disability/ mental retardation is present in about 1 in 5 of all individuals affected by an autism spectrum disorder, but some degree of peculiar cognitive development is present in all. There is a substantial body of evidence regarding the brain-neuropsychology-behaviour relationships in autism, even though no unitary basic cause has been established. Genetic factors are very important in the pathogenesis of autism, but environmental risk factors of various kinds also play a role. A lot of medical, developmental and psychiatric disorders are overrepresented in autism, and these always need to be taken into account in the diagnostic process. Outcome is variable but psychosocially very restricted in a majority of cases. Effective interventions for specific problems are available, but there is no one treatment that will lead to a cure at the present time. This paper will review some of the most recent evidence in terms of autism prevalence, genetics, neuropsychology, intervention and outcome. Future developments will be briefly discussed.

ML-004   Topic: 44, 25
The biosocial roots of mind and brain
Chairperson: Lionel Hersov, London, United Kingdom,
child+family@tavi-port.org

ML-004-004   Topic: 44, 25
The biosocial roots of mind and brain
Leon Eisenberg, Harvard Medical School,
Dept. of Social Medicine, Boston, MA, USA,
leon_eisenberg@hms.harvard.edu

Abstract: The Biosocial Roots of Mind and Brain by Leon Eisenberg, MD Two and a half millennia ago, a physician of the Hippocratic school wrote: "Men ought to know that from the brain and the brain alone arise our pleasures, joys, laughters, and jests, as well as our sorrows, pains, griefs, and tears." When those words were written, they were a testimony of faith; today, scientific evidence underpins this assertion, but with modifications. The brain is the organ of the mind, but we have learned that the very structure of the brain is itself modified by inputs from the environments, biological and social, to which the individual is exposed. Biology matters; inheritance matters; but so does learning. Nature and nurture stand in reciprocity, not in opposition. Offspring inherit, along with their parents' genes, their parents, their peers, and their neighborhoods. The ontogenetic niche is a crucial link between parents and offspring, an envelope of life chances. Development is at one and the same time a social, a psychological, and a biological process. Advances in neuroscience have revealed that the gross structure of the brain follows a genetic blueprint, but the refinement of precise connections is guided by environmental stimuli, in turn modified by the behavior of the organism itself, in an interactive cascade. New synapses result from experience. In experience-expectant synaptogenesis, synapses form after minimal experience; the prototype is the development of stereoscopy. It requires normal visual input, but because that input is an expectable part of the environmental niche, synapses require minimal reinforcement. In contrast, in experience-dependent synaptogenesis, adaptation to relatively unique features of the environment is optimized by fashioning new connections to deal with features that vary from one environment to the other and must be learned. The substrate of experience-expectant learning is the pruning back of surplus synapses which do not receive appropriate excitation. Experience-dependent neural activity selects a functionally appropriate subset out of the abundant connections already present in the infant brain. The dependence of human infants on parenting for sheer survival creates the social context in which we become human. Not only does the growth of the child's social intelligence result from social relationships, but do does the organization of its neuroendocrine axis. Infant homeostasis is an outcome of a collaborative process. Infant body temperatures are regulated by caretakers when they respond to signals such as crying or changes in color by holding the infant more closely. Maternal touch and warmth modify infant hormone production. Early experience determines the rate at which the brain ages. The amount of stimulation the young receive from their parents modulates their cortisol production. Soma, as well as psyche, is a social no less than a biological construct.

ML-005   Topic: 24
Environmentally mediated risks for psychopathology
Chairperson: Per-Anders Rydelius, Karolinska Institutet
Woman and Child Health, Stockholm, Sweden,
per-anders.rydelius@ks.se

ML-005-005   Topic: 24
Environmentally mediated risks for psychopathology
Michael Rutter, Institute of Psychiatry, SGDP Centre,
London, United Kingdom, j.wickham@iop.kcl.ac.uk

The testing of hypotheses regarding the environmental mediation of risks for adverse psychological outcomes has to be preceded by a clear conceptualisation of the postulated risk factor – as illustrated by findings on parent-child separation and the involvement of fathers in childrearing. The identification of the points on the dimension where the risks arise may help in that connection – as shown by findings on early childcare, parental age at the child|s birth, and physical punishment. The testing of environmental risk hypotheses ordinarily requires the use of designs that pull apart variables that usually go together; the measurement of within-individual behavioural change in relation to timed and measured environmental change; the use of natural experiments that can differentiate between environmental and genetic risk mediation, as well as between-person effects on the environment and environmental effects on the person; and the use of statistical techniques that can take account of measurement error. A range of examples that illustrate the success of these strategies will be described. The importance of taking account of gene-environment interaction will be considered in relation to both quantitative and molecular genetic evidence. Gene-environment correlation and a broader group of person effects on the environment will be discussed in relation to the origin of individual differences in environmental risk exposure. The huge individual differences in response to environmental risk will be noted, and finally the need to put together findings into an overall causal model will be discussed.

ML-006   Topic: 47
Impacts of rapid social and family changes on the mental health of children in Asia

Chairperson: Barry Nurcombe,
University of Queensland Dept. of Psychiatry, Brisbane,
Australia, bnurcombe@psychiatry.uq.edu.au

ML-006-006   Topic: 47
Impacts of rapid social and family changes on the mental health of children in Asia

K. Michael Hong, Cheju National University,
College of Medicine, Cheju, Republic of Korea,
kmhong@cheju.ar.ky

During the latter half of the 20th century, almost all countries in Asia went through their own form of "modernization" in which drastic economical, political, and social changes occurred to various extents and at varying rates. This modernization involved industrialization, urbanization, family nuclearization (which resulted in the breakdown of the traditional family system), and "westernization" (which resulted in the introduction of a western ideology in value orientation included the introduction to democracy, capitalism, individualism, human/gender equal right issues and freedom of choice issues). While these changes certainly brought about improvements in many areas of Asian life, such as the standards of living, sanitation, nutrition, education and physical health, they seem to be accompanied by a disconcerting increase in the number of mental health problems in children and adolescents. These mental health problems include: developmental, emotional, and behavioral disorders, cases of child abuse and neglect, school violence, delinquency, and suicide. In this paper, clinical observations and epidemiological-empirical studies are presented, psycho-pathogenic mechanisms and processes are formulated, and the impacts and implications on the mental health of children are discussed from developmental, ecological, and ethological perspectives. The author suggests that one of the most critical pathogenic factors could be the rapidness and swiftness of change rather than the change itself. This compressed form of modernization occurred within the span of only 30-40 years in most Asian countries, but was accomplished gradually over 200-300 years in western countries. The important mediating pathogenic processes are the breakdown of the traditional value orientation, nuclearization of the family system and a sharp increase in the number of divorces (with a subsequent weakening of the major support network), and the growing number of child rearing problems associated with rapid social changes. The author suggests that there are crises and grave problems in child rearing in most Asian countries, based on the following observations: avoidance of pregnancy and an increase of unwanted children, avoidance and refusal of child rearing and abandonment of young children, confusion and inappropriateness in early child rearing, inappropriate or inadequate discipline (over-protection and over-control), changes in gender roles and attitudes, and preoccupation with intellectual capability and an endless pressure on scholastic achievement. The author also presents the following phenomena, which must have significant implications on the mental health of children in many countries in Asia: marked changes of the family system and the alarming increase in the number of divorces, the reduction in the number of children in a family, the rising number of working mothers and women's equal right movements, the lack of opportunities for parents to learn how to raise a child, the steep competition and exclusive emphasis on scholastic achievement in school, the marked change in value orientations from traditional to modern, the confusing and often contradictory pieces of advice given by "experts" and "professionals" on child rearing and child education, the new tides of globalization and the confounding co-existence of multi-cultures in most countries and the emergence of a virtual world, IT and BT industry in some advanced countries. The author concludes with a discussion, from a developmental, ecological and ethological point of view, of the implications of these findings on interventions and preventions for mental health of children in developing countries. The critical importance of early child rearing and the quality of the mother-infant attachment for the future mental health of children in the 21st century is emphasized. The need for new guidelines and new paradigms to bring up mentally healthy children in this complex and ever changing world is advocated. Perhaps a solution can be found in integrating the Old and the New as well as the East and the West.

ML-007   Topic: 24
The place of development in child and adolescent psychiatry. The Donald Cohen Memorial Lecture

Chairperson: Peter Jensen, Columbia University Center for Advancement Child MH, New York, USA,
pj131@columbia.edu

ML-007-007   Topic: 24
The place of development in child and adolescent psychiatry. The Donald Cohen Memorial Lecture

Helmut Remschmidt, Universität Marburg,
Kinder- und Jugendpsychiatrie, Marburg, Germany,
remschm@med.uni-marburg.de

There is no doubt that the developmental perspective is of great importance for the understanding of psychopathological disorders in children and adolescents. Developmental physiology, developmental neurology and developmental psychology are basic sciences of child psychiatry. The developmental perspective can be looked upon a kind of bridge between different disciplines and as a unifying concept (Eisenberg, 1977) integrating different scientific and practical approaches to normality and psychopathology, not only for children but also for adults. This is particular true for the discipline Developmental Psychopathology aiming at the study of the effect of all kinds of influences upon psychological functioning and behaviour. Research fields and – strategies in developmental psychopathology cover numerous areas like the developmental process itself, brain maturation, sex differences and individual differences, continuity and change of behaviour, the importance of risk factors and protective factors, the classification of disorders based on developmental principals as well as studies of the course of disorders and the possibility of prediction. Finally it seems important to integrate and structure the existent knowledge in terms of development-related models that allow the derivation of new eye possessies for the complex process of individual growth and maturation in the context of the family and other components of the psychosocial system This lecture is devoted to the memory of the late Donald Cohen, former director of the Yale Child Study Centre and President of IACAPAP who contributed substantially to the field of developmental psychopathology not only by profound scientific achievements but also by his personal example as a researcher, physician, mentor, teacher and world wide advocate of troubled children and their families.

ML-008   Topic: 28, 24
Primary parental preoccupation:
Circuits, genes and the crucial role of the environment
Chairperson: Martin H. Schmidt, Zentralinstitut für Seelische Gesundheit, Mannheim, Germany, schmidt@zi-mannheim.de

ML-008-008   Topic: 28, 24
Primary parental preoccupation:
Circuits, genes and the crucial role of the environment
James Leckman, Yale University, Child Study Center, New Haven, USA, james.leckman@yale.edu

Parental caregiving includes a set of highly conserved behaviors and mental states that may reflect both an individual's genetic endowment and the early experience of being cared for as a child. This review first examines the mental and behavioral elements of early parental caregiving in humans. Second, we consider what is known about the neurobiological substrates of maternal behaviors in mammalian species including some limited human data. Third, we briefly review the evidence that specific genes encode proteins that are crucial for the development of the neural substrates that underlie specific features of maternal behavior. Fourth, we review the emerging literature on the 'programming' role of the intrauterine environment and postnatal caregiving environment in shaping subsequent maternal behavior. We conclude that there are critical developmental windows during which the genetically determined microcircuitry of key limbic-hypothalamic-midbrain structures are susceptible to early environmental influences and that these influences powerfully shape an individual's responsivity to psychosocial stressors and their resiliency or vulnerability to various forms of human psychopathology later in life.

State-of-the-Art-Lectures

ST-001   Topic: 6
Cognitive behaviour therapy:
Development and current issues
Track: Therapy and intervention
Chairperson: Andreas Warnke, Universitätsklinik Würzburg Kinder- und Jugendpsychiatrie, Würzburg, Germany, warnke@kjp.uni-wuerzburg.de

ST-001-001   Topic: 6
Cognitive behaviour therapy:
Development and current issues
Philip Graham, London, United Kingdom, pjgraham1@aol.com

The aim of this presentation is to provide an account of a relatively new therapeutic approach, so that those who are unfamiliar with it will be encouraged to investigate its possibilities further. In this state of the art lecture I aim to provide an account of the development of cognitive behaviour therapy from both behavioural and psychoanalytic approaches. I shall summarise the main issues relating to evidence for effectiveness in comparison to other forms of treatment. I shall then discuss the prospects for the use of this form of psychotherapy in the future.

ST-002   Topic: 41
Current issues in adolescent psychiatry
Chairperson: Ernesto Caffo, University of Modena Dept. of Neuroscience, Modena, Italy, caffo@unimo.it

ST-002-002   Topic: 41
Current issues in adolescent psychiatry
Philippe Jeammet, Université Paris VI, Psychiatrie de l'Enfant, Paris, France, philippe.jeammet@imm.fr

Most adolescents are healthy individuals. They are dynamic, enthusiastic and above all have a capacity to adapt to a constantly changing world that many adults envy. This makes it all the more unacceptable to see that some adolescents, about 15%, slip into self-destructive behaviour and sabotage their potential. Suicide and attempted suicide are the most prefect examples of this behaviour, but the same holds true for all self-destructive behaviour such as alcoholism, drug addiction, eating disorders, school refusal and other attitudes of opposition or active passivity. This is all the more tragic and outrageous when we realize that only a minority among these adolescents suffer from declared mental disorders (about 20/30%). However, while these self-destructive attitudes are not necessarily pathological, they are pathogenic, which is to say that the adolescent bound up in such behaviour, winds up becoming truly ill. Yet clinical practice shows us that adolescents with similar risk factors and vulnerability do not necessarily follow the same path. The future of these adolescents who function on an all or nothing basis, often depends on the quality of their relationships with adults. They are as capable of enthusiasm as they are sensitive to deception. Adolescence is precisely the passing from a state of infantile dependency to one of more autonomy. The adolescent has to construct a new distance in his relationships with adults, especially with those adults on whom he was formerly the most dependent: parents and close relations. Those who attain adolescence with the least sense of secur-

ity and self-esteem are the ones who are going to be the most in need of adult support. Yet they are the very ones who are the most unwilling to accept it. Oppositional behaviour, becomes a way to affirm one's difference and to create the "negative identity", described by the famous adolescent psychiatrist, Eric Erikson. The problem is that once this negative behavior is installed it takes on an aura of fascination. It becomes the major way to free one's self of adults, to no longer depend upon their judgement. In reality it only serves to reinforce a deeply rooted dependency. Unfortunately we end up with a vicious circle: the more we try to help the adolescent, the more he refuses and opposes us. And so we come to the tragic paradox: those adolescents who most need help are the very ones who refuse it the most vigorously. How can we help them? How can we create the conditions for a positive nourishing relationship with adults which they will be willing to accept? First we must try to understand what motivates their attitude and behaviour.

ST-003   Topic: 35
Neuroimaging: Psychiatric disorders
as information processing disorders
Chairperson: James Leckman, Yale University Child Study Center, New Haven, USA, james.leckman@yale.edu

ST-003-003   Topic: 35
Neuroimaging: Psychiatric disorders
as information processing disorders
Alexander C. McFarlane, University of Adelaide, Queen Elizabeth Hospital, Woodville, Australia, alexander.mcfarlane@adelaide.edu.au

One of the most remarkable capacities of the human brain involves the ability to collect and interpret the mass of information from the environment and then convert this into a world of reality. Critical to making sense of the present, is the ability to access memory. The clinical conceptualizations involve the process of registration, short term and long term memory. However, organizing the present, involves a more complex process described as working memory. This involves the ability to organize current perceptions, to manipulate them and to make sense of them using a variety of information from long term memory. It is the disruption of this process which is central to understanding the experience and phenomenology of psychiatric disorders. Neuroimaging has provided a series of windows into the processes of working memory and the various neuro anatomical systems that contribute to the developing humans capacity to make sense of their world. In this presentation the potential for the disruption of the normal developmental progressions in neural development because of traumatic life experience, as well as biological vulnerabilities will be highlighted. Neuroimaging studies of psychiatric disorders in adulthood, demonstrate the importance of fluid integration of the dorsal lateral hippocampul systems involved in defining context and meaning and those of the medial prefrontal cortex and the amygdala in defining emotional salience. Hence neuroimaging can provide a model of how developmental disruption can lead to the disorganisation of the stability of the monitoring systems of the brain. Using methods that combine an analyse of measurement of the temporal dynamics of the brain with peripheral arousal, it is now possible to use these methods of measurement to establish the impact of treatment and the ability to normalise the disturbed information processing associated with particular disorders.

ST-004   Topic: 53
Caring for children exposed to war, disaster and terrorism

Chairperson: Ronald Feldman, Columbia University School of Social Work, New York, NY, USA, raf1@columbia.edu

ST-004-004   Topic: 53
Caring for children exposed to war, disaster and terrorism

Nathaniel Laor, Tel Aviv University, Faculty of Medicine, Tel Aviv, Israel, nlaor@netvision.net.il

War, terrorism and disasters are serious threats to the physical existence and the identity of individuals and communities at large. They generate general confusion, political instability, social disarray, intra- and inter-group conflict and collapse of regulative ideologies. This presentation focuses on psycho-social processes taking place in the children's community under such events, and the role of mental health professionals working with exposed children and adolescents. We present terrorism and the response to it as a case study in children's psycho-social reaction to massive violence exerted on their community. We describe the multiple faces of terrorism and its aims, and the various responses observed in children and adolescents. We also examine the important role played by ideology as regulatory factor in regard to the resilience as observed individually as well as in communities. We present data (psychological symptoms, ideology parameters and personal resilience) of a large sample of adolescents exposed to continuous stress due to war and terrorist attacks and discuss it in terms of a multi-dimensional process that needs to take place in parallel to the trauma relief efforts: the facilitation of reconciliation through transcending ideologies of hate and the enhancement of coexistence between groups in conflict (ethnic, religious, political).

ST-005   Topic: 84, 24
Developmental psychopathology of ADHD
Track: ADHD

Chairperson: Sam Tyano, Geha Mental Health Center, Petah Tiqva, Israel, styano@post.tau.ac.il

ST-005-005   Topic: 84, 24
Developmental psychopathology of ADHD

Hans-Christoph Steinhausen, ZKJP Universität Zürich, Kinder- und Jugendpsychiatrie, Zürich, Switzerland, steinh@kjpd.unizh.ch

Developmental issues in ADHD are apparent on various levels. On the level of aetiology genetic disposition and acquired biological factors interact with modulating psychosocial factors so that ADHD is frequently representing in a complex condition with additional problems due to coexisting disorders and burden on the patient, family and society. These patterns unfold over time with changes in behaviour and functioning that are not sufficiently captured by the diagnostic criteria of ADHD, which are adequate for boys aged 6–12 years with normal intelligence and less adequate for girls, preschoolers, adolescents, adults and those with mental retardation. Precursors of ADHD in infants and toddlers focus on temperament variation whereas in preschoolers it is difficult to differentiate ADHD from the normal range of behaviours. Recently, adaptations of diagnostic criteria of ADHD to the preschool age period have been proposed and research is underway addressing the specific issues of assessment and treatment of ADHD in preschoolers. Our own longitudinal studies in late childhood to early adolescence assessed the change in behavioural symptoms, neuropsychological functioning, and neurophysiological functioning. Whereas a sizeable proposition of patients did not fulfil diagnostic criteria at follow-up there was less reduction of behavioural symptoms over time. Changes in neuropsychological functioning were dependent on timeframe and measures, and neurophysiological findings were incompatible with the assumption of brain maturation within the observed time period. Long-term outcome studies underline the poor and disabling course of ADHD in a sizeable proportion of patients with a number of unfavourable prognostic factors including clinical features and family characteristics, whereas the effects of intervention on the long-term course are less clear. Only a better understanding of the complex aetiology and more refined interventions will ultimately result in better prognosis of ADHD.

ST-006   Topic: 51
The psychopathology and treatment of child sexual abuse

Chairperson: Ian Goodyer, Cambridge University Dept. Developmental Psychiatry, Cambridge, United Kingdom, ig104@cam.ac.uk

ST-006-006   Topic: 51
The psychopathology and treatment of child sexual abuse

Barry Nurcombe, University of Queensland, Dept. of Psychiatry, Brisbane, Australia, bnurcombe@psychiatry.uq.edu.au

Methods: Critical review of literature. **Results:** Retrospective studies have linked child sexual abuse (CSA) with later emotional disorders, low self esteem, suicidal behaviour, substance abuse, eating disorder, borderline personality disorder, early pregnancy, risky life styles, sexual dysfunction, and dissociative and somatoform disorders. There have been 14 RCT studies of treatment in CSA. Group therapy and cognitive behaviour therapy have generally been found superior to no treatment or non-specific treatment. **Conclusion:** CSA is typically associated with other family pathology. An eclectic approach to therapy is required.

ST-007   Topic: 30, 31
Molecular mechanisms of learning and memory
Chairperson: Ernesto Caffo, University of Modena Dept. of Neuroscience, Modena, Italy, caffo@unimo.it

ST-007-007   Topic: 30, 31
Molecular mechanisms of learning and memory
Paul Lombroso, Yale University, Child Study Center,
New Haven, CT, USA, paul.lombroso@yale.edu

The underlying mechanisms by which normal learning and memory occur will be reviewed. This topic is at the interface between psychiatry and neuroscience, and those of us who care for children and their families should become familiar with this area of research. Areas to be reviewed will be the various domains of memory, the regions of the brain that are critically involved in the consolidation of memories, and the molecular mechanisms that lead to synaptic morphological changes and that underlies all learning. The lecture will then proceed to a discussion of how disruptions to normal learning can arise when mutations occur in genes required for normal learning. Fragile X syndrome will be used as an example of a disorder in which a mutation has occurred to a critical gene in this pathway. The type of mutation [triplet repeat expansion] and the normal function of the FMR protein will be reviewed. This discussion will clarify how disruptions to activity dependent strengthening of synaptic morphology is able to compromise normal learning and memory formation. The lecture will also discuss how these issues can be studied in the laboratory using animal models of learning. This is an area in psychiatric research that we as clinicians and researchers should be interested in and embrace as our own.

ST-008   Topic: 3, 23
Evidence-based psychotherapeutic treatments
for children and adolescents
Track: Therapy and intervention
Chairperson: Helmut Remschmidt, Universität Marburg
Kinder- und Jugendpsychiatrie, Marburg, Germany,
remschm@med.uni-marburg.de

ST-008-008   Topic: 3, 23
Evidence-based psychotherapeutic treatments
for children and adolescents
John Weisz, University of California, Dept. of Psychology,
Los Angeles, CA, USA, weisz@psych.ucla.edu
Kristin Hawley

Objective: To describe and critique the state of knowledge on the effects of psychotherapies for children and adolescents, with an emphasis on treatments for anxiety, depression, ADHD, and conduct disorder. **Methods:** Findings from meta-analyses and task force reviews of youth psychotherapy research will be presented, with attention given to the nature of the evidence in general and the types of interventions for which evidence is strongest and weakest, in particular. The most robust treatments will be described and illustrated. Strengths and limitations of the evidence base will be noted, and new directions will be proposed for research and practice, and their interaction. **Results:** Effect sizes for most structured treatments using manuals fall within the medium to large range (i.e., 0.5 to 0.8 SD), larger than effect sizes for some well-known medical interventions for some physical conditions. In addition, the evidence shows specificity of effects, with treatments producing larger effects for targeted problems and disorders than for other problems and disorders not targeted in treat-

ment. Treatment effects are also generally durable, holding up well over the 6–7 month average lag between end of treatment and follow-up outcome assessment. The strengths of the evidence notwithstanding, significant gaps remain in our knowledge of the boundary conditions within which treatment works (i.e., moderators), the reaons why they work (i.e., mediators), and their effectiveness in clinically representative contexts and conditions. **Conclusion:** Five decades of youth psychotherapy research have produced a substantial evidence base encompassing multiple efficacious treatments, some quite robust. However, important gaps remain, suggesting a rich agenda for research in the decades ahead.

ST-009   Topic: 78
Eating disorders in childhood and adolescence
Track: Eating disorders
Chairperson: Kari Schleimer, University of Lund
Child & Adolescent Psychiatry, Akarp, Sweden,
kari.schleimer@telia.com

ST-009-009   Topic: 78
Eating disorders in childhood and adolescence
Beate Herpertz-Dahlmann, RWTH Aachen,
Kinder- u. Jugendpsychiatrie, Aachen, Germany,
bherpertz-dahlmann@ukaachen.de

Objective: The lecture tries to present an overview on three main topics: childhood and adolescent anorexia and bulimia nervosa as well as obesity-linked binge eating and night eating. **Methods:** It covers epidemiology, diagnostic issues and new insights into etiology including genetic and sociocultural causes. The results of an epidemiological study in preschool children on obesity, binge eating and night eating are presented. Metabolic changes emphazising findings on abnormalities in the leptin axis and bone turnover are discussed. The importance of diagnosing comorbid disorders like OCD, depression and anxiety disorders will be stressed. **Results:** The focus of the treatment issues are behavioral family therapy including psychoeducational groups for parents,nutritional counselling, body oriented therapy and individual and group cognitive-behavioral therapy strategies for the patients and the treatment of comorbid disorders. **Conclusion:** At last an overview on long-term research is given and adult-onset and adolescent-onset eating disorder outcome compared. The lecture will be practise and clinician-oriented.

ST-010   Topic: 51, 54
Street children as a world wide problem:
Perspectives from the Philippines
Chairperson: Peter Riedesser, UKE Hamburg-Eppendorf
Abt. Psychiatrie, Hamburg, Germany,
riedesser@uke.uni-hamburg.de

ST-010-010   Topic: 51
Street children as a world wide problem:
Perspectives from the Philippines
Cornelio Banaag, Medical City Hospital, Psychiatry, Pasig
City, Philippines, cjrpbanaag@mydestiny.net

The term street children was coined in the early 1980's to identify children who had chosen to spend majority of their time in the streets trying to earn a living. The United Nations estimate the population of street children worldwide at 150 million, with the number increasing every day. The WHO estimates a wide range of 10 to 100 million depending on the exact definition used. The interweaving political, economic and psychosocial conditions that drive children to the streets are too complex to explain this worldwide phenomenon. Poverty, and all its associated adversities, is the most commonly cited leading cause. The average age of street children is 3 to 18 years. With some variations in different countries, 40% of these children are homeless and 60% are involved with various work to support their families. Life on the streets ex-poses these children to illnesses, physical injuries, street fights, sexual exploitation, high levels of violence, substance abuse, and mental health problems. Many gov-ernment and non-government organizations are involved in providing a helping net-work. A study in the Philippines suggests that many street children are resilient. Mul-tiple factors make for their resilience.

ST-011   Topic: 42
Longitudinal studies in child and adolescent psychiatry
Chairperson: K. Michael Hong, Cheju National University College of Medicine, Cheju, Republic of Korea, kmhong@cheju.ar.ky

ST-011-011   Topic: 42
Longitudinal studies in child and adolescent psychiatry
Frank C. Verhulst, Erasmus MC-Sophia, Child & Adolescent Psychiatry, Rotterdam, Netherlands, m.engel@erasmusmc.nl

Objective: To give an overview of existing studies on child-adult continuities and discontinuities of child psychopathology and to illustrate the longitudinal course of child psychopathology by findings from a longitudinal general population study. **Methods:** Existing studies on the long-term continuity and discontinuity of child and adolescent psychopathology are reviewed. The longitudinal course of child psychopathology is illustrated by findings from a 14-year follow-up of a general population sample. Both rating scales and psychiatric interviews were used to assess psychopathology. Both traditional statistical techniques as well as more advanced techniques were used, including multilevel growth curve analyses, to identify individuals who follow deviant developmental trajectories. **Results:** Child and adolescent psychopathology tends to persist into adulthood. Especially children and adolescents with chronic high levels of problems tend to have problems in multiple areas of functioning. Using multilevel growtrh curve analyses it is possible to identify children in the general population with extremely deviant developmental trajectories. Deviant trajectories of externalizing behaviors were predictive of various forms of antisocial behavior as well as of multiple forms of adult psychiatric disorders. **Conclusion:** When psychopathology is chronic from childhood or adolescence into adulthood, the consequences for overall adaptive functioning reach beyond the mere level of psychopathology but extends to a broad range of maladaptive functioning. Using growth curve anayses makes it possible to identify individuals with extremely deviant developmental trajectories. This type of approach will have an enormous impact on both etiological research as well as on prevention research.

ST-012   Topic: 24, 43
**The Biology of childhood experience
(Dedicated to the memory of Richard Harrington)**
Chairperson: Savita Malhotra, FAMS Dept. of Psychiatry, Chandigarh, India, savitam@sancharnet.in

ST-012-012   Topic: 24, 43
**The Biology of childhood experience
(Dedicated to the memory of Richard Harrington)**
Ian Goodyer, Cambridge University, Dept. Developmental Psychiatry, Cambridge, United Kingdom, ig104@cam.ac.uk

There is clear evidence that children's genetic makeup affects their own behavioural characteristics. Heritability estimates for a given trait vary widely across samples, and no one estimate can be considered definitive. Knowing only the strength of genetic factors, is not a sufficient basis for understanding vulnerability process for psychopathology. Indeed behavioural 'genetic' studies demonstrate that environments are markedly important in determining the liability for common emotional and behavioural disorders in young people. Recent advances in molecular genetics have begun to provide 'genetic variables' for inclusion in behavioural studies. Gene-environment (G-E) interactions are beginning to be demonstrated that point to how nature and nurture may operate to influence the liabilities for common emotional and behavioural disorders. In addition non-genomic physiological processes are also being elucidated whose role in gene-social environment relations remains to be determined. Characterising the distal processes of genetic vulnerabilities and early parenting adversities for psychopathology and relating these to the intermediate biology of psychiatric disorder in childhood and adolescence is a key research area for the 21st century. This lecture illustrates with examples from selected G-E findings, studies of early maternal adversity, genetic influences on biochemistry and hormonal effects on mood and cognition, how the brain is a social organism and mind states arise from the biology of personal experiences. The implication of these biological experiences for psychopathology and clinical practice will be discussed.

ST-013   Topic: 82
Dyslexia
Chairperson: John Sikorski, UCSF Dept. of Child Psychiatry, San Francisco, CA, USA, jbsikor@itsa.ucsf.edu

ST-013-013   Topic: 82
Dyslexia
Gerd Schulte-Körne, Universitätsklinik Marburg, Kinder- und Jugendpsychiatrie, Marburg, Germany, schulte1@med.uni-marburg.de

Dyslexia is characterized as a specific impairment of reading and or spelling ability despite adequate intelligence an a normal IQ, no obvious sensory deficits, and adequate sociocultural opportunity. Dyslexia occurs in all languages and especially spelling disorder often persists into adulthood. Dyslexia is known to be a hereditary disorder that affects about 5% of school-aged children, making it the most common of childhood learning disorders. Several diagnostic methods were used also there is continuing controversy concerning the diagnostic criteria for dyslexia. Dyslexia is a clinically heterogeneous disorder with a complex neurobiological aetiology. Despite decades of investigation, including studies of neuropsychology, neurophysiology, neuroimaging, and moleculargenetics specific causal mechanisms underlying dyslexia are still obscure. Several therapeutic methods were applied but therapeutic standards have to be developed. Whereas in irregular languages like English remediation is based on teaching phonics and training phonological awareness in regular languages like German training of orthographic processing is very common.

ST-014
Bipolar disorders

Chairperson: Per-Anders Rydelius, Karolinska Institutet Woman and Child Health, Stockholm, Sweden, per-anders.rydelius@ks.se

ST-014-014   Topic: 70
Bipolar disorders

Luis Augusto Rohde, UFRGS-HCPA-Brazil, Dept. of Psychiatry, Porto Alegre, Brazil, lrohde@terra.com.br

ST-015   Topic: 78
Causes of childhood obesity and therapeutic implications

Track: Eating disorders

Chairperson: Martine Flament, University of Ottawa Inst. Mental Health Research, Ottawa, ON, Canada, mflament@rohcg.on.ca

ST-015-015   Topic: 78
Causes of childhood obesity and therapeutic implications

Johannes Hebebrand, Universitätsklinik Essen, Kinder- und Jugendpsychiatrie, Essen, Germany, johannes.hebebrand@uni-duisburg-essen.de

Obesity results if energy intake exceeds energy expenditure for a prolonged period of time. Several mechanisms can independently or jointly contribute to an excessive gain in fat mass. Among these, genetic factors play an important role; heritability is assumed to account for at least 50% of the variation of the body mass index (BMI; kg/m^2). Mutations in the melanocortin-4 receptor gene can be detected in between 2 and 6% of extremely obese children. The first polygenes have been identified, which in concert act to either protect or predispose an individual to develop obesity. A low parental socio-economic status is an independent risk factor. Recent longitudinal studies have shown that high depression scores in childhood and adolescence predict future overweight and obesity. The implications of these etiological factors for the treatment of obesity are difficult to assess. In general, the strong physiological counter-regulation upon weight loss applies to both the juvenile and adult organism. Evidence for the long-term effectiveness of therapeutic interventions is scanty; despite the increasing prevalence rates of overweight and obesity in children only single small randomised control trials have been performed. Currently, pharmacological and surgical interventions are not routinely recommended for this age group. Prevention studies are similarly scarce; it is assumed that targeting the reduction of sedentary activities is possibly the most successful preventive measure. More empirical studies are urgently required to identify promising approaches for both therapy and prevention. Possibly, the delineation of the molecular genetic basis of obesity will allow a more individualized treatment. Within child and adolescent psychiatry future research should address the relevance of psychological factors in the development of obesity.

Symposia

S-001 Topic: 12, 34
What is the role of second-generation antipsychotics in the treatment of children and adolescents with major psychiatric disorders?

Track: Therapy and intervention

Chairperson: Christoph Correll, The Zucker Hillside Hospital Dept. of Psychiatry Research, Glen Oaks, NY, USA, ccorrell@lij.edu

What is the role of second-generation antipsychotics in the treatment of children and adolescents with major psychiatric disorders?

Christoph Correll, The Zucker Hillside Hospital, Dept. of Psychiatry Research, Glen Oaks, NY, USA, ccorrell@lij.edu

Goal: The goal of this symposium is to identify 'state-of-the-art' strategies for the use of antipsychotic medications in the management of children and adolescents with major psychiatric disorders. Learning objectives: 1. Define pediatric populations for whom second-generation antipsychotics are indicated 2. Identify the role of second-generation antipsychotics in the management of major psychiatric disorders in children and adolescents 3. Describe the level of evidence for the effectiveness of second-generation antipsychotic use in youth 4. Discuss risk-benefit ratios of individual second-generation antipsychotics in pediatric populations 5. Use treatment algorithms and practice guidelines for the safe and effective use of second-generation antipsychotics in children and adolescents Background: Second-generation antipsychotics are increasingly prescribed to children and adolescents targeting a variety of psychotic and non-psychotic disorders. This is mainly due to lower rates of neuromotor side effects compared to conventional antipsychotics. In addition, second generation antipsychotics may also have superior and broader effectiveness than traditional antipsychotics. Content: This symposium will focus on the evaluation of the evidence base for the safety and effectiveness of second generation antipsychotics in the treatment of children and adolescents with major psychiatric disorders. Furthermore, treatment guidelines and algorithms will be presented to help guide clinician's treatment decisions.

S-001-001 Topic: 12, 34
Second-generation antipsychotic treatment of youth with schizophrenia-spectrum disorder

Stanley P. Kutcher, Dalhousie University, Halifax, Nova Scotia, Canada, stan.kutcher@dal.ca

Objective: To review the literature on the the use of second generation antipsychotic medications in young people. Methods: The world literature was reviewed to identify papers published regarding the use of second generation antipsychotics in youth and well as personal communication with researchers in the area. Results: A small number of papers usually of small sample numbers and open studies were identified and their results summarized. Conclusion: There is limited evidence to support the use second generation antipsychotics in youth from properly conducted trials, however the available evidence is "better" than that of for first generation componds. Clinical use of these medications is discussed.

S-001-002 Topic: 12, 34
Practice guidelines for the use of second-generation antipsychotics in youngsters with bipoal disorder

John McClellan, University of Washington, Dept. of Psychiatry, Seattle, WA, USA, drjack@u.washington.edu

Objective: To review the current literature supporting the use of atypical antipsychotics in youth with bipolar disorder. Methods: The existing literature was reviewed using Medline, focusing the key words bipolar disorder, children, adolescents and antipsychotics. Studies using randomized controlled designs were prioritized for making treatment recommendations. Results: There are no well-designed controlled trials examining the use of atypical antipsychotic as monotherapy for juvenile bipolar disorder. Open trials and retrospective chart reviews support the effectiveness of olanzapine (Frazier et al., 2001) and risperidone (Frazier et al., 1999) for juvenile mania. A double blind controlled trial found that quetiapine plus valproate worked better than valproate alone for adolescent mania (Delbello et al., 2002). Conclusion: Controlled trials in adults support the use of atypical antipsychotics as first line treatments for acute mania. To date, studies are generally lacking in juveniles, thus the use of these medications in youth with bipolar disorder is justified based on the adult literature. When used as mood stabilizers, the atypical antipsychotic agents are prescribed using the same dosage ranges, and have the same spectrum of side effects as when used for psychotic illnesses. Weight gain in youth has been a particular concern for this class of agents.

S-001-003 Topic: 12, 34
Evidence base for the effectiveness of second-generation antipsychotics in youngsters with subaverage IQ and autism-spectrum disorders

Jan Buitelaar, University Medical Center, Psychiatry & Adolescent, Nijmegen, Netherlands, jb@psy.umcn.nl

Objective: No first-line medication treatment was available for children with severe Disruptive Behavior Disorders and subaverage intelligence, and for children with Autism Spectrum Disorders (ASD). Atypical antipsychotic agents, which block postsynaptic dopamine and serotonin receptors, have advantages over traditional antipsychotic medications. Objective. To review data on the safety and efficacy of atypical antipsychotic agents in children with DBD and ASD. Methods: The results of recent controlled trials and extension studies will be reviewed and discussed. Results: Two large randomized placebo-controlled trials with risperidone (0.02-0.06 mg/kg/day) in children with DBD and subaverage IQ documented clinically significant decreases on the primary outcome measure, the Conduct Problem subscale of the Nisonger Child Behavior Rating Form (NCBRF). The most common side effects included somnolence, headache, appetite increase, and dyspepsia. Side effects related to extrapyramidal symptoms were reported in (13.2%) and (5.3%) of the subjects in the risperidone and placebo groups (n.s.). In an extension study long-term risperidone appeared to be generally safe, well tolerated, and effective for treating severely disruptive behaviour. In another multisite, randomized, double-blind trial of risperidone as compared with placebo for the treatment of ASD accompanied by severe tantrums, aggression, or self-injurious behaviour, response to risperidone was 69% as compared to 12% in the placebo group. Two-thirds of the children with a positive response to risperidone at eight weeks maintained benefits at six months. **Conclusion:** Atypical antipsychotics like risperidone appear to be effective and safe in controlling severe behavior problems in children with DBD and subaverage IQ and in children with ASD.

S-001-004   Topic: 12, 34
Treatment recommendations for the use of antipsychotics for aggressive youth
Elizabeth Pappadopulos, Columbia University/NYSPI, CACMH, New York, USA, pappadoe@childpsych.columbia.edu

Objective: To identify typical patterns of adjustment problems in girls with severe antisocial problems. **Methods:** A person-oriented approach is applied, with a focus on syndromes of problems in the individual. A broad array of problems is hereby considered, including alcohol and drug abuse, criminality, oval aggression, psychological health and somatic complaints. Data are taken from a unique data base at the Swedish National Board of Institutional Care, which includes data from 780 13–19 years old girls who have been admitted to specially approved institutions in accordance with the Swedish Care of Young Persons Act (LVU) since 1997. The girls were interviewed at intake with the Adolescent Drug Abuse Diagnosis (ADAD). The data base covers almost the entire population of Swedish girls with the most severe antisocial problems. **Results:** A ten-cluster solution was chosen for behavior problems. Four different clusters (97 girls) included drugs and crime. Two clusters (95 girls) had high values in vandalism and alcohol. 303 girls distributed in three clusters included overt aggression. One large cluster with 217 girls did not have any of the measured behaviour problems. Seven clusters with inner problems were found. Three of the clusters including 250 girls had very serious problems including high suicidal and self-destructive behaviour. Totally there was 517 (73 percent) girls having some kind of inner problem. There were low correlations between inner and behavior problems. **Conclusion:** The study is still in progress. Conclusions will be presented at the conference.

S-001-005   Topic: 12, 34
Novel antipsychotics for children and adolescents with tic disorders
Aribert Rothenberger, Universität Göttingen, Göttingen, Germany, arothen@gwdg.de
Tobias Banaschewski; Veit Roessner

Objective: Drug treatment is still the most promising intervention to reduce motor and vocal tics in intensity and frequency. Since many years neuroleptics like haloperidol and pimozide play a major role worldwide, while benzamides like sulpiride and tiapride are in use mainly in Europe. Objective: With the advent of novel neuroleptics these were also used to treat tic disorders, with the hope of better efficacy and safety. Hence, the level of evidence of second-generation antipsychotics for children and adolescents with tic disorders has to be evaluated. **Methods:** Review of the empirically based literature on novel antipsychotics like risperidone, ziprasidone, quetiapine, olanzapine and amisulpride. **Results:** Sofar, risperidone shows the broadest empirical basis, while reports on the other

compounds come from a limited number of studies (mostly case reports or open-label). **Conclusion:** Risperidone seems to be clinically helpful and safe. Thus it may become the first-line drug in the treatment of tic disorders. But the other novel antipsychotics can also reduce tics in some cases.

S-001-006   Topic: 12, 34
Risk benefit evaluation of early interventions with second-generation antipsychotics for youth at high risk for psychosis
Christoph Correll, The Zucker Hillside Hospital, Dept. of Psychiatry Research, Glen Oaks, NY, USA, ccorrell@lij.edu

Objective: To evaluate the evidence base for the effectiveness and safety of interventions in youth who are considered to be in the prodromal, i.e., prepsychotic, phases of a psychotic disorder. **Methods:** Systematic review of published and presented results from studies reporting on the effectiveness of pharmacologic and non-pharmacologic interventions for subjects at ultra-high risk for the development of psychosis. **Results:** Information on the design of 11 ongoing or completed prodromal intervention studies was available. In five of these studies with reported results, a combination of psychotropic and psychotherapeutic interventions (n=3), second-generation antipsychotic treatment alone (n=1) or cognitive behavioral therapy alone (n=1) was effective for the amelioration of prepsychotic and subsyndromal psychotic psychopathology. Moreover, preliminary evidence suggests a potential usefulness of early interventions for the prevention of progression to full blown psychosis. Information on the safety of second-generation antipsychotic treatment and on the effectiveness of non-antipsychotic medications in this population is limited. Finally, data is missing regarding the effect of early interventions on the course of illness after a conversion to psychosis has occurred. **Conclusion:** Early detection and intervention programs, employing pharmacological and non-pharmacological treatments, have been shown to reduce prepsychotic symptomatology in high-risk individuals. More information is needed to evaluate the effect on delaying or preventing the progression to psychosis, and to document an impact on the symptomatic and functional outcome in individuals who have developed a psychotic disorder. Finally, the feasibility of transferring early detection and intervention programs from research to community settings requires further study.

S-002   Topic: 23
Treatment evaluation under realistic clinical conditions
Track: Therapy and intervention
Chairperson: Helmut Remschmidt, Universität Marburg Kinder- und Jugendpsychiatrie, Marburg, Germany, remschm@med.uni-marburg.de

Treatment evaluation under realistic clinical conditions
Helmut Remschmidt, Universität Marburg, Kinder- und Jugendpsychiatrie, Marburg, Germany, remschm@med.uni-marburg.de

There are remarkable differences with regard to treatment success between experimental/controlled treatment studies and treatment studies under realistic clinical conditions. It is essential to find out which treatment matters are effective in which patients and under which conditions. Recent studies investigating this question have focused on empirical supported psychotherapeutic and combined treatment methods carried out in efficiency and effectiveness studies. The current trend of treatment evaluation is towards studies performed under natural every day treatment conditions. This is the major aim of this Symposium which includes four presentations, two more general ones devoted to a multi-component approach of treatment and two more specific ones aiming at the treatment of conduct disorders and depression.

S-002-007   Topic: 3
The component model of treatment in child and adolescent psychiatry

Helmut Remschmidt, Universität Marburg, Kinder- und Jugendpsychiatrie, Marburg, Germany, remschm@med.uni-marburg.de

Objective: To describe the theoretical concept and practical realization of the component model of treatment in child and adolescent psychiatry. **Methods:** The treatment procedures in a department of child and adolescent psychiatry are analyzed based of more than 4500 patients in different settings (inpatient, day patient, and outpatient settings) with regard to the application of five different treatment components (individual psychotherapy with the patient, functional therapies, parent- and family-oriented interventions, other environmental interventions and psychotropic medication). These five treatment components were applied in variable combination to different disorders and in various settings. **Results:** Treatment success based on therapists' ratings revealed effect sizes in the outpatient setting around one for normal completers vs. drop-outs, 1.27 for normal completers vs. non-beginners, and 0.34 for non-beginners vs. drop-outs. Similar effect sizes were found for inpatient treatment. **Conclusion:** In spite of some methodological restrictions, the results demonstrate that the component approach of treatment can be looked upon as a useful and effective procedure under realistic clinical conditions.

S-002-008   Topic: 19, 26
Which diagnostic groups can be treated effectively? Results from research and from real-life clinical services

Fritz Mattejat, Universitätsklinik Marburg, Kinder- und Jugendpsychiatrie, Marburg, Germany, mattejat@med.uni-marburg.de

Objective: In recent years the research to identify evidence based treatments increased substantially. The most important method of efficacy research is the randomized controlled trial (RCT). This design often cannot be applied in real-world clinical settings with severely disturbed patients. The majority of efficacy studies is conducted with recruited patients with mild disturbances (not with referred patients) in specific research settings (not within real-life clinical settings). The kind how therapies are conducted in efficacy studies differs considerably from how treatment is conducted in real-life clinical practice. In the presentation the question is investigated, whether the results from "research therapies" can be replicated when clinical representative therapies are evaluated. **Methods:** A complete sample of severely disturbed patients which were referred to inpatient treatment in the Marburg child and adolescent psychiatric inpatient unit was investigated at admission, discharge and at a 1.5-year follow-up (three-point-measurement longitudinal design). Evaluation criteria were: Symptoms, level of functioning and quality of life. Data are analyzed for different diagnostic groups separately. The results of each diagnostic group is compared with results from efficacy research. **Results:** There are a number of accordances and similarities between our findings and the results in the efficacy research literature. Furthermore, in addition to RCT-findings some of our the results give more specific and more realistic information about the course of treatment and recovery in different diagnostic groups. **Conclusion:** The results from clinically representative evaluations provide additional informations, which complement the knowledge which is generated by efficacy studies from RCTs. This information can be used in order to inform patients and their parents about prognosis so that decisions about interventions can be made on a better informed basis.

S-002-009   Topic: 85
Making interventions work in real life settings: How much does the level of therapist skill matter?

Stephen Scott, King's College of London, Maudsley Hospital, London, United Kingdom, s.scott@iop.kcl.ac.uk

Objective: To examine the impact of therapist skill and adherence to a manualised treatment on child symptom outcome. **Methods:** In a multi-centre controlled trial in real life clinical conditions, we showed that severe anti-social behaviour (above the 98th percentile) in children aged 3–8 referred to clinics could be substantially reduced (effect size 1.06 standard deviations) using a Webster-Stratton's Incredible Years Parenting Programme. However, one of the four centres had considerably smaller effects than the others. Independent ratings were made of treatment fidelity from video tapes of therapy sessions. **Results:** Treatment fidelity was shown to be an important predictor of outcome, with the centres with lowest fidelity not improving child outcome at all. The key element was the extent to which the therapist followed the specific skills based elements of the programme. Findings will be related to other predictors, such as initial severity of ADHD, and presented in the framework of phenotype-environment interactions. **Conclusion:** For the effective translation of developmental science interventions into real world everyday practice, it is crucial that high standards of implementation are adhered to; it is not enough to send staff a short training course and expect the results to be good.

S-002-010   Topic: 6, 70
Cognitive-behavioral therapy for youth depression in community mental health clinics

John Weisz, University of California, Dept. of Psychology, Los Angeles, CA, USA, weisz@psych.ucla.edu

Objective: To describe an effectiveness test of cognitive-behavioral therapy (CBT) for youth depression in community mental health clinic settings. **Methods:** Depressed youths aged 8-15 who were referred to community mental health clinic were randomly assigned to receive either CBT or the usual care (UC) provided by the clinic. Therapists in each clinic had also been randomly assigned to learn and use

CBT or to continue providing their own form of UC. Pre-treatment, post-treatment, and follow-up assessments provide evidence on the outcomes experienced by youths in the two treatment conditions. **Results:** At this time, not all youths have completed treatment in the UC condition; its duration is free to vary, and some youths have been in UC treatment for more than a year. Because this means that final outcome data are not available yet, the presentation will focus primarily on the experience of bringing CBT into community mental health clinics, conducting a clinical trial in such settings, working with clinic administrative staff and with community families, and arranging the training and clinical supervision of clinic-employed therapists for their roles as providers of treatment procedures not previously familiar to them, and adapting and refining treatment procedures to fit community-referred clients and their situations. Some preliminary outcome findings may also be presented. **Conclusion:** Bringing structured, manual-guided treatment procedures into clinical practice settings is challenging but important work that may yield important benefits to our field.

S-003   Topic: 80, 93
Borderline disorder in children and adolescents
Chairperson: Eberhard Schulz,
Universität Freiburg Kinder- und Jugendpsychiatrie,
Freiburg, Germany, schulz@psyallg.ukl.uni-freiburg.de

Borderline personality disorder in children and adolescents
Eberhard Schulz, Universität Freiburg,
Kinder- und Jugendpsychiatrie, Freiburg, Germany,
schulz@psyallg.ukl.uni-freiburg.de

BPD is a serious mental disorder with a characteristic pervasive pattern of instability in affect regulation, impulse control, interpersonal relationships, and self-image. BPD affects approximately 2% of the general population, 11% of psychiatric outpatients and up to 20% of psychiatric inpatients. BPD is characterised by severe psychosocial impairment and a high mortality rate due to suicide of up to 10% of patients. Borderline personality disorder (BPD) with early onset is usually considered to have a poor or extremely poor prognosis. Forty-two adolescents with BPD were followed over the course of 10 years. Sociodemographic, psychosocial, and treatment variables appear to be influenced by gender. Data on course and outcome will be presented. Follow-up studies did not support continuity between the borderline syndrome of children and borderline personality disorder in adults, e.g. the pattern of neuropsychological profiles and neurological soft-signs (e.g. motor development) is not present in "borderline personality disorder". But there is some overlap between multiple complex developmental disorder (MCDD) and children presenting with symptoms of early-onset borderline disorder in terms of affect regulation and irritability, sense of reality and identity, interpersonal relationship and attachment, impulsivity and self-harming behaviour, instability and fluidity of the symptoms and the high rate of psychosocial stressors, e.g. abuse and neglect. In the light of these findings, follow-up data from a sample of children with MCDD will be presented. An additional contribution deals with a study on the impact of borderline personality disorder on parenting. In this regard, treatment and preventive issues will be discussed from a child psychiatric perspec-

tive. Finally psychotherapy with Dialectical-Behavioral Therapy for Adolescents (DBT-A) will be described and data from an ongoing prospective clinical trial in a sample of adolescents with borderline disorder will be discussed.

S-003-011   Topic: 80, 47
Impact on parenting of borderline personality disorders
Wilhelm Felder, Kinder- und Jugendpsychiatrie, Bern,
Switzerland, wilhelm.felder@gef.be.ch

The aim of the lecture is to present and discuss the following two questions: – what does it mean for a child to have a mother and/or a father with a borderline personality disorder? – What does it mean for a mother/a father to have a child with a borderline personality disorder? In the lecture will be presented findings from the Child and Adolescent psychiatry (inpatient and outpatient-units) and the psychiatric inpatient-unit for adults of the University of Berne. The review of the current literature to both above mentioned questions deals manly with the implications for therapy/counselling.

S-003-012   Topic: 80, 19
Dialectical behavioral therapy for adolescents: Evaluation of the concept
Christian Fleischhaker, Universität Freiburg, Kinder- und
Jugendpsychiatrie, Freiburg, Germany,
fleischhaker@psyallg.ukl.uni-freiburg.de
R. Böhme; B. Sixt; Eberhard Schulz

Objective: Dialectical-Behavioral Therapy (DBT) had been developed by M. Linehan specifically for the outpatient treatment of chronically parasuicidal patients who where diagnosed with borderline personality disorder (BPD). DBT is one of the two empirically supported treatments for suicidal multi-problem adult patients. A. Miller and J. Rathus adapted DBT for suicidal adolescents with borderline personality traits because of its focus on reducing suicidal and quality of life reducing behaviors, as well as keeping adolescents and their families engaged in treatment. Preliminary open trial data of DBT-A by Miller and colleagues are promising. DBT for adolescents (DBT-A) was adapted for an outpatient treatment setting in Germany by Fleischhaker and colleagues. **Methods:** DBT-A consists of 16 concomitant weekly individual and group therapy sessions. The group therapy consists of 16 psychoeducational multi-family skills training sessions. After agreement on goals and commitment to change the individual therapy is used to work one-to-one with the therapist to reduce factors that interfere with the ability to use the learned skills and ensuring that generalization occurs via in vivo intervention. Family sessions or meetings with school-teachers or other treatment providers are performed, so that the patient does not have to get worse to get additional help. Following the completion of the 16-week program, individual therapy is discontinued and the adolescent is given the opportunity to participate in individual bimonthly post-therapy sessions for three months. **Results:** In this open clinical trial the effectiveness for the German Version of DBT-A could be shown in parasuicidal adolescents (n = 12) with a pre- and post-therapy comparison. Subjects who have received DBT-A showed a significant reduction of parasuicide acts in the months after the end of treatment compared with the months before treatment. Second, DBT-A retained 75% of patients in therapy.

Finally the treatment is effective in improving patients global psychopathology and psychosocial adaptation. Data from 1 year follow-up revealed a significant decrease in self-injuries behavior and psychopathology. **Conclusion:** The German Version of DBT-A seems to be effective in the treatment of parasuicidal adolescents in an open clinical trial. The promising results from this ambulant pilot study suggest that further evaluation of DBT-A outpatients in a randomized, controlled clinical trial appears warranted.

S-003-013   Topic: 80, 24
Borderline disorders in childhood: A misleading term for serious developmental psychopathology

Rutger Jan van der Gaag, UMCN ACKJON Nijmegen, Child & Adolescent Psychiatry, Nijmegen, Netherlands, rutger.jan.van.der.gaag@skjpon.nl

Borderline disorders in childhood have been well described in a series of studies. The clinging in social contact, the lack of fine tuned social sensitivity, the extreme mood and behavioural swings and distorted cognitions share resemblance with those described in Borderline Personality Disorders in adults. Yet in follow up studies there is no evidence for any continuity between the two conditions. The trauma hypothesis does not hold for the condition in children. The late Donald Cohen proposed to study this clinically so difficult to manage and yet important group of children in developmental terms. In this presentation evidence will be presented for the validity of the developmental vulnerability of this group and a plea shall be made to drop the term that leads to misunderstandings that are neither beneficial to the patients, nor their parents let stand the professional dealing with these complex cases.

S-003-014   Topic: 93, 23
Effectiveness of dialectical behavior therapy for suicidal adolescent inpatients

Laurence Y. Katz, University of Manitoba, Dept. of Psychiatry, Winnipeg, Manitoba, Canada, lkatz@exchange.hsc.mb.ca
Brian J. Cox; Shiny Gunasekara; Alec L. Miller

Objective: To evaluate the effectiveness of dialectical behavior therapy (DBT) implementation in a general child and adolescent psychiatric inpatient unit and to provide preliminary outcome data on DBT versus treatment-as-usual (TAU). **Methods:** Sixty-two adolescents with suicide attempts or suicidal ideation were admitted to one of two psychiatric inpatient units for an average of eighteen days. One unit utilized a DBT protocol and the other unit relied on TAU. Assessments of depressive symptoms, suicidal ideation, hopelessness, parasuicidal behavior, hospitalizations, emergency room visits and adherence to follow-up recommendations were conducted pre and post-treatment and at one-year follow-up for both groups. In addition, behavioral incidents on the units were evaluated. **Results:** DBT significantly reduced behavioral incidents during admission when compared with TAU. Both groups demonstrated highly significant reductions in parasuicidal behavior, depressive symptoms and suicidal ideation at one-year. **Conclusion:** DBT can be effectively implemented in acute care child and adolescent psychiatric inpatient units. Short-term, acute care psychiatric hospitalization leads to symptom reduction in parasuicidal adolescents. The promising results from this pilot study suggest that further

evaluation of DBT for adolescent inpatients appears warranted.

S-004   Topic: 53
The impact of trauma and disaster on children

Chairperson: Nathaniel Laor, Tel Aviv University Faculty of Medicine, Tel Aviv, Israel, nlaor@netvision.net.il
Peter Riedesser, UKE Hamburg-Eppendorf Abt. Psychiatrie, Hamburg, Germany, riedesser@uke.uni-hamburg.de

S-004-015   Topic: 51, 3
Developmental psychopathology model and multiagency approach for traumatized children and adolescents

Ernesto Caffo, University of Modena, Dept. of Neuroscience, Modena, Italy, caffo@unimo.it

Objective: Each year millions of children are exposed to some form of extreme traumatic stressor such as natural disasters, motor vehicle accidents, life-threatening illnesses, physical abuse, sexual assault, witnessing domestic or community violence. Mental health professionals are increasing their understanding about what factors are associated with increased risk (vulnerability) and affect how children cope with traumatic events. Telefono Azzurro is a non-profit organization, dedicated to enhancing children and adolescents' well-being and health, especially for those living situations of developmental difficulties, trauma and emergency. The mission of Telefono Azzurro is to promote children and adolescents' rights and developing good practices for their care. **Methods:** Telefono Azzurro is composed by several different structures (Call Center, Emergency Team, Tetto Azzurro, Training and Study Center) and is involved in primary prevention, emergency intervention, treatment, research and training. The theoretical model and data concerning Telefono Azzurro activities are reported. Issues and difficulties in building an interagency response and adopting a developmental psychopathology model are discussed. **Results:** Managing a case of childhood maladjustment or abuse, is a complex process, demanding collaboration between different and specific agencies (school, social services, court, law enforcement) and different professionals (doctors, psychologists, social workers, lawyers, judges and policemen). In this direction, Telefono Azzurro has developed, over the past decade, partnerships and collaborative ways of working with health and non-health sectors, such as police, schools, community services and courts. **Conclusion:** Developmental psychopathology and multiagency approach open important challenges to researchers and practitioners in the field of mental health services for children and adolescents. Specific services should address risk and protective factors, empower caregivers, promote well-being and use evidence-based and network intervention strategies.

S-004-016   Topic: 28
The intrapsychic and intergenerational legacy of fear, anger and retribution

James Leckman, Yale University, Child Study Center, New Haven, USA, james.leckman@yale.edu

Terrorism and war promotes group cohesion. By standing "united," the victims of an attack re-enforce their affiliative bonds and enhance their sense of security. This is an important aspect of recovery. Obsessive-compulsive-like thoughts and behaviors aimed at threat detection and appraisal and habitual harm avoidant behaviors are another by-product of these events, as societies take steps to protect themselves and regulate their fear. Terrorism and war also naturally promote externally directed anger and the preparation for counter attacks in retribution – the current War on terrorism is a clear and compelling example. Unfortunately, these acts invite a self perpetuating cycle of violence and retribution as well as encouraging the development of hostile and distorted narratives about the "enemy" that left unchecked can extend across generations. This presentation focuses on the limitations of these "adaptive" responses and speculates about the usefulness of educational interventions aimed at exploring the self defeating aspects of these responses. Although doubtless naive, this presentation ends with a consideration of the possible benefits for the self and society that are based on generosity and idealization of the "enemy."

S-004-017   Topic: 53, 48
Trauma, attachment and personality disorders

Massimo Ammaniti, Univ. Roma La Sapienza,
Psicologia Dinamica e Clinica, Rome, Italy,
maammani@tin.it
Giampaolo Nicolais; Mario Speranza

Objective: More recently the attachment theory has deepened the impact of Trauma on attachment system which can produce disorganization, dissociation and defensive mechanisms which could lead to personality disorders. This theoretical framework is discussed through clinical evidences in abusive parents who present disorganization of attachment and personality disorder. Results: The research has evidenced the significant connection between traumatic experiences and personality disorder, especially borderline personality disorder. Conclusion: The pathogenic effect of Trauma can be explained using different perspectives, like the neurobiological one or the psychopathological one, which puts a special emphasis on the storage of trauma in memory system.

S-004-018   Topic: 52, 57
The relationship between trauma, violence and delinquency

Hans Steiner, Stanford University, School of Psychiatry,
Stanford, CA, USA, steiner@stanford.edu
Laura Delizonna; Belinda Plattner; Astrid Schallauer;
Margo Thienemann

Objective: We will summarize a series of investigations documenting what we currently know of the developmental psychopathology in delinquents. Clinical studies will be integrated with new findings from neuroscience indicating trauma specific pathways from abuse to perpetration of crime. Methods: A selective review of the literature of trauma, subtypes of aggression and the neuronal architecture underlying these manifestations of trauma. Results: Earlier studies relied on questionnaire data and clinical descriptions. More modern approaches bring to bear cutting edge methods of assessment, such as structured interviews, standardized inventories and in process measures, assessing trauma, types and severity and chronicity of trauma, types of psychopathology and functioning under allostatic load. These studies provide a convergent picture.

Posttraumatic Stress Disorder is extremely prevalent in delinquent youths (between 12 and 60 %). Traumatized youths are significantly more impulsive than their non-traumatized comparison delinquents. Personality fragmentation and severe forms of dissociative disorders are very prevalent in delinquents as well. Biological underpinnings of maladaptive aggression are beginning to emerge. A recent report suggests possible genetic vulnerability to trauma in certain aggressive children. Conclusion: Maladaptive reactive-affective-defensive-impulsive (RADI) aggression is extremely common in psychopathological delinquents. Psychiatric trauma causes dysregulation in this important system of self regulation. Modern treatments of delinquents will need to address this problem.

S-004-019   Topic: 35, 53
The effects in adult life of exposure in childhood to a natural disaster

Alexander C. McFarlane, University of Adelaide, Queen
Elizabeth Hospital, Woodville, Australia,
alexander.mcfarlane@adelaide.edu.au
Miranda van Hooff; Michael Sawyer

Objective: To examine the long term consequences of exposure to a natural disaster in childhood on adult psychological adjustment. Methods: In 1983 a population of 808 primary school children were exposed to a major bushfire disaster. A comparison population of 705 children who had not been exposed to the disaster were examined simultaneously. The original sample involved the collection of data at three time points in the first two years after the disaster, examining the relative impact of property damage, personal loss and family functioning on the emergence of psychological symptoms. This population has been tracked down some 20 years later when they have reached adulthood. They have been assessed using the CIDI to examine patterns of psychological morbidity. A range of intercurrent traumas, including forms of childhood abuse, have been documented. The individual's perceptions of their parenting and their general attitudes to life have also been assessed. Results: The patterns of adult psychological morbidity will be defined. The interaction between exposure to the disaster and other adversity in childhood will be documented. The patterns of family functioning reported by the parents will be compared with the individual's perception of the patterns of parenting in adulthood. Conclusion: This project represents one of the first longitudinal studies which is able to control for the severity of childhood symptomatology following a natural disaster as a predictor of adult psychiatric morbidity as well as examining the impact of intercurrent stressors.

S-005   Topic: 69
Schizophrenia and other psychotic disorders I
Track: Psychotic disorders

Chairperson: Carlo Cianchetti, University of Cagliari Dept.
of Child Neuropsychiatry, Cagliari, Italy, cianchet@unica.it

S-005-020   Topic: 69
Neurodevelopmental hypothesis in schizophrenia: comparative study of obstetric complications and morbidity in childhood in a Tunisian sample

Naoufel Gaddour, CHU F Bourguiba, service de psychiatrie, Monastir, Tunisia, naoufelgaddour@historique.zzn.com
Mokni Sana; Mechri Anouar; Letaief Mondher; Gaha Lotfi

Objective: Very few studies from emerging countries are published concerning the neurodevelopmental aspects of schizophrenia. However, meteorological, demographic and health factors in most of these countries are very different from the thoses in western countries, and can make studies in this field bring more findings. Our objective was to compare the prevalence of obstetric complications and morbidity in childhood in a schizophrenic patients group in relation to two groups of first degree relatives and healthy controls. **Methods:** It is a retrospective case-control study. A schizophrenic adult patients group (N = 55) (SP) was compared to a group of healthy relatives (N = 40) (HR) and to healthy controls without familial psychiatric history (N = 38) (HC), all matched according to age and sex. Obstetric complications have been collected at home at the time of one visit, from the biologic mothers, using the McNeil-Sjostrom questionnaire. Morbidity in childhood was evaluated through a questionnaire about anterior morbid situations and about former hospitalisations. **Results:** The middle total obstetric complications score was significantly higher in the schizophrenic group: 1.52 ± 1.47 versus 0.8 ± 1.77 (HR) and 0.5 ± 0.97 (HC), $p < 0.001$. Obstetrical complications were more frequent during the delivery period. Schizophrenic patients had significantly more hospitalisations during childhood (SP: 27.3%/HR: 5%/HC: 18.4%, p = 0.02) and presented more enuresis (SP: 29.1%/HR: 12.5%/HC: 7.9%, p = 0.001). **Conclusion:** Our results support the role of obstetric complications and morbidity in childhood in the etiopathogeny of schizophrenia. Further studies assessing influence of weather, specific infectious agents, and demographic factors can be relevant too.

S-005-021   Topic: 69, 30
Visual working memory deficits in adolescents suffering from schizophrenia studied with EEG and fMRI

Fabian Härtling, Universität Frankfurt, Kinder- und Jugendpsychiatrie, Frankfurt, Germany, f.haertling@em.uni-frankfurt.de
Robert Bittner; Corinna Haenschel; Marcus Cap; Tanja Goncharova; David E.J. Linden; Fritz Poustka

Objective: Deficits in working memory (WM) are an important feature throughout the course of schizophrenia. Abnormalities in brain function which underlie these deficits and contribute to the development of the illness can be investigated with functional neuroimaging techniques. While this has been done extensively in adults, evidence for neurophysiological correlates of WM deficits in adolescents is still lacking. **Methods:** We used electroencephalography (EEG) and functional magnetic resonance imaging (fMRI) in a group of 11 adolescent patients with early onset schizophrenia (EOS) (mean ± SD age, 18.1 ± 1.3 years; range 16 to 20 years) with the ICD-10 diagnosis of schizophrenia or schizoaffective disorder (3 females, 8 males) and 11 age, sex-, hand- and IQ-matched normal controls, performing a delayed discrimination task (DDT). We var-

ied WM load by presenting one to three visual objects. A probe stimulus was shown after a 12 second delay. Our design allowed us to separate encoding, maintenance and retrieval related activity. Whole-brain fMRI (1,5 Tesla, repetition time TR = 2 s) and high density EEG (64 channels) were acquired in separate sessions. **Results:** In the fMRI, patients showed more prefrontal activity than controls doing the memory delay in the easiest memory load condition. Conversely they showed less prefrontal activity than controls in the more difficult conditions. The EEG data revealed abnormalities in the visual event related potential in the patient group. **Conclusion:** Results indicate a dysfunction of the working memory network in patients during all task phases including early visual areas as well as higher order areas especially in the prefrontal cortex. Our data provide first evidence for widespread neurophysiological dysfunction in adolescents suffering from EOS. The prefrontal hyperactivity in lower load conditions would be compatible with models of reduced cognitive capacity in EOS, which have so far proposed for adult onset schizophrenia.

S-005-022   Topic: 69, 12
Efficacy, subjective well-being and safety of Olanzapine in adolescent patients with schizophrenia: Findings from a prospective open-label multicenter study

Ralf Dittmann, Lilly Deutschland GmbH, Medical Department, Bad Homburg, Germany, dittmann@lilly.com
Ulrich Hagenah; Jenny Junghanß; Iris Linde; Anneliese Maestele; Claudia Mehler; Eberhard Meyer

Objective: To present results of the entire sample from a study of olanzapine in the treatment of young patients with schizophrenia. **Methods:** This is an open-label multicenter trial of olanzapine (5–20 mg/day) in adolescents and young adults (12–21 years) with DSM-IV diagnosis of schizophrenia. We used BPRS0-6 (response criterion at Week 6: = 30% reduction), CGI-S and -I, and Subjective Well-Being (SWN, short form) scales to assess the efficacy of olanzapine. Safety was assessed based on spontaneous adverse events (AEs), laboratory analytes, weight, and Simpson-Angus Scores. **Results:** 100 patients entered the study, 96 were treated with olanzapine, 80 reached Week 6, and 34 of 60 responders completed the 6-month observation period. The response rate at Week 6 was 62.5% (N = 60/96). Mean length of olanzapine treatment (mean maximum dose = 16.7 mg) was 97.2 days. Mean BPRS0-6 score decreased from baseline to Week 6 by 17.0 ± 14.4 points ($p < 0.001$). There were also improvements in CGI-S ($p < 0.001$) and CGI-I scores. Mean changes from baseline to Week 6 in the SWN score were 7.5 ± 16.4 ($p < 0.01$) for all patients, and 11.7 ± 16.4 ($p < 0.01$) for the responders. Three patients had serious adverse events (infection (1); rehospitalization (N = 2)); four different patients discontinued early for non-serious AEs. The most common spontaneously reported treatment-emergent AEs were weight gain (N = 29, 30.2%) and increased prolactin (N = 24, 25.0%). Leukopenia was documented in 6 patients (6.3%). Mean weight gain was 5.1 kg; mean change in Simpson-Angus score was 0.2 (entire sample, LOCF up to Week 6). **Conclusion:** Data revealed the following: 1. Olanzapine was effective in this age group. 2. Subjective well-being improved statistically significantly, in parallel to BPRS results. 3. Olanzapine was well tolerated, there were only few dropouts due to AEs.

S-005-023   Topic: 69, 26

One-year prevalence of auditory hallucinations in 7 years old primary school children in a Dutch province

Jack A. Jenner, University Hospital Groningen,
Voices Outpatient Dept., Groningen, Netherlands,
j.a.jenner@acggn.azg.nl

Objective: To examine the on-year prevalence of auditory vocal hallucinations, their correlation with behaviour problems in children attending primary school and to study their predictive value for adolescent schizophrenia. **Methods:** The municipal health service Groningen requested parents of all 7-year old children attending primary school to consent in writing for testing vision and hearing of their child. Additional written consent was obtained for testing auditory vocal hallucinations with the Auditory Hallucination Rating Scale (adjusted for age), and filing out the Children Behaviour Checklist. A cohort is being constructed of all voice hearing children and non-voice hearers matched for gender, age, urbanity and type and religious denomination of their school. This cohort will be followed over the years to study the predictive value of auditory hallucinations. **Results:** About 80% (5000 children) have been assessed with AHRS. One-year prevalence is 8.2%, a substantial number of these appeared severely handicapped due to voicehearing. **Conclusion:** One-year prevalence is in line with other international studies. Analysis is still in progress; further results as to prevalence, burden, control and distress of hearing voices and their correlation with abnormal behaviour measured with the CBCL will be presented at the conference.

S-005-024   Topic: 69, 1

Disability and need in adolescent onset psychosis

Leonie Boeing, Lothian NHS Young Peoples Unit,
Royal Edinburgh Hospital, Edinburgh, United Kingdom,
leonie.boeing@lpct.scot.nhs.uk
Val Murray; Anthony Pelosi; Robert McCabe;
Douglas Blackwood; Robert Wrate

Objective: Early Intervention Services advocate the implementation of assertive multi-modal intervention for young people with first episode psychosis. Little is known of care needs in adolescent onset psychosis. We examine the prevalence, disability and needs for care of a heterogeneous group of young people with adolescent onset psychosis as seen by mainstream mental health services. **Methods:** Cases were identified from multiple sources, OPCRIT retrospective examination of case notes identified 101 subjects. Opt-out design for cross-sectional interview of 53 subjects, their carers and keyworkers using outcome measures and a developmentally appropriate version of the Cardinal Needs Schedule. **Results:** Twenty-one (20%) were not in contact with the mental health services, and five could not be located. 80% of first admissions were to adult acute psychiatric wards. Interviewees had high levels of symptomatic and social morbidity and substance misuse. Despite high levels of clinical input 20% had five or more unmet needs and 17% had intractable problems. Care provision was better for 'clinical' than for 'social' domains. **Conclusion:** Young people with adolescent onset psychosis have a low-prevalence disorder with potentially poor prognosis that requires an assertive multi-agency approach. The findings pose a major challenge to policy makers and clinicians to improve the provision of age-appropriate psychological, social and medical interventions sensitive to their developmental needs.

S-005-025   Topic: 69, 42

Early-onset psychotic disorders: Diagnostic stability over a 3-year period

Carlo Cianchetti, University of Cagliari,
Dept. of Child Neuropsychiatry, Cagliari, Italy,
cianchet@unica.it
Maria Giuseppina Ledda; S. Pellerano; M. Pintor;
G. L. Mellis; T. Piroddi

Objective: The problem of the stability of the diagnosis after the first psychotic episodes was posed for adolescents in 1991 by Werry et al. We evaluated the modification of the first diagnosis at a follow-up in a group of patients with onset of the disorder in adolescence. **Methods:** The study concerns 43 adolescents (26 males and 17 females). All subjects were hospitalized due the presence of a disorder with psychotic features, that is, presence of delusions or hallucinations or both; none of them presented depressive disorder with psychotic features. Diagnoses were made according strict DSM-IV criteria. Mean age at onset of symptoms was 15.1 (±1.9). The first diagnosis was made after 6 months from the first symptoms; a second diagnosis after 12 months, taking in account clinical features between 6 and 12 months; a third diagnosis after at least 3 years on the basis of clinical features after 12th month (in some cases follow-up arrives to 7 years, but in none the diagnosis after 3 years did change). All were initially treated with neuroleptics (classic or atypical), in some cases associated with mood stabilizers. **Results:** The first diagnosis, after 6 months from the first symptoms, was as follows: schizophrenic disorder (SPh) in 17, schizoaffective (SA) in 17 and bipolar disorder (BP) in 9. After 12 months, diagnosis was changed in 2 SPh (to SA), in 5 SA (2 to SPh and 3 to BP) and in 2 BP (to SA). After 3 years, the diagnoses made at 6 months changed as follows: 3 SPh to BP, 5 SA to SPh and 4 SA to BP, 3 BP to SA. Therefore, diagnostic change at 3 years occurred in 4/17 (24%) SPh, in 9/17 (53%) SA and in 3/9 (33%) BP. Overall, change of diagnosis after 3 years occurred in 16/43 (37%) cases. **Conclusion:** Our data show that a consistent part of the initial diagnoses are unreliable in psychotic adolescents. Particularly SA disorders change to SPh or BP disorders. This confirms that SA diagnosis is somewhat hybrid between SPh and BP. SPh and BP disorders seem to have similar degree of diagnostic stability at follow-up.

S-006   Topic: 3

Models of treatment and prevention I

Track: Therapy and intervention

Chairperson: Alan Flisher, University of Cape Town
Psychiatry and Mental Health, Observatory, South Africa,
aflisher@curie.uct.ac.za

S-006-026   Topic: 3, 23

The effectiveness of the positive thinking program in preventing internalising disorders in 8–9 year old children

Monique Nesa, Curtin University, School of Psychology,
Perth, Australia, m.nesa@curtin.edu.au
Rosanna Rooney; Clare Roberts; Robert Kane; Sven Silburn;
Lisbeth Pike

Objective: Research has investigated the possibility of preventing depression and anxiety in adolescents, but very few studies have investigated this phenomenon in children.

Internalising problems are common mental health problems experienced by this group with prevalence rates of 12% found in a recent Australian survey of child mental health (Sawyer et al., 2000). Middle childhood is a developmental period where cognitive systems relating to self and attributions for life events have not yet become stable (Nolen-Hoeksema, Girgus & Seligman, 1992; Cole & Turner, 1994), and also a period where the prevalence of anxiety problems is increasing. Hence, early intervention in middle childhood may hold promise for reducing the incidence of disorders such as anxiety and depression. The Positive Thinking (PT) program (Rooney et al. 2000), is a school-based intervention aimed at preventing internalising disorders among 8–9 year old children utilising a universal approach and delivered as part of the school health curriculum. The sessions focus on building positive self-cognitions, optimism and self-esteem. **Methods:** An initial pilot study involved 120 (72 in intervention; 48 in control) eight and nine-year old children from four low-socio-economic schools in Perth, Western Australia. A series of paired t-tests, z tests and ANCOVAS were conducted to analyse pre-, post-test and 9-month follow-up scores for the intervention and control groups. **Results:** Nine month follow-up data showed a significant prevention effect for Major Depression Disorder and Dysthymic Disorder for children in the intervention group compared to those in the control group. **Conclusion:** Following from the significant results, a larger randomised control study is presently being conducted with eight and nine-year old children from twenty state primary schools in low socio-economic areas of Perth. If the program is shown to be effective, it can be used as part of the health education curriculum as a non-stigmatising method of addressing mental health issues in childhood. Funding for the pilot study was provided by Edith Cowan University.

S-006-027   Topic: 4, 25

Consulting for daycare in the inner city

Helge Staby Deaton, Anna Freud Center, Princeton, NJ, USA, he.stabyd@verizon.net

Objective: As consultant I was requested to work in an inner city daycare with 84 children age 21/2 to 5 to provide support for parents and staff in dealing with developmental issues including treatment for those children who needed it. **Methods:** Overall I used a psychoanalytic approach in my work. **Results:** 1. The turnover of staff has stopped. 2. Some teachers have become confident in discussing either difficult classroom situations concerning group interaction among children, the teacher and a specific child, discrete difficult behaviors of individual children, as well as concerns about emotions such as prolonged sadness or anger of a child. 3. Conferences have been called between director, parents, teachers and myself before a child is dismissed from school. 4. The director has consulted with me about specific requests made by parents. 5. Most children that I worked with gained in their ability to interact more age adequately socially, to communicate better with both adults and other children, to enjoy and use the available activities more and to continue in their growth. 6. The overall atmosphere in the center has improved considerably. **Conclusion:** Psychological intervention and consultation in the daycare setting has proved to be important and necessary in furthering the early childhood development of children who would otherwise have had no access to such support.

S-006-028   Topic: 3, 2

The World Health Organisation (WHO) Mental Health Policy Project: Child and adolescent mental health

Alan Flisher, University of Cape Town, Psychiatry and Mental Health, Observatory, South Africa, aflisher@curie.uct.ac.za
Stuart Lustig; Michelle Funk; Myron Belfer

Objective: The purpose of the Child and Adolescent Mental Health module is provide guidelines for the development of policies and plans to improve the mental health of children and adolescents, based on the most recent evidence for cost-effective mental health care. The module is part of the World Health Organisation (WHO) Mental Health Policy and Service (MHPS) Guidance Package. **Methods:** The module was drafted with the main target audiences in mind, namely: a) policy makers and public health professionals in ministries of health or health departments of countries and large administrative divisions of countries; and b) international, regional and national policy and advocacy organisations. A range of individuals and organisations provided feedback on the first a draft of the module, which was incorporated into later drafts. **Results:** The module follows a step-by-step format, with numerous practical examples from specific countries to illustrate particular aspects. It contains the following sections: a) context of child and adolescent mental health; b) developing a child and adolescent mental health policy; c) developing child and adolescent mental health areas for action; d) developing a child and adolescent mental health plan; and e) implementation of policies and plans. There is extensive cross-referencing to other modules in the WHO MHPS package. The module will be published and available on the WHO website during 2004. **Conclusion:** A module on child and adolescent mental health has been developed which can be used as: a) a training package for mental health policy-makers and planners or as educational material in university or college courses; b) a framework for technical consultancy by a wide range of international and national organisations providing support to countries that wish to reform their child and adolescent mental health policy and/or services; and c) an advocacy tool by consumer, family and advocacy organisations.

S-006-029   Topic: 4, 24

An investigation of the effect of a home based program on the outcome of children with developmental delay and their families

Anne Rickards, Melbourne, Australia, alaviniarickards@hotmail.com
Dinah Reddihough; Roslyn Wright-Rossi; Jacqui Simpson

Objective: There is ongoing debate about the type and intensity of service that is most helpful to assist children with developmental delay. This study aimed to investigate whether the provision of a home based program in addition to the program at a Centre improves development in the children and the coping ability of their families. **Methods:** The subjects were 57 children, aged between three and five years who had mild to moderate developmental delay but no physical disability. All attended one of two early intervention centres in Melbourne, Australia; half of the group were randomised to receive an additional program at their homes. A special education teacher provided 40 visits over 12 months helping the families to carry out the Centre's program at home. All children were assessed before and immediately after the completion of the intervention. At both times families completed questionaires assessing family stress, support and empowerment Differences in change over time between the intervention and control group were analysed by T-Test for Independent Samples. **Results:** Change in cognitive development over time favoured the children who received the extra intervention and the difference between intervention and control groups was highly significant (p=0.002). Results on behaviour measures for the children and parent measures also favoured the intervention group but were not statistically significant. **Conclusion:** Results suggest that as well as providing a preschool type intervention for children with developmental delay it is important to involve their families so that parents have the opportunity to continue the program at home.

S-006-030   Topic: 3, 73
'Anger sux real bad':
A five step model of trauma treatment
Dieter David Seuthe, Fachklinik Ederbergland, Psychologie u. Psychotherapie, Hatzfeld-Eifa, Germany, dseuthe@web.de

Objective: 'Tom', 10, had been severely emotionally, physically and sexually abused. He presented with extreme anger attacks, putting himself and others at risk. During our first session at a New Zealand Child & Adolescent Mental Health Service, Tom did a drawing (http://www.saltkrokan.de/drawingtom.jpg): a boy with eyes closed, fists clenched and teeth gritted, lost in helpless rage. He titled it 'Anger sux real bad'. Tom's drawing made me re-think and research better ways of trauma treatment. Psychotherapists can't make past traumata go away but we can help making the scars smaller and the hurting bearable. **Methods:** Working with numerous severely traumatised young clients at Child & Adolescent MH Services in New Zealand, I found out that post-traumatic treatment most successfully follows a specific pattern of five steps. **Results:** Revisiting the trauma needs to be carried out in the least intrusive way, with a reliable support network and/or MH staff involved, in case relived emotions become too overpowering. Externalising is substantial for a favourable outcome. Trauma contents need to be put into external objects like drawings, music, sculptures. Externalising the internalised pain takes the destructive power of traumata out of a person. If a client can touch, see or hear their pain in an external object they can gain control again. Reframing means to find out what strength may lie in having survived the trauma, how this process can empower a young client. Integrating involves finding hope in the strength of a survivor and creating hope for others. Consolidating describes the process of taking control again, becoming strong enough to move on. **Conclusion:** This five step trauma treatment reliably works in clinical practice. My presentation at an international MH congress hopefully would initiate discussion and research on this approach.

S-006-031   Topic: 78, 41
Acute care of adolescents suffering
from Anorexia Nervosa (AN)
H. Vielhaber, Kinderklinik Dritter Orden, München, Germany; H. Backmund; M. Gerlinghoff

Anorexia nervosa is a severe, potentially life-threatening disease usually starting at an age of about 14 years. Early treat-

ment is known to improve prognosis (Zipfel et al., 2000). Despite this adequate treatment is often delayed for years due to an initial gain in well-being and a strong bias of adolescents and their parents against psychotherapy. To improve compliance we started to stress medical complications when consulted in our center of eating disorders (TCE). In addition we recommend admission to a pediatric ward to any patient at a bmi of < 16. The following objectives were aimed at: 1. medical examination and observation to recognize medical complications; 2. nutritional treatment should be started via liquid formula given p.o. exclusively. Gavage feeding should be avoided whenever possible; 3. Patients should be motivated to start subsequent psychotherapy. Within 2 years 35 patients at an average age of 15.9 years (range 12–18) were admitted to a pediatric ward of the hospital of the 3rd order in Munich. BMI range was 11.7 to 16.7. Medical complications (e.g. pericardial effusion, mitral valve prolapse, bradycardia) and weight gain are reported. Acceptance to subsequent psychotherapy is discussed; experience made in dealing with anorectic patients on a general pediatric ward is described. In conclusion all patients and their families accepted acute admittance to a pediatric ward, most of them accepted subsequent psychotherapy; gavage feeding could be completely avoided.

S-007   Topic: 5, 43
Risk behaviors and mental health
Track: Therapy and intervention
Chairperson: Mary Schwab-Stone,
Yale University School of Medicine, New Haven, CT, USA,
mary.schwab-stone@yale.edu

S-007-032   Topic: 5, 37
The international social and health assessment
Mary Schwab-Stone, Yale University, School of Medicine, New Haven, CT, USA, mary.schwab-stone@yale.edu
Vladislav Ruchkin; Robert Vermeiren

Objective: This talk will introduce the International Social and Health Assessment project and will provide an overview of the history of this cross-cultural collaborative study of adolescent psychopathology, problem behavior, as well as factors that shape developmental outcomes. **Methods:** Over the past decade a school-based epidemiological study has been conducted with adolescent students in a Northeastern urban public school system in the U.S. The Social and Health Assessment (SAHA) is a survey measure that covers a range of domains of functioning, including psychopathology, conduct problems and substance use, daily activities, attitudes toward school and other aspects of family, school and community life that bear on psychiatric and behavioral risk. In 2002–2003, the SAHA was administered to large samples of students from the US, Russia, Belgium, Surinam, South Korea, and the Czech Republic, totaling more than 10 000 students. **Results:** Specific examples of the use of these data, both within and across countries will be presented to illustrate the utility of this method for understanding the correlates of psychiatric symptoms and problem behaviors and their dynamics over time. **Conclusion:** The potential contributions of this type of collaborative project will be discussed from pragmatic, theoretical and policy perspectives, noting the challenges of this type of collaboration and emphasizing the relevance of this work in our increasingly interconnected global era.

S-007-033   Topic: 5, 68
Substance use and mental health:
An international school-based study
Ine Jespers, University of Antwerp, Child & Adolescent Psychiatry, Antwerp, Belgium, ijespers@hotmail.com
Robert Vermeiren; Mary Schwab-Stone; Vladislav Ruchkin

Objective: To investigate patterns of substance use and the relationships between substance use and mental health in cross-cultural samples of adolescents. **Methods:** The Social and Health Assessment (SAHA), a school survey that investigates risk-taking behavior (e.g. substance use) and psychopathology (e.g. PTSD, depression), was used for this purpose. For this presentation, patterns of relationship will be compared for student samples in the US, Russia, and Belgium. **Results:** Although patterns of substance use differ by country, similarities in the relationship between substance use and mental health characteristics prevails. With regard to internalizing problems (depression, posttraumatic symptoms), hard drugs users showed the highest levels, whereas marijuana users and alcohol users differed only slightly from non-users. Externalizing problems increased from the no-substance use group over the alcohol use group to the marijuana use group and, finally, the hard drug use group. **Conclusion:** Cross-cultural studies can offer important insights into differences and similarities of the relationships between substance use and mental health across varying social contexts. The presentation will focus on the patterns of relationships, explore different explanations for these findings, and suggest topics of public health importance for future cross-cultural research.

S-007-034   Topic: 5, 45
Mental health characteristics of antisocial adolescents across different countries
Robert Vermeiren, University of Antwerp,
Child & Adolescent Psychiatry, Antwerp, Belgium,
robert@vermeiren.name
Mary Schwab-Stone; Vladislav Ruchkin

Objective: To investigate in adolescents the cross-cultural relationship between type of antisocial behavior (no antisocial behavior, status offenders, non-violent offenders and violent offenders) and mental health characteristics. **Methods:** The Social and Health Assessment (SAHA) is a self-report questionnaire that investigates risk-taking behavior (e.g. antisocial behavior) and psychopathology (e.g. PTSD, depression, anxiety), which offers a unique opportunity for cross-national comparisons. The SAHA was administered to large samples (each > 2500) of 11 to 18 year old adolescents from three middle to large-size cities (New Haven, US; Arkangelsk, Russia; Antwerp, Belgium). **Results:** Results from this project demonstrate that for both genders and in all three countries, mental health problems differ by type of antisocial behavior. With respect to internalizing problems, depression was higher in all three offender groups compared to controls, although differences by country were noted. Post-traumatic symptoms were generally higher in violent offenders than other offender groups. Externalzing symptomatology gradually increased from the non-antisocial group to the status offending group to the non-violent and finally the violent group. Although patterns of relationships are comparable, differences between countries were noted. **Conclusion:** The school-based SAHA survey adds to the knowledge on mental health problems

in antisocial youths and puts these insights into an international context.

S-007-035   Topic: 5, 26
Depression and internalizing and externalizing behaviors: A three country comparison
Vladislav Ruchkin, Yale Child Study Center, New Haven CT, USA, vladislav.ruchkin@yale.edu
Mary Schwab-Stone; Robert Vermeiren

Objective: To compare cross-cultural trends for comorbid internalizing and externalizing psychopathology, prosocial beliefs, and perceptions of risk in adolescents with and without clinical levels of self-reported depressive symptoms. **Methods:** A self-report survey was conducted in a representative sample of 3,309 14 to 17 year old adolescents from urban communities in the US (n = 1,343), Belgium (n = 946) and Russia (n = 1,009). **Results:** In all three countries, girls reported higher levels of depressive symptoms than boys. The findings also demonstrate that in both genders depressive symptoms were associated with increased levels of internalizing and externalizing problems, as well as lower levels of prosocial beliefs and low perceptions of harm from risk-taking behavior. Depressed boys had relatively higher levels of externalizing problems than depressed girls. Greater levels of internalizing problems observed in depressed youth, as compared to their non-depressed counterparts, were not gender-specific. **Conclusion:** Current findings suggest that the relationships between depression and comorbid psychopathology are not culture specific and have similar patterns in different populations.

S-007-036   Topic: 5, 85
Antisocial behavior, community violence exposure, and substance abuse in youth in Czech Republic: Preliminary results
Marek Blatny, Academy of Sciences, Inst. of Psychology, Brno, Czech Republic, blatny@psu.cas.cz
Michal Hrdlicka; Tomas Urbanek; Martin Jelinek;
Veronika Balastikova; Vladislav Ruchkin;
Mary Schwab-Stone

Objective: To investigate the relationships between antisocial behavior, exposure to community violence (witnessing and victimization), and substance abuse (cigarettes, alcohol, and illegal drugs) in the national sample of urban adolescents in Czech Republic. **Methods:** The Social and Health Assessment (SAHA), a school survey, was conducted with 3023 adolescents (age 12–14 years old) in Prague and 12 regional capitals of the Czech Republic. **Results:** K-means cluster analysis was used to identify the main clusters of antisocial behavior. Subsequently, adolescents from different clusters were compared on the levels of their violence exposure and substance use. Four major clusters of children were identified. The first cluster (53.6% of the sample) comprised non-problematic children with the lowest levels of antisocial behavior, as well as the lowest levels of violence exposure and substance use. Children in the second cluster (16%) were characterized by mild conduct problems. They reported higher levels of witnessing and victimization, as compared to non-problematic children from the first cluster, as well as greater levels of smoking, and marijuana and alcohol use. The third cluster (24.4%) included children with moderate aggressive behavior (fistfights and shoving) and no other expressions of antisocial behavior, with low levels of violence exposure, and low substance abuse. Finally, adolescents from the fourth cluster (1.6%) reported the highest levels of all types of antisocial behavior, as well as the highest levels of exposure to violence and substance abuse. **Conclusion:** Our research revealed various forms of disturbed behavior in Czech urban youth, with diverse associations to exposure to violence and substance abuse. Not all forms of disturbed behavior were connected with substance abuse. Further analyses are needed to clarify context of these relationships.

S-008   Topic: 48
Attachment and interaction
Chairperson: Philippe Jeammet,
Université Paris VI Psychiatrie de l'Enfant, Paris, France,
philippe.jeammet@imm.fr

S-008-037   Topic: 48
Ways of attachment and internal working models among some young psychotic adolescents when they leave day hospital
Alain Frottin, CPR, Senlis, France, cprns@wanadoo.fr
Andjelka Filipovic; Eric Albert

Objective: The young teenagers, after leaving day hospital to join suitable institutions according with their age and disturbances can show different kind of development: enlarged interest about knowledge with better social integration and ability to learn a job, persistent deficiency which needs specialized reception places, and the worst one but fortunately seldom observed event, emergence of a psychiatric illness such as acute delusion psychosis, major depressive syndrome, psychopathy. The hypothesis: precocious ways of attachment to parental figures and internal working models linked to them may represent a sensitivity factor, or on the contrary a protective one. **Methods:** The different sorts of attachment in ten young teenagers older than twelve were explored with the stories to complete test. This method, theoretically used with little children gave the opportunity of testing many youngsters unable to read, either completely, or not fluently enough. **Results:** Despite of the small number of children assessed in this study, two groups were made out. In the first group, the major kind of attachment found was the one described as avoiding. But paradoxically, the youngsters in this group were best able to seek some help from somebody, to attract fellowship, to develop intellectual knowledge. We consider this kind of attachment as a positive factor, allowing a better evolution over adolescence and thereafter. In the second group, ambivalent and disorganized types of attachment were found out as prominent. These adolescents need for their futures more containing institutions. **Conclusion:** Exploration of attachment and internal working models may represent a forecasting element, inviting to prepare with a special care the moment when adolescents leave day hospitals, taking into account any revival of traumatic separation. Loss and mourning have to be symbolized.

S-008-038   Topic: 48, 41
The attachment of adolescent parents and their babies
Dora Musetti Schelotto, Montevideo, Uruguay,
bacviruy@mednet.apc.org

Objective: 1) To study the different types of relationships that can be observed between adolescent parents and their babies. 2) To assist these parents and help them to develop healthy raising up strategies. **Methods:** Being members of the staff of a specialized clinic that deals with infant mental troubles, we receive adolescent parents referred from Montevideo Children's Hospital. In order to know the existent bonds we focused: 1) the personality of the parents, the way in which pregnancy and birth had affected it, the feelings that emerged in these events 2) their capacity to take care of the baby, to understand his/her needs 3) the developing features of the baby, his ability to interact with others, to play; the way he slept and fed. Considering these aspects, we used initially and every six months the "Parent Perception Interview" (C. R. Tissot, S. Busconi, J. P. Bachmann, G. Besson, B. Cramer) for evaluating the changes in the "internal representation" of parents about the babies and about themselves, and applied the "Symptom Checklist" of the same authors to follow the evolution of the baby's Health quality. To assist improvements, we worked weekly with parents and their baby, stressing successes and suggesting new ways of handling unresolved situations. **Results:** These parents showed an impairment to understand the needs of their babies; they had feelings of rivalry and competition towards them, of guilt and unfitness for performing their role. They felt that adults did not respect their right to be parents, and that they needed help in their task of sustaining the growth of their children. After a few months of attention, they learned fairly sound strategies of baby care, and managed to improve their relationship with their children.

S-008-039   Topic: 48, 53
Mother's perception of child's emotions in the context of intrafamily problems caused by some war events
Mladen Knezevic, University of Zagreb, Dept. of Social
Work, Zagreb, Croatia, mladen.knezevic@pravo.hr
Milivoj Jovancevic

Objective: The purpose of the study was to investigate possible differences in mother's perception of child's emotions in the context of intrarfamilial problems. The cause of intrafamilial problems was a disturbance in father's behavior due to his traumatic war experiences. **Methods:** An IFEEL test was used to research mother's perception of child's emotions. Questionnaire were used to collect data about father's behavioral problems. Interviews with mothers and fathers was used to collect data. Some statistical procedures were used to analyze data, among them method of polar taxons. Sample: Sample consisted of 185 women who were settled in the refugee camps in Croatia and Bosnia and Herzegovina, or were settled in abandoned houses. All of them have had different war experiences. And almost all of their partners have had different war experiences. **Results:** It was obvious that mothers whose husbands or partners have had serious psychological problems caused by war events have had different perceptions of emotions on the faces of their children. Normally, they were dealing with their children in accordance with perception of their child's emotions. **Conclusion:** Different traumatic experiences (war) changed the way how mothers perceived emotions of their babies, and how they were dealing with them. Moreover, traumatic war experiences in their partners are changing the way of perception of child's experiences. Mothers, whose partners have had the most traumatic experiences, tend to perceive emotions in the faces of their children in different way.

S-009   Topic: 55
Children of sick parents I
Chairperson: Jonathan Hill, University of Liverpool
Dept. of Psychiatry, Liverpool, United Kingdom,
jonathan.hill@liverpool.ac.uk

S-009-041   Topic: 55, 11
Parents with Psychiatric Illness.
The feasability of offering a preventive group intervention to their children
Maria Lawlor, NEHB Child and Family Centre,
Dept. of Child Psychiatry, Drogheda, Ireland,
maria.lawlor@nehb.ie

Objective: The children of parents with psychiatric illness are vulnerable to mental health problems. Targeting interventions at this population seems an ideal opportunity for primary and secondary prevention. Adult psychiatric patients may be unwilling to involve their children with mental health services. This study was undertaken to assess if it was clinically indicated and feasable to offer the children a preventive group intervention. **Methods:** Children (aged 5–17) of a sample of ten adult psychiatric patients were screened for mental health problems. The attitudes of adult psychiatric patients to parenting, to the impact of the illness on their parenting and on their children, and to the involvement of their children in a therapeutic psychoeducational support group was explored using a questionnaire and semistructured interview. **Results:** This study found that 79% of the children were in the clinical range on the SDQ. Parents described how the illness impacted on their parenting. Most parents described difficulties with parenting and child behaviour management. Most parents were willing for the children to attend a group to help them cope with the parents' illness. **Conclusion:** Parents and children need help in coping with parental psychiatric illness. Child mental health problems are an additional stress to parents who are coping with their own psychiatric illnesses. It is both feasable and clinically indicated to offer a group intervention to the children of adult psychiatric patients. Parents would benefit from support with parenting and behaviour management. Adult psychiatric services need to take account of the impact of parenthood on their patients. Adult and child psychiatric services should work together in the interests of improving family mental health.

S-009-042   Topic: 55, 22
First experiences with the implementation of a counselling service for children of somatically ill parents
Christian Kienbacher, Wien, Austria,
christian.kienbacher@univie.ac.at
Carolin Prause; Margit Stöckl; Gertrude Bogyi;
Max H. Friedrich

Objective: We examined the conditions under which families are able to accept a preventive counselling service for chil-

dren of somatically ill parents. We approached the target group in three ways. 1: With an on spot service at an oncological unit, 2: As a counselling service at a child and adolescent psychiatry, 3: Via public relations (mass media, folder, homepage, patient workshops, posters, lectures). **Methods:** We recorded the number of implementation activities and how many families contacted us. Over a period of 18 months we recorded the problems that turned up, and after that we made a content analysis. In order to find out more about the mental health status of our clients we also used standardized questionnaires. **Results:** Of the 85 families 35 families got a counselling at the oncological unit. At the beginning the oncological staff had reservations about using the questionnaires. Doctors and families were often opposed to a service located at a psychiatric ward. The counselling service at the child and adolescent psychiatry was often approached because the child displayed psychological disorders and not because of the illness of the parent. Some children developed eating disorders, anxiety disorders or pain disorders under the strain of the parental illness. 11 out of 18 youths complained about headaches. **Conclusion:** In order to establish such a counselling service, extensive networking activities and plenty of time are necessary in order to raise awareness for the necessity of such a preventive care for children of physically ill parents.

S-009-043   Topic: 55, 25
Children of untreated addicted parents
Michael Klein, Forschungsschwerpunkt, Sucht KFH, Köln,
Germany, mikle@t-online.de
Katrin Kürschner

Objective: International research has impressively shown that children of alcoholics (COAs) are a high risk group for many mental and physical health problems. They have an up to sixfold increased risk for addictive disorders and stem from addicted families in more than a third of all cases. Parental alcohol and drug problems have an intensive impact on development in childhood and adolescence. There seem to be adverse effects in affective, cognitive, and behavioral domains. Though there is a vast amount of research, especially on children of alcoholics in treatment, there is little known on the situation and developmental trajectories of children of untreated addicted parents. **Methods:** Our project has focussed on these children by selecting children of untreated parents with an alcohol problem (screening questionnaires given to a community sample of more than 8,000 students aged 11 to 16). As a result of the screening procedure there have been 151 children in the study group for in-depth-interviews. Results were analyzed by comparing the COAs to 150 non-COAs (control group) and the COAs of untreated to the COAs of treated parents. **Results:** The COAs had more violence experience, exhibited more co-dependent behavior, had less self-esteem. But they also had positive resources, e.g. good sibling relationships. The COAs of untreated parents had worse social conditions than the COAs of treated parents. In addition, they had more affective and expressive problems, less self-efficacy and more pessimistic attitudes. Especially those children were strained in many ways whose parents were comorbid on addictive and mental disorders at the same time. **Conclusion:** In order to reduce the risk of addictive and mental disorders in future, children of untreated addicted parents are in special need of early interventive measures. As with COAs in general, there has to be an distinct increase in efforts to help those children and their families.

S-009-044   Topic: 55

An examination of deficits in mentalising as a vulnerability for adjustment problems at age 5 in children of mothers with post-natal depression

Jonathan Hill, University of Liverpool, Dept. of Psychiatry, Liverpool, United Kingdom, jonathan.hill@liverpool.ac.uk
Lynne Murray; Victoria Leidecker; Helen Sharp

Objective: To test whether deficits in mentalisation, assessed using a doll's house procedure, in 5 year olds exposed in infancy to post-natal depression are associated with adjustment problems; and to examine the role of insecure attachment assessed at 18 months. **Methods:** Findings to be reported in this paper come from a prospective longitudinal study of child development following post-natal depression (Murray et al. 1996), with comprehensive assessments in infancy, childhood and adolescence. These included the Strange Situation Test with mothers at 18 months, and a doll's house play procedure and teacher rated adjustment at 5 years. The video tapes of 87 children (50 post-natal depression, 38 controls) were rated with new scales of mentalising (intentionality and coherence). Intentionality reflected the extent to which the story was told in terms of characters' motives or feelings, and coherence the quality of the story. Analyses focussed on the emotionally challenging 'Bad and Nasty Time' doll's house scene. **Results:** Insecure attachment at 18 months was associated with lower mentalising at 5 years (intentionality, $p < 0.001$; coherence, $p = 0.005$). Lower mentalising was associated with adjustment problems, but this effect was greater in the children of mothers with post-natal depression (intentionality $r = -0.44$, $p = 0.001$; coherence $r = -0.34$, $p = 0.016$) than controls (intentionality $r = -0.11$, $p = 0.52$; coherence $r = -0.10$, $p = 0.56$). Increased teacher rated adjustment problems in the post-natal depression group were confined to children with both low intentionality and low coherence, defined as below the median on both ($t = 2.81$, $p = 0.009$; group by low intentionality/coherence interaction $p = 0.001$). **Conclusion:** Insecure attachment in infancy is associated with deficits in mentalising at 5 years via mechanisms yet to be identified. Deficits in mentalising confer vulnerability to adjustment problems in the presence of risks associated with post-natal depression.

S-009-045   Topic: 55

Factors associated with maternal prenatal depressive symptoms and subsequent child adjustment

Ilona Luoma, Tampere University Hospital, Dept. of Child Psychiatry, Tampere, Finland, ilona.luoma@pshp.fi
Pälvi Kaukonen; Tuula Tamminen

Objective: The aim of the study was to explore which factors are associated with maternal prenatal depressive symptoms and predict subsequent emotional/behavioural symptoms in the child. **Methods:** The original sample consisted of 349 first-time mothers and was gathered from maternal health clinics in Tampere, Finland, 1989–90. Mothers' depressive symptoms were screened during the third trimester of pregnancy by the Edinburgh Postnatal Depression Scale (EPDS). Maternal demographic factors and reports of health, family relationships and psychological well-being were gathered by questionnaires. Emotional and behavioural symptoms of the firstborn children at the age of 8 to 9 years were assessed by the Child Behavior Checklists (CBCLs) completed by the mothers (n = 186). **Results:** Of the mothers participating in the follow-up 10.8% had high levels of depressive

symptoms prenatally. Many factors describing the mother's psychological well-being, health habits (for example smoking and alcohol consumption) and satisfaction with social conditions were associated with high level of depressive symptoms. Of these factors, maternal history of mental health problems, low level of life satisfaction during pregnancy, feelings of depression, and poor relationships with partner and own mother were associated with high level of child's emotional and behavioural problems at the age of 8 to 9 years. In logistic regression, maternal history of mental health problems remained the only variable predicting child's high symptom level in middle childhood. **Conclusion:** To promote the well-being of the unborn child, it is important to note that factors describing maternal psychological well-being and the quality of the relationships with significant others are associated with maternal depressive symptoms during pregnancy and may have long-term consequences for subsequent child adjustment. The numbers of mothers who had smoked or used alcohol during pregnancy were low, which may explain the finding that these factors were not statistically significant predictors of child well-being.

S-010   Topic: 3

Three prevention programs from Australia

Track: Therapy and intervention
Chairperson: Barry Nurcombe, University of Queensland Dept. of Psychiatry, Brisbane, Australia, bnurcombe@psychiatry.uq.edu.au

Three prevention programs from Australia

Barry Nurcombe, University of Queensland, Dept. of Psychiatry, Brisbane, Australia, bnurcombe@psychiatry.uq.edu.au

Objective: To introduce the audience to the impact the Australian National Mental Policy has had on the promotion of mental health in Australia. **Methods:** Professor Graham Martin will open the discussion by describing the purpose and effects of the National Mental Health Policy. Professor Martin will then go on to describe the design, implementation, and results of suicide prevention projects in Australia. Professor McDermott will describe the rationale, implementation, and effectiveness of an intervention program for children following a natural disaster: bushfire. Professor Nurcombe will describe an experimental project comparing the effectiveness of cognitive behavior therapy and family therapy for sexually abused children, with spesial reference to the problem of self-termination. **Results:** The National Mental Health Polcy has had a considerable effect on the stimulation of promotion and prevention projects. **Conclusion:** Other countries should consider the adoption of a National Mental Policy.

S-010-046   Topic: 93, 3

Public health approaches to suicide prevention: Is the rhetoric of national strategy more important than the reality of evidence in shaping effective programs?

Graham Martin, The University of Queensland, Child & Adolescent Psychiatry, Herston, Australia, g.martin@uq.edu.au

Objective: To explore the impact of a national strategy for suicide prevention and the evidence base which may have driven it. **Methods:** Professor Martin was a member of the Australian National Youth Suicide Prevention Advisory Group from 1995 to 1999, a member of the Evaluation Working Group (EWG) subcommittee reviewing evaluation for over 70 funded programs, and a member of the writing group for the Australian National Action Plan for Suicide Prevention 1999–2003. He is currently a member of the National Advisory Committee for the Australian Suicide Prevention Strategy, a member of the National Media and Mental Health Reference Group, and Immediate Past National Chairman of Suicide Prevention Australia. Three national evidence-based reviews related to risk factors for suicide in young people were commissioned for the first National Strategy (Patton & Burns, Cantor, and Beautrais). **Results:** The findings of these reviews will be synthesized to provide an overview of the evidence for suicide prevention together with other major reviews and papers (for instance Gunnell & Frankel, 1994) which have shaped our thinking about what might be possible in suicide prevention. Recently there has been a shift away from emphasis on best practice in clinical settings following attempted suicide, toward development of broad community programs using Public Health Approaches and Mental Health Promotion. The evidence for Public Health approaches will be reviewed, and set into the context of the last 10 years of the Australian National Suicide Prevention Strategy. Changes in Australian suicide rates will be reviewed against the changes in policy and strategy. **Conclusion:** As scientist practitioners we are increasingly evidence-driven, yet there is often a time lag between available evidence being published and its appearance in policy and strategy. Conversely, the rhetoric of policy often challenges researchers to closely examine proposed new directions, leading to the development of novel paradigms.

S-010-047   Topic: 53, 3
Children and natural disasters: A selective prevention program utilizing population-based screening

Brett McDermott, University of Queensland, Mater Child and Youth Mental, South Brisbane, QLD, Australia,
brett_mcdermott@mater.org.au

Objective: There is robust evidence that children and adolescents experience PTSD, anxiety and depressive psychopathology following natural disasters. This paper will detail how proactive, school-based screening after a natural disaster facilitated a selective psychological intervention. **Methods:** Following devastating Australian wildfire disasters, school children, age range 6–18 years completed standardized measures of psychopathology, and measures of trauma exposure, separation experience and perception of threat. Interventions, a guided trauma workbook for children and group therapy for adolescents, were offered based on test results. **Results:** Over 2500 children (mean 13.43 ± 2.5 years) were screened. 13% of students were identified with significant emotional distress 6 months following the disaster. Significant, independent predictors of emotional distress were: persisting depressive symptoms; perception of threat to self or to parents; evacuation experience; and school grade; but not gender. Non-linear relationships between depression, emotional distress and school grade were found. Student and parent satisfaction with the school-based screening and subsequent treatment modalities was high. **Conclusion:** School-based post-disaster case identification by screening was a well accepted, economic and effective modality for case identification of

children with persisting post-disaster psychopathology. Both guided trauma workbooks and group therapy were useful responses to providing an intervention to the large numbers of children with persisting post-disaster emotional distress.

S-010-048   Topic: 51, 3
The Queensland child sexual abuse treatment study

Barry Nurcombe, University of Queensland,
Dept. of Psychiatry, Brisbane, Australia,
bnurcombe@psychiatry.uq.edu.au

Objective: To compare the relative effectiveness of cognitive behavioural therapy (CBT) and family therapy (FT), delivered by trained community clinicians, in the treatment of sexually abused children and adolescents. **Methods:** 91 sexually abused subjects, aged 6-16 years, were randomly assigned to two 18-week, manualized treatment programs, CBT and FT, delivered by trained, supervised, community clinicians throughout Queensland. The fidelity of implementation was checked by audit of sessional audiotapes. Extensive psychological assessments of the children and parents were completed at 0, 18, and 52 weeks. **Results:** Both treatment groups improved significantly to below the clinical level in regard to child dissociation, depression, anger, post-traumatic stress symptoms, and avoidant coping style. Parents did not improve in depression or anxiety. There were no significant differences in effectiveness between CBT and FT. Premature self-termination was predicted by maternal depression. **Conclusion:** More attention should be given to the engagement of families, the treatment of maternal depression, and the provision of assistance to families with practical problems before focussed treatment is begun.

S-011   Topic: 69, 24
Detection and intervention in early onset psychosis: The VESPA project

Track: Psychotic disorders

Chairperson: Franz Resch, Universität Heidelberg
Kinder- und Jugendpsychiatrie, Heidelberg, Germany,
franz_resch@med.uni-heidelberg.de
Dieter Bürgin, Universitätsklinik Basel
Kinder- u. Jugendpsychiatrie, Basel, Switzerland,
dieter.buergin@unibas.ch

Detection and intervention in early onset psychosis: The VESPA project

Franz Resch, Universität Heidelberg,
Kinder- und Jugendpsychiatrie, Heidelberg, Germany,
franz_resch@med.uni-heidelberg.de

Early onset schizophrenia represents a major challenge for child and adolescent psychiatry. The duration of untreated psychosis has a strong impact on clinical and social prognosis of the patient. The VESPA-Study (Verbundstudie Psychosen der Adoleszenz) of German speaking countries (Austria, Germany and Switzerland) in cooperation with the Melbourne Early detection team (Australia) addresses this problem. Early detection of prodromal signs and incipient psychosis may include subjective experiences operationalized in the concept of basic symptoms. Problems of the diagnostic process and prognostic factors of therapeutic relationship, personality and risk behaviour will be discussed.

S-011-049   Topic: 69, 24

Diagnostic changes 18 months
after a first-admission diagnosis of psychosis

Benno Graf Schimmelmann, UKE Hamburg-Eppendorf,
Kinder- und Jugendpsychiatrie, Hamburg, Germany,
bschimme@uke.uni-hamburg.de
Philippe Conus; Jane Edwards; Patrick D. McGorry;
Martin Lambert

Objective: Diagnostic changes may reflect evolution of an illness, emergence of newly disclosed information, or unreliability of assessment. This study evaluates the stability of research diagnoses in a heterogeneous first-admission sample with psychosis. **Methods:** The Early Psychosis Prevention and Intervention Centre (EPPIC) in Melbourne, Australia, has admitted 786 first-episode psychosis (FEP) patients, age 14–29, between 1998–2000. Of those, 230 subjects were included in prospective studies receiving a SKID I interview on admission. 115 patients were randomly assigned to the current study. The DSM-IV consensus diagnoses at baseline and at discharge (18 month later) were formulated by psychiatrists blind to previous research diagnoses. **Results:** Only 56% of the 18-month-diagnoses were congruent. The most temporally consistent 18-month categories were schizoaffective disorder (n=5, 100%,) and schizophrenia (87%, n=34). The most frequent shift in diagnosis at 18 months was to schizophrenia spectrum (n=38). As expected, the most incongruent diagnosis was schizophreniform disorder (n=45). Of those 24 (53%) received a diagnosis of schizophrenia, 7 (16%) of affective psychoses. **Conclusion:** The findings support the need for a longitudinally based diagnostic process in first episode psychotic patients in order to meet their therapeutic, especially psychopharmacological requirements.

S-011-050   Topic: 69, 24

Correlates of substance misuse in 668 patients
with first-episode psychosis treated
at the Early Psychosis Prevention
and Intervention Centre (EPPIC) in Melbourne/Australia

Martin Lambert, UKE Hamburg-Eppendorf, Hamburg,
Germany, lambert@uke.uni-hamburg.de
Philippe Conus; Benno Graf Schimmelmann;
Patrick D. McGorry

Objective: Previous studies about psychosis and comorbid substance abuse disorder (SUD) have several limitations: (1) mainly focus on multiple episode patients, (2) selection bias through informed consent design and (3) lack of investigation of the course of SUD. **Methods:** The Early Psychosis Prevention and Intervention Centre (EPPIC) in Melbourne, Australia, has admitted 786 first-episode psychosis (FEP) patients between 1998–2000. Data were collected from patients' medical records (MR) using a systematic comprehensive approach (Early Psychosis File Questionnaire). 82 MR were not available for the study. Of the remaining 704 MR that were assessed, 36 patients did not meet diagnostic inclusion criteria. **Results:** 61% of the 668 FEP patients met criteria for SUD (410 with SUD cf. 258 without SUD). The most prevalent current SUD at baseline were cannabis-related (67%). 72% of patients with SUD fulfilled criteria for dependence, while 35% also met criteria for a secondary SUD. At baseline, FEP with comorbid SUD had significantly higher severity of illness scores (CGI-S; $p < 0.001$) and lower levels of functioning (GAF and SOFAS; $p < 0.001$). After 18 months of treatment, SUD outcomes were highly correlated with increased rates of loss to follow-up ($p < 0.001$), higher number of relapses during the treatment period ($p < 0.05$), lower rates of remission ($p < 0.001$), higher psychopathology scores at endpoint (CGI-S: $p < 0.001$), increased suicidal attempts during treatment ($p < 0.01$) and lower level of functioning as measured by the GAF ($p < 0.001$), SOFAS ($p < 0.001$), and the Vocation and Location Index (both $p < 0.001$). **Conclusion:** SUD in FEP patients is an important clinical variable associated with increased morbidity and poor symptomatic and functional outcome. Early intervention strategies that target comorbid SUD in FEP are clearly warranted.

S-011-051   Topic: 69, 24

Duration of untreated psychosis and course of child
and adolescent psychotic disorders

Ulrich Preuss, Universitätsklinik Bern,
Kinder- und Jugendpsychiatrie, Bern, Switzerland,
ulrich.preuss@kjp.unibe.ch
Heiner Meng; Dieter Bürgin; Wilhelm Felder; M. Günter

Objective: To examine the development of course in childrens' and adolescents' first and early-onset psychotic illness in relation to duration of untreated period before the first clinical diagnosis and initiation of psychiatric treatment. **Methods:** These data are from a one year longitudinal, prospective, cooperative study from different sites in Austria, Switzerland, and Germany. 69 subjects were drawn from a 1-year observational study on individuals ages 11-18 with early onset psychotic disorders, schizophrenia, schizophrenia spectrum disorders, and affective disorder with psychotic symptoms. Diagnosis was derived from SCID I interviews and on basis of DSM-IV criteria for schizophrenia. Participant's development was observed 3 times while treatment and after release. **Results:** Youths with schizophrenia (sz: n=24), schizophrenia spectrum disorders (sp: n=27), affective disorder, psychotic symptoms (af: n=7) were included. DUP measured in estimates of patients, parents and investigators showed various seizes between informants and raters. Correlations between parents' and raters' estimates of DUP and a limited range of predictive value of DUP for symptoms and general measures for over all outcome after one year characterized the relevance of the duration of the untreated period in young first episode individuals, but only small predictive value from Duration of untreated psychosis on one outcome could be found. Other disorders were clearly differentiated from psychotic disorders in symptoms, course, and outcome. Small samples limited prove in this domain. **Conclusion:** The concept of DUP is very general and may be of relevance for outcome, but Dup estimated retrospectively. This limits the evidence derived from analyses of DUP in relation to measures of course and outcome. Clinicians must be careful in overrating the length of DUP, but early recognition of psychotic disorders stays in first line tasks, until it is resolved whether DUP is of absolute relevance for severity and long-term outcome in psychosis or less important as considered today. Key Words: childhood, adolescent schizophrenia; schizophrenia spectrum disorders; affective disorder; psychosis; gender differences, DUP; early onset schizophrenia; first episode psychosis.

S-011-052   Topic: 69, 24
Cooperate, don't just collaborate
Monika Strauss, KJPD, St. Gallen, St. Gallen, Switzerland,
monika.strauss@kjpd-sg.ch
Peter Parzer; Joachim Jungmann; Franz Resch

Objective: This study was designed to get more information of the course of the schizophrenic disorder as well as to verify some hypothesis on the conditions influencing the outcome. **Methods:** 32 out of a group of 36 patients who had suffered their first episode of a schizophrenic psychosis during their adolescence were interviewed on the phone after 3 years. 16 out of these 32 patients could also be interviewed both in a clinical interview using the PANSS and some items of the BSABS and in a family interview. The cooperation was rated on the basis of data found in the patient treatment files. **Results:** App. 40% of the patients had a favourable outcome, with only 19% considered healthy. App. 60% had an unfavourable outcome. The overall very low scores of psychopathological symptoms seemed to contradict with quite a serious level of social impairment. Most patients showed some basic symptoms such as impaired cognition or increased susceptibility to emotional stress. The classical outcome predictors found by previous authors were confirmed. Yet the most striking predictor for a good outcome was the cooperation of the patients and their families with the therapeutic team, the predictive value of this item being 40% (pseudo r2). The medication compliance did not define the cooperation item, since the patients were compliant for medication. Cooperation was defined by a 8 item description of the patient-therapist relationship. **Conclusion:** Considering the generally poor outcome of young schizophrenics the finding of a strong influence of a good cooperation between doctors and patients should be further examined by a prospective study design.

S-011-053   Topic: 69, 24
Subtyping adolescents with a first schizophrenic episode using a person centered approach
Georg Spiel, Landeskrankenhaus Klagenfurt,
Neurologie und Psychiatrie, Klagenfurt, Austria,
georg.spiel@kabeg.at
C. von Korff; H.-A. Ballin; R. Gößler; M. Günter;
Heiner Meng; G. Sange

Objective: The group of adolescents suffering psychosis challenges us with regard to diagnosis, treatment and prognosis. The high risk of early disability in this group of patients is evident. Undoubtedly essential progress has been achieved in diagnostic and treatment issues, but nevertheless we face many unresolved scientific questions. Up to now our knowledge bases on the one hand on samples of patients with a psychotic disorder and on the other hand on single case-informations. The aim of the study is to overcome this apparent discrepancy in approaching the topic by using the so called person centered methodological approach. Instead of focusing on single symptoms as isolated variable in a group of patients, we concentrate on typical and atypical symptom constellations. Using this theoretical background accidental co-occurrence of psychopathological features in the single case can be differentiated from comorbidity as the expression of a nosological entity. **Methods:** Using the data basis of the Vespa study (Verbundstudie Erstmanifestierte juvenile Psychosen in der Adoleszenz) psychopathological symptoms - documented

by the AMDP system - and the BSABS of the entire cohort is analyzed by the Configurable Frequency Analysis (KFA, Lienert). **Results:** Within the AMDP data 5 subtypes of the group can be delineated from one to another. Within the BSABS in which the patients' subjective experiences are evaluated two subtypes can be found showing different symptom intensivity. All types differ in age structure and specific psychopathological features. **Conclusion:** The intention of the study was to identify subtypes in the group of psychotic patients as described above. In a next step these cross sectional results should be combined with longitudinal data looking for specific anamnestic and prognostic features of the subtypes of psychotic adolescents found by using KFA.

S-011-054   Topic: 69, 24
Basic symptoms as indicator of a risk for psychosis in adolescence?
Heiner Meng, JPA Basel, Kinder- und Jugendpsychiatrie,
Basel, Switzerland, heiner.meng@unibas.ch
Beat Mohler; Eginhard Koch; Peter Parzer; M. Günter;
Ulrich Preuss; Georg Spiel

Objective: The need for early intervention in (adolescent) psychosis is in opposition to the difficulty of early detection. Due to the low incidence of juvenile psychosis, primary prevention is not yet possible. What we can do is to identify adolescents at a high risk for psychosis. The concept of basic symptoms will be presented and its applicability for the identification of adolescents at a high risk for psychosis will be discussed. **Methods:** Retrospective, cross-sectional and prospective longitudinal data will be presented from the VESPA study, the Basel Adolescent Project (BAP) and a sample of the university clinic of Heidelberg. In these projects, n=108 psychotic patients, n=116 non-psychotic adolescents and n=99 normal controls have been compared from the point of view of the prevalence of basic symptoms. Longitudinal data will be presented in order to see how basic symptoms develop in a one year follow-up period. **Results:** Normal adolescents display significantly fewer basic symptoms than nonpsychotic psychiatric patients, who in turn show significantly fewer symptoms than psychotic adolescents. Basic symptoms as subjective experiences are difficult to detect unless they have been systematically investigated. After one year, basic symptoms went back towards normal. **Conclusion:** The assessment of basic symptoms proved to be helpful to differentiate between normal adolescents and those at the beginning of severe psychopathology. Basic symptoms seem to represent rather a state than a trait factor. It might be an element for identification of adolescents at ultra high risk (UHR) for psychosis.

S-012   Topic: 89, 45
Attachment, malnutrition and corporal punishment of young children: Universals and cultural differences in parenting
Chairperson: Klaus Minde, Montreal, QC, Canada,
klaus.minde@mcgill.ca

Attachment, malnutrition and corporal punishment of young children: Universals and cultural differences in parenting

Klaus Minde, Montreal, QC, Canada,
klaus.minde@mcgill.ca

Objective: There is significant agreement on parental behaviors associated with a secure and insecure attachment pattern and with malnutrition in young children in the Western world. Likewise, corporal punishment is viewed as a problematic form of discipline. In this symposium, 4 teams of investigators from 6 countries will examine the validity of these "Western" findings in the context of specific non-Western cultural traditions. **Methods:** In 3 studies from Africa (Côte d'Ivoire, Mali, South Africa) samples of preschool children and their mothers were observed and videotaped, some repeatedly, and interviewed using various standardized instruments. The aim was to obtain information on attachment and general psychosocial variables. In 2 data sets, a subgroup of the children was also malnourished. Corporal punishment data were based on a qualitative literature review and dealt primarily with practices in Latin and Pacific cultures as African data do not exist. **Results:** Most children were classified as securely attached in all 3 African studies, supporting key hypotheses of attachment theory. Children also showed more distress when mothers withdrew from reciprocal contact. Infant malnutrition was likewise associated with underinvolved and relatively unresponsive caretaking, However, there were also significant culture specific findings. In contrast to Western data, children showed no insecure-avoidant but disorganized or disorientated behaviors. Specific maternal behaviors associated with insecure attachment in western countries (e.g. child does not put arm around mother when picked up) were not found in Africa. Mothers of secure children also did not reflect on their children's qualities. The association in western cultures between spanking and later aggression or depression was not demonstrated in Latino or Afro-American children. **Conclusion:** Interactional behavior of children everywhere is guided by universally valid attachment patterns. Cultural traditions affect maternal verbal representations more than behavioral interactions The effect of corporal punishment is culture specific.

S-012-055   Topic: 45, 48
Infant-mother attachment among the Dogon of Mali: Findings on the universal and culturally specific dimensions of infant attachment and the relationship between infant undernutrition and maternal responsiveness

Mary True, Saint Mary's College, Psychology, Moraga, USA,
mtrue@stmarys-ca.edu
L. Pisani; F. Oumar; J. Padilla

Objective: A large majority of attachment research involves samples from Western or industrialized cultures. In this study we examined the central hypotheses of attachment theory among the Dogon of rural Mali. We also investigated the relationship between infant undernutrition and maternal responsiveness; approximately 20% of Dogon infants die before 1 year and 35% before the fifth year. **Methods:** We observed 49 Dogon mothers and infants. Half were from two small traditional, agrarian villages where there was little exposure to Western or global culture. The other half were from a semi-urban provincial capital, where there was some Western influence. The mothers and infants were observed five times across three contexts: during two well-infant exams, in the Strange Situation, and in the home. **Results:** Findings supporting the universality of attachment theory were: a) a significant correlation (p < 0.01) between infant exploration and maternal responsiveness, b) a majority of infants (68%) were classified as secure, and c)infant disorganization was related to maternal frightened and frightening behavior (p < 0.05). Findings supporting the role of culture in the development of infant attachment were: a) the lack of insecure-avoidant infants – the most common type of insecurity in Western samples; b) the average maternal latency to response to infant distress was 1/3 of that in Western samples, and c) a significant correlation (p = 0.02) between infant undernutrition and latency of maternal responsiveness. **Conclusion:** The findings of cultural differences are reflective of Dogon childrearing practices and the environment of risk.

S-012-056   Topic: 45, 48
Assessing child caring practices associated with inadequate nutrition in Côte d'Ivoire

Jean-François Bouville, Paris, France, jbouvil@yahoo.com

Objective: In environments with limited food and health resources, child growth and development may depend to a greater extent on the caring behaviors, defined as the caregivers provision of time, attention and support extended to meet the child's physical, psychological and social needs. Psychosocial aspects of "care for nutrition" include specific characteristics of the child-caregiver relationship, feeding styles and support system associated with the child's nutritional status. Although many studies suggest that malnutrition in young children occurs in conditions where overall psychosocial care is inadequate, no consensus has been reached to date on specific indicators or pathways linking nutritional status and traditionally used "care for nutrition" behaviours. In this presentation we provide data on a longitudinal study of the functional home environments (daily interactions, feeding patterns, and family context) of 32 children aged 6 months to 2 years in Abidjan, Côte d'Ivoire. **Methods:** Thirty-two children aged 6 to 24 months were observed for 10 hours on 2 consecutive days every 6 months, recording parent-child interactions, feeding patterns and aspects of family functioning. Twenty-five of these children developed moderate malnutrition during the course of the study and 7 required hospitalization because of severe malnutrition. **Results:** Four sets of attachment-based psychosocial care indicators associated with specific types of child nutritional development were observed. Children with moderate malnutrition had primarily unresponsive, underinvolved mothers while those with severe malnutrition showed little fear of strangers and did not behave as if they were ever hungry, hence lacking interest in food. **Conclusion:** Child malnutrition in developing countries may be specifically associated, in certain circumstances, with child caring practices. Intervention may benefit from an improved assessment of "care for nutrition" behaviours in high risk populations.

S-012-057 Topic: 45, 48

The cultural meaning of specific attachment behaviours of toddlers in a South African township

Klaus Minde, Montreal, QC, Canada,
klaus.minde@mcgill.ca
Wendy Vogel

Objective: The concordance between attachment categories (secure vs insecure) in mothers and their infants living in Western cultures is about 85%. This is remarkable since attachment classifications in young children are based on observed mother-child interactions while adults are evaluated by a semi-structured interview. Based on experience with recently immigrated families from developing countries, the present study examined the possible relevance non-Western cultural traditions have on these concordant attachment patterns. **Methods:** The sample consisted of 46 children, aged 18–40 months, and their Northern Sotho speaking mothers who lived in a township of Johannesburg. Families had 4 home-visits by local research assistants. Mothers were assessed using a 70 item semi-structured demographic interview and the SCL-90-R. Visit 3 consisted of a 2 hour observation of mother-child interaction, which was analyzed using the Attachment Q-Sort (AQS) criteria of Waters (1995). During visit 4 mothers were given the Working Model of the Child Interview (WMCI) (Zeahnah and Benoit, 1995) which assesses the attachment status of the mother. **Results:** Agreement between home observations and WMCI ratings was only 29% on secure and 65% on insecure attachment when the US developed scoring criteria of the WMCI were used. Agreement increased to 81% for secure and 79% for insecure attachment when the same WMCI protocols were re-scored, using a modified scoring system developed by local cultural experts. Analyses of home observations also showed some behaviors associated with secure attachment in the West (e.g. sharing things with mother) not to differentiate the Northern Sotho attachment groups. **Conclusion:** Results suggest that interview based representations of attachment patterns are more profoundly influenced by cultural traditions than are actual parent-child interactions.

S-012-058 Topic: 45

Cultural issues in the corporal punishment of children

Martin Maldonado-Duran, Family Service and Guidance,
Child Psychiatry, Topeka, USA, maldo2000mor@aol.com

Objective: Corporal punishment is a controversial form of disciplining children and there are differing views about its long-term consequences on children in different cultures. The present paper will examine: 1) the prevalence of corporal punishment, 2) the reasons why some children are punished, 3) underlying parental beliefs and social/cultural factors, 4) short and long term effects on child behaviour. **Methods:** The available scientific literature on physical punishment in different countries/cultures was reviewed. Studies included surveys of prevalence, parental beliefs, retrospective recall by children/adolescents, and the association between childhood discipline and emotional behavioral disturbances in children and adults. **Results:** Prevalence: reports of physical punishment vary from 30% to 80% of all children and cultures. In the US 90% of parents endorse physical discipline and even young children are spanked. Age: younger children are spanked/hit more often than adolescents, and boys more than girls. Difficult children are spanked/hit more. Mothers generally spank more often than fathers. Parental beliefs: In several Western countries parents believe children have to be spanked to curb their negative inclinations while Latino parents, and those in other traditional societies, spank their children for disobedience and to teach them to be less uncooperative, selfish or disrespectful vis-a-vis their families. Effects: In the US an association between spanking and aggressive behavior, depression and other emotional disturbances has been established although Afro-American children may perceive physical discipline as parental involvement or love. In many other cultures children are taught to believe spankings are good for them. **Conclusion:** Corporal punishment is widely practiced by parents everywhere, although its severity and underlying reasons relate to sociocultural factors outlined in this presentation. Its effects depend on its severity and social meaning. Parents often repeat their own experience from childhood.

S-013 Topic: 80

The role of basic personality traits in child psychiatric disorders

Chairperson: Klaus Schmeck, Universitätsklinik Ulm
Kinder- und Jugendpsychiatrie, Ulm, Germany,
klaus.schmeck@medizin.uni-ulm.de

The role of basic personality traits in child psychiatric disorders

Klaus Schmeck, Universitätsklinik Ulm, Kinder- und
Jugendpsychiatrie, Ulm, Germany,
klaus.schmeck@medizin.uni-ulm.de

Basic personality traits like temperament and character can play a crucial role in our understanding of the development of many psychiatric disorders. This is not only true for personality disorders but also for externalizing disorders like ADHD or conduct disorder, internalizing disorders like overanxious disorder or social phobia and different types of eating disorders. The most frequently used instrument to assess personality is the NEO-PI of Costa & McCrae. In psychiatric samples Cloninger's Temperament and Character Inventory TCI is also often used. In this symposium speakers will present empirical studies that used Junior TCI and NEO-PI-R to assess basic personality traits of adolescents with different psychiatric disorders. We will discuss the stability of personality in adolescence and the possible etiologic role of these personality traits in the development of psychopathology. A special focus will be on personality factors that are associated with different subtypes of eating disorders.

S-013-059 Topic: 80, 42

Stability of the relationship between adolescent personality and psychopathology

Kirstin Goth, Universität Frankfurt,
Kinder- und Jugendpsychiatrie, Frankfurt, Germany,
k.goth@em.uni-frankfurt.de
Fritz Poustka

Objective: Cloninger's biopsychological model of personality provides the possibility of valid diagnostic decisions. The stability of the specific covariations between Personality and Psychopathology and the possibility of prognostic decisions were checked in a longitudinal study. **Methods:** Subjects were 80 patients with mixed diagnoses of our

Child Psychiatric Department (Frankfurt, Germany), who completed the JTCI 12-18 and the YSR at their admission (t1) and the JTCI and SDQ after an average interval of 1.8 years (SD 0.7; t2). Stability of personality and psychopathology was evaluated by retest-correlations and contingency analysis, dependent stability by MANOVA with repeated measures. Diagnostic and prognostic validity was tested by stepwise discriminant analysis. **Results:** Personality showed a high stability over time (retest-correlations 0.64 –0.82), with exception of HA (0.55) and SD (0.30) 0.35 out of the 80 participants could be classified as recovered at t2. At both times pathology could be explained by the variation of personality dimensions. For t1 79.1% could be correctly classified through SD, HA and NS, for t2 73.8% through SD and HA, while distinct weights of personality occurred in subgroups by pathology-type (SD and HA for internalizing, NS and CO for externalizing disorders). The prediction of future psychopathology by personality at t1 was not possible. But systematic differences in changes of personality over the time in dependence of future psychopathology (decrease in HA and increase in SD in the recovered subgroup) and additionally in interaction with pathology-type at t1 (internalizing: increase in SD and NS, externalizing: increase in CO, mixed: increase in HA in the recovered subgroups) were obtained. **Conclusion:** The stable diagnostic potential of Cloninger's model of personality could be demonstrated. The specific changes in the character and temperament dimensions over time may indicate an indirect relationship between personality and development of psychopathology, but concerning the direction and additional influences further investigation is needed.

S-013-060   Topic: 78, 10

Personality, coping and parental bonding in anorexic adolescents: A family study

Diane Purper-Ouakil, Paris, France
Véronique Dessons; Catherine Doyen; Fernando Perez-Diaz; Marie-Christine Mouren-Simeoni

Objective: Several personality traits have consistently been related to anorexia nervosa. These patients generally show high levels of harm avoidance, persistence and perfectionism and low scores of novelty seeking. Their particular personality style may be related to the selection of poor coping strategies and the high stress reactivity reported in this population. Modalities of attachment and bonding might also be related to stress vulnerability in young anorexics. Main objectives of our study were: 1) to examine personality, coping strategies and parental bonding in anorexic adolescents and controls, 2) to compare personality traits and coping style between parents of anorexics and parents of controls. **Methods:** Sample: twenty anorexic girls (mean age 14.6), their parents and twenty control adolescents matched for age and socio-economic status and their parents. Assessments were carried out with the NEO-Personality Inventory revised, the Coping Inventory for Stressful Situations and the Parental Bonding Inventory. **Results:** Our study revealed lower neuroticism (especially for the sub-scale impulsivity), lower extraversion, higher agreeability and conscientiousness in anorexics compared to controls. Anorexics also obtained higher task oriented coping and reported lower maternal and paternal overprotection. Mothers of anorexic adolescents were higher in agreeability and lower in impulsivity than mothers of controls, whereas patient's fathers showed more conscientious-

ness and higher task oriented coping. **Conclusion:** Anorexics share with their mothers a tendency towards strong emotional control and with their fathers a propensity for empathy and active coping.

S-013-061   Topic: 78

J-TCI in patients with eating disorders

Andreas Karwautz, Universitätsklinikum Wien,
Abt. Neuropsychiatrie, Wien, Austria,
andreas.karwautz@univie.ac.at
Gudrun Wagner; Klaus Schwienbacher; Maria Haidvogl; Gerald Nobis; Janet Linda Treasure; David Andrew Collier

Objective: The aim of this study was to retrospectively identify pre-morbid personality characteristics of patients with later eating disorders. Whereas personality is well described in persons during or after the period of illness, none of these studies has addressed the period before eating disorder onset. **Methods:** Temperament and character of 91 sister-pairs discordant for an eating disorder history were judged by their parents using the Junior Temperament and Character Inventory (J-TCI) regarding the time before eating disorder onset. 40 patients of those fulfilled the strict criteria for lifetime anorexia nervosa restricting type (without binging or purging behaviour for at least 3 years), 51 patients fulfilled the criteria for binge-purging anorexia nervosa or bulimia nervosa. Eating disorder patients were compared with their healthy sisters. The 4 main scales of temperament are novelty seeking, harm avoidance, reward dependence, and persistence; the 3 character scales are self-directedness, cooperativeness, and self-transcendence. **Results:** The personality profile of patients with anorexia nervosa restricting type were characterised by lower novelty seeking, lower reward dependence, and higher persistence. Patients with binge/purging behaviour were characterized by higher harm avoidance, lower reward dependence, lower self-directedness, and lower cooperativeness compared with their healthy sisters. Regression analyses showed that high persistence in childhood and adolescence is the predominant factor in patients developing anorexia nervosa restricting type (as retrospectively rated by the parents), whereas for the development of binge/purging behaviour all 4 temperament scales and 2 of the 3 character scales are relevant. **Conclusion:** The results on these pre-morbid personality characteristics are compared with prevailing findings regarding personality during the eating disorders. The relevance of pre-morbid personality profiles for prevention and therapy for restricting anorexia, binge/purging anorexia, and bulimia nervosa are discussed.

S-013-062   Topic: 78, 23

Temperament and character profile of female adolescent patients with eating disorders: A pretreatment evaluation with the Junior Temperament and Character Inventory

Romuald Brunner, Universität Heidelberg,
Kinder- und Jugendpsychiatrie, Heidelberg, Germany,
romuald.brunner@med.uni-heidelberg.de
A. Hueg; Johann Haffner; Peter Parzer; Franz Resch

Objective: The current study aimed to examine differences in personality-related factors between restricting anorexia nervosa (RAN), binging/purging anorexia nervosa (BPAN), and bulimia nervosa (BN) patients. **Methods:** Subjects were

73 consecutively admitted female eating disordered patients, 12 to 18 years old. The German version of the Junior Temperament and Character Inventory was administered to 29 RAN (mean age: 14.7), 16 BPAN (mean age: 15.8), and 28 BN (mean age: 15.8) patients. The Junior Temperament and Character Inventory (JTCI) consists of the following main constructs: Novelty Seeking, Harm Avoidance, Reward Dependence, Persistence, Self-Directedness, Cooperativeness, and Self-Transcendence. **Results:** Differences in temperamental factors were most pronounced between RAN and BN patients, whereas BPAN patients exhibited a personality profile between RAN and BN. BN patients scored higher on Novelty Seeking and lower on Persistence compared to RAN patients. In contrast to RAN patients lower scores on Self-Directedness could be found in BN as well as BPAN patients. **Conclusion:** The current results of differential temperamental dimensions in adolescent eating disordered patients are similar to those findings of patients in adulthood, which strengthens the assumption of distinct personality factors underlying the different subtypes of eating disorders.

S-013-063   Topic: 24
Temperament and character traits of children and adolescents in a German residential care population

Marc Schmid, Universitätsklinikum Ulm,
Kinder- und Jugendpsychiatrie, Ulm, Germany
Lutz Goldbeck; Jakob Nützel; Klaus Schmeck; Jörg M. Fegert

Objective: Multiple risk factors for the development of mental disorders (e.g. abuse, neglect, genetic predisposition) are common in children and adolescents in residential care. Beside other important factors "difficult" temperamental traits increase children's risk of being brought up in an institution. The aim of this study is to assess the relationship between temperament and character traits and mental disorders of children and adolescents in residential care. **Methods:** In this epidemiologic study we assessed 691 children and adolescents (age 4–18 years, mean age 13.8, SD = 3.29) who live in 20 residential care institutions of various sizes. In a first step the children and adolescents and their residential caregivers answered a standard symptom checklist (CBCL/YSR, Achenbach) and a personality questionnaire (Junior Temperament and Character Inventory JTCI) (adolescents only). In the second step those participants scoring more than one standard deviation above the mean of the German norms were assessed with a standardized clinical examination to check for ICD-10 diagnoses using the DISYPS-KJ (Diagnostik System für Psychische Störungen im Kindes- und Jugendalter nach ICD-10 und DSM IV). **Results:** There are some characteristics in the JTCI-Profile of residential care children. This population achieve low scores in self directness (T-Score 42.7, SD 10.5). Correlations between CBCL-subscales and JTCI-subscales are in the medium to high range (r = 0.4–0.5). Furthermore there are interactions between JTCI Subscales and ICD-10 diagnoses some subscales defer well between children with and without diagnosis (low Self Directness/high Novelty Seeking). Adolescents with ADHD and Conduct disorders achieve significant higher scores in the subscale Novelty Seeking and lower scores in the subscale Persistence. **Conclusion:** Children and adolescents in residential care have difficulties to establish a reliable and self-confident personality. This goes in line with a high amount of behavioral and emotional problems.

S-013-064   Topic: 80, 24
The influence of personality on internalizing and externalizing disorders

Volkmar Höfling, Universität Frankfurt, Frankfurt,
Germany, vhoef@gmx.de
Karin Schermelleh-Engel; Helfried Moosbrugger;
Klaus Schmeck; Fritz Poustka

Objective: Cloninger's model of personality was developed to explain psychopathological syndromes. This study examined the influence of the temperament and the character on internalizing (withdrawn, somatic complaints and anxiety/depression) and externalizing (delinquent/aggressive behavior) disorders. It was assumed that Cloninger's temperament dimensions novelty seeking (NS), harm avoidance (HA) and persistence (P) and the character dimensions self directedness (SD) and cooperativeness (C) are significant determinants of these psychic disorders. Furthermore, SD and C were expected to moderate the effects of NS and HA on specific disorders (anxiety/depression, delinquent and aggressive behavior). **Methods:** 120 German adolescent in-patients filled in the German versions of the Junior Temperament and Character Inventory (JTCI 12–18) and the Youth Self Report (YSR/11–18). For the analysis of overall effects of the personality factors on psychopathology two linear structural equation models were performed using the LISREL program. The moderator effects of the character dimensions on the relation between temperament dimensions and psychopathology were analyzed by Quasi-ML. **Results:** Our results showed that the temperament dimensions NS and HA had positive effects on internalizing disorders, while NS had a positive and SD had a negative effect on externalizing disorders. Furthermore, the relationship between NS and delinquent and aggressive behavior depended on the levels of the character dimensions SD and C, while the relation between HA and anxiety/depression depended on the levels of SD. Figure 1 illustrates two of these moderator effects. **Conclusion:** As we expected, temperament and character dimensions influence psychopathology: High scores in NS and HA and low scores in SD increase the risk to suffer from internalizing and externalizing disorders. Adolescents with high scores in NS or HA compensate this risk with high scores in SD and C, while low scores in SD and C intensify this risk. Implications of these findings for further research and limitations of this study are discussed.

S-014   Topic: 52, 34
Aggressiveness and violence in children and adolescents

Chairperson: Josep Tomàs, Autonomous University of
Barcelona, Barcelona, Spain, cornella@comg.es

Aggressiveness and violence in children and adolescents

Josep Tomàs, Autonomous University of Barcelona,
Barcelona, Spain, cornella@comg.es

Aggressiveness and violence constitute a serious problem. Children and adolescents are not immune to that. We have the perception that we live in a society every time more violent, where the problems are solved through the conflict. From the Child and Adolescent Psychiatry we should undertake actions of prevention, precocious detection and appropriate treatment. In this symposium we outline the

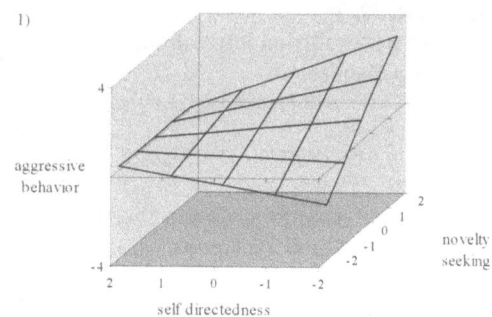

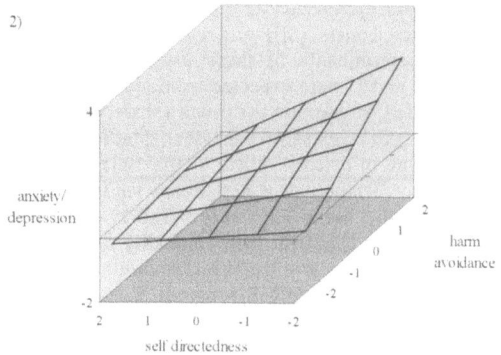

1) illustrates the moderator effect of self directedness on the relation between novelty seeking and aggressive behavior, 2) the moderator effect of self directedness on the relation between harm avoidance and anxiety/depression. All variables are standardized.

clinical outcomes of aggressive and violent behaviours and their evolution through the age. We also consider the differential diagnosis and the evident relationship between despair and aggressiveness, especially in adolescents. Finally we make a reflection on the therapeutic strategies, both pharmacological and psychological therapies.

S-014-065   Topic: 52, 34
Aggressiveness and violence in children and adolescents – clinical diagnosis
Josep Cornellà, Girona, Spain, cornella@comg.es
Alex Llusent

Objective: The aggressiveness and violence in adolescents and young people increase. During year 2002, in Spain, almost 7000 adolescents (10–16 years of age) were put under judicial trusteeship due to the commission of criminal acts. Objectives. The objective of this presentation is to analyse the factors Related to this increase of violence acts, with the purpose of being able to design preventive programs. **Methods:** Descriptive analysis. **Results:** The greater frequency corresponds to masculine sex (92%), in ages between 15 and 16 years (89%). The internal conditioners are analysed (distresses and other mental health disorders, fear to the passivity in the adolescent, internal tensions and verbal language deficits) as well as the external ones (precarious economic conditions, school failure, familiar deficits in the ethical and moral formation and conflicts). The impact of mass media and the videogames is also considered. Between the psychiatric disorders associated to

aggressiveness we consider the negativist defiant disorder, the dissocial disorder, and the intermittent explosive disorder. As prediction factors emphasize hyperactivity, low level of scholastic preparation, having delinquent friends, and drug availability. At age 14, these factors are centred in little familiar control, familiar conflicts, bad school adaptation and little aspirations in the life. The forms of expression of the aggressiveness and violence in the adolescents can be: crises of the adolescence, criminal behaviours and masked depressions. **Conclusion:** It is necessary a greater investigation around the phenomena of the aggressiveness and violence among adolescents and young people, in order to establish the suitable guidelines of prevention.

S-014-066   Topic: 52, 34
From despair to aggressiveness
Alex Llusent, Girona, Spain, alexllusent80@hotmail.com
Josep Cornellà

Objective: From the consultation with adolescents there is the perception of increasing levels of aggressiveness and despair that increase the suicide risk. The detection of these risk factors should help to design strategies of prevention. To evaluate the risk toward the aggressiveness and the levels of despair among students finishing the secondary school, in views to plan actions of prevention. **Methods:** The study includes the 188 students of fourth course of Secondary Education of the three 'State Secondary School' where we carry out preventive activities and health attention. The Student Questionnaire of the High Risk Action Council has been used (Sumter, SC, USA) to value the risk of aggressive behaviours, and the Scale of Despair of Beck to evaluate the negative expectations regarding the future and to its well-being. The punctuations of this scale are a watering predictor to the suicide. **Results:** The level of aggressiveness is high, with a punctuation of 13.21 (±5.011). The half punctuation of the Scale of Despair is located in 5.34 (±3.2). Suicidal risk is not present in 31.7%, is low in 55%, moderated in 11,67%, and is high in 1.67% of the interviewed students. The future appears uncertain for more than the third part of the adolescents of our study. Significant differences have not been observed according to the sex. **Conclusion:** The fourth course of Secondary Education represents, in many occasions, the last opportunity to make a preventiveactivity with the adolescents. The results of this survey force us tooutline strategies of prevention in mental health.

S-014-067   Topic: 52, 34
Conduct disorders: Treatment
Anna Bielsa, Janssen Cilag Lab, Psichiatry, Madrid, Spain, amex.c.viajes@aexp.com
Josep Tomàs

We analyse the different aspects of Conduct Disorders (CD) treatment, considering our experience with a group of adolescents with CD in special school due to their social problems. Few treatments with proven efficacy are available. Early intervention with young children is crucial. Treatment takes a variety of forms: a) Family interventions b) Social support c) Behaviour modification d) Psychopharmacology e) Legal sanctions Complex cases require multimodal treatment. Creating and reinforcing "limit setting" for the child require counselling of parents, treatment of parent's psychiatric problems, increased supervision at home, surveillance at school, or use of legal mechanisms Hospitalisation is only useful for containment and intensive evaluation, for medical trials or for the treatment of other psychiatric disorders. Psychotherapeutic Interventions: Several treatments on cognitive, behavioural, and family systems principles have shown efficacy. The Intensive cognitive problem-solving skills training is useful for generating the use of alternative solutions to manage interpersonal problems. Parental involvement is very important. The Pharmacotherapy can include any psychotropic drug depending on the individual patient's target symptoms. a) In patients with ADHD: stimulants, clonidine, alone or in combination: bupropion. b) If CD is secondary to a major depression: SSRIs. c) In severe impulsive aggression: Lithium. d) In bipolar disorder: Lithium. e) To reduce aggression we can use trazodone. f) Severe impulsive aggression, emotional liability and abnormal EEG with low or non-response to the Lithium: carbamazepine or valproate. g) In uncontrollable rage reactions and impulsive aggression with evidence of organicity: propanolol. h) In clinical psychosis: antipsychotic drugs. i) In severely aggressive children: atypical antipsychotic (risperidone). The interdisciplinary work on each adolescent is very important. In our group the treatment at the family by child psychiatrists in their home and psychologists with the educator in their school has been very useful.

S-015 Topic: 2
Systems of care in a world wide perspective
Track: Therapy and intervention

Chairperson: Myron Belfer, Harvard Medical School
Dep. of Social Medicine, Boston, MA, USA,
myron-belfer@hms.harvard.edu

S-015-068 Topic: 2, 45
Systems of care in Africa

Brian Robertson, University of Cape Town,
Psychiatry and Mental Health, Constantia, South Africa,
brian@curie.uct.ac.za
Custodia Mandlhate; Amira Seif El-Din; Birama Seck

Objective: To describe the context, characteristics and future direction of child and adolescent mental health care systems in Africa. **Methods:** Key informants representing major constituencies of child and adolescent mental health care in Africa were given a draft outline of the topic, and asked to contribute from their collective experience and research. A review of local and international literature was conducted. **Results:** Rapid change against a background of complex diversity is the most prominent feature of Africa today. Approximately 800 million people live in seven Arab North African countries, and 46 French (20), English (20), Portuguese (5) and Spanish-speaking (1) subSaharan countries. Although subSaharan Africa constitutes 11% of the world population, it accounts for only 1.3% of the income. Only 40% of countries have special programmes in mental health for children. Child and adolescent mental health in Africa is mediated by differing world-views, challenging social contexts, and significant social capital. A selection of epidemiological studies spanning the past three decades is referenced, and their limitations in measuring the burden of mental health problems discussed. Formal and informal systems of care in Africa are described. Informal systems include the family and community, indigenous healing systems, and nongovernmental organizations.

Existing formal systems of care are largely European in origin. In addition to primary, secondary and tertiary mental health services provided by the health sector, the maternal and child health, education, and social welfare sectors make significant contributions to child mental health care in Africa. Existing training and research activities are described. Policy development and implementation is critical for sustaining mental health care systems in the future. Recommendations regarding additional initiatives are discussed. **Conclusion:** The future of child and adolescent mental health care systems in Africa will be greatly enhanced with increased support from the international community.

S-015-069 Topic: 2, 45
Undertreatment of behavioural problems in non-native children in the Netherlands

Barbara Zwirs, UMC Utrecht, Dept. of Child Psychiatry,
Utrecht, Netherlands, b.zwirs@wkz.azu.nl
Huib Burger; Tom Schulpen; Jan Buitelaar

Objective: Attention-deficit hyperactivity disorder (ADHD) is the most common psychiatric disorder in children (3-5%). In these children comorbid psychiatric disorders like oppositional defiant disorder (ODD) and conduct disorder (CD) are highly prevalent. At present, there is substantial evidence that accurate detection and treatment of ADHD is lacking. Overdiagnosis and overtreatment seem to occur mainly in western children and underdiagnosis and undertreatment in non-western children. The aim is to investigate the relationship between ethnicity, behavioural problems and treatment in children of different ethnic origins in the Netherlands. **Methods:** The study population included Dutch, Moroccan, Turkish and Surinamese children aged 6 to 8 years attending mainstream schools in 2 large cities in the Netherlands. Teachers completed a scale consisting of all 30 items of the teacher version of the Dutch Strengths and Difficulties Questionnaire, 5 DSM-IV items on ADHD, CD and ODD and 5 items regarding impairment and treatment of the child. **Results:** Teachers reported more problem behaviour among Moroccan children than among Dutch, Turkish and Surinamese children ($p < 0.01$). After adjusting for gender, age, problem scores and impairment level, Moroccan, Turkish and Surinamese children were approximately 70% less likely to be treated for their problem behaviour than Dutch children ($p < 0.01$). **Conclusion:** Non-native children in the Netherlands are less likely to be treated for behavioural problems than native children even when accounting for differences in problem behaviour and impairment level.

S-015-070 Topic: 2, 45
Child psychiatric services in Iraq

A. Karem Salman Al-Obedy, Central Child Hospital,
Psychiatric Clinic, Baghdad, Iraq, abd_karem60@yahoo.com

Objective: Mesopotamia (Iraq) is the land of antiquity and the cradle of civilization on the earth. The evolution of psychiatry and that of medicine as a whole in Mesopotamia was ascending and declining with the political situations, and during the last three decades, health services including psychiatric services in general affected by the bad policy of the previous reign. The aim of this study was to evaluate the facts regarding the child psychiatric services in this country. **Methods:** The present data collected by interviews with a number of practitioners were attached with child psychiatry, and through reference to hospital statistics and other relevant literatures, in addition to the authors clinical experience. **Results:** The results show, that there were limited number of general psychiatrists in Iraq (around 70, 0.2 per 100,000 population), with no qualified child psychiatrist, and there was no child psychiatric center at all, while the services were admitted in inappropriate ways, through a number of general psychiatric departments or hospitals and child institutes, while the size of the problem was significant, and training program in child psychiatry was inefficient. **Conclusion:** We conclude that child psychiatric services in Iraq still underdeveloped, and the recommendations were to initiate child psychiatric units in general hospital of pediatrics and child psychiatric center, communication with other similar centers in the world for training of professions in this field is of great importance.

S-015-071   Topic: 2, 45
Mental health problems in disabled children and their families: Developing preventive programs in East-European Countries

Oleh Romanchuk, Early Intervention, Lviv, Ukraine, olerom@ukr.net

Objective: The objective of the research was to study adjustment reactions of parents to the birth of a disabled child and their interaction with professionals and with the surrounding social system. The aim was to find the greatest challenges for families and most important prognostic factors that facilitate/impede the adjustment process. Knowing these factors is important for developing preventive programs that are integrated into the east-european cultural context and not just copied from Western models. **Methods:** 100 families with children with intellectual and physical disabilities from 3 to 10 years of age were studied using the method of semi structured interview. **Results:** High prevalence (68%) of persistent negative adjustment reactions was revealed. In 71% of the families absence of a trusting and a supporting partnership with professionals was discovered. 55% of the families reported that the experience of getting information about the child's disability from professionals was extremely traumatic for them. They quoted examples like advices to abandon their child and highly negative presentation of the child. Stigmatizing experience and absence of human, community-based programs were another major factors leading to social isolation of families. 63% of them reported loneliness and lack of social support. Other interesting findings concerned peculiarities of east-european cultural context: strict gender roles in families – making adjustment process especially difficult for fathers; "cult" of professionals – that prevents equal partnership; believes in "magical" cure by paramedical professionals and "healers" – that supports unrealistic hopes for cure. **Conclusion:** The research shows the importance of the development of educational programs for professionals, need for general society awareness-raising campaigns and demand of the development of new models for programs that are family-centered and community based. One of the most important programs is Early Intervention that should support the family adjustment process, promote positive parent-child relations, empower parents, educate them and provide opportunities for social support.

S-015-072   Topic: 1, 40
Mental health of children and adolescents in the period of transformations in Poland

Irena Namyslowska, Inst. of Psychiatry-Neurology, Dept. Adolescent & Psychiatry, Warsaw, Poland, namyslow@ipin.edu.pl

Objective: To examine and analyze the influence of the profound socio-economical and cultural changes in Poland during transformation period on families and subsequently on mental health of children and adolescents. **Methods:** Available data on mental health of children and adolescents such as admissions to mental hospitals and out-patient clinics, depression and suicide rates, criminal aggressive acts of minors, as well as alcohol and psychoactive substances consumption are presented and the changes in recent 10 years are analyze in the context of the burden put by the transformation on Polish families. **Results:** In the difficult period of transformation in every area of life in Poland one may observed several trends concerning mental health of children and adolescent such as growing number of depressed adolescents and its correlation with the lack of paternal authority, lowering age of initiation of alcohol consumption, increase in the use of psychoactive substances. At the same time the increased of sexual and physical abuse of children and adolescents in Polish families was observed. **Conclusion:** The transformation period in Poland in the recent years has brought profound stress in every area of life of Polish families. Special emphasis is put on the unstable value systems, which may have important implication for the mental health of children and adolescents.

S-015-073   Topic: 1, 41
Factors associated with local vs. specialty mental health service use among adolescents: What differs?

Björn S. Reigstad, Nordlandssykehuset, Child & Adolescent Psychiatry, Bodø, Norway, bre@nlsh.no
Kirsti Margrethe Jørgensen

Objective: To investigate whether adolescents referred to specialty mental health services from local professionals differ from adolescents who only have received help for psychiatric problems locally. **Methods:** Adolescents (n = 76) from an adolescent population sample (N = 2.538) who had received help during the last year for mental problems from local professionals were compared to a clinical sample of adolescents (N = 129) referred to specialty mental health services from such local professionals. Comparisons were made according to scores on the Youth Self-Report (YSR); depressive symptoms; family functioning; attachment to parents; self-concept; coping styles; response styles; dysfunctional attitudes; negative life events; daily hassles; sociodemographics. **Results:** As compared to adolescents receiving help locally, adolescents in specialty mental health care scored higher on YSR internalizing syndrome; YSR rule breaking; YSR thought problems; suicidality; knowing someone who had attempted suicide; parental divorce; substance use; recent moves; living in lodgings; lost a pal or boy/girlfriend; and lower on attachment to parents. Multivariate logistic regression analysis identified four factors predictive of receiving specialty mental health care: low family functioning; moved previous year; knowing someone who had attempted suicide; own suicidality. **Conclusion:** Family functioning as reported by the adolescents, and not mental health problems except for suicidality, was found to be the strongest predictor of referral to specialty mental health services. Contrary to findings from many other studies, referral was associated with internalizing problems, not externalizing ones.

S-016   Topic: 6, 85
Prevention and treatment of conduct disorders

Track: Therapy and intervention

Chairperson: Walter Matthys, University of Utrecht Child & Adolescent Psychiatry, Utrecht, Netherlands, w.matthys@psych.azu.nl

Prevention and treatment of oppositional defiant and conduct disorders

Walter Matthys, University of Utrecht, Child & Adolescent Psychiatry, Utrecht, Netherlands, w.matthys@psych.azu.nl

Walter Matthys (Utrecht) as chairman will first briefly introduce major issues in research on the effects of psychotherapy, i.a. effectiveness, cost-effectiveness, mediators, moderators and predictors of treatment outcome. Steve Scott (London) will present an indicated prevention study of conduct disorders and school failure in children aged 5 and 6 years. John Lochman (Alabama) will present recent studies on indicated prevention among children aged 8 to 12 years using the Coping Power Program. Marjo Zonnevylle-Bender (Utrecht) will present 4 year follow-up data with respect to substance use and antisocial behaviour from a study in which the Coping Power Program was adapted for use in the outpatient treatment of children aged 8 to 12 years with oppositional defiant and conduct disorders. Angela Wagner (Mannheim) then will present a study on the outcome and on the predictors of outpatient and inpatient treatment of children with conduct disorders. Finally, Irene van Bokhoven (Utrecht) will present a study on the predictive value of neurobiological child characteristics, psychological child characteristics and family characteristics on the outcome of in-patient and day-treatment with oppositional defiant and conduct disordered children.

S-016-074   Topic: 85, 10
Prevention of antisocial behaviour and academic failure through a parenting programme delivered in primary schools

Stephen Scott, King's College of London, Maudsley Hospital, London, United Kingdom, s.scott@iop.kcl.ac.uk

Objective: To see whether a parenting programme delivered in schools to a high risk population would get a reasonable level of take up, and improve reading and antisocial behaviour. **Methods:** *Design* Randomised controlled trial with 110 5 and 6 year old children 1sd or more above the mean on combined teacher and parent SDQ, about the worst 15% of the population. *Setting and Intervention* The intervention package was delivered in 8 primary schools over three school terms. In term 1 there was a basic 12 week parenting course (Incredible Years) addressing the parent-child relationship and how to handle difficult child behaviour, in term 2 there was a 10 week reading programme (new, In house), and in term 3 a 6 week combined course. Controls received a telephone helpline for accessing regular services. **Results:** *Attendance* 53% of eligible parents enrolled, going to a mean of 16 out of 26 avail-

able sessions. *Antisocial behaviour* On the PACS interview the effect size was 0.51 standard deviations, substantial for a prevention trial. The reduction in antisocial behaviour corresponds to an improvement for the participants from being within the worst 15% of antisocial children to being outside the most antisocial 35%. The effect size for hyperactivity was also significant, 0.43. Hyperactivity is an important independent risk factor for social exclusion. *Parent Satisfaction* 93% of parents said they were well or extremely satisfied with the programme. *Child Literacy* The intervention group gained seven months in reading skills, an effect size of 0.43. This result held up unchanged after multiple regression correction for age and gender. Race, parent education, parent income, and child age and gender did not affect degree of change, suggesting that the programme is robust and suited to disadvantaged populations. **Conclusion:** This study showed that a programme to support parents was improved substantially two crucial aspects of child development, social behaviour and reading. Parent satisfaction was very high. The programme was successfully delivered in an everyday community setting, the local primary school, which contributed to its being seen as non-stigmatising.

S-016-075   Topic: 6, 85
Prevention and treatment of oppositional defiant and conduct disorders

John Lochman, University of Alabama, Psychology, Tuscaloosa, AL, USA, jlochman@gp.as.ua.edu

Objective: This study uniquely examines the effects of indicated and universal preventive school-based interventions at the middle school transition with aggressive children who are at risk for later delinquency and substance use, using two samples. Moderate to high risk children were identified by fourth grade teachers' ratings of students' aggressiveness. The Coping Power program is based on a contextual social-cognitive model. **Methods:** Sample 1 consists of 183 aggressive 4th–5th grade boys in 11 elementary schools, and sample 2 consists of 245 aggressive 5th grade boys and girls in 17 elementary schools. Children in both samples were randomly assigned to a Coping Power intervention or to a control condition. In the second sample, some classrooms were also randomly assigned to a universal teacher-training intervention. Self reports of children's delinquency and substance use are obtained at a one-year follow-up, along with measures of parenting practices and children's social cognition. **Results:** Significant Coping Power intervention effects are found on self-reported delinquency (both samples), parent-rated substance use (sample 1), and self-reported substance use (sample 2 only). Results also indicate that the greatest effects are apparent on the combined parent-and-child intervention, and that the universal intervention has direct effects on child substance use and enhances the Coping Power effects on delinquency. **Conclusion:** Both indicated and universal preventive interventions can affect children's antisocial behavior at the time of transition to middle school. The study has implications for screening of at-risk children, and for inclusion of teacher training as an universal preventive intervention.

S-016-076 Topic: 68, 85

Substance abuse and antisocial behavior in disruptive behavior disorder (DBD) children –

A 4-year follow-up study of outpatient treatment

Marjo Zonnevylle-Bender, University Medical Center, Child & Adolescent Psychiatry, Utrecht, Netherlands, m.zonnevylle-bender@psych.azu.nl
Nicolle van de Wiel; Walter Matthys

Objective: Since research indicated that anti-social behavior in children served as a risk predictor for substance abuse in adolescence (e.g. Lochman & Wayland, 1994), the long term effects of treatment on substance abuse and antisocial behavior in DBD children were determined in this 4-year follow-up study. **Methods:** DBD children (58) received either manualized behavior therapy (Utrecht Coping Power Program; UCPP) or "Care as Usual" (CU). Prior to treatment and in a follow-up period of 4 years a total of 5 measurements were performed measuring reduction in adolescent externalizing behavior (aggression and delinquency). During the last measurement substance abuse was also determined. The Child Behavior Checklist (CBCL; Achenbach, 1991) and the National Youth Survey Questionnaire (NYS; Elliott et al., 1985) were used to measure respectively aggressive behavior, delinquent behavior and substance abuse. Statistical analyses: Repeated measurement analysis of variance (ANOVA) with treatment as between subjects factor (UCPP versus CU) and time as within subjects factor was used to assess changes in CBCL externalizing behavior. One-factor analyses of variance (ANOVA's) were performed to assess the effect of treatment (UCPP versus CU) on the NYS. **Results:** CBCL externalizing scores revealed a main effect of time, no main effect of treatment and no time by treatment interaction, with both groups having significantly higher CBCL externalizing scores prior to treatment. Between the two treatment groups no differences were seen, neither in substance abuse nor in delinquency, with both groups being comparable to normative data. **Conclusion:** In this 4-year follow-up study the beneficial long-term effects of treatment in DBD children persisted; both groups showed substantially lower externalizing behavior compared to prior to treatment. Moreover, for both groups substance abuse and delinquency was within normative levels.

S-016-077 Topic: 6, 85

How effective is the treatment of children and adolescents with conduct disorder in a clinical setting?

Angela Wagner, Uni. Pittsburgh Medical Center, Dept. of Psychiatry, Pittsburgh, USA, wagnera@upmc.edu
Christine Jennen-Steinmetz; Christopher Goepel; Martin H. Schmidt

Objective: Conduct Disorder is one of the most frequently diagnosed conditions in outpatient and inpatient mental health facilities for children. The course of Conduct Disorder is variable, but in a majority of individuals the disorder remits by adulthood. The purpose of this study was to analyze the effectiveness of interventions in a clinical setting and to find possible predictors. **Methods:** We assessed 821 outpatients and 744 inpatients with Conduct Disorder. The sample was divided into three groups according to the ICD 10 subtypes ('Impulsive': F90.1; 'Emotional': F91.2, F92; 'Antisocial': F91.1, F91.3). All subjects received a parental training in addition to a behavioral psychotherapy on an individual basis. The outcome was defined as an improvement in psychosocial functioning (SGKJ) at the end of the treatment. **Results:** In terms of outcome, the 'Impulsive' subgroup (87.3%) responded significantly better to treatment in an inpatient setting than the 'Emotional' subgroup (76.0%) and the 'Antisocial' subgroup (64.4%). In comparison, for outpatient treatment, 43.2% of the 'Impulsive' subgroup, 32.0% of the 'Emotional' subgroup, and 29.4% of the 'Antisocial' subgroup had a good response to treatment. Cooperation of parents and children during the treatment, low severity of disease at the beginning, a small amount of psychosocial risk factors and additional pharmacotherapy were found to be the most important predictors for a good response. **Conclusion:** Patients who met criteria for the 'Impulsive' subtype could be treated most successfully in both inpatient and outpatient therapy. Behavioral therapy on an individual basis seems to be insufficient. Effectiveness of the treatment of children and adolescents with Conduct Disorders can be increased by training of parents, home treatment or pharmacotherapy.

S-016-078 Topic: 23, 85

Prediction of treatment outcome in children with disruptive behaviour disorders:

A study of neurobiological, neuropsychological and psychosocial factors

Irene van Bokhoven, UMCU Utrecht, Child & Adolescent Psychiatry, Utrecht, Netherlands, I.vanBokhoven@azu.nl
Walter Matthys; Stephanie van Goozen; Herman van Engeland

Objective: Although the short-term effectiveness of various behavioural intervention strategies in children with disruptive behaviour disorder (DBD) children has been demonstrated, it is clear that some children benefit more than others. In this study we explored the predictive value of family characteristics, psychological and demographic child characteristics, and neurobiological child characteristics, on treatment outcome. **Methods:** Existing data on child characteristics were combined with case-records concerning family characteristics in a sample of 52 DBD children who were treated in in-patient and day-treatment units. Treatment consisted of a comprehensive and integrated programme based on cognitive behavioural and operant procedures, including pharmacotherapy. Externalizing problem scores, using the parent-rated Child Behavior Checklist, served as outcome measure. We used linear regression analyses to examine the predictors of post-treatment externalizing problems, adjusted for pre-treatment problems. **Results:** A larger discrepancy between verbal IQ (VIQ) and performance IQ (PIQ), with VIQ being lower than PIQ, and a lower skin conductance level (SCL) were found to predict a less favourable treatment outcome. **Conclusion:** Only two factors (SCL and VIQ-PIQ) were found to have a predictive influence on the effect of treatment. These results support the fearlessness theory according to which low activity of the autonomous nervous system, as manifested in low skin conductance, is related to the effectiveness of conditioning and accordingly to poor treatment outcome.

S-017   Topic: 61, 66
Breaking down the barriers to effective care and treatment for children with emotional and behavioral disorders: A citizen advocacy perspective
Chairperson: L. Patt Franciosi, World Federation for Mental Health, Meguon, WI, USA, pgarrison@wfmh.com

Breaking down the barriers to effective care and treatment for children with emotional and behavioral disorders: A citizen advocacy perspective
L. Patt Franciosi, World Federation for Mental Health, Meguon, WI, USA, pgarrison@wfmh.com

This symposium will focus attention on the need for increased public awareness and understanding of child and adolescent behavioral disorders, and on the importance of promoting accurate portrayals of these disorders, the children who experience them, and their families. The information will be presented from the perspective of citizen mental health advocates, family members, and leaders of national and international mental health education and advocacy organizations. The symposium will call attention to the need for mental health professionals working in the field of child and adolescent mental health to understand and support the involvement of citizen advocates and families in reducing stigma and discrimination about emotional and behavioral disorders that impact young people. In this symposium, Dr. Franciosi will discuss how lack of accurate knowledge about child and adolescent emotional disorders, public misperception, and stigma can be overcome through enhanced public education and awareness, and by greater sensitivity by mental health professionals and the media. She will describe the development and dissemination of a set of guidelines encouraging accurate reporting on ADHD, "ADHD: The Hope Behind the Hype," which were developed by WFMH for presentation at the European Society for Child and Adolescent Psychiatry Conference in September 2003. She and other members of the panel will discuss how these guidelines and other public education tools such as the World Mental Health Day 2003 campaign materials that focused on emotional and behavioral disorders of children and adolescents can be used by both professional and citizen advocacy organizations to inform and enlist the support of writers and journalists to promote accurate and supportive coverage of child and adolescent emotional health disorders and issues.

S-017-079   Topic: 66
Why citizen advocacy makes a difference in the lives of children and adolescents with emotional and behavioral disorders
L. Patt Franciosi, World Federation for Mental Health, Meguon, WI, USA, pgarrison@wfmh.com

S-017-080   Topic: 47
The climate for effective family and citizen mental heath advocacy for child and adolescent mental health in Europe
Leo de Graaf, Acquoy, Netherlands, leodegraaf@wanadoo.nl

Objective: To offer a conceptual framework for parents who feel blamed for the behavioural and emotional problems of their children. **Methods:** Reflections on the impact of some crucial factors that influence the start and subsequent course of child & adolescent behavioural and emotional disorders, from which the role of parents on the course of these disorders can be deducted. **Results:** First some considerations are given to the nature/nurture dichotomy. On the Nature side the role of heritability for some personality traits and common disorders is clarified. On the Nurture side the importance of a safe attachment and "good-enough" care is discussed, but also the importance of other influences in the upbringing of children, like siblings, peers and schools are stressed, which dilute the role of parents. Next some old and new myths are discussed: the schizophrenogenic mother, the cold, aloof mother of the autistic child and the idea of the irreparable early damage of children. Finally some reflections are given about the mad/bad dichotomy: the historical and geographical vicissitudes in the interpretation of the same problematic behaviour of children and adolescents: sometimes as bad, sometimes as mad, i.e. as a mental health problem. **Conclusion:** 1. Parents are only to a very limited extent responsible for the mental health problems of their children; 2. It still remains a matter of debate if certain behaviour is seen as a symptom of madness or a sign of badness; 3. These findings should be brought to the attention of the parents, professionals, the media and the public at large in order to remove the blame from the parents, under which blame still many parents are suffering.

S-017-081   Topic: 66, 84
Advocacy begins at home: Establishing a support and advocacy Group for parents of children with ADHD
Anne Tischlinger, World Federation for Mental Health, Wien, Austria, anne.tischlinger@utanet.at
B. Pharm

Objective: To establish an effective support and advocacy group for parents of children with ADHD in Austria. **Methods:** A support and advocacy association for ADHD known as VEREIN ADAPT was founded by a group of parents of children with the disorder in Vienna, Austria in 1999. Activities to date have included lectures, members' meetings, parent-educator and adult groups, further education for parents and professionals, publication of a newsletter, attendance at national and international congresses, and cooperation with similar organizations abroad. **Results:** A small team of dedicated volunteer parents has succeeded in obtaining approximately 300 members all over Austria, the association's newsletter is sent to 1300 parents, educators and professionals, the ADHD further education program has benefited various types of professionals as well as parents and stimulated many other institutions and groups to follow suit, and successful cooperation takes place with other parent support groups within Austria, with professionals from all over the country, and with sister associations abroad. **Conclusion:** VEREIN ADAPT has succeeded in providing effective support and advocacy for families of children with ADHD in Austria by bringing relevant, state-of-the-art information to a variety of people, who are involved in the diagnosis, therapy and daily lives of children with this disorder.

S-017-082   Topic: 84
Strength in numbers: Building a global network to support families of children with ADHD
Knut Halvard Bronder, Norwegian ADHD Association, Lysaker, Norway

Objective: To increase the knowledge and acceptance of ADHD in all countries around the world by forming an international advocacy support group. **Methods:** Providing correct information to the national advocacy groups will ease their work. A World advocacy group will connect national advocacy group so they can interact and share correct, scientific information. The National advocacy groups can provide correct information and support to its members. **Results:** In many societies will a psychiatric disorder lead to social exclusion. To obtain support from others who have managed to break down these barriers will make it easier to accept the diagnose, and obtaining correct informational material from the ADHD World Group will ease their work burden and economy in the early phases of forming an advocacy group. **Conclusion:** The Executive Committee are in process preparing an international advocacy group for ADHD. Thoughts and situation report will be given.

S-017-083   Topic: 61, 59
The roles of mental health professionals, citizen advocates and the media in reducing public misperception and stigma about child and adolescent emotional and behavioral disorders
L. Patt Franciosi, World Federation for Mental Health, Meguon, WI, USA, pgarrison@wfmh.com

Objective: To focus attention on the need for increased public awareness and understanding of child and adolescent behavioral disorders, and on the importance of promoting accurate portrayals of these disorders, the children who experience them, and their families. **Methods:** The symposium will be presented as a panel discussion to present the perspective of internationally recognized mental health advocates, professionals, and family members of children with emotional and behavioral disorders to address issues relating to public misperception, stigma and in sensitivity about child and adolescent behavioral disorders in the media and general public. **Results:** The workshop will provide guidance and strategies to the participants for undertaking public awareness activities to overcome the effects of stigma, discrimination and public misperception of child and adolescent behavioral disorders, and will present a set of guidelines developed by the World Federation for Mental Health to encourage accurate reporting by the media on ADHD – ADHD: The Hope Behind the Hype," and will summarize the impact of the WFMH 2003 World Mental Health Day global mental health education campaign. **Conclusion:** Well-planned and implemented public awareness campaigns can help to reduce barriers to effective care and treatment for children with emotional and behavioral disorders by promoting collaboration among advocates, parents, and mental health professionals.

S-018   Topic: 73, 93
Children in needs: Post-traumatic Stress Disorder (PTSD) and prevention of suicide in children and adolescents
Chairperson: Kari Schleimer, University of Lund Child & Adolescent Psychiatry, Akarp, Sweden, kari.schleimer@telia.com

Children in needs: Post-traumatic Stress Disorder (PTSD) and prevention of suicide in children and adolescents
Kari Schleimer, University of Lund, Child & Adolescent Psychiatry, Akarp, Sweden, kari.schleimer@telia.com

With regard to the effects of the Civil War, Aids, and social trasition on Children in Mosambique offered psychotherapeutic help. The evolving infrastuctural need healing systems will be described and discussed versus a system relying on mainly traditional healing systems. Prevention of suicide in children and adolescents working with guiding principles for the prevention of suicidal tendencies in Sweden is presented. The principles will be compiled and recognized on a national basis and will comprise all staff members working within child and adolescent psychiatry. The consequences for children concerning prevention and psychiatric treatment are discussed. A general way of preventing violence, suicide is to improve the quality of life in children/adolescents in the most important aspects. The collegues from Nishnij Novograd, Russia, are convinced, that with the aim of treatment of affective disorders and suicide prevention for children and adolescents it is important to help such children and these families in a multidisciplinary way. Early recognition of developmental problems and disorders is necessary before any behavioural programm or therapy and prevention takes place. Under the topic "working with street children" the authors from Lübeck, Germany, tried to know, in a deeper way, the mental universe of the "street children", employing a phenomenological approach. 100 children were interviewed, in groups of five, during one year.

S-018-084   Topic: 54, 53
Childhood in Mosambique: Effects of the Civil War, Aids, and social transition on children offered psychotherapeutic help
Joachim Walter, Luisenklinik, Bad Dürrheim, Germany, drjoachimwalter@web.de
Boia Ephraime

Objective: As in many countries of Africa inspite of high prevalence of experiences of violence, AIDS radically changing social circumstances contributing to social disorganisation, abuse and neglect, Mozambique can only offer very limited child and adolescent psychotherapeutic and psychiatric help. However, many different NGO's have been trying to establish systems of psychosocial and psychotherapeutical support systems. **Methods:** Comprehensive research has not been conducted to a slowly developing research infrastructure. The authors present case vignettes of patients treated within a psychotherapeutical curricular project. **Results:** The evolving infrastuctural need will be described and discussed versus a system relying on mainly traditional healing systems.

S-018-085   Topic: 93
Prevention of suicide in children and adolescents in Sweden
Kari Schleimer, University of Lund, Child & Adolescent Psychiatry, Akarp, Sweden, kari.schleimer@telia.com

Objective: The incidence of suicides in Sweden has decreased constantly over a period of the last two decades except for the group of individuals up to the age of 18 years. Annually about 30–40 young people aged 15–19 years take their lives. In a population of schoolchildren (up to 9th grade) 5–6% confirmed having tried to take their life at least once. Even if every suicidal attempt seems to be all of a sudden and surprising to those close to the child or adolescent, quite a few earlier signs usually can be recognized in retrospective. These signs should lead to preventive measures. In 1997 Sweden got a national center for research in suicidology and prevention of bad-health. **Methods:** A report about the center's work is given with its research and development, analysis and follow-up of epidemiological data, information, teaching and education. An overview of measures is also presented. **Results:** The national center has become a WHO collaborating center with overall objectives: – to reduce the number of suicides and suicidal attempts in the country – to reduce circumstances that may lead to young people taking their life – to detect at an early stage and to try to break off raising trends of suicide and suicidal attempts in vulnerable groups – to increase general knowledge about suicide in order to create supportive methods in society for those contemplating suicide. Locally every department and clinic is working with guiding principles for the prevention of suicidal tendencies in children and adolescents. These principles will be compiled and recognized on a national basis and will comprise all staff members working within child and adolescent psychiatry.

S-018-086   Topic: 93, 70
Affective disorders and suicide prevention in treatment of children and adolescents in Russia

Tatjana Dmitrieva, Center for Mental Health, of Children and Adolescents, Nizhny Novgorod, Russia, tndmitr@sandy.ru

Objective: During the last ten years in Russia some of negative consequences of perestroika such as sharp socio-economic changes and the ideological vacuum have been apparent. The difficult situation for children can be shown by the increased number of suicides, which rose about twice during the last ten years. There are narrow relations between aggressive and affective disorder. About 25% depressive children also show conduct disorder. The number of conduct disorder also increased markedly over the last ten years. **Methods:** The consequences for children concerning prevention and psychiatric treatment are discussed. **Results:** A general way of preventing violence, suicide is to improve the quality of life in children/adolescents in the most important aspects. Early recognition of developmental problem and disorder is necessary before any behavioural and suicidal act takes place. That is important to help such children and these families in the multidisciplinary way. School is a very significant area for depression/suicide prevention and mental health promotion. School specialists should cooperate with parents in preventing violence and suicidal behavior in school children and adolescents. Training in identifying distress, possible violence, affective disorders is important way to prevent suicidality. **Conclusion:** Psychiatric health services should be used as approachable, attractive and non-stigmatizing for children.

S-018-087   Topic: 49, 3
Working with street children

Alvaro Seligman Silva, Vorwerker Fachklinik, Kinder- und Jugendpsychiatrie, Lübeck, Germany, seligmann-silva@vorwerker-diakonie.de

Objective: The theme street children has been greatly discussed. However, these discussions have always deported from ideas based on external references to the life conditions of the children themselves. In this paper, the authors tried to know, in a deeper way, the mental universe of the street children, employing a phenomenological approach. Therefore, it aims to know how these children think, feel and express their own life experiences. **Methods:** 100 children were interviewed, in groups of five, during one year. **Results:** The children's reports are discussed here, as well as some reflexions of the authors, which bring some light on practical aspects on dealing with this group by different professionals.

S-019   Topic: 68
Alcohol and cannabis consumption:
Policy and consequences

Chairperson: Katja Becker, Zentralinstitut für Seelische Gesundheit, Mannheim, Germany, kbecker@zi-mannheim.de

Alcohol and cannabis consumption:
Policy and consequences

Katja Becker, Zentralinstitut für Seelische Gesundheit, Mannheim, Germany, kbecker@zi-mannheim.de

Alcohol and cigarettes are the most widely used and abused substances, followed by cannabis. Their use often starts in adolescence and substance use disorders may be linked to immediate factors such as accidents, violence and school dropout. Only a subset of adolescent drug users meets the criteria for abuse or dependence. Multiple factors play a role in the etiology, e.g. different individual risk and protective factors, genetic and other biological factors, individual characteristics, family factors, peer influences, resilience, and psychiatric comorbidity. The aim of the symposia is to provide an overview of international studies on alcohol use and cannabis consumption in adolescence from various perspectives: Hans-Christoph Steinhausen and C. Winkler Metzke (Switzerland) will talk about developmental psychopathology of alcohol use in adolescents, presenting findings from a Swiss epidemiological study. They studied 624 high-risk subjects with alcohol use and matched controls at mean ages of 13, 16 and 20 years. Stability and outcome of alcohol use were examined as well as the influence of a large series of psychosocial variables. Transversal studies have indicated a higher rate of psychiatric problems among children of alcoholics. Erikson F. Furtado (Brazil) will therefore report on behavioral problems in children of alcoholic fathers, presenting two-generation data from a longitudinal study from birth to puberty. The results indicate a higher vulnerability for psychopathological manifestation in the offspring of alcoholic fathers, mainly for expansive symptoms. Availability of legal and illegal drugs, national laws and national drug politics are important factors in substance use. Oliver Bilke (Germany) will talk about the influence of European cannabis politics on mental health care and show us a binational clinical perspective. Petra Zimmermann et al. (Germany) investigated the impact of cannabis use on the availability of ecstasy and on the subsequent first onset of ecstasy use in a large representative German community sample (n = 3021) of adolescents and young adults aged 14 to 24 years. Finally, Helga Hannesdottir and T. Thyrfingsson (Iceland) will present data on psychosocial factors among substance-abusing Icelandic adolescents.

S-019-088   Topic: 68, 24
Developmental psychopathology of alcohol use in adolescents.
Findings from a Swiss epidemiological study

Hans-Christoph Steinhausen, ZKJP Universität Zürich, Kinder- und Jugendpsychiatrie, Zürich, Switzerland, steinh@kjpd.unizh.ch
C. Winkler Metzke

Objective: To examine the stability and outcome of alcohol use in a large community study of adolescents. **Methods:** In a prospective longitudinal study (N = 624) high-risk subjects with alcohol use and matched controls were studied at mean ages of 13, 16 and 20 years. Stability of alcohol use in adolescence, prediction of alcohol use by a large series of psychosocial variables, and course of various types of alcohol use were studied. **Results:** Stability of alcohol use varied according to a recently etablished typology of the authors that consider abstainers, social drinkers, heavy drinkers, and problem drinkers. There are clear associations with mental disorders and psychosocial functioning in young adulthood. **Conclusion:** Alcohol use in adolescence has clear implications for mental and psychosocial functioning in young adulthood. Screening in the community for risk subjects is feasable at relatively low costs in order to implement preventive measures.

S-019-089   Topic: 55, 68
Behavior problems in children of alcoholic fathers from pre-school age to puberty

Erikson F. Furtado, University of Sao Paulo, Med. School of Ribeirao Preto, Ribeirao Preto, Brazil, efurtado@fmrp.usp.br
Martin Schmidt; Manfred Laucht

Objective: Paternal alcoholism has been implicated as a psychopathological condition importantly related to high rates of emotional suffering in the offspring. Transversal studies have indicated a higher rate of psychiatric problems among children of alcoholics (COAS). Relative few prospective longitudinal child psychiatric studies have been conducted on this subject up to now. **Methods:** From the Mannheim Study of Risk Children, an ongoing prospective high-risk population study, data of 219 children (26 COAS and 193 Non-COAS) were analyzed from birth to 11 years. Demographic data and number and severity of behavior problems have been investigated. The COAS family status was characterized by father's lower educational level, economic difficulties and more adverse life events. Other psychosocial problems, such as marital conflict and lack of coping mechanisms, were found to be more frequent in the COAS families. **Results:** Two years old COAS showed significant more frequently temper attacks, disobedience, inattention and hyperactivity. Four and half years old COAS presented more eating behavior problems, impulsivity, temper attacks and shyness. Eight years old COAS were found with more impulsivity, aggressive behavior, distractibility, oppositional behavior in the family, and

lying behavior. Eleven years old COAS showed more bulimia, hyperactivity and oppositional behavior in the family. **Conclusion:** The results indicated a higher vulnerability for psychopathological manifestation, mainly for expansive symptoms, in the offspring of alcoholic fathers. Further research is necessary to elucidate the pathways and the moderate factors in this high-risk group. Keywords: Paternal alcoholism, Longitudinal prospective study, Developmental psychopathology, Expansive symptoms.

S-019-090   Topic: 68, 3
National drug politics and their influence on mental health care in adolescents – a binational clinical perspective

Oliver Bilke, Humboldt-Klinikum, Kinder- und Jugendpsychiatrie, Berlin, Germany, oliver.bilke@vivantes.de

Objective: To evaluate the relevance of national drug politics on the clinical treatment of adolescent drug users we analysed the different drug politics of Switzerland and Germany in relation to three mental health institutions near the lake of Constance (1) and in Berlin (2). **Methods:** Official statements of governments, drug controlling agencies and state-funded research institutes are compared. They are related to the regular in-patient population of two hospitals with mandatory referral of all adolescent psychiatric emergencies in their area of responsibility. The rural areas of eastern and central Switzerland with their particularly easy access to illegal drugs are compared to Berlin metropolitan inner city areas well known as drug centres. Qualitative interviews (CH: y2003, Berlin: y2004) and treatment data are compared. **Results:** The incidence of Cannabis-related disorders in the in-patient population was much higher in Switzerland due to the easy access. Most patients were of Swiss origin, there were only a few cases of polytoxicomania. Almost all patients were well oriented in national drug politics, they knew the public discussion and tried to defend their behavior. In Berlin there is a majority of intensive polytoxicomaniacs with along history of heroine, cocaine and other toxic substances. THC is not seen as a problem in itself and there were only a few mere THC-users. Knowledge about the poltical aspects of drug use was very small. **Conclusion:** Liberal and openly discussed consistent drug politics such as in Switzerland supports therapeutic contact with patients. In inner city areas with a low level of interest in these political aspects other more structural aspects dominate. In the first case, psycho- and socio-therapeutic interventions are useful, in the second emergency procedures are requested. Further public health details are discussed.

S-019-091   Topic: 68
Availability of ecstasy as potential mechanism between prior cannabis use and subsequent first onset of ecstasy use

Petra Zimmermann, Max-Planck-Institut für Klinische Psychologie, München, Germany, pzimmer@mpipsykl.mpg.de
Hans-Ulrich Wittchen; Roselind Lieb

Objective: To investigate the impact of cannabis use on the availability of ecstasy and on the subsequent first onset of ecstasy use (MDMA) in a representative community sample of adolescents and young adults. **Methods:** Baseline and four-year-follow-up data from the Early-Developmental-Stages-of-Psychopathology-Study (EDSP), a prospective-longitudinal community study of originally 3021 adolescents and young adults aged 14–24 years at baseline are used. Data were assessed with the M-CIDI (Munich-Composite-International-Diagnostic-Interview) and its DSM-IV algorithms. Prospective multiple logistic regressions controlling for age, gender, regular alcohol, and regular nicotine use as well as survival analyses were performed. **Results:** Respondents who had used cannabis at baseline, but never ecstasy in their life reported more often ecstasy availability at follow-up than cannabis non-users (the higher the frequency of cannabis use at baseline the more likely the subsequent availability of ecstasy at follow-up). Regarding cannabis use and drug availability at baseline jointly as predictors for actual first onset of ecstasy use during follow-up cannabis use emerged to be the dominant predicting factor. Even cannabis use without drug availability was markedly linked to onset of ecstasy use. **Conclusion:** Overall, our results provide evidence that cannabis use is a risk factor for a higher availability of ecstasy and for subsequent first onset of ecstasy use. Thus, other pathways than ambient drug availability seem to play an important role.

S-019-092   Topic: 68
Drug and alcohol abuse among adolescents admitted for drug and alcohol withdrawal treatment in Iceland: Insights from demography, sociology, psychology, trauma and clinical implications of basic research findings

Helga Hannesdottir, University Hospital Landspital,
Dept. of Psychiatry, Reykjavik, Iceland,
helhann@landspitli.is
Thorarinn Tyrfingsson

Objective: Alcohol and drug addiction is a form of compulsive behavior, resulting from the interplay of chronic alcohol and drug exposure, genetic, educational and environmental factors. Addiction is a complex brain disease marked by recurring events (intoxication, withdrawal and craving) that let to the relapsing nature of the disorder. **Methods:** 213 adolescents admitted in 2002–2003, aged 14–19 years were assessed during admission to the National Center for Addiction Medicine, Vogur Hospital. **Results:** The presentation discusses the epidemiological, psychological, social, and environmental findings contributing to alcohol and drug abuse. **Conclusion:** There are reasons to consider psychological, social and environmental factors as well as educational and family factors and psychiatric comorbidity when treating adolescents for addiction.

S-020   Topic: 3
Prevention of behavioral and emotional problems in childhood

Track: Therapy and intervention

Chairperson: Manfred Döpfner, Universität zu Köln
Psychiatrie und Psychotherapie, Köln, Germany,
manfred.doepfner@t-online.de

Prevention of behavioral and emotional problems in childhood

Manfred Döpfner, Universität zu Köln,
Psychiatrie und Psychotherapie, Köln, Germany,
manfred.doepfner@t-online.de

Prevention research has become an important new frontier in the study of mental disorders. The prevention of behavioral and emotional problems in childhood and adolescence is one of the most demanding and probably most promising research areas. National Advisory Boards recommended that prevention research be reflected in all phases of research (pre-intervention, intervention, and services); across disciplines (biological, psychological, social); across levels of intervention (individual, psychological, social); across types of intervention research (prevention and treatment); and across disorders. Several recent European prevention research projects are presented in the symposium. Both methodological strategies and problems as well as empirical results are discussed. According to NIMH suggestions the integration across prevention and treatment research is stressed. The importance of both efficacy and effectiveness trials will be discussed. Efficacy trials test the extent to which a specific intervention produces positive results under near-ideal conditions. Effectiveness trials test the extent to which efficacious interventions have a beneficial effect when deployed in natural settings.

S-020-093   Topic: 10
Parent training: The long-term efficacy of a program to prevent child behaviour problems on a universal basis

Kurt Hahlweg, Tech. Universität Braunschweig,
Inst. für Psychologie, Braunschweig, Germany,
k.hahlweg@tu-bs.de
Annett Kuschel; Heike Bertram; Nina Heinrichs

In the US, behavioral parent training is known to be most efficacious in treating and preventing child behavior problems. In Germany, a lack of prevention programs for child behavior problems is evident. In a randomized, controlled, and prospective two-site study, we are currently investigating the efficacy of the Triple P parent group training as a universal prevention program. Parents of children between 3 and 6 years were randomly assigned to either the Triple P group program or a no-intervention control group. A multimethod and multimodal assessment was conducted pre- and post-treatment, and 1 and 2 years after the initial assessment. In sum, 280 families participated. 143 received the Triple P program and 137 were assigned to the control group. This presentation will report on the post and 1-year outcome. Implications of these results will be discussed, particularly with their meaning for the dissemination of effective prevention programs into the field.

S-020-094   Topic: 3
Efficacy of indicated prevention with pre-school children: The prevention program for externalizing problem behaviour (PEP)

Manfred Döpfner, Universität zu Köln,
Psychiatrie und Psychotherapie, Köln, Germany,
manfred.doepfner@t-online.de
Inez Freund-Braier; Gabriele Brix; Christopher Hautmann;
Julia Plück

Objective: Disruptive disorders (conduct disorders and hyperkinetic disorders) have a high stability from preschool age to adolescence. Therefore, an early prevention and intervention program which is effective in reducing problem behavior and applicable in routine care is needed. Prevention and intervention programs which aim to modify parent-child and teacher-child interactions haven been proven to be effective in reducing externalising problem behavior. Based on a clinical treatment program for hyperkinetic and oppostional problem behaviour we developed such a prevention program for parents and pre-school teachers of children aged 3–6. Focussing on specific situations, participants detect ineffective reinforcement processes and learn about favourable strategies to modify the child's behaviour. **Methods:** n = 128 Children aged 3 to 6 with disruptive behaviour problems were identified via screening with parent and teacher ratings and randomly assigend either to parent and teacher prevention program or to a no prevention control group. Behaviour problems of the children in the family, the kindergarten and in a play situation as well as parenting behaviour were assessed by rating scales and behavioural observation before and after the prevention. The prevention program consisted of 10 two-hour sessions with parent groups (mean 5 parents per group) and 10 two-hour session with pre-school teacher groups. **Results:** The prevention program was effective on parent ratings of ADHD and oppositional defiant behaviour problems. On teacher ratings of the child behaviour problems reductions in the prevention group and the control group were found.

S-020-095   Topic: 6, 3

Preventing disruptive behavior in elementary school-children: The effectiveness of the good behavior game

Alfons Crijnen, Erasmus University, Child & Adolescent Psychiatry, Rotterdam, The Netherlands,
a.crijnen@erasmusmc.nl
Pol van Lier; Patricia Vuijk

Objective: Childhood aggression is a strong predictor of later antisocial and criminal behavior, and substance abuse. The more serious and the greater the variety and frequency of early aggressive behavior, the greater the risk that antisocial and criminal behavior will continue into later adolescence and adulthood. It is widely acknowledged that emphasis should be given to prevention rather than treatment of aggressive behavior and conduct disorder. Preventive interventions should interrupt the developmental trajectory towards conduct problems at an early age because the malleability is greater at younger ages than at older age. Interventions must take place before the behavioral patterns become broad and diversified, before they become well learned and reinforced, and before peers and adults will respond with counter-aggression or rejection, which serves to maintain the antisocial behavior pattern. Prevention is the more important because for established conduct disorder or related antisocial behavior patterns no treatment approach has been demonstrated to be effective in the long run. In this presentation, results of a randomized controlled trial examing the effectiveness of the Good Behavior Game (GBG) in reducing disruptive behavior will be discussed. **Methods:** The GBG is a well-known classroom intervention which uses positive and negative behaviors of each child to produce systematic consequences for all members of his or her group. Children are consistently given rewards for positive behavior regardless of how troublesome they are perceived by their teachers. Negative behavior is neglected as much as possible. The GBG and

control condition were randomly assigned to 666 children in 33 classes and the intervention was introduced to these children over a period of 2 years. **Results:** The prevention program was effective in reducing attention deficit/hyperactivity behavior. Furthermore, children differing in the risk for developing disruptive behavior were identified. It was found that the program was most effective for children with intermediate levels of attention deficit/hyperactivity, oppositional behavior and aggressive behavior. For high risk children, a significant reduction in aggressive behavior was observed. Risk factors predicting predicting risk status as well as intervention effect were identified. Knowledge about these risk factors is very informative for screening purposes as well as for the development of targeted interventions. **Conclusion:** Universal preventive interventions in elemenatry schools are effective in reducing disruptive behavior. For high risk children, these universal interventions should be accompanied by interventions targeted more specifically to their needs.

S-021   Topic: 22, 67

Consultation from child and adolescent psychiatry and psychotherapy

Track: Therapy and intervention

Chairperson: Reiner Frank, Med. Universität München
Kinder- und Jugendpsychiatrie, München, Germany,
reiner.frank@med.uni-muenchen.de
Inger Helene Vandvik, Rikshospitalet Nat. Hospital
Child & Adolescent Psychiatry, Oslo, Norway,
i.h.vandvik@medisin.uio.no

Consultation from child and adolescent psychiatry and psychotherapy

Reiner Frank, Med. Universität München,
Kinder- und Jugendpsychiatrie, München, Germany,
reiner.frank@med.uni-muenchen.de

The aim of the workshop is to bring together child and adolescent psychiatrists engaged in consultative work with a focus on empirical data. It begins with an overview on developmental aspects and proceeds to specific questions encountered on intensive care units. Schedule Chair Frank, Munich, Vandvik, Oslo Speakers Schäfert/Frank, Stuttgart, Munich – A developmental perspective in child and adolescent psychiatric and psychosomatic consultation Vandvik, Oslo Assessment of patients with somatic symptoms without organic findings van Weel, The Hague Behaviour changes in seriously ill children – psychological or organic? Schieveld, Maastricht Delirium and pre-delirious state at the Paediatric Intensive Care Unit and at the paediatric ward Steiner, Stanford Somatisation in cancer survivors.

S-021-096   Topic: 22

A developmental perspective in child and adolescent psychiatric and psychosomatic consultation in a children's hospital

Rainer Schäfert, Bürgerhospital Stuttgart,
Abt. Psychosomatik, Stuttgart, Germany,
rainer.schaefert@t-online.de
Reiner Frank

Objective: To describe the developmental characteristics of psychiatric and psychosomatic consultations in a children's hospital, focusing on age-typical reasons for referral.

Methods: The notes of all consultations delivered by the 'Institute for Child and Adolescent Psychiatry' to the 'Dr. von Hauner Children's Hospital' of the Ludwig-Maximilians-University of Munich between 1986 and 1997 were coded retrospectively. 521 consultations were documented. Compared to the age distribution of the hospital population, which shows a continuous decline from the 1st year of life towards adulthood, in the consultation group infancy and preschool age are underrepresented, school age and adolescence are overrepresented. The developmental perspective is brought in by analysing reasons for referral by age groups. **Results:** Reasons for referral were as follows: Infancy (0–3 years) (n = 89): child abuse (60%), parent-child-problems (33%), developmental disorders (27%), chronic disease (19%), feeding disorders (12%). Preschool age (3–6 years) (n = 58): developmental disorders (38%), chronic disease (33%), abnormal behaviour (29%), child abuse (26%), sexual abuse (19%), psychosomatic disorder (19%). School age (6–12 years) (n = 164): psychosomatic disorder (44%), abnormal behaviour (30%), chronic disease (27%), parent-child-problems (27%), developmental problems (21%). Adolescence (12–18 years) (n = 171): psychosomatic disorder (46%), chronic disease (29%), parent-child-problems (28%), suicide attempts (22%), coping problems (21%), abnormal behaviour (21%). Young adults (over 18 years) (n = 23): chronic disease (65%), coping problems (48%). **Conclusion:** Consultative work as well as psychotherapy should be developmental oriented. Age-specific developmental tasks and age-typical health problems encountered in consultation should be incorporated in training programs.

S-021-097   Topic: 22
Assessment of patients with somatic symptoms without organic findings

Inger Helene Vandvik, Rikshospitalet Nat. Hospital, Child & Adolescent Psychiatry, Oslo, Norway, i.h.vandvik@medisin.uio.no

Objective: To present an overview of the most common somatic symptoms and disorders without clear physical findings in children and adolescents and ways of assessment. Reasons why these patients are underrepresented in child psychiatric practice will be discussed. **Methods:** Case histories will serve to illustrate the need for a multi-professional bio-psycho-social assessment. The use of semi-structured interviews, questionnaires, psychological and pedagogical testing and a family sculpture will be presented. **Results:** Physical problems often trigger the symptoms. Concerns about school work (poor results or high expectations) and/or stressful events are common. The child may be conscientious, sensitive or anxious and have concerns related to pain/physical discomfort. A minority has a coexistent psychiatric disorder. Health problems and focus on diseases, high demands on parenting and hostility towards psychological explanatory models may characterise the families. **Conclusion:** Assessment and treatment are best accomplished by a trusting relationship between the somatic doctors and the child psychiatric team. This makes it possible to shift the focus from the physical to the psychosocial issues in a tempo the family can accept.

S-021-098   Topic: 67
Behaviour changes in seriously ill children – psychological or organic?

Jeanne van Weel, De Jutters, Center for Mental Health, The Hague, Netherlands, e.vanweel@dejutters.com

Objective: To help the clinician differentiating between psychological and organic behaviour changes in children in (paediatric) hospital. **Methods:** An overview of the clinical picture of 30 patients referred for acute behaviour changes: reasons for referral, clinical presentation (to nurses, doctors and parents) and presence of symptoms of delirium, etiological factors, treatment and outcome. **Results:** (1) the reasons for referral varied from isolated psychiatric symptoms (anxiety, hallucinations), bizarre behaviour, to help in dealing with traumatic experiences. In time recognition of delirium raised, possibly by the education of the consulted psychiatrists. (2) From the symptoms of delirium, disorder of attention and impairment of memory were seldom recognised by referring doctors. Nurses usually give a more accurate picture of the child's dysfunctioning prior to referral: they mention their inability to comfort the child, that the child is irritable and their cry has changed, pain sensitivity is in- or decreased. (3) 2/3 of the children were suffering from central nervous system pathology. (4) 80 % was treated by the consulted psychiatrist – a) when possible by identifying and reversing the reason for delirium – b) with haloperidol and environmental manipulation (decrease of sensory input, re establish day-night rhythm). (5) 4 children died in hospital, no systematic follow up on their cognitive functioning was done. **Conclusion:** Paediatricians do not always recognise the clinical picture of organic behaviour changes in seriously ill children, a delirium. Prompt psychiatric consultation upon request and education about the clinical picture can help recognition and earlier referral. Delirium is a fearful experience for child, parent and professional. Recognition is necessary for appropriate intervention. Acute changes in behaviour and emotions are very common in children in hospital. Recognition of either psychological or organic aetiology is important since the treatment is different. Very little research on children with organic behaviour changes, delirium, exists. Delirium is a clinical diagnosis, rating scales and psychological tests have limited value.

S-021-099   Topic: 22, 67
Delirium and pre-delirious state at the PICU (Pediatric Intensive Care Unit) and at the pediatric ward. A prospective study on 25 cases in two years (2002–2003)

Jan Schieveld, University Hospital Maastricht, Psychiatry and Neuropsychology, Maastricht, Netherlands, kirsten_venrooij@spsy.azm.nl

Objective: To investigate the incidence and to describe the population and patient characteristics, the clinical presentations of (pre-)delirious states, the treatment modalities, the outcome and follow-up in a severely ill pediatric university hospital population. **Methods:** The detailed description, prospectively of a consecutive series of referred children in exactly 2 years from the PICU, the medium care and the ward. **Results:** 25 children, 7 from the ward, 18 from the PICU. 19 children with a mean PIM score: 15.35%, a mean PRISM score: 28.55%. 11 girls and 14 boys, ages: 3 months–16 years. 18 full-blown delirium (9 hypo, 8 hyper), 8 pre-delirious state (anxiety–moaning–agitation). Incidence: at the PICU 3/100/year, at the ward 0.5/100/year. All got either haloperidol or risperidone, 22 responded very well, there were 3 treatment drop-outs. 4 children died. **Conclusion:** There exists an organic mental spectrum disorder in child neuropsychiatry; one pole is delirium and the other one is "organic substance related mental disorder": anxiety–moaning; the clinical picture fluctuates over time and over the spectrum. Haloperidol and risperidone are both excellent drugs for both poles at all childhood ages (and haloperidol also < 4 years of age). Considering the treatment reasons there should be and a systematically search for the spectrum disorder and a neuro-psychological follow-up after 3 months. Keywords: Delirium, PIM and PRISM scores, haloperidol, risperidone, child neuropsychiatry.

S-021-100   Topic: 67, 22
Somatization in survivors of juvenile cancer

Hans Steiner, Stanford University, School of Psychiatry, Stanford, CA, USA, steiner@stanford.edu

Objective: The study of the psychological and psychiatric impact of surviving cancer often yields conflicting results. We intended to show the complex impact of surviving a life threatening illness by conducting interviews and collecting self report measures. We were particularly interested in the role somatization as a defense and as a syndrome plays in this context as it complicates medical management. **Methods:** We studied a cohort of non-clinical high school students and young adults (N = 1500; mean age 16, SD 1, 535 women; ethnically diverse) and conacer survivors (at least 5 years status post cancer treatment; N = 50; mean age 18; SD 1; 70% women; ethnically diverse). Both samples were obtained locally in Northern California. We emplyed semi-structured interviews (Davidson PTSD) and self report instruments (REM-71; WAI-84, SCL-90), yielding measures of PTSD, psychiatric symptoms and personality traits and defenses. **Results:** Both full syndromal PTSD and partial PTSD were seen in cancer survivors at higher rates than would be expected by chance (> 3%). Associated with PTSD status were increased somatization as a defense and as a symptomatic cluster. **Conclusion:** We discuss the implications of these findings for the diagnosis and management of the psychiatric complications of cancer survival. In all likelihood, we can extend these findings to other dramatic, life saving and high tech medical interventions, such a transplantation procedures and intubation.

S-022   Topic: 51
Child abuse and neglect

*Chairperson: Jörg M. Fegert,
Universität Ulm Kinder- und Jugendpsychiatrie, Ulm, Germany, joerg.fegert@medizin.uni-ulm.de*

S-022-101   Topic: 51, 55
Sex abuse victims as mothers:
Relationship to attributions, discipline practices and behavior problems

William Friedrich, Mayo Clinic, Psychiatry and Psychology, Rochester, MN, USA, friedrich.william@mayo.edu

Objective: To examine the relationship of a maternal history of sexual abuse to parenting behaviors that are related to child outcome. These include discipline practices, family sexuality, traumas that their child has experienced, negative perceptions of the child, and behavior problems in the child, including sexual behavior. **Methods:** A consecutive sample of 391 mothers of predominately Caucasian children and adolescents (M Age 12.7, SD = 3.6) admitted to an inpatient psychiatric unit completed measures assessing the following: their child's level of behavior problems, traumatic history, family sexuality, conflict tactics, attributions of their child, their social relationship quality, current depression, and also their experience with emotional, physical and sexual abuse **Results:** Victimization history was variably related to their child having experienced more trauma, a higher level of a variety of behavior problems, a lower quality of parenting, reduced satisfaction with social support, greater depression, and more negative attributions of their child. A maltreatment history in the mother was also significantly associated with a greater likelihood of their child being sexually abused. **Conclusion:** These results point to the need to focus on both maternal issues as well as the mother-child relationship in any clinical intervention with families characterized by maltreatment in the parental generation

S-022-102   Topic: 51
Maltreated children's family representations:
About maintaining emotional security

*Smadar Celestin-Westreich, Vrije Universiteit Brussel VUB, Developmental Psychology, Brussels, Belgium, smadar.westreich@vub.ac.be
Leon Patrice Celestin; Ingrid Ponjaert-Kristoffersen*

Objective: Research has increasingly documented the deleterious developmental effects of child maltreatment. Yet, partly due to the complexity of this specific disclosure context and associated methodological difficulties (widespread use but limited systematisation of projective techniques), relatively few studies have directly investigated maltreated children's experiences of family relations. Gaining insight into maltreated children's family representation nevertheless remains critical to adequate assessment and therapeutic intervention. This presentation analyses a set of studies into maltreated children's family representations within the context of the emotional security hypothesis. **Methods:** The population comprised children aged 5–12 (mean = 7.3, sd = 2.3), from Family & Child Maltreatment Evaluation Centers. Quantitative and qualitative analyses including extensive background variables were processed on data set (a) (N = 70) including 35 maltreated children and 35 pair-wise matched controls, who took the 'Animal Family Drawing' (AFD) test and data set (b) of 48 children whose 'Family Relations Test' (FRT) responses were compared to norms. Both instruments are standardized validated self-expression measures of self- and family-representations. **Results:** Besides showing negative developmental impacts in drawing patterns, maltreated children differed significantly (p < 0.05) from controls through defensive disclosure, lack of positive self- & parental representations and signs of "mental frozenness" (AFD-test). Differentiated response patterns appeared on the Family Relations Test with either significant (p < 0.05) avoidance or excess of (negative) emotional expressions along with tendencies to idealise non-offending parents. Furthermore, number of family transitions and combination of maltreatment types were linked to family representations according to age groups. **Conclusion:** Importantly, these results underscore specificities of maltreated children's family experiences that reflect a set of differentiated modalities as regards attachment pathways. From the perspective of maintaining emotional security throughout complex endangering family contexts, processes like affective polarization, coping through idealisation and overcompensation are revealed in these data. Discussion further details these maltreated children's family representations in relation to vulnerability and resiliency factors.

S-022-103   Topic: 51
Trauma experience: Its incidence, feature and clinical issues in adolescents in Japan

Keizo Nagao, Sakakibara Hospital, Dept. of Psychiatry, Japan, gzb06665@nifty.ne.jp
M. Kisida; M. Okuno; E. Shindo

Objective: The chance to be bleached to the trauma is different according to the culture and the age. Then, what is easy to damage adolescents in recent Japan, and the frequency and extent of it was investigated. Objects are 104 nursing students (the second school year). **Methods:** Answer was obtained in shape of one of the authors to read out the question items though the investigation was a questionnaire method. **Results:** It consists that A criteria of DSM-4 is 8 (8%), "there is a strong stress experience though it does not arrive at A criteria" is 52 (50%), "the trauma experience in the tremble" is 23 (22%), and no traumatic experience is 21 (20%). Cause of sixty of the former two groups mainly comprise of bulling and distressed personal relationship in 24 (40%) and bereavement by intimate friend or near relatives in 18 (30%). These are thought to be the maximum cause which can become PTSD at this age in our country. Next, to see the feature of the main symptoms seen in bullying, compared with those who experienced the loss. Bullying of the self-reproach idea was dominant higher though there was no difference in the PTSD symptoms compared with the loss experience. The related clinical issue would be discussed at the congress.

S-022-104   Topic: 51, 47
Childhood sexual abuse and psychological disturbance in a national youth sample

Helmer Bøving Larsen, University of Copenhagen, Dept. of Psychology, Copenhagen S, Denmark, helmer.larsen@psy.ku.dk
Karin Helweg-Larsen

Objective: This study was designed to ascertain the prevalence, correlates, and psychological consequences of childhood sexual abuse (CSA) in a Danish representative sample of more than 6,000 adolescents studied at age 15. **Methods:** An anonymous computer assisted self interview (CASI) was employed, providing information on prevalence rates, types of abuse, ages of victims, relationship to the abuser, and rates of anxiety and depression. **Results:** Nearly 12% reported having experienced CSA before the age of 15 years. Most of the abusers were young men, disclosure of the abuse was infrequent, and seldom ever officially reported. There were consistent relationships between the extent of CSA and risk of psychological disturbance, with those reporting CSA involving intercourse having the highest rates of symptoms of anxiety and depression. These results persisted when findings were adjusted

for childhood family and related factors. **Conclusion:** The findings sugggest that CSA is associated with increased risk of psychological disturbance in adolescence even when allowance is made for confounding factors. Key words: Childhood sexual abuse, childhood and family factors.

S-022-105   Topic: 51, 24
Effects of childhood physical trauma on brain development

Ramón Lindauer, De Bascule – Child and, Adolescent Psychiatry, Amstelveen, Netherlands, rjl.lindauer@12move.nl
Jan Booij; Miranda Olff; Gerard den Heeten; Berthold Gersons; Frits Boer

Objective: To investigate the effects of childhood physical trauma and PTSD (posttraumatic stress disorder) on brain circuits which are involved in emotion and memory with functional brain imaging. **Methods:** We assessed the effects on brain blood flow with [99mTc]HMPAO SPECT (single photon emission computerized tomography) in patients with PTSD and childhood physical trauma (n=6), in patients with PTSD without childhood physical trauma (n=17), and traumatized control subjects (n=15) in reaction to symptom provocation using personalized narratives. Before scanning each subject listened to an audiotape with a description of his/her own traumatic event and the accompanying sensory information (script). MRI scans were used to co-register in SPECT scans and to make a ROI map (region of interest). **Results:** Brain blood flow in both PTSD groups was significantly higher in the medial temporal, ventromedial prefrontal, orbitofrontal, and occipital cortex compared to the traumatized control group. Brain blood flow in these brain areas was higher in the patient group with PTSD and childhood physical trauma compared to the patient group with PTSD without childhood physical trauma. Positive correlations were found between PTSD symptoms and brain blood flow in the medial temporal and orbitofrontal cortex. **Conclusion:** Changes in brain blood flow were found in patients with PTSD and especially in patients who experienced childhood physical trauma. Changes were found in brain areas which are involved in emotion and memory.

S-022-106   Topic: 51, 24
The mediating influence of personality characteristics on the development of psychopathology in sexually abused children

Eric Schoentjes, University Hospital Ghent, Child & Adolescent Psychiatry, Gent, Belgium, eric.schoentjes@ugent.be
Sarah Bal; Dirk Deboutte

Objective: The study of the mediating effect of personality characteristics on the development of trauma-related psychopathology in children has been hampered by the lack of adequate instruments to assess personality in children. In this preliminary study we want to examine whether correlations exists between the personality of the sexually traumatized child and the presence of psychopathology. **Methods:** 53 sexually abused children aged 6 to 15 years were assessed for the presence of psychopathology with a semi structured diagnostic interview, the Child Assessment Schedule and a parent-report questionnaire, the Child Behavior Checklist. Children's personality was assessed with the Hierarchical Personality Inventory for Children (Mervielde, I. & Defruyt, F. 1999). Children were categorized according to the presence or absence of psychopathology and to their levels in 5 broad domains (and 18 facets) of personality (i.e. Conscientiousness, Benevolence, Extraversion, Imagination and Emotional Stability). Chi-square analyses were performed to examine whether certain personality characteristics were significantly more associated with the presence of psychiatric impairment. **Results:** The presence of psychiatric disorders was related to certain personality characteristics, such as Expressiveness, Intellect, Irritability and Self-Confidence. **Conclusion:** Further study of the influence of personality on the development psychopathology in sexually or otherwise traumatized children is warranted, as it appears that these characteristics can play a mediating role in the development of psychopathology following the sexual abuse (Mervielde, I. & De Fruyt, F. 1999). 'Construction of the Hierarchical Personality Inventory for Children' (HiPIC). In I. Mervielde, I. Deary, F. De Fruyt, & F. Ostendorf (Eds.) 'Personality psychology in Europe' (Vol. 7, pp. 107–127). Tilburg University Press.

S-023　Topic: 55
Children of sick parents II

Chairperson: Michael Schulte-Markwort, UKE Hamburg-Eppendorf, Hamburg, Germany,
schulte.markwort@uke.uni-hamburg.de

S-023-107　Topic: 55, 3
Experiences of the Beardslee preventive and the brief parent intervention: Preliminary results of a randomized controlled study in Finland

Tytti Solantaus, STAKES, Dept. of Mental Health, Helsinki, Finland, tytti.solantaus@stakes.fi
Sini Toikka; Maarit Alasuutari

Objective: Children of the mentally ill have an increased risk to develop mental problems themselves. In Finland, a nationwide project (The Efficient Family Project) was established to develop and implement evidence based means to prevent children's disorders in families with mentally ill parents. Clinicians working in mental services were trained to carry out the Beardslee Preventive Family Intervention and the brief Parent Intervention. **Methods:** A study was initiated to compare the effectiveness and special indications of the two interventions in 12 different mental health clinics. Patients with depressive diagnoses and children of 8–15 are included in the study. The recruitment is going on and will continue until 180 families are included. The families are randomized into one of the intervention groups. The study is carried out by means of questionnaires at baseline, 4, 10 and 18 months. The families' experiences of the interventions are inquired immediately after the intervention is over. **Results:** First results of the families' experiences will be reported in the presentation. **Conclusion:** Preliminary conlusions of the feasibility of the two interventions are discussed.

S-023-108　Topic: 55, 22
Gender-specific differences in the process of coping in families with a parent affected by a chronic somatic disease (e.g. Multiple Sclerosis)

Barbara Steck, Universitätsklinik Basel,
Kinder- und Jugendpsychiatrie, Basel, Switzerland,
barbara.steck@unibas.ch
Andrea Grether; M. Ehrensperger; Felix Amsler; L. Kappos;
Dieter Bürgin

Objective: Multiple Sclerosis (MS) confronts patients and their partners with a wide array of challenges. The aim of this study was to investigate how coping is affected by such variables as gender, the degree of disability, cognitive impairment and any associated depression. **Methods:** Based on the investigation of 45 families and their offspring (4–26 years old), the coping capacities of the MS affected, the healthy parent, the couple and their children are quantitatively evaluated by means of semi-structured interviews The disability of the affected parent is assessed by the Kurtzke EDSS, the cognitive impairment by neuropsychological testing, depression by the BDI. Correlations between the coping capacities of each family member and the degree of physical disability as well as cognitive impairment and depression are measured. **Results:** Coping of the parents is gender specific and related to the degree of disability and depression. Offspring's coping is influenced by their gender and by the coping capacities of the healthy parent. Cognitive impairment and depression of the MS patient have a greater impact on the coping abilities of children than the more visible physical symptoms. **Conclusion:** Comprehensive care of a patient with MS involves the entire family. The evaluation of the MS patient, his partner and their children show significant gender-specific interactions between coping, the level of neurological disability, cognitive impairment and depression.

S-023-109　Topic: 55, 22
Conzeptualization and evaluation of a preventive intervention for children of somatically ill parents

Rina Saha, UKE Hamburg-Eppendorf,
Kinder- und Jugendpsychiatrie, Hamburg, Germany,
rsaha@uke.uni-hamburg.de
Bela Paschen; Christiane Baldus; Miriam Haagen;
Martina Pott; Georg Romer

Objective: Serious somatic illness in a parent is a recognized risk factor for psychic maladjustment in children and adolescents. Since July 2000, a preventive out-patient counselling service for children of somatically ill parents was implemented at our department, since 2002 cooperating in a 3-year transnational multisite research project funded by the EU (COSIP: Children of Somatically Ill Parents). Developing and evaluating the counselling service should inform future preventive programs. **Methods:** A descriptive analysis was made of all families seen for counselling (n = 70) covering sociodemographic and illness-related data. A specifically tailored evaluation-design was developed to measure process quality, satisfaction and goal attainment in the short-term preventive interventions based on standardized interrogations of parents, children up from age 11 and therapists involved in counselling. **Results:** Most parents as well as most children experienced the short-term intervention as helpful and supportive in coping with the multiple stressors of the situation. In the therapist's perspective, anticipation of possible losses appears to be a major issue in counselling these children and their families. Parents emphasize the importance of support in their sense of parental competence, whereas children seem to benefit most from support in active coping behaviour. Moreover results from differential analyses are considered as source of further improvement of the counselling. **Conclusion:** Preventive interventions for this target group should be provided on a low-threshold base. The evaluation of the intervention offers data to enhance the specific intervention.

S-024   Topic: 51, 2
Child and adolescent psychiatry in relation to child/welfare/child protection
Chairperson: Yoshiro Ono, Wakayama Prefecture Children Disabled Person's Center, Wakayama, Japan, onoyoshiro@jtw.zaq.ne.jp

Child and adolescent psychiatry in relation to child welfare/child protection
Yoshiro Ono, Wakayama Prefecture Children, Disabled Person's Center, Wakayama, Japan, onoyoshiro@jtw.zaq.ne.jp

Child and adolescent psychiatry is a multidisciplinary practice by nature, and has a close relation to child welfare. Recently, as the interest in the psychiatric aspect of child abuse & neglect has been increased, the practices of child and adolescent psychiatry in the field of child welfare/child protection come to be recognized to be more important. In this symposium, we will address the role and necessity of child and adolescent psychiatry in the practices of child welfare/child protection, and discuss from the international perspective. Two papers from Japan will address the involvement of child and adolescent psychiatrists in the child protective practices at the Child Welfare Centers in Japan. A Turkish child psychiatrist will address clinical characteristics of cases of child abuse and neglect in relation to cultural factors. Finally, a Finnish child psychiatrist will talk about the collaboration with child welfare in the clinical practices for families with inadequate parenting and parents with psychiatric problems.

S-024-110   Topic: 40, 66
Involvement of child and adolescent psychiatry in the practice of child welfare/child protection in Japan
Yoshiro Ono, Wakayama Prefecture Children, Disabled Person's Center, Wakayama, Japan, onoyoshiro@jtw.zaq.ne.jp
H. Homma; Y. Ishida; H. Ide; M. Okamoto; S. Kameoka; Hiroshi Nakayama

Objective: Although child and adolescent psychiatry is essential in the practice of child welfare and protection, involvement of child psychiatrists is extremely limited in Japan. The purpose of the current study was to delineate the roles and necessity of child psychiatrists in these fields by reevaluating the child welfare systems in Japan. **Methods:** A national survey of child psychiatrists involved in the Child Welfare Centers in Japan was conducted in which the numbers of child psychiatrists and their practice were investigated. **Results:** Of the 155 public child welfare cen-

ters that responded to the survey, only 18 (11.6%) reported having at least one psychiatrist working on a full-time basis. In the remainder of the child welfare centers, part-time psychiatrists were providing psychiatric evaluation and treatments. Moreover, there was a great difference in the involvement of child psychiatrists between child welfare centers located in urban areas and those in rural areas. In the small centers located in rural areas, involvement of the child psychiatrists in the practice of child welfare/child protection was meager at best. **Conclusion:** It was revealed that there was an absolute lack of involvement of child and adolescent psychiatry in the Japanese child welfare/child protection system. To provide effective protection and treatment for the victims of child maltreatment, a special field of child and adolescent psychiatry within the child welfare system needs to be proposed.

S-024-111   Topic: 51, 66
The medico-legal-ethical issues in provision of mental health services for victims of child abuse and neglect in Japan
Hiroshi Nakayama, Kawasaki City, Children's Consultation Ct., Kawasaki, Japan, nakayama-hiro@city.kawasaki.jp
Yoshiro Ono; H. Homma; H. Ide; S. Kameoka; A. Yamamoto

Objective: Due to the fact that interventions for abused children have, to date, centered solely on protection in Japan, our systems to provide psychiatric treatment for them is wholly inadequate. The purpose of the current study was to clarify the problems of the current system to treat abused children from the medico-legal-ethical point of view. **Methods:** A two-day conference was held in order to build a consensus on the inpatient care for abused children. Seventeen professionals, including child psychiatrists working in the public child welfare centers, with adequate experiences participated. **Results:** The following problems and opinions were raised. 1) Problems in the introduction for inpatient treatment: When we wish to provide psychiatric treatment for abused children, it is necessary to obtain parental consent. Although parents often refuse to consent to the treatment, the legal means with which to bypass such parental decisions have not been established in Japan. 2) Problems during inpatient care: There is an absolute lack of psychiatric facilities with which to provide special care for abused children in Japan. Those hospitals that are providing treatment face serious difficulties in staffing, casework, and costs. 3) Problems of follow-up-care after discharge: For most of the abused children, integration into the original families after discharge has proven difficult. Therefore child welfare centers are responsible for both residential care and follow-up psychiatric care after discharge. **Conclusion:** It was unanimously agreed that there is an urgent and crucial need to establish a system that provides psychiatric treatment for abused children in Japan. As child welfare centers are primarily responsible for protection and treatment of abused children, we have reached a consensus that employment of full-time working child psychiatrists is essential at all child welfare centers throughout the country.

S-024-112   Topic: 40, 66

Child psychiatry and child welfare:
Collaboration at the family ward

Ilona Luoma, Tampere University Hospital,
Dept. of Child Psychiatry, Tampere, Finland,
ilona.luoma@pshp.fi

Objective: To describe a model of collaboration between professionals in child psychiatry and child welfare. This model is applied at the Family Ward at Tampere University Hospital, Finland. **Methods:** Family Ward is a child psychiatric day ward for infants and young children and their families. The ward has a capacity for three families at the same time. The family inpatient period lasts three weeks and includes child psychiatric evaluation and treatment of children and the families. The staff consists of a multidisciplinary team. Problems in parenting, family violence, parental psychiatric disorders, and conflicts between parents over contact or the residence of their child are common among the families, and in many cases these are also the causes of referral. Therefore the collaboration with child welfare is needed. **Results:** In the majority of cases both practical support and guidance or treatment of parents is necessary. Case conferences with child welfare workers are held in over 90% of cases before, during and after the family inpatient period. An intervention plan including both clinical care of the child and the family (provided by health services) and supportive measures (provided by child welfare) is made for each family. Recommendations for foster care are made if treatment and supportive measures are not adequate or appropriate (in about 10% of cases). **Conclusion:** Collaboration between professionals in child health and welfare services is important particularly in the evaluation and treatment of infants and young children because of their dependency on parental care and vulnerability to deficiencies in parenting. Treating and supporting parenthood by means of interdisciplinary collaboration is a way to promote child mental health and development.

S-024-113   Topic: 89

Children with Reactive Attachment Disorder (RAD)
in Turkey: Sociodemographic, clinical characteristics
and response to treatment

Nahit Motavalli Mukaddes, Istanbul University, Istanbul,
Turkey, nmotavalli@yahoo.com

Reactive attachment disorder is disturbance of social interaction and relatedness based on grossly pathogenic caretaking. DSM-IV specifies that before the age of 5, developmentally inappropriate behaviors are due to a large degree of pathogenic care. It was first described as a diagnostic category in DSM-III in 1980, however, earlier studies in the twentieth century described social-emotional problems, language impairment, and cognitive delay in institutionalized children using terms like "Hospitalism", "maternal deprivation", "anaclitical depression". In the recent century, the field has been witnessed an increasing number of studies conducted with children who were exposed to minimal levels of social and perceptual stimuli. These studies mentioned that frequent change of caregiver, poverty, mental retardation of parents, long separation from caregiver, broken home, and premature parenthood as the most common risk factor that leads to neglect. Most of the studies were done in institutions, while there is a lack of data about risk factors leading to pathogenic care in chil-

dren who live with their parents. The aim of this presentation is: a) to call attention to hidden neglect in clinic-referred children who live with their parents with special focusing in assessment of environmental risk factors and discuss the cultural characteristics of neglect in this group: b) to discuss the clinical symptoms and their similarity with Pervasive Developmental Disorder: c) to summarize our previous studies on treatment program of this group.

S-025   Topic: 24

Track: Psychotic disorders

Formal thought disorder in children: A developmental
phenomenon, a pragmatic language impairment
or a precursor of severe adult psychopathology?

Barry Nurcombe, University of Queensland
Dept. of Psychiatry, Brisbane, Australia,
bnurcombe@psychiatry.uq.edu.au

Formal thought disorder in children: A developmental
phenomenon, a pragmatic language impairment
or a precursor of severe adult psychopathology?

Sam Tyano, Geha Mental Health Center, Petah Tiqva,
Israel, styano@post.tau.ac.il
Rutger Jan van der Gaag; Franz Resch; Tamar Mozes;
R. Caplan

Toddlers do no tune into the listeners needs. Their parents help them by explaining the context of what they are telling to the listener in order to help them understand. Gradually children take over these pragmatic considerations and stop changing topic's without informing the listener and keep their thoughts "on track" in order to helping others understand what they are trying to convey. So normally developing children present with "formal thought" disorders in their preschool period of development. Some children with severe developmental disorders (autism; McDD) persist in formal thought disorder, beyond the age one would expect, given their developmental age and intelligence. The question is if their formal thought disorder are precursors of severe psychopathology e.g. schizophrenia, or whether they represent pragmatic language impairments related to the core features of autism spectrum disorder. In this presentation this issue will be approached both from a theoretical point of view and an empirical perspective presenting data from a pilot study in which the both formal thought disorder as pragmatic skills are evaluated in typically developing children as compared to children with autism, McDD and externalizing and internalizing disorders.

S-025-114   Topic: 69, 42

Early detection of psychosis in adolescents –
A prospective study

Franz Resch, Universität Heidelberg,
Kinder- und Jugendpsychiatrie, Heidelberg, Germany,
franz_resch@med.uni-heidelberg.de
P. Parzer; Fritz Poustka

Objective: Early detection and prevention has become a major topic in schizophrenia research. In adult samples, basic symptoms seem to present as a practicable clinical tool for early detection of schizophrenia. In this study, we examined the relevance of basic symptoms for psychiatric disorders in adolescent patients with special focus on early detection of psychosis. Furthermore we aimed to investigate the association of basic symptoms and personality traits, as both are influenced by biologically-based mechanisms and indicate vulnerability. **Methods:** >From 90 adolescents, who were consecutive inpatients with adolescent psychiatric disorders in 1995 and 1996, 54 were followed up 4.7 years later. Patients were examined with the Bonn Scale for the Assessment of Basic Symptoms (BSABS) at t1 and t2 and the Junior Temperament and Character Inventory (JTCI). **Results:** None of the participants developed a psychotic disorder, although 50% had presented with high scores of basic symptoms at initial assessment. Indirect minus symptoms turned out to be the most valid predictor for a persisting psychiatric diagnosis. In addition, Indirect minus symptoms correlated significantly with the personality dimensions harm avoidance and self-directedness. **Conclusion:** In adolescents, basic symptoms in association with personality traits present as non-specific indicator of psychopathology rather than as an indicator of vulnerability for schizophrenia.

S-025-117   Topic: 69

Formal thought disorder in children: A developmental phenomenon, a pragmatic language impairment or a precursor of severe adult psychopathology?

Rutger Jan van der Gaag, UMCN ACKJON Nijmegen, Child & Adolescent Psychiatry, Nijmegen, Netherlands, rutger.jan.van.der.gaag@skjpon.nl

Toddlers do no tune into the listeners needs. Their parents help them by explaining the context of what they are telling to the listener in order to help them understand. Gradually children take over these pragmatic considerations and stop changing topic's without informing the listener and keep their thoughts "on track" in order to helping others understand what they are trying to convey. So normally developing children present with "formal thought" disorders in their preschool period of development. Some children with severe developmental disorders (autism; McDD) persist in formal thought disorder, beyond the age one would expect, given their developmental age and intelligence. The question is if their formal thought disorder are precursors of severe psychopathology, e.g. schizophrenia, or whether they represent pragmatic language impairments related to the core features of autism spectrum disorder. In this presentation this issue will be approached both from a theoretical point of view and an empirical perspective presenting data from a pilot study in which the both formal thought disorder as pragmatic skills are evaluated in typically developing children as compared to children with autism, McDD and externalizing and internalizing disorders.

S-026   Topic: 69

Schizophrenia and other psychotic disorders II

Track: Psychotic disorders

Chairperson: Savita Malhotra, FAMS Dept. of Psychiatry, Chandigarh, India, savitam@sancharnet.in

S-026-119   Topic: 69

Clinical features of the first psychotic episode: correlation with the final diagnosis

Maria Giuseppina Ledda, University of Cagliari, Child & Adolescent Psychiatry, Cagliari, Italy, emmegielle@yahoo.com
Al Fratta; S. Pellerano; S. Mannino; Simona Corona; A. Zuddas; Carlo Cianchetti

Objective: Clinical studies show the difficulty of predict the evolution of a first psychotic episode in adolescents. We attempted to correlate the clinical features of a first psychotic episode with the final diagnosis, in order to individuate predictory elements of the final diagnosis. **Methods:** A group of 36 subjects (22 males and 14 females), aged 15.0 ± 1.9 years at onset, presenting with psychotic features was studied. Clinical data were registered according to the Kiddie-SADS-PL and PANSS at time of first admission and at a follow-up. Final diagnoses [schizophrenic disorder (SPh in 15, schizoaffective (SA) in 10, bipolar disorder with psychotic features (BP) in 11] were made according the DSM-IV criteria after at least 36 months (up to 7 years) from the index episode. **Results:** The group of patients with final diagnosis of SPh significantly differed from that of BP having higher rates or values on the following parameters: familiarity for SPh disorders (less for BP disorder), preceding difficulties in the relationship with mates and adults, difficulties in the studies, graduality of the onset, longer duration of the first episode, affective flattening, isolation, avoiding, disorientation, hostility, mannerism, auditory and tactile hallucinations, delusions of thought insertion and message from TV. The same group of SPh subjects significantly differed from that of SA for higher familiarity for SPh disorder and lower for BP disorder, more isolation and mannerism, higher presence of thought transmission delusions and less excitement. The group of SA subjects significantly differed from that of BP for the more graduality of onset, less delusions of grandiosity and more affective flattening and isolation. **Conclusion:** The above individuated clinical features can orient the differential diagnosis between SPh, SA and BP disorders.

S-026-120   Topic: 69, 79

Psychosis in deaf children and adolescents: A review and a clinical case

Macarena Marin Olalla, Torrecardenas Hospital, Almeria, Spain, bernamaca@hotmail.com
Ruth Garcia; Bernardo Perez Ramirez; Ross Campion; Peter Hindley

Objective: Psychotic Manifestations are subjective experiences, difficult to quantify in all patients, most especially in deaf children and adolescents. The aim of this paper is to illustrate this, describing a case of a prelingually deaf patient who experienced visual hallucinations and to conduct a detailed review of the relevant literature. **Methods:** A literature search was performed in Medline using the following key words: deafness, psychosis, hearing impairment, child adolescent, and hallucinations. In an attempt to clarify diagnosis the case report was prepared using a detailed psychiatry history and neurological examination. **Results:** A total of 1506 articles on psychosis and 2418 on schizophrenia in children/adolescents were found and contrasted with 15 articles on psychosis or schizophrenia in deafness/hearing impairment (HI) children/adolescents. Five reports on deafness/HI children/adolescents were published in Non-English, and 3 had been published after 1990. Some 56 articles on visual hallucinations in children/adolescents were found and one of them from deafness/HI. In the case report, visual hallucinations, thought disorder and suspiciousness were the main manifestations of psychosis. Epilepsy and brain damage were excluded. **Conclusion:** To date, there is still very little information in the available literature about specific symptoms of psychosis in deaf children/adolescents. So deafness, in addition to the usual phantasy and imaginative world of children/adolescents, contributes to the difficulty of accurately diagnosing psychosis. It is important to acknowledge that deaf people communicate differently, using a different language and a different skill set. As described in our clinical case, deaf children/adolescents use mainly the visual channels of communication (e.g. sign language). For this reason, in those suffering psychosis, visual hallucinations arise more commonly in deaf people than in hearing people. In conclusion, speech and language provide invaluable information in considering a diagnosis of psychosis. However, it is not difficult to appreciate the complex challenge of confidently making such a diagnosis in deaf children/adolescents. A most important clues lies in an awareness and understanding of deaf people and their language.

S-026-121   Topic: 69

Study of childhood onset schizophrenia (cos) using spect and neuropsychological assessment

Savita Malhotra, FAMS, Dept. of Psychiatry, Chandigarh, India, savitam@sancharnet.in
Nitin Gupta; Anish Bhattacharaya; Mehak Kapoor

Objective: To study the brain dysfunction using SPECT and neuropsychological functioning in patients with COS. **Methods:** It was a cross-sectional study of 12 COS patients with onset at or before 14 years of age, diagnosed as per ICD-10 DCR criteria attending a tertiary care centre in North India. All the patients were assessed on sociodemographic, clinical profile sheet, PANSS and Edinburgh Scale of handedness. For the neuropsychological assessment Wisconsin Card Sorting Test was used. Single Photon Emission Computed Tomography (SPECT) was done on all patients. **Results:** 5 (41.6%) patients showed perfusion anomaly on SPECT scan specifically in the left temporo- parietal area of brain. On WCST score these 5 patients showed a higher percentage of errors (65.15% ± 8.91) as compared to the remaining 7 patients (54.08 ± 15.27) who showed no abnormality on SPECT scan. **Conclusion:** The results from WCST show that COS patients have problems in executive functioning which is a frontal lobe function. Also patients had perfusion anomaly in the left parieto-temporal region. Thus this study suggests that deficits found in Childhood Onset Schizophrenia could be due to fronto–temporo–parietal localization of pathology in the brain.

S-026-122   Topic: 69

Results of integrated treatment (HIT) in early psychoses: a pilot study

Jack A. Jenner, University Hospital Groningen, Voices Outpatient Dept., Groningen, Netherlands, j.a.jenner@acggn.azg.nl
G. van de Willge

Objective: Feasibility and effectiveness of HIT were tested as early intervention in a naturalistic, retrospective pilot study of 14 adolescents with auditory hallucinations consecutively referred to Groningen Voices Outpatient Department. **Methods:** Independent assessors collected diagnosis, sociodemographics, psychiatric history, former treatment and current treatment status from medical files. Auditory Hallucinations Rating Scale, Groningen Social Disabilities Scale and 5-point rating scales on characteristics and subjective burden of voices, and satisfaction with therapy were scored with semi-structured interview. **Results:** Good compliance and high satisfaction with HIT-treatment in most cases; 65% free of voices; majority demonstrates substantial improvement on mastery, anxiety, interference with thinking and social functioning; none worsened. **Conclusion:** Results suggest HIT to be effective beyond auditory vocal hallucinations to other domains of psychopathology, subjective burden and mastery, and social functioning. Similar results have been demonstrated in chronic patients with persistent hallucinations. Introduction: HIT, Hallucination focused Integrative Treatment, integrates motivational interviewing, cognitive behaviour treatment, coping training, single family treatment and rehabilitation training with routine treatment. HIT was found significantly ($p < 0.05$) better than routine treatment in a RCT with 76 adult schizophrenics on: – Psychopathology (PANSS-dimensions: positive; disorganisation; depression; total) – Subjective burden (AHRS-dimensions: distress; interference; negative content; control) – Quality of life (WHOQOL) – Social functioning (GSDS). Significant improvements in favour of HIT were retained upon 18-month follow-up. In another naturalistic study, effects remained at 4 years follow-up; 69% retained improvement, whilst 26% were further improved.

S-026-123   Topic: 69, 31

Niacin sensitivity in juvenile patients and first-degree-relatives of patients with schizophrenia – a potential vulnerability marker of an endophenotype of schizophrenia characterised by altered phospholipid-eicosanoid metabolism

Silke Klemm, Universität Jena, Kinder- und Jugendpsychiatrie, Jena, Germany, silke.klemm@med.uni-jena.de
S. Smesny; M. Stockebrand; S. Grunwald; Bernhard Blanz

Objective: Altered flush response to niacin (vitamin B3) skin stimulation was repeatedly found in patients with schizophrenia recently being considered as potential biological marker of an endophenotype of schizophrenia characterised by altered membrane lipid metabolism and prostaglandin formation, respectively [Horrobin DF (1998) Schizophrenia Research 30(3): 193–208]. Limited data of first-degree relatives of psychosis patients [Waldo MC (1999) Schizophrenia Research 40: 49–53] are suggestive that impaired niacin sensitivity might reflect also a genetically determined metabolic vulnerability to develop schizophrenia. Our aim was to investigate niacin sensitivity in prodromal and first episode schizophrenia patients (n = 23), children and siblings of schizophrenia patients (n = 24) and healthy controls (n = 26) matched for age and gender. **Methods:** Niacin was applied in 0.001 M, 0.01 M, and 0.1 M concentration to the inner forearm skin. Skin flushing was assessed before and at 3-min intervals up to 15 minutes after stimulation starting 90 sec after removal of niacin patches using optical reflection spectroscopy [Smesny S et al. (2001) Biomed Technik 46/10: 280–286]. **Results:** In the lowest niacin concentrations a significantly weaker skin flushing could be detected in patients compared to controls. A diminished sensitivity in risk subjects compared to the controls was revealed only in male subjects. **Conclusion:** Preliminary results of an ongoing study corroborate previous findings of altered niacin sensitivity in first episode patients with schizophrenia. Findings are suggestive that altered niacin skin response might indicate a metabolic feature associated with the risk to develop schizophrenia, possibly more pronounced in men than in women.

S-027 Topic: 3
Cycles of disadvantage
Track: Therapy and intervention
*Chairperson: Klaus Schmeck, Universitätsklinik Ulm
Kinder- und Jugendpsychiatrie, Ulm, Germany,
klaus.schmeck@medizin.uni-ulm.de*

Cycles of disadvantage
*Klaus Schmeck, Universitätsklinik Ulm,
Kinder- und Jugendpsychiatrie, Ulm, Germany,
klaus.schmeck@medizin.uni-ulm.de*

In children and adolescents with psychiatric disorders, a longitudinal transmission of disorders over the generations is often encountered. This transmission is partly based on a genetic contribution from parents to off-springs. To a substantial part, however, it is due to the effects of disadvantageous living conditions that continue from generation to generation. In this symposium speakers will focus on the effects of different abnormal living conditions on behavioural and emotional problems of children and adolescents. Presented are (a) effects of an early intervention program to support adoptive parents, (b) effects of a preventive program with teenage mothers, (c) prevalence of psychiatric problems of adolescents living in residential care and the need for psychiatric and psychotherapeutic interventions in this setting (d) a longitudinal study using a new instrument to predict the course of juvenile delinquency. In all these living conditions, interventions are necessary to break the vicious cycle of disadvantage.

S-027-124 Topic: 50, 42
A longitudinal study of adopted children:
Early intervention in parent-child relationships
*Femmie Juffer, Leiden University, Child & Family Studies,
Leiden, Netherlands, juffer@fsw.leidenuniv.nl
Marinus H. van Ijzendoorn;
Marian J. Bakermans-Kranenburg*

Objective: Several studies found that adopted children present more behavior problems and are overrepresented in clinical and mental health services. In our study an early intervention was designed to support adoptive parents. We examined the effects of this intervention on disorganized infant attachment, as insecure disorganized attachment is a serious risk factor for later child psychopathology. **Methods:** In a randomized study involving 130 families with 6-months-old infants adopted from Sri Lanka, South Korea, and Colombia, two intervention programs based on attachment theory were tested. The study consisted of two subsamples: 90 families with a first (adopted) child, and 40 'mixed' families with birth children and a first adopted child. In the first intervention program, mothers were provided a perso-

nal book, and in the second program mothers received the same book and three home-based sessions of video feedback. The third (control) group did not receive intervention. The intervention programs aimed at enhancing parental sensitive responsiveness, with the ultimate goal of promoting secure infant-parent attachment relationships and infant competence. **Results:** The intervention with video feedback and the personal book resulted in enhanced maternal sensitive responsiveness (d = 0.65). Children of mothers who received this intervention were less likely to be classified as disorganized attached at the age of 12 months compared to their control counterparts (6% vs. 22%; d = 0.46). In the book-only group no effect on the number of infants with disorganized attachment classifications was found. Positive long-term effects of the video-feedback intervention were found in one subsample: adopted children in 'mixed' adoptive families presented fewer internalizing behavior problems, and adopted girls scored higher on ego-resiliency and social competence compared to controls at age 7. In the total sample, early parent-child relationship and parental sensitivity predicted adopted children's socio-emotional and cognitive development, and rate of behavior problems in middle childhood. **Conclusion:** A short-term video-feedback intervention in adoptive families in early childhood was effective in the domain of parent-child relationships. Early intervention in adoptive families may support parents and children and prevent later problems.

S-027-125 Topic: 41, 3
Secondary preventive intervention
in adolescent mothers and their newborn infants
*Ute Ziegenhain, Universitätsklinik Ulm,
Kinder- und Jugendpsychiatrie, Ulm, Germany,
ute.ziegenhain@medizin.uni-ulm.de
B. Derksen; R. Dreisörner*

Objective: Adolescent and single mothers and their infants are a high risk group. The accumulation and the interaction of multiple risk factors have an adverse effect on the quality of mother-infant interaction and are related to later behavioral problems. The study investigates the effects of attachment-based intervention on maternal sensitive behavior. In addition, the influence of the mother's attachment representation is related to the effectiveness of the intervention. Sample: 29 adolescents from child welfare institutions in Berlin were recruited when pregnant. Mean age was 17 (15–20). **Methods:** In a quasi-experimental-control design adolescent mothers and their infants received attachment-based and video-based intervention (n = 10). They were compared to a group of mothers who received intervention based on counselling (n = 5). The interventions repeatedly took place during the first three months of the infants' life. Three months after the interventions ended (age six months), both intervention-groups and a group of mothers without intervention (n = 14) were evaluated. Assessments utilized were the Ainsworth sensitivity scale (videotaped mother-infant interaction) and the Adult Attachment Interview (maternal attachment representation). **Results:** The sensitive behavior of mothers with attachment-based intervention eventually improved compared to the counselling-group and compared to the group with no intervention. In addition, the quality of the mothers' mental representation (dichotomized as moderate vs. extreme incoherent) influenced their sensitive behavior in interaction with the infant during the interventions, and up to three months later. **Conclusion:** Attachment based intervention seems to promote early infant-parent relationships. However, the effect of the intervention is significantly influenced by maternal representations. The success of interventions can be enhanced by systematically integrating the knowledge about maternal representation in the therapeutical work with parents.

S-027-126   Topic: 26

Prevalence of mental disorders among children and adolescents in a German residential care population

Marc Schmid, Universitätsklinikum Ulm,
Kinder-und Jugendpsychiatrie, Ulm, Germany
Lutz Goldbeck; Jakob Nützel; Jörg M. Fegert

Objective: Multiple risk factors for the development of mental disorders (e.g. abuse, neglect, divorce; genetic predisposition) are common in children and adolescents in residential care. In this study we assess the prevalence of behavioral and emotional symptoms and mental disorders in a German residential care population. Sample: This epidemiologic study takes place in 20 residential care institutions including about 691 children and adolescents (age 4–18 years, mean age 13.8 SD = 3.29). This sample comprises institutions of various sizes and therefore represents a good cross section of the whole "residential care situation" in Germany. **Methods:** A two-step design is performed. First, the children and adolescents and their residential caregivers answer a standard symptom checklist (CBCL/YSR Achenbach). For those participants scoring more than one standard deviation above the age- and gender-related mean of the German population reference groups, a standardized clinical examination is performed to confirm an ICD-10 diagnosis using the DISYPS-KJ (Diagnostik System für Psychische Störungen im Kindes und Jugendalter nach ICD-10 und DSM-IV). **Results:** The study population reaches high average scores in almost all scales and subscales of the CBCL and YSR, between 1 and 1.5 standard deviations above the mean of the normal control population (means Total-T-Score 64.36 (SD = 9.9) INT-T-Score 60.23 (SD = 9.9) EXT-T-Score 64.36 (SD = 11.89)). There is a high prevalence (over 50%) of mental disorders. The most frequent diagnoses are conduct disorder, ADHD with conduct disorder and dysthymia with high rates of comorbidity. **Conclusion:** Children and adolescents in residential care can be described as high-risk population. Multiple symptoms and comorbid disorders might indicate the risk to develop a personality disorder. Therapeutic options in cooperation between residential care institutions and child and adolescent psychiatry should be taken including appropriate diagnostic procedures, continued psychotherapy, staff counseling and/or medication.

S-027-127   Topic: 57, 42

Results of the 2 year follow-up of a 25 year prospective longitudinal study on delinquent adolescents

Daniel Gutschner, IFB-Institut für forensische,
Kinder- und Jugendpsychiatrie, Bern, Switzerland,
daniel.gutschner@ifkjb.ch

Objective: In this presentation we will discuss the results of the 2-year follow-up of our longitudinal study on delinquent adolescents. **Methods:** The adolescents had been referred to us by juvenile courts for assessment. The first as-

sessment was made in a multi-informant setting: Standardized tests for intelligence (Hamburg-Wechsler; CFT 20) and attention (FAIR), the Rey complexe figure and a list of other questionnaires (Achenbach CBCL, TRF, YSR; Giessen-Test self- and objective (teachers, parents) report; FAF) were used. Furthermore, structured interviews were held to gain information about socioeconomic data and psychopathology. At the second time of measurement (2 years later) the assessment on the same adolescents was made with questionnaires (Achenbach CBCL, TRF, YSR; Giessen-Test self- and objective (teachers, social worker, parents) report; JTCI, FAF and REF-F(m)) and a structured interview on socioeconomic data and psychopathology. **Results:** We assessed 87 juveniles, 87%males and 13% females in the ages of 12–20 years. We found positive associations between certain psychiatric disorders and delinquency. Furthermore, there seems to be an association between psychiatric disorder and recidivism but also between intervention measures and recidivism. We found also that objective reports from teachers or social workers are more reliable than the self reports or objective reports from parents. **Conclusion:** This results show that early assessment of conspicuous behaviour in juveniles, including objective reports by teachers or social workers, is very important. Also the choice of further intervention should be considered carefully and be in accord with the results of the psychological/psychiatrical report.

S-028   Topic: 45

Cultural and transcultural Issues in the diagnosis and treatment of children and adolescents in different countries

Chairperson: Martin Maldonado-Duran,
Family Service and Guidance Child Psychiatry, Topeka,
USA, maldo2000mor@aol.com

Cultural and transcultural issues in the diagnosis and treatment of children and adolescents in different countries

Martin Maldonado-Duran, Family Service and Guidance,
Child Psychiatry, Topeka, USA, maldo2000mor@aol.com
Manuel Fernandez Criado

Objective: Examination of differences between countries/cultural groups on prevalence, diagnostic criteria and cultural understanding of emotional/behavioral disorders and treatment in children. Analysis of recent cultural trends in evidence-based psychiatry and its consequences, particularly in psychopharmacological treatent. Finally, description of these factors in operation in a transcultural clinical setting dealing with immigrant children/families. **Methods:** Clinicians from three countries (France, US, Spain) review the relevant literature on the above topics. Differences in diagnosis and treatment approaches based on cultural beliefs, economic factors and pressures on child psychiatrists are described. Controversies surrounding psychopharmacological treatment of children are explored, particulary tendencies based on evidence-based medicine and the construction of children as a collection of symptoms. Data from a transcultural clinic in Paris, where immigrant children are treated examining the narratives of migration, transgenerational transmission of trauma and parental representations of their children. **Results:** There are important differences in the prevalence of a number of disturbances, owing to different diagnostic criteria, cultural factors leading to under-recognition of some disorders and overdiagnosis of others. Some can be understood as culture-bound (e.g. attention deficit disorder in the US). Cultural factors are also crucial in the use of pharmacological agents, owing to pressures on child psychiatrists for quick treatments, evidenced-based approaches to diagnosis and treatment and economic factors. Often the individual child is only understood with a simplistic "engineering approach" in treatment. The findings from the transcultural clinic illustrate the usefulness of such approach to diagnosis and intervention, taking culturally-based parental beliefs and preferences in the treatment of children. **Conclusion:** It is necessary for our discipline to continue focus on the individual child/family, and to examine culturally based factors (psychodynamic, economic, "therapeutic traditions") in diagnosis and treatment. Further comparisons between cultural groups are necessary to expand the view of children in their context and to provide a more comprehensive and culturally informed intervention strategy.

S-028-128   Topic: 7, 17
Psychodynamic considerations in the pharmacological treatment of children and adolescents
Manuel Fernández-Criado, Consulting Office, Dept. of Psychiatry, Madrid, Spain, fdezcriado@terra.es

Objective: To explore the psycho-cultural dimension in the pharmacological treatment of children from a review of the relevant scientific literature. Understand the psychocultural factors in operation when using pharmacological treatment with children. **Methods:** From a review of the relevant psychodynamic, psychocultural and pharmaocological literature we enumerate the main factors that affect decisions about whether the physician should recommend using medications, for what disorders and in what circumstances. We look at the question of pressures to prescribe and discuss the contribution of the individual child and family to the presenting situation. We consider the effect of "evidence-based" approaches on the understanding and treatment of the individual child. **Results:** The evidence-based approach tends to reduce at the child as a collection of symptoms and leads to a danger of using an "engineering approach" to the treatment of individual persons. There are intense cultural and economic pressures on psychiatrists to use pharmacological agents: this risks reducing the person to a "brain chemistry" entity. A hundred years of psychodynamic formulations on child-rearing, family relationships and psychic functioning of the child are increasingly being ignored or overlooked in this "assembly line" approach. **Conclusion:** The implications of these pressures are discussed and alternatives in education and clinical practice suggested.

S-028-129   Topic: 47, 11
Culturally based psychosocial interventions in immigrant families. Transmission and trauma
Felicia Heidenreich, Médecins sans Frontières, Hôpital Avicenne, Bobigny Cedex, France, felicia.heidenreich@avc.ap-hop-paris.fr
Marie Rose Moro

Objective: In clinical work with children and families we are more and more often confronted with families of cultures different of our own. Some have been in France for a long time, other have arrived just recently fleeing violence or poverty. **Methods:** We have developed a specific approach in dealing with cultural codations in psychotherapy. Through the elaboration of a narrative of the family's migration, we access representations of the the child and the difficulties encountered. Analyses of psychotherapeutic sessions allow for a better understanding of mecanisms involved in the evocation of traditional etiologies. **Results:** We find a discrepancy between the massive transmission of effects of traumatic experiences and a deficient transmission of protective cultural representations. **Conclusion:** The use of psychodynamic and anthropological elements in a complementarist approach on the basis of the work of Georges Devereux helps us to work in a coherent way in retelling a story about the disorder which makes sense to the family.

S-028-130   Topic: 86, 45
Cultural differences in the definition, prevalence, clinical approach and treatment of emotional-behavioral disturbances in children
Martin Maldonado-Duran, Family Service and Guidance, Child Psychiatry, Topeka, USA, maldo2000mor@aol.com
Charles Millhuff; Kirby Pope

Objective: To review the relevant literature about differences in definition, prevalence, conceptualization and intervention strategies with various emotional and behavioral disturbances in children. Analyze the clinical implications of this in various cultural contexts. **Methods:** Through a review of the available scientific literature, the authors explore differences in the prevalence of disorders like attention deficit hyperactivity, and other behavioral disturbances. We review available literature as to the use of pharmacological agents, emphasizing psychostimulants and antidepressants. **Results:** There are wide discrepancies on the prevalence of a number of disorders in children and adolescents reported from various countries. These discrepancies can be due to a different definition as well as to varying cultural expectations of what is normal and how children should behave. There are also differences in what intervention approaches are acceptable in various cultural contexts, industrialized societies favoring pharmacological agents and brief therapies. **Conclusion:** The cultural dimension is important in the definition of pathology. Similarly, we review differences in treatment strategies, for example with the use of psychopharmacological agents. We explore socioeconomical influences and pressures on clinicians to use brief strategies in industrialized countries.

S-029   Topic: 12
Antipsychotic induced body weight change and associated metabolic changes
Track: Therapy and intervention
Chairperson: Frank Theisen, Universitätsklinik Marburg Kinder- und Jugendpsychiatrie, Marburg, Germany, theisen@med.uni-marburg.de
Alan Apter, Schneider Childrens Medical Dept. of Psychiatry, Petah Tikva, Israel, eapter@clalit.org.il

Antipsychotic induced body weight change and associated metabolic changes
Frank Theisen, Universitätsklinik Marburg, Kinder- und Jugendpsychiatrie, Marburg, Germany, theisen@med.uni-marburg.de

After a brief introduction by the Chairman, Hubertus Himmerich will introduce into general possible mechanisms leading to weight gain including neurotransmitter and immunoendocrine systems and report on major consequences on health and treatment compliance. Alan Apter will present results of a clinical comparative study on weight gain under olanzapine, risperidone and haloperidol under consideration of caloric intake and energy expenditure. Yuval Bloch will consider severe metabolic derangements in patients treated with atypical antipsychotics and discuss therapeutic options and suggested guidelines. Michael Haberhausen will present recent results on weight changes and associated metabolic abnormalities including glucose dysregulation and dyslipidemias upon use of clozapine and olanzapine. Daniel Müller will give a brief introduction into general pharmacogenetic aspects which will be followed by a review of the literature with particular reference to recent candidate gene approaches related to antipsychotic-induced weight gain.

S-029-131   Topic: 12, 26
Epidemiology, possible mechanisms and consequences of psychopharmacologically induced weight gain

Hubertus Himmerich, Max-Planck-Institut für Psychiatrie, München, Germany, himmerich@mpipsykl.mpg.de
T. Kraus; A. Schuld; T. Pollmächter

Objective: Weight gain occurs during treatment with psychopharmacological drugs of different chemical structure and is an important problem when patients are treated with antidepressants, antipsychotics, or mood stabilizers. **Methods:** The clinical relevance of drug-induced weight changes is due to increased rates of morbidity and reduced treatment compliance. Also laboratory parameters change during psychopharmacologically induced weight gain. In the framework of a clinical study we could show that body mass index (BMI) changes from baseline to the end of treatment week five correlated significantly with ALAT and ASAT changes. **Results:** Regarding the underlying causes, the important role of neurotransmitter systems and in particular the blockade of serotonin and histamine receptors has been discussed since decades. Only recently, however, research has been started on the effects of psychotropic agents on neuroendocrine systems (leptin, ghrelin and TNF-alpha) involved in appetite and weight regulation. To assess whether carbamazepine and lithium have effects on weight and the circulating levels of leptin and TNF-alpha we weekly measured plasma levels of TNF-alpha, leptin and weight in patients receiving lithium or carbamazepine suffering from different psychiatric disorders during the first four weeks of treatment. Carbamazepine and lithium treatment lead to an increase of weight across four weeks, associated with a significant increase of TNF-alpha and its soluble receptors p55 and p75 within the plasma. These results support the notion that the activation of the TNF-alpha cytokine system is an early marker of weight gain induced by psychotropic agents. **Conclusion:** But according to our data, immunoendocrine parameters do not reliably predict weight changes in individual patients. In contrast, weight changes very early during psychopharmacological treatment significantly correlate with further weight development.

S-029-132   Topic: 12
Weight gain associated with antipsychotic medications in adolescent schizophrenia inpatients: Physiological mechanisms and risk factors

Alan Apter, Schneider Childrens Medical,
Dept. of Psychiatry, Petah Tikva, Israel, eapter@clalit.org.il
D. Gothelf; A. Brand-Gothelf; Gidi Ratzoni; L. Kikinzon;
A. Weizman

Objective: 1. To evaluate weight gain associated with olanzapine, risperidone and haloperidol treatment and its clinical risk factors in adolescent patients. 2. To study energy balance in olanzapine-treated patients. **Methods:** Weight and body mass index (BMI) of adolescents treated with olanzapine (n = 21), risperidone (n = 21) or haloperidol (n = 8) were prospectively monitored for the first 12 weeks of treatment. In addition, caloric intake and energy expenditure of 10 males treated with olanzapine were measured at baseline and after 4 weeks of treatment. **Results:** Average weight gain was higher for the olanzapine (7.2 kg) than for the risperidone (3.9 kg) and haloperidol (1.1 kg) groups. Gender (male), low concern about gaining weight (females), and low baseline BMI positively correlated with weight gain. The increase in BMI was due to increase caloric intake without change in diet composition. Olanzapine had no significant effect on resting energy expenditure. Activity energy expenditure was very low before and after treatment. **Conclusion:** Olanzapine and risperidone are associated with higher weight gain than that reported in adults. Olanzapine-induced weight gain is associated with general increased caloric intake.

S-029-133   Topic: 69, 12
Metabolic derangements during atypical antipsychotic therapy – a therapeutic dilemma

Yuval Bloch, Shalvatal Mental Health Center,
Child & Adolescent Outpatient, Hod-Hasharon, Israel,
blochy@netvision.net.il

During therapy with atypical antipsychotic agents, patients develop severe metabolic derangements including weight gain and disturbances in glucose and lipid metabolism. What are the therapeutic options? What is more hazardous – switching medication, or treating the newly evolved side effect? The importance of this dilemma can be highlighted, by a calculation made in the adult psychiatric literature. Fontaine and colleagues, using data from the Framingham Heart Study, indicate that in a population of 100,000 patients with schizophrenia, clozapine treatment could prevent approximately 492 deaths due to suicide but could cause an estimated 416 additional deaths because of coronary heart disease related to weight gain. The effects on self esteem and compliance must be weighed as well. We will review the relevant literature and present a prolonged follow-up of some of the cases. A discussion and suggested guidelines will be presented.

S-029-134   Topic: 34, 12
Alterations of glucose and lipid metabolism under treatment with atypical antipsychotics

Michael Haberhausen, Universitätsklinik Marburg,
Kinder- und Jugendpsychiatrie, Marburg, Germany,
haberhau@med.uni-marburg.de

Objective: Recent studies have demonstrated a high prevalence of hyperglycemia and dyslipidemia upon treatment with atypical antipsychotics in adult patients. The aim of this study was to investigate the effects of clozapine and olanzapine on lipid and glucose metabolism parameters in hospitalized adolescent patients with schizophrenia spectrum disorders over a period of 6 weeks. This young group of patients is not as frequently pretreated with diverse other antipsychotics including atypical drugs as adult patients. **Methods:** In this prospective longitudinal study of consecutively ascertained inpatients lipid and glucose metabolism parameters (cholesterol, triglycerides, HDL, LDL, VLDL and glucose) were assessed prior to and 1, 2, 4 and 6 weeks after initiation of clozapine or olanzapine treatment. Statistical analysis will include the absolute and relative changes in these parameters in relationship to baseline and a comparison between clozapine and olanzapine. **Results:** Preliminary data of this ongoing study (so far we included n=12 adolescent patients) show that a proportion of patients displays alterations in the investigated lipid and glucose metabolism parameters. **Conclusion:** Our preliminary findings suggest that adolescent patients treated with clozapine or olanzapine may be at risk to develop hyperglycemia and/or dyslipidemia.

S-029-135   Topic: 34, 12
Pharmacogenetics of antipsychotic-induced weight gain

Daniel Müller, University of Toronto, Dept. of Psychiatry, Toronto, Canada, daniel_mueller@camh.net

Objective: To investigate genetic variation in the neurotransmitter and appetite/energy/fat regulating system in antipsychotic induced weight gain. **Methods:** A population of 139 chronic schizophrenic patients deriving from two study-samples (A=80, B=59) and being mainly treated with clozapine were followed up for weight changes for up to 14 weeks. Over 20 genetic variants are currently being investigated in fourteen candidate genes (SNAP-25, COMT, MAO-A, ACE, 5-HT1, 5-HT2, DRD2, HRH2, GNB3, BDNF, TNF-alpha, leptin, CCK, and MC4-R). **Results:** Analyses with ANOVA revealed that the DdeI and MnlI polymorphisms of the SNAP-25 were associated with weight gain $(F[2, 125]=8.06, p <0.01;$ and $F[2, 125]=4.23, p=0.01)$. Similarly, the 2548A/G polymorphism of the leptin gene regulatory region was associated with weight gain, where patients with A/G or G/G genotype showed on average less weight gain $(F[2, 119]=3.38, p=0.04)$. Statistical trends were found with the GT(n) repeat and the Val66Met polymorphism of the BDNF gene $F[11, 62]=1.64, p=0.10$ and $F[2, 96]=3.15, p=0.05)$. **Conclusion:** Our preliminary results indicate that antipsychotic in-duced weight gain may depend on genetic variants that modulate neurotransmitter release through SNAP-25 associated presynaptic vesicle trafficking, energy balance through the MC4-R/BDNF axis and body fat regulation through leptin regulation. The association with leptin is particularly interesting as this result is in accordance with recent findings from an independent sample (Reynolds et al., 2003), thus lowering the likelihood of a false positive finding.

S-030   Topic: 3
Models of treatment and prevention II
Track: Therapy and intervention

Chairperson: John Fayyad, St. George Hospital Psychiatry and Psychology, Beirut, Lebanon, jfayyad@inco.com.lb

S-030-136   Topic: 25, 81
A song about mental retardation: Sexuality aspects

Altino Bessa Marques Filho, Medicine College FAMERP, Psychiatry and Psichology, São José do Rio Preto, SP, Brazil, hospitalbezerra@terra.com.br
Adolfo Bezerra de Menezes

Objective: Verify if main points of sexuality aspects, reported in verses, have didactic function, i.e., teach students and community members how a teenager boy with mental retardation could think about his limitations, handicaps, desires and expectations about relationships and sex. **Methods:** In a quality form and based in the knowledge from doing assistance to mental retarded people by the first author for seventeen years in a brazilian institution for children and teenagers whose IQ does not exceed 70; the same writer has also taught Psychopathology at local Medicine School since 1980 and he is a music composer too. Therefore, lyrics are a outcome of the three activities. **Results:** The adolescent narrates perceptions of his personal defectiveness, differences, slowness in confrontation with normal contemporaneous people; he can admit that is lacking something in his head as a explanation for the life events related before; to compensate the misinformation that majority of mental retarded carriers is submitted to, about important existences facts, enclosing relationships, love and sex, the adolescent-narrator just follow his impulses and try to disguise them with his unsatisfactory motor coordination, enjoying life on his own way, learning, right or wrong, from television, replacing parents and teachers. **Conclusion:** Popular song's words can be employed as a significative pedagogical recourse in classes and conferences; musical compositions reporting conspicuous aspects in Psychiatry of children and adolescents should be encouraged and published.

S-030-137   Topic: 25, 3
Managing pediatric mental disorders in primary care: A stepped collaborative care model

John Campo, Western Psychiatric Institute, Psychiatry, Pittsburgh, PA, USA, campojv@msx.upmc.edu
Sheree Shafer; Jennifer Strohm; Amanda Lucas; David Shaeffer; Harold Altman; Christine Gelachek

Objective: To describe a working model of pediatric mental health service delivery in a rural primary care practice using a stepped collaborative care model. **Methods:** Mental health (MH) triage and referral patterns in 2002 were examined for 31,352 office visits to a rural primary care practice with a multidisciplinary collaborative care team (CCT) that includes a nurse care manager (CM), a social worker, and a part-time pediatric psychiatrist that supports primary care clinicians (PCCs) in the management of common pediatric mental disorders. Children identified with behavioral health issues are triaged to three levels of care according to predetermined guidelines: routine services, on-site CCT services, and off-site specialty MH referral. **Results:** PCCs requested triage assistance during 789 primary care visits (2.5% of annual visits); 279 (35%) were first time MH contacts. Of these, 187 (67%) were triaged to routine services delivered by the PCC with CM support, 52 (19%) to on-site management by the CCT, 36 (13%) to specialty outpatient MH referral, and 4 (1%) to emergency psychiatric evaluation. Family compliance with a scheduled initial assessment and triage visit was 91%. Functional somatic symptoms were the reason for referral in 336 triage visits (43%). **Conclusion:** Enhanced primary care management of pediatric mental disorders using a stepped collaborative care model is feasible and has potential to improve access to MH services for children and adolescents in primary care medical settings. Future research to improve the quality of primary care based pediatric mental health services is needed.

S-030-138 Topic: 22, 58

Mental support team activities in Ikeda incident

Naoyasu Motomura, Osaka, Japan,
motomura@cc.osaka-kyoiku.ac.jp
Yozo Takino; Masahiro Iwakiri

Objective: On June 8, 2001, 23 children and teachers were killed or injured in Ikeda elementary school attached Osaka Kyoiku University. On that day the mental support team (MST) was promptly organized and the mental support activities for victims have started. The aim of this study was to clarify our activities. **Methods:** The victims were bereaved families, childrens parents and teachers. We showed our mental support activities chronologically and have checked the merits and demerits of our activities. **Results:** Mental support activity was 24-hour hotline, outreach program, free counseling for children and psycho-education for parents. These activities were assessed very useful for victims. However, as the safe or crisis management of elementary school was accused by parents or bereaved families and the needs for support was various among the victims, mental support for victims have been very complicated. **Conclusion:** As we do not have school crisis management organization in publicly or privately in Japan, we discussed the school crisis management organizations, which fit for Japanese school system.

S-030-139 Topic: 21, 70

LARS & LISA – a school-based universal primary prevention program of depressive symptoms in adolescents: A 12-month follow-up

Patrick Pössel, Universität Tübingen, Klinische Psychologie,
Tübingen, Germany, patrick.poessel@uni-tuebingen.de
Simone Seemann; Martin Hautzinger

Objective: Depressive disorders in adolescents are a widespread problem with extensive psychosocial consequences. Based on the "social information processing model of social competence" of Dodge (1993) a universal primary prevention program of depression among adolescents was developed and successfully evaluated in our research group. Beyond, a second study showed positive effects on conduct behaviour. Based on these results we explore the effects of LARS&LISA on a wide range of psychopathological symptoms. **Methods:** The LARS&LISA is a school-based cognitive-behavioral universal primary prevention program. It was administered once a week over a 10-week period in the context of regular school lessons. One session took two lessons, i.e., a total of 1.5 hours. During this time the control classes attended their usual lessons. Training classes were divided into two groups according to gender, because our pilot study has shown more cooperation between students when the genders were segregated. Each group was coached by one trainer and one co-trainer. Thus, each school class required a total of four trainers, who were either psychologists (M.A. level) or graduate students experienced in working with adolescents. **Results:** We were

able to show positive effects of LARS&LISA for the self- and teacher-reports of depression but not for conduct behaviour already within the pre-measurement 12-month follow-up comparison. **Conclusion:** LARS&LISA is a effective prevention program against self- and other-reported depressive symptoms but earlier founded positive effects on conduct behaviour are not replicable in this study.

S-030-140 Topic: 23, 41

RAMBO – the evaluation of a risk assessment and risk management program in a UK adolescent psychiatric secure inpatient unit

Theodore Mutale, St. Andrews Hospital, Lowther Adolescent Service, Northampton, United Kingdom, afrilion@aol.com

Objective: To evaluate the impact on antisocial, dangerous and self harming behaviour of a structured risk management program targetted at risk and protective factors identified by a semistructured risk assessment schedule. **Methods:** Consecutive mentally disordered young offenders (admissions and discharges) admitted to author's unit between 1998 and 2004 had a RAMBO (Risk Assessment and Management of Behavioural Outcomes) risk assessment schedule completed in the first and last weeks of admission. Risk and protective factors identified in the first week assessment were targeted by a structured group, family or individual manualised RAMBO program. The RAMBO program is essentially a responsive cognitive behavioural program. A Behavioural Monitoring Program organised independantly of the RAMBO program recorded all antisocial, dangerous or self harming behaviour in the 4 weeks leading up to admission and during the inpatient period. **Results:** The number of risk factors was significantly reduced and this decrease was associated with a significant reduction in antisocial, dangerous or self harming behaviour. At least 80% of previously severely disturbed young people were discharged safetly directly back into the community. **Conclusion:** A structured risk management program targeted at risk factors identified by a risk assessment schedule was an effective adjunct to managing mentally disordered young offenders.

S-030-141 Topic: 23, 41

Interpersonal problems of youth psychiatric inpatients during the course of therapy

Christian Haase, Universität Kiel,
Kinder- und Jugendpsychiatrie, Kiel, Germany,
ch.haase@kiju-psych.uni-kiel.de
Renate Kühl

Objective: The "Inventory of Interpersonal Problems" (IIP-C, Horowitz et al. 1994) was developed on the basis of interpersonal personality models to record subjective interpersonal problems of individuals. In psychotherapy research of adults the IIP-C is an important method of measurement in the evaluation of prognosis and the progress and results of treatment (Strauß, 1996). **Methods:** 90 adolescent inpatients were tested with the IIP-C. The sample consisted of patients with predominant internalising disorders and patients with Anorexia nervosa. Parallel to the self ratings the therapeutic teams evaluated the interpersonal problems of the patients with a from the IIP-C derived inventory (IIP-C-F). The measurement followed a pre post design. **Results:** For both questionnaires satisfactory reliability and validity scores were calculated. We present the results of a multivariate analysis of variance with repeated measurements. Changes during the course of treatment in reference to diagnostic criteria and success of therapy are described. The different progress for the clinical subgroups will be interpreted. Difference between self estimations and ratings of the ward can be discussed according to success of therapy and diagnosis: e.g. unsuccessfully treated adolescents are described by the team already at the beginning of treatment as more dominant, aggressive, quarrelsome and obstructive contrary to the self estimates of the patients. **Conclusion:** The results of the IIP-C and IIP-C-F are relevant for the indication, evaluation and prognosis of inpatient treatment.

S-031   Topic: 68
Substance related disorders
Chairperson: Oliver Bilke, Humboldt-Klinikum Kinder- und Jugendpsychiatrie, Berlin, Germany, oliver.bilke@vivantes.de

S-031-142   Topic: 68, 45
Pattern of substance abuse among the street children of Karachi
Majid Ali Abidi, Hamdard University Hospital, Dept. of Psychiatry, Karachi, Pakistan, majidabidi@hotmail.com
Shehla Raheem

Objective: Karachi is the largest city of Pakistan with 12 millions peoples living there which includes about 13 thousand street children spending their life on the streets of city. This study aims to find patterns of substances abused by these street children. **Methods:** The study includes those children who are living on street more than one year and matching the diagnostic criteria of substance related disorder according to DSM-IV. A structured questionnaire was applied to children on streets. This questionnaire includes demographic data, data regarding being street children and data regarding substances using by them. **Results:** Among those who fulfil the criteria of substance related disorder almost all were male children with 10–12 years as commonest age. Inhaling of fume of 'Samad Bond' (an adhesive chemical containing Ethanol) found to be the commonest substance of used followed by poly drug marijuana and heroin respectively. **Conclusion:** The data show that a large number of street children are victims of substances related disorder which is creating a number of psycho-social consequences. There is dire need to take serious measurement to this issue in country like Pakistan where literacy rate is very low with its unique politico-social environment.

S-031-143   Topic: 68, 23
A multidimensional implementation evaluation of a residential treatment center for adolescent substance abuse
Leyla Faw, National Clinical, Assessment Authority, London, United Kingdom, lfaw@ncaa.nhs.uk
Aaron Hogue; Howard Liddle

Objective: The study had three purposes: (1) to measure treatment implementation in a contemporary residential treatment center for adolescents with substance abuse problems; (2) to measure the variability in program implementation across clients, and (3) to perform exploratory analyses on the relation between treatment implementation and five important pre-treatment client variables (internalizing, externalizing, motivation for treatment, cooperation, and empathy. **Methods:** Subjects were 43 adolescents (mean age 15.4) enrolled in a residential treatment program for comorbid substance abuse in Miami, Florida. The sample was mostly Hispanic (72%) or African American (17%), and male (74%). Conduct disorder was comorbid in 84% of cases. To measure implementation, adherence to the prescribed parameters of weekly service provision was calculated for each adolescent, and the therapeutic milieu of the program was rated weekly by each adolescent. Statistical Process Control (SPC) was employed to measure variability in treatment implementation across clients. Pre-treatment client predictors of therapeutic milieu were analyzed using regression. **Results:** Adherence to the weekly parameters of service provision was moderate, while clients rated the milieu as highly therapeutic. SPC control charts revealed that implementation was consistent across clients. Both motivation for treatment and externalizing scores negatively predicted client ratings of therapeutic milieu ($r = -0.42$, $p = 0.07$; $r = -0.37$, $p = 0.09$; alpha $= 0.10$ to allow detection of trends). **Conclusion:** The finding that different treatment components were implemented with varying fidelity to the treatment model suggest that residential treatment implementation should be measured multi-dimensionally. Findings that program implementation was consistent across participants are the first of their kind, and have implications for future studies aiming to measure implementation in real time. The ability of pre-treatment externalizing and motivation scores to negatively predict adolescents' perceptions of therapeutic milieu suggests that (1) motivation may not function in the same way in adolescents as for adults and (2) externalizing problems may impact an adolescent's response to treatment.

S-031-144   Topic: 80, 23
Effectiveness of an inpatient treatment program for adolescents with developing personality disorders
Kirsten Catthoor, De Viersprong, Youth Department, Halsteren, Netherlands, kirsten.catthoor@deviersprong.nl
Joost Hutsebaut

Objective: In the field of research on adolescent psychiatry, research standards like standardised treatment packages or psychometrically sound research instruments have yet to be developed. Nevertheless, questions about the outcome of treatment being offered within a naturalistic setting remain highly relevant in today's development towards an evidence-based treatment. In this presentation we discuss the treatment approach at the adolescent ward of 'De Viersprong' and we offer the first results of a long term outcome research. The Youth Clinic of 'De Viersprong' is a highly specialised psychotherapeutic centre for the treatment of adolescents, aged between 14 and 19, with a developing personality disorder. The institute offers a long term inpatient treatment program which is multidisciplinary organised and guarded by the milieutherapy serving to establish a safe environment. An individually developed treatment plan, including six contextual levels and seven modes of expression, directs the treatment approach of each patient following different phases throughout treatment. **Methods:** In discussing the outcome results we rely on the data collected within the context of the nation wide STEP (Standard Evaluation Project). Measurements, including general complaints (SCL-90) and quality of life (EQ-5), take place at the start and end of treatment, and in follow-up after six and twelve months. **Results:** Results collected in the last three years show that the level of complaints at the start of treatment is high, but decreases significantly after treatment. Further on, this improvement shows to be very stable in time. Although there is a small increase in complaints within the first 6 months after the end of treatment, the overall improvement after 12 months reaches again the level at dismissing. The same pattern of results is being seen for quality of life. **Conclusion:** Further research will extend these findings by collecting data, more sensitive to basic personality changes thought to be effected by treatment, and by complementing individual measures with measures of family functioning.

S-031-145   Topic: 68, 16
Abuse liability assessment of atomoxetine in a drug-abusing population
Donald Jasinski, Johns Hopkins Bayview Medical, Center for Chemical Dependence, Baltimore, USA, drjasins@jhmi.edu
Douglas Faries; Rodney Moore; Albert J. Allen

Objective: Atomoxetine is a non-amphetamine approved to treat attention-deficit/hyperactivity disorder (ADHD) in children, adolescents, and adults. Abuse of methylphenidate and other amphetamines used to treat ADHD is common and is a recognized public health problem. This study examines the liability of atomoxetine to produce subjective effects that lead to abuse. **Methods:** Following consent and screening, 48 experienced, stimulant-preferring drug abusers on an inpatient unit were randomized and received double-blind, single doses of 8 treatments using a balanced Latin square design. Treatments were placebo, 90 mg methylphenidate, 60 mg phentermine, 100 and 200 mg desipramine, and 45, 90, and 180 mg atomoxetine. Forty subjects received all 8 doses. The Drug Rating Questionnaire-Subject (DRQS), and subscales of the Addiction Research Center Inventory (ARCI) were collected for 24 hours after each dose. Six-hour areas under the curve (AUC) were compared using analysis of variance (ANOVA) with Dunnett's correction. **Results:** Methylphenidate and phentermine produced amphetamine-like effects and euphoria, with significant scores on the DRQS liking scale, the MBG Scale (euphoria), and the Amphetamine and Benzedrine Group Scales (amphetamine-like effects). In contrast, no dose of desipramine or atomoxetine produced amphetamine-like subjective effects or euphoria as evidenced by lack of effect on these same scales. **Conclusion:** Atomoxetine is not a euphoriant and does not produce amphetamine-like subjective effects. Therefore, atomoxetine has significantly less abuse liability than methylphenidate (CSII) or phentermine (CSIV), and no greater abuse liability than desipramine or placebo. Overall, atomoxetine is judged to be a psychotropic, not liable to abuse like that of methylphenidate and other amphetamines. Funding Source: Research funded by Lilly Research Laboratories.

S-032   Topic: 7
Psychoanalytic/Psychodynamic treatment
Track: Therapy and intervention
Chairperson: Annette Streeck-Fischer, NLKH Tiefenbrunn Psychotherapie von Kindern, Rosdorf, Germany, annette.streeck@t-online.de

S-032-146   Topic: 7, 41
'Marilyn Manson or The Identification with Evil' – The imaginative psychotherapy of a severely physically ill adolescent
Renate Sannwald, Berlin, Germany, ruediger.sannwald@cducsu.de

Objective: How to achieve emotional restoration of a severely physically ill adolescent **Methods:** Imaginative Psychotherapy. **Results:** I intend to show how a 15 year-old adolescent tries to stabilize himself emotionally after a life-threatening physical illness in a type of identification with evil similar to the 'identification with the aggressor' that Anna Freud described. In a 30 hour short-time imaginative psychotherapy he succeeds to resolve this 'early defence mechanism' and to get a new grip on his own emotional resources. **Conclusion:** Imaginative psychotherapy is an excellent method in the treatment of emotional disorders resulting from severe physical illness.

S-032-147   Topic: 7, 11
Different ways of art therapy and their effects on diagnosis and therapy
Gottfried Maria Barth, University of Tübingen, Child a. Adolescent Psychiatry, Tübingen, Germany, gottfried.barth@uni-tuebingen.de
Christoph Schwarz; Monika Staigle; Gunther Klosinski

Objective: In child and adolescent psychiatry creative approaches are important ways of diagnosis and therapy. Very frequently art therapy is applied. There are very different ways in handling and interpretation of pictures. Some efforts are made in systematically evaluation and diagnosis depending discrimination of pictures. **Methods:** Different ways of art therapy and interpretation of pictures are demonstrated. Inpatient treatment in the department of child and adolescent psychiatry in Tübingen applies art therapy to nearly all adolescents. This integration of all severe disturbed patients needs an authoritative frame and careful interpretation. **Results:** It was possible for all patients to participate in art therapy. Most patients were engaged in this way of creative work. Interpretation could create artefacts in intensive inpatient therapy. Art therapy without verbal interpretation proved of value. Some basic forms of painting can be recognized depending on diagnoses and advance of therapy: regressive form, pseudo-maturation, high degree of symbolisation. Ways of systematically comprehending pictures can be developed. **Conclusion:** By an especial protection of patients and their pictures severe disturbed patients as well can be included in art therapy. Avoiding simple interpretations opens the possibility of integration art therapy in psychoanalytic conducted inpatient psychiatric treatment. Pictures show the developmental phase of patients. In this way art therapy can be used in a therapeutic and an evaluating perspective.

S-032-148   Topic: 11, 10
Taking care of adolescent inpatients' parents. Etablishing a therapeutic alliance between families and healthcare providers
Manh-Hiep Pham, Hop. Universitaire de Genève, Psychiatrie Enfant Adolescent, Chene-Bourg, Switzerland, manh.h.pham@hcuge.ch
Dario Balanzin; Joelle Materi

Objective: A positive therapeutic alliance between patient and therapist is a major determinant in therapeutic compliance and in the evolution of a treatment, often resulting in a favorable prognosis in many kinds of diseases. Moreover, the role and support of parents and family is particularly important in the well-being and outcome of young hospitalized patients. **Methods:** In order to sustain an effective therapy for the adolescent, we propose to take care of families as well, in a way that maintains a clear boundary between our various therapeutic functions. Allocating a resident as the main therapist for the patient, and the chief resident to work primarily with the family, separates these functions distinctly. **Results:** This creates a positive partnership with the parents, while fostering an individual therapeutic relationship with the adolescent. We discuss the benefits and drawbacks of separating these roles. **Conclusion:** It is therefore necessary to extend the notion of a therapeutic alliance to the parents and family, including them in a medical discussion and decision making for the benefit of their child's healthcare. There is not any existence of financial interest or other affiliation with a funding organization or with a commercial supporter of the session and/or provider of commercial services.

S-032-149 Topic: 7, 85
Psychotherapy with children who have disruptive disorders
Pia Eresund, NLPO, Child & Adolescent Psychiatry, Stockholm, Sweden, pia.eresund@bup.sll.se

Objective: Development of technique in child psychotherapy. **Methods:** Supportive expressive play psychotherapy, a psychodynamically based technique for children with conduct disorders, will be described and illustrated with clinical vignettes from a research project and also from ongoing therapies. **Results:** This technique was used with nine latency age boys in a clinical research project. The child therapists in the project worked simultaneously with the parents. All the boys had DSM IV diagnoses of either oppositional defiant disorder (ODD) or conduct disorder (CD) and in addition three boys had neuropsychiatric diagnoses (DAMP, ADHD). Progress was made in all the cases and after treatment only one boy still qualified for the criteria of ODD or CD. Play therapy worked best for those boys who did not have co-morbid neuropsychiatric disorders, but with the addition of more structure and pedagogic interventions it also worked well for one boy with ADHD. Collaborative meetings with teachers were associated with positive effects, especially on the behaviour at school. **Conclusion:** Process and outcome of supportive expressive psychotherapy should be evaluated on a broader scale.

S-032-150 Topic: 11, 41
Gestalt therapy of psychache in suicidal adolescents
Alexander Mokhovikov, Odessa National University, Dept. of Clinical Psychology, Odessa, Ukraine, alexm@te.net.ua

Objective: In suicidology unbearable psychological pain (psychache) is considered the common stimulus in suicidal behaviour, but its importance is not limited by that. In the field of internal phenomenology the appearance of psychache is indicative of an experience of value, for example a feeling, a need or a relationship. At the level of relations with other people psychache is a signal that tolerance of feelings, frustrated needs or real relationships has reached its limit. The objective of this investigation was to single out principal directions of phenomenological work in Ge-

stalt therapy of suicidal adolescents. **Methods:** Methods used were Gestalt therapy of 80 suicidal clients and qualitative process analysis of its results. **Results:** The following directions of phenomenological work were singled out: 1) correction of the phenomena of the actual suicidal vector in the client, and 2) therapeutic reconstruction of psychache in his/her life history (relieving the basic frustrated meta-needs). The actual suicidal vector is presented in the phenomena of introjection, projection, retroflexion and confluence. Therapeutic help in introjection consists in promoting a feeling in the client, that choice is possible for him/her, and in enhancing his/her awareness of the difference between…

S-032-151 Topic: 7
Dreams as important diagnostic means in psychotherapy of adolescents
Sandra Stankovic, Institute for Mental Health, Belgrade, Serbia and Montenegro, imz@imh.org.yu

The idea that one can learn about inner world of a client through free associations, fantasies, dreams, relationship they build with us in therapy with help of counter-transfer, is old as psychotherapy itself. Dreams not only represent inner realities of our clients but also what happens in therapeutic relationship. If these are adequately understood and interpreted they can be a reliable guide in therapy. It is my intention to point to their diagnostic importance within this work, through the presentation of dreams and the therapeutic process of an adolescent. Depending on the phase of psychotherapy in which these appear, with which anxieties they are colored, in which way they are understood by dreamer and therapist, dreams can be important diagnostic means that direct us further on in traveling through the world of adolescents.

S-033 Topic: 2
International perspectives on development of child mental health and disability policies in the aftermath of a disaster
Track: Therapy and intervention
Chairperson: Kerim Munir, Children's Hospital Boston Division of General Pediatrics, Boston, USA, kerim.munir@childrens.harvard.edu

International perspectives on development of child mental health and disability policies in the aftermath of a disaster
Kerim Munir, Children's Hospital Boston, Division of General Pediatrics, Boston, USA, kerim.munir@childrens.harvard.edu

Objective: We report on the international collaborative work of university centers in three different countries in providing technical advice for development of a national policy in child mental health and disability in the aftermath of a major disaster. **Methods:** Dr. Munir will describe the chronology of two major earthquakes in northwestern Turkey in 1999, UNICEF relief efforts, and the World Bank and Ministry of Health efforts for development of a national mental health policy. Dr. Erol will report on the findings of the Child Mental Health Survey funded by the UNDP, World Bank and the World Health Organization describing the distribution and "profile" of behavioral and emotional problems in a nationally representative sample of Turkish children. Dr. Cuhadaroglu will summarize the views of the Turkish Child Psychiatry Association with respect to national policy and future training needs. Dr. Hassiotis will incorporate the mental health needs of individuals with serious developmental and intellectual disabilities within varying national mental health policy frameworks. **Results:** The models described demonstrate significant improvements in capacities at the national level in mental health, disability and public health systems. **Conclusion:** Disasters not only highlight grave costs in terms of long-term psychological, social, and economic effects but represent opportunities for cross-national collaboration and sustainable change in mental health policy.

S-033-152   Topic: 9, 25

An opportunity and promise for the transformation of mental health services after two major earthquakes

Kerim Munir, Children's Hospital Boston,
Division of General Pediatrics, Boston, USA,
kerim.munir@childrens.harvard.edu

Objective: To describe an international and interdisciplinary collaborative work by university centers in three different countries for the development of national mental health and developmental disability policy in the aftermath of a major disaster. **Methods:** We report on the chronology of two major earthquakes that hit the northwestern industrial Marmara region of Turkey in which 25,000 people died, 45,000 were injured and half a million in immediate need of shelter. The limitation in available mental health services in the affected earthquake provinces reflected a major flaw in the organization of mental health services within primary and general health care. We review and discuss the youth-oriented mental health services in Turkey with respect to: (1) the pre-disaster organization of mental health services in the context of basic reforms in primary health care in 1961; (2) the post-disaster recovery plan for children launched by UNICEF with special reference to the psychosocial intervention project in schools in collaboration with the Ministry of National Education; (3) the post-disaster Marmara Earthquake Emergency Reconstruction (MEER) mental health policy project sponsored by the Ministry of Health and the World Bank ostensibly to address mental health needs equitably within the country's 81 disparate provinces; and (4) the post-disaster research capacity building efforts in child mental health and developmental disabilities sponsored by the Fogarty International Center and National Institute of Mental Health in collaboration with the Children's Hospital Boston, Harvard Medical School and leading university centers in Turkey. **Results:** The earthquake emergency magnified the country's pre-existing mental and public health problems. The post-disaster era has provided an opportunity for the Government, national professional associations and universities to strengthen the country's mental health services. As the country continues its transformation with an ever increasing pace of urbanization, public education, economic and constitutional reforms for European Union entry, there is a demand for better quality mental health services within general health care. **Conclusion:** Disasters highlight grave costs in terms of economic, social and psychological effects but represent important windows for political action and interdisciplinary and international partnerships.

S-033-153   Topic: 24

Mental health profile of Turkish children

Nese Erol, Ankara University, Dept. of Child Psychiatry,
Ankara, Turkey, erol@medicine.ankara.edu.tr

Objective: Carried out within the framework of "The Mental Health Survey of Turkey" to investigate the prevalence, distribution and characteristics of behavioral and emotional problems in a nationally representative sample of Turkish children 4–18 years of age as reported by their parents teachers and themselves. **Methods:** We conducted a cross-sectional population based survey using a self-weighted, equal probability sample. Data was collected from N = 3889 selected households sponsored by the General Directorate of Primary Health Care of Ministry of Health, through the collaboration of Child Psychiatry Department of Ankara University Medical Faculty and Hacettepe University Institute of Population Studies. Field staff and local süpervisors included social workers, psychologists, midwives, nurses and health educators. The internal consistency and test-retest reliability coefficient measures were satisfactory for all the checklists. **Results:** The prevalence of total problems were 10.7 % based on parent, 10.3 % based on teacher information and 10.2 % based on youth self reports. Although a considerable proportion of children are reported to have behavioural and emotional problems, very few children (0.2%) in the 4–18 age group were referred to mental health services. Although 5 % of the 11–18 age group reported perceived need for help for behavioural and emotional problems, only 0.3 % were referred. **Conclusion:** This is the first epidemiological study on childhood mental disorders using a national representative sample in Turkey. Although the youth constitute a major portion of the national population they received disproportionately inadequate care for their psychological suffering. Implications of the study in terms of the national mental health policy is discussed. There is a need to raise mental health consciousness among professionals, to identify mental health-related problems in childhood and adolescents; and to develop targeted outreach programs aimed at families and teachers of children with early behavioral and emotional problems. Research and capacity building programs sponsored by WHO, UN, Fogarty International Center/NIH, and EU agencies in collaboration with universities and national/international non-governmental organizations is urgently needed to sustain such efforts.

S-033-154   Topic: 2

Mental health policy for children and adolescents: Views of the Turkish child psychiatry and mental health association

Füsun Çuhadaroğlu Çetin, Hacettepe University,
Child & Adolescent Psychiatry, Ankara, Turkey,
fusunc@hacettepe.edu.tr

Objective: To present the salient views of the Turkish Child Psychiatry and Mental Health Association on the child and adolescent mental health plans, programs and policies within the national mental health policy framework sponsored by the Marmara Earthquake Emergency Reconstruction (MEER) project of the General Directorate of Health Care in the Ministry of Health. **Methods:** Children and adolescents need to be considered uniquely in the policy studies. About 40 percent of Turkey's population are children and adolescents in the 0–18 age group. The policy implications for care of children (ages 0–1, 2–3, 4–6, 7–11) and adolescents (ages 12–18) are discussed. **Results:** We describe a vision on the national mental health policy framework with respect to the: (1) organization and financing of services; (2) promotion of psychologically healthy development of youth within the context of preventive and public health services; (3) evaluation of needs and the barriers facing youth oriented services; (5) personnel and training needs; (6) establishment of service units in the community; (5) provision of diagnostic and treatment services; (6) integration of special education, rehabiliatation and inclusion services; (7) improvement of service quality; and (8) development of support systems and advocacy. **Conclusion:** As in many other developing regions, the national mental health policy framework needs to be based on the true conditions prevailing within a given country. For this purpose, data obtained from prior scientific research and from programs put into effect in countries with similar conditions ought be taken into considerartion. In recognising the facts pertaining to a given country, the mental health policy needs to develop a set of targeted plans and programs to address the public's urgent and long-term needs.

S-033-155   Topic: 2
Mental health needs of adolescents with intellectual disabilities (ID): Implications for policy development

Angela Hassiotis, University College London, Dept. of Psychiatry, London, United Kingdom, a.hassiotis@ucl.ac.uk

Objective: To address the mental health and developmental needs of adolescents with intellectual disability (ID) as a distinct group. To investigate the prevalence and presentation of mental health problems in adolescents with ID in a geographical catchment area and to explore the pathways to available care. **Methods:** A cross sectional survey of adolescents with ID (N = 75) 12–19 years old from specialist and community services. Structured interviews conducted with adolescents and their carers and where possible their teachers. A social and health care questionnaire. **Results:** Majority of subjects (42%) had severe/profound ID. 24% had a history of epilepsy/seizures and 10% cerebral palsy. 50.7% had a MH problem as reported by parents that increased to 66.7% following clinical assessment. The commonest ICD-10 diagnoses were conduct disorder (21.4%), atypical autism (16%) and hyperkinetic disorder (14.7%). There was moderate agreement between parental reports and clinical diagnoses (kappa=0.51). Significant negative correlations were found between subdomain scores of the Vineland Adaptive Behaviour Scale and the Developmental Behaviour Checklist. In terms of service utilisation, the majority of subjects (94.7%) were receiving health and social care. Almost half of all visits to General Practitioners in the past year were due to the parent seeking help for a subject's behavioural problem. 15% were receiving psychiatric medication. **Conclusion:** Prevalence of mental health problems in adolescents with ID are high. Adolescents with a diagnosis of autism and low adaptive skills are most at risk of comorbid mental disorders. Parents and primary health care providers need targeted mental health promotion and education to recognise problems early and to seek specialist help. Services should co-ordinate their referral and assessment processes better in order to meet current and future needs, particularly at the time of transition. Policy implications are discussed.

S-034   Topic: 6
Behavioural and family therapies

Track: Therapy and intervention

Chairperson: Martine Flament, University of Ottawa Inst. Mental Health Research, Ottawa, ON, Canada, mflament@rohcg.on.ca
Michael Scholz, Technische Universität Dresden Kinder- und Jugendpsychiatrie, Dresden, Germany, ki.jugendpsych@mailbox.tu-dresden.de

S-034-156   Topic: 10, 4
Changes in family relationships after Multifamily Therapy

Michael Scholz, Technische Universität Dresden, Kinder- und Jugendpsychiatrie, Dresden, Germany, ki.jugendpsych@mailbox.tu-dresden.de
Maud Rix; Franziska Nestler; Annegret Selisko

In controlled studies Eisler and Dare found family therapy to be more successful in the treatment of anorexia in adolescents than any other therapy. An even greater improvement can be reached by employing the multifamily therapy (MFT) due to group dynamics and individual effects reinforcing the effects of family therapy. In Dresden MFT has been used for treatment of eating disorders as well as emotional and behavior disorders in a day clinic setting since 1998. The significant better treatment results of family therapy in anorectic patients can be reproduced with other childhood disorders and can also be improved through use of MFT. MFT costs less and produces lower relapse rates than inpatient treatment. The main focus of treatment, using systemic approach, is enforcement and strengthening of specific coping strategies which help to overcome the symptomatology. Patient's and control families of all age groups differ in innerfamiliar emotional attachment and autonomy (Scholz, Rix, Nestler, Selisko). Results show disorder specific intrafamiliar relationship patterns in families with depressive (N = 33), behavior disordered (n = 36), and anorectic adolescents (n = 56) in comparison to a control group (n = 66). Changes in intrafamiliar relationships of patients receiving in-patient-treatment or MFT were compared. The most significant changes happen in MFT. In successfully treated families the structure of family relationship is coming close to normality (Thömke, 2004). Emotional connectedness and autonomy in families play an important role in the seriousness of psychiatric disorders and the outcome of therapy.

S-034-157   Topic: 10, 78
18 months results of a family therapy research in Anorexia Nervosa (AN)

Nathalie Godart, Institut Mutualiste Montsouris, Psychiatrie, Paris, France, nathalie.godart@imm.fr
Fabienne Perdereau; Zoé Rein; Florence Curt; Martine Flament; Philippe Jeammet

Objective: We have undertaken, in January 1999, a research project on the efficacy of the adjunction of family therapy in the treatment of anorexia nervosa. We will outline here this study and discuss the first results. There have been some evaluative treatment studies (1) about family therapy for anorexia nervosa in the literature but there has been none about combining family therapy to the other forms of treatment. The aims of our project are: – to assess the efficacy of combining family therapy to the usual treatment currently provide for Anorexia Nervosa, – to assess the evolution of the family functioning. Our hypotheses are – combining family therapy to the usual treatment in Anorexia Nervosa leads to better outcome for the patient in regard to the eating disorder symptoms, the other psychiatric symptoms, psychosocial adaptation and rapidity of recovery; – family functioning will be improved by the family therapy **Methods:** We include Anorexia Nervosa female in-patients at the end of their hospitalization in our department. The patients are randomized for the treatment group (usual treatment with family therapy or usual treatment without family therapy). We defined indicators of efficacy according to the literature. In summary these indicators are presence and severity of the eating disorder symptoms, other psychiatric symptoms, psychosocial adaptation, hospitalizations, rapidity of recovery, and family interactions. **Results:** We will describe here the results of this study.

S-034-158   Topic: 10, 40

Parenting: Support for families with pre-school children

Jane Akister, APU, Social Work, Cambridge,
United Kingdom, j.akister@apu.ac.uk

Objective: Home-Start is the UK's leading family support organisation. Our approach is simple. We provide trained, parent volunteers to help any parent, with at least one child under five who is finding it hard to cope. Established in 1973, Home-Start now works alongside 21,000 families and 48,000 children each year (www.home-start.org.uk). **Methods:** There is an increasing 'focus' on parenting by government and welfare providers. Home-start offers support to parents identified as 'at risk' in the parenting task. Services offered can range from support or therapeutic groups to a volunteer visiting scheme. Types of intervention offered to children and families are largely determined by the judgements of professionals' about what is best for them. This, small scale, study investigated service users views about the help they receive. **Results:** The study determines the concerns of parents using Home-Start and whether they differ from a community sample of parents with similar age children. **Conclusion:** A questionnaire survey of parents with some interviews was administered. Home-Start is viewed positively by over 80% of its users. There was marked preference for Parent Volunteers, to visit homes, over Parenting Groups. This paper will report on the findings and explore the implications for policy and service delivery in supporting parents with young children.

S-034-159   Topic: 6, 10

The cognitive-behavioral based parent-child interaction group for children with attention deficit with or without hyperactivity and their parents

Pei-Chin Peggy Lee, Chung Shan Medical University,
Dept. Occupational Therapy, Taichung, Taiwan,
peggy@csmu.edu.tw
Sho-Man Susan Tsai; Lai-Shiun Ho; Su-Chun Wu

Objective: The purpose of this study is to develop a treatment program of cognitive-behavioral therapy (CBT) for children with attention deficit with or without hyperactivity (AD or ADHD) and to preliminarily test its efficacy. The treatment program includes a child-parent interaction group and a parent group. **Methods:** Children diagnosed as AD or ADHD at the ages between 7 to 9 years old and their parents were included in this study. Four Taiwan developed scales for children with AD or ADHD (Hung, 2001) were used to measure changes in children's problematic behaviors and adaptive function in the home context and in the school context as evaluated by their parents and teachers. A Chinese version of Parenting Stress Index (Wong, 2003) was used to measure parental stress. These rating scales were administered prior to the group, one week after the group and two months after the group. Data were analyzed with ANOVA procedures using SPSS11.0 package. a level of 0.05 was set. **Results:** Eight children were included in this research. Their average age is 97.25 months (range: 86–108 months). A CBT based treatment manual was developed. This CBT program consists of ten treatment sessions. Each session includes a one-hour child-parent interaction group and a one-hour parent group. Data analysis found children's problem behavior and adaptive function in the home context and school context improved. Parents stress decreased. However, none of them reach statistical significance. A parent-initiated reading and support group was formed after the treatment groups ended. **Conclusion:** A CBT program of child-parent interaction group and parent group were developed for children with AD or ADHD and their parent. Preliminary results showed progress in children's adaptation and parental support, but didn't proved to be statistically significant. More treatment sessions and more sensitive measurement might be needed to detect treatment effect.

S-034-160   Topic: 6

Empirically-supported psychotherapies for children and adolescents: An expert review from the French National Institute of Health and Medical Research (Inserm)

Martine Flament, University of Ottawa, Inst. Mental Health Research, Ottawa, ON, Canada, mflament@rohcg.on.ca
Jacques Miermont; Joel Swenson; Mardjane Teherani;
Bruno Falissard; Jean Cottraux

Objective: In 2002, the Inserm assembled a group of experts to review the empirical support of efficacy, for the treatment of mental disorders, of three forms of psychotherapies: psychodynamic psychotherapies, cognitive behavioral therapies and family therapies. A publication resulted in 2004. The evidence collected regarding children and adolescents is presented. **Methods:** An independent search of scientific databases was conducted by the Inserm Collective Expertise Center, and each expert completed the retrieved bibliography in his/her area of expertise. Empirical evidence of efficacy was based on: (i) patient populations defined according to international diagnostic classifications (DSM, ICD); (ii) standardized outcome measures targeting symptoms or syndromes; (iii) efficacy of therapies established preferably by meta-analyses, or by randomized controlled trials, or by cohort studies/open trials. Two levels of evidence were defined: "well-established efficacy" and "probable efficacy". **Results:** For psychodynamic psychotherapies: 3 retrospective studies were retrieved on one cohort of children/adolescents, indicating general improvement and best outcome for emotional disorders and younger subjects. For cognitive-behavioral treatment: there is well-established efficacy for short-term treatment of depression of moderate severity in adolescents (2 meta-analyses) and short-term treatment of bulimia nervosa (4 meta-analyses); probable efficacy for anxiety disorders (6 controlled trials) and prevention of relapse in weight-restored anorexics (1 controlled study). Specific forms of family therapies have well-established efficacy for the treatment of autism (7 controlled studies), hyperactivity (5 controlled studies), conduct disorders (8 controlled studies), and there is possible efficacy of family therapy for anorexia nervosa (5 controlled studies). **Conclusion:** Empirical support for efficacy of specific psychotherapies for distinct psychiatric disorders of youth is still partial. More research is needed in this area. Consumers' information and clinicians' training need to be based on the scientific evidence for efficacy of available psychological treatments.

S-034-161 Topic: 10, 3
Recruitment in an indicated prevention program parental participation decisions

Julia Plück, Medizin. Universität zu Köln, Kinder- und Jugendpsychiatrie, Köln, Germany, julia.plueck@medizin.uni-koeln.de
Gabriele Brix; Inez Freund-Braier; Christopher Hautmann; Manfred Döpfner

Objective: Externalizing behavior problems are the most frequent ones in childhood. Additional problematic social circumstances make more severe disorders increase, requiring intensive professional help. As known from epidemiological surveys only a small part of those parents that describe problems in their child even in a high degree, look for such help in an active way. **Methods:** The efficacy of the indicated "Prevention Program for Externalizing Problem Behavior" (PEP) offers professional help for children at risk and is currently investigated in a randomized controlled trial funded by the German Research Foundation. It is focusing preschool children aged 3 to 6 are related to most closely: Their nurses in kindergarten and their parents. Therefore the process of recruitment of the sample includes several steps of parental choice concerning their participation. The training consists of 10 meetings and is based on well-established therapeutic methods in treatment of hyperactive and oppositional problem behavior (identifying specific problem situations, detecting ineffective reinforcement processes, practicing favorable strategies etc.). **Results:** Parents and kindergarten teachers of 2123 Children in public kindergartens in the City of Cologne completed a screening questionnaire selected from CBCL. The 85th percentile of a general externalizing-score was defined to indicate children at risk. Parents and kindergarten teachers of 160 children took part in a multidimensional assessment battery. The presentation focuses on the recruitment of the sample, analyses percentage of and reasons for dropout at different steps of the study including rates of participation during the training. **Conclusion:** Getting personal contact with the project is an important point of decision. Strategies for keeping the families in the study will be discussed.

S-035 Topic: 69
Schizophrenia and other psychotic disorders III

Track: Psychotic disorders

Chairperson: Robert Oades, Universitätsklinik Essen Kinder- und Jugendpsychiatrie, Essen, Germany, oades@uni-essen.de

S-035-162 Topic: 69, 41
Parameters of social functioning in adolescents at high risk for psychosis

Mirjam Simons-Sprong, University Medical Center, Child & Adolescent Psychiatry, Utrecht, Netherlands, m.sprong-2@psych.azu.nl
P.F. Schothorst; J.T. Swaab-Barneveld; Herman van Engeland

Objective: Abnormal social behavior and social cognitive deficits have been found in schizophrenic patients as well as in subjects at high risk for psychosis. However, little is known about the relationship between social cognition and social functioning and the role of social cognition in the development of psychosis. In this study parameters of social functioning are explored in subjects at high risk for psychosis and the predictive validity of these parameters for the transition to psychosis will be analyzed. **Methods:** 100 Ss at high risk for psychosis displaying putatively prodromal symptoms (i.e. brief, limited and intermittent psychotic symptoms, attenuated positive symptoms, basic symptoms and/or a combination of genetic risk and decline in general functioning) will be compared with 40 Ss displaying primarily social functioning and social information processing impairments (i.e. Multiple Complex Developmental Disorder) who are also considered at risk for psychosis. They will be compared on measures of social cognition and social functioning. Social cognitive measures include facial emotion recognition and mentalising abilities, the ability to recognize visual stimuli as social stimuli and general cognitive abilities. During a follow-up period of 2 years transition to psychosis and the evolution of social impairment will be monitored. **Results:** The design of the study, the preliminary results and conclusions on approximately 20 high risk and 20 MCDD SS will be presented.

S-035-163 Topic: 69, 36
Mismatch negativity (MMN) sources in the frontal and temporal lobes of adolescent patients with schizophrenia: an ERP- and MR-imaging study

Robert Oades, Universitätsklinik Essen, Kinder- und Jugendpsychiatrie, Essen, Germany, oades@uni-essen.de
Nele Wild-Wall; Stephanie Juran; Matthias Weisbrod; Eric Chen; Bernd Röpcke

Objective: MMN is an electrophysiological measure of automatic auditory change detection. A smaller MMN in patients with schizophrenia may reflect altered frontal activity (Oades et al. 1995 EEG Clin Neurophysiol 44, 428–438). We sought dipole sources in newly ill adolescent and older residual patients. **Methods:** Following our report on the coordinates for frontal and temporal lobe dipole-loci contributing to normal MMN (Jemel et al. 2002 Brain Topogr 15, 13–27) we replicated this result using brain electrical source analysis (BESA) and MR-images of the brain in healthy teenagers (mean age 17 y) and adults (mean age 34 y) and compared it with adolescent patients with a first episode of schizophrenia, and a group 15 years after the onset of schizophrenia in adolescence. **Results:** For MMN associated with a frequency deviant tone asymmetric loci in the superior-temporal and left anterior-cingulate gyri were replicated, while that in the right inferior-frontal gyrus moved to the mid-frontal border (residual variance

[RV] <1%). Healthy subjects showed maturational changes between the second and fourth decades that included a changed orientation of the left cingulate dipole and a more dorsomedial location of the right frontal dipole in older subjects. Patients showed a modest MMN reduction, a weaker left temporal lobe source but essentially similar loci (RV~1%). Discrete changes in the locus of left temporal and cingulate sources were illustrated by plotting volumes around the group solution for individual's data to 4% RV, with the radius illustrating the standard deviation of the distance to the solutions for other subjects' loci. The left temporal lobe source was marginally more medial in patients (5 mm, p<0.01), while the left cingulate was more rostral (10 mm, p<0.0001). **Conclusion:** The data show a degree of compensation of function, despite altered source locations in the left hemisphere that were evident even at onset in adolescence.

S-035-164   Topic: 69, 12
Novel antipsychotics in treatment of childhood onset schizophrenia – Case reports

Smiljka Popovic-Deusic, Institute for Mental Health, Belgrade, Serbia and Montenegro, imz@imh.org.yu
Olivera Aleksic; Milica Pejovic-Milovancevic

Objective: Childhood onset schizophrenia is very rare disorder, affecting children 50 times less than adults. Diagnostic criteria for childhood onset schizophrenia and adult schizophrenia are the same. There is no separate diagnostic category for children, but there is a clear distinction with pervasive developmental disorders. The rare opportunity to treat childhood onset schizophrenia at our Department (8 cases that met the diagnostic criteria for this specific disorders in last ten years) is the reason why we are presenting these case studies. **Methods:** To present 5 clinical cases of preschool boys with early childhood schizophrenia treated with new antipsychotic drugs (clozapine, risperidone). **Results:** We discuss and compare previous treatment schemes with classical antipsychotis (haloperidol, thirodazine) and experienced efficacy and side effects on children with novel antipsychotics. **Conclusion:** There is great evidence of the advantage of new antipsychotic drugs (clozapine, risperidone) as a first choice of therapeutic agents able to prevent many side effects and improve children's functioning.

S-035-165   Topic: 69
Basic symptoms in early onset psychosis

Franz Resch, Universität Heidelberg,
Kinder- und Jugendpsychiatrie, Heidelberg, Germany,
franz_resch@med.uni-heidelberg.de
Peter Parzer; Luise Poustka

Objective: Early detection and prevention has become a major topic in schizophrenia research. In adult samples, basic symptoms seem to present as a practicable clinical tool for early detection of schizophrenia. In this study, we examined the relevance of basic symptoms for psychiatric disorders in adolescent patients with special focus on early detection of psychosis. Furthermore we aimed to investigate the association of basic symptoms and personality traits, as both are influenced by biologically- based mechanisms and indicate vulnerability. **Methods:** From 90 adolescents, who were consecutive inpatients with adolescent psychiatric disorders in 1995 and 1996, 54 were followed up 4.7 years later. Patients were examined with the Bonn Scale for the Assessment of Basic Symptoms (BSABS) at t1

and t2 and the Junior Temperament and Character Inventory (JTCI). **Results:** None of the participants developed a psychotic disorder, although 50% had presented with high scores of basic symptoms at initial assessment. Indirect minus symptoms turned out to be the most valid predictor for a persisting psychiatric diagnosis. In addition, Indirect minus symptoms correlated significantly with the personality dimensions harm avoidance and self-directedness. **Conclusion:** In adolescents, basic symptoms in association with personality traits present as non-specific indicator of psychopathology rather than as an indicator of vulnerability for schizophrenia.

S-035-166   Topic: 69, 36
Auditory change detection sources in the brain: An ERP-Study in early-onset, adolescent patients at the outbreak of schizophrenia and 15 years later

Nele Wild-Wall, Universitätsklinikum Essen, Kinder- und Jugendpsychiatrie, Essen, Germany, nele@wild-wall.de
Stephanie Juran; Robert Oades; Matthias Weisbrod;
Eric Chen; Bernd Röpcke

Objective: More illness, poorer prognosis and impaired brain structure are reported for patients with an onset of schizophrenia in adolescence. Is this reflected in early stimulus processing? **Methods:** This study compares an electrophysiological measure of automatic, auditory attention-related function and its sources in the brain for 19 patients (17.5 years) at onset, and 17 patients 15 years after an early onset with age-matched healthy subjects. Mismatch Negativity (MMN), recorded from 32 sites during a simple visual vigilance task, was associated with a rare tone shorter than the standard. **Results:** Brain electrical source analysis (BESA) confirmed bilateral frontal and temporal lobe dipoles (Jemel et al. 2002 Brain Topogr 15, 13–27). Both patient groups showed a smaller MMN than the controls. There were several signs of illness progression in the older patient group: a) a visual vigilance decrement was only evident in the older patients, b) the left superior temporal source was weaker, c) the left cingulate source changed orientation, d) the right inferior frontal source was active later. **Conclusion:** This illness-related progression of a cognitive impairment is consistent with a poorer prognosis for patients with an onset of psychosis in adolescence, with a neurodevelopmental hypothesis, and that there may often be initial structural impairments in young patients in contrast to the more variable, sporadic changes in those with a later onset.

S-036   Topic: 39
Disorders of behavioral and emotional regulation in infancy: From research to clinical applications

Chairperson: Martin Maldonado-Duran,
Family Service and Guidance Child Psychiatry, Topeka,
USA, maldo2000mor@aol.com

Disorders of behavioral and emotional regulation in infancy: From research to clinical applications

Martin Maldonado-Duran, Family Service and Guidance,
Child Psychiatry, Topeka, USA, maldo2000mor@aol.com
Mechthilde Papousek; Sandra Maestro

Objective: To compare and contrast findings from a number of empirical studies of infants with behavioral and emotional dysregulation in the first three years of life. The comparisons include symptom patterns, characteristics of the relationship with primary caregivers, issues of sensory integration and diagnoses. Each group discusses the clinical implications of their findings particularly focusing on what they have learned regarding therapeutic interventions. **Methods:** Teams of researchers from four countries (Germany, Israel, Italy and the US) present their findings regarding the above-named categories, with a large number of infants/caregivers (900, 414, 45, 200) the data comprehend problems like excessive crying, feeding difficulties, sleeping disturbance, problems in sensory integration, language development and the capacity to relate to others, particularly primary caregivers. **Results:** The Munich group finds "regulatory difficulties" usually underlying problems in feeding, sleeping and excessive crying. Similar findings are obtained by the group in Topeka (US). These regulatory difficulties are met with caregiving practices that may or may not be suitable to help the baby become organized. The group from Israel finds difficulties in the parent/infant relationship in infants referred for feeding difficulties (less touch and less affectionate interactions). The group from Pisa presents the diagnostic boundaries between regulatory and more severe disturbances (multisystem developmental disorder). In general, the presence of emotional difficulties in caregivers adds to the difficulties in promoting a "good fit" with the infant's characteristics. **Conclusion:** The various groups provide recommendations on clinical interventions given those research findings. The importance of the caregiving environment is highlighted, in terms of helping the infant regulate states, cope with the environment and the challenges of sleeping, eating, and maintaining a state of contentment. Early detection and intervention are crucial in order to assist the baby and the caregivers with tools to promote a better developmental and adaptive path.

S-036-167   Topic: 39
Regulatory disturbances in infancy:
Clinical features and diagnostic boundaries,
implications for intervention

Martin Maldonado-Duran, Family Service and Guidance, Child Psychiatry, Topeka, USA, maldo2000mor@aol.com
Charles Millhuff

Objective: To analyze findings from two infant groups and study the clinical characteristics and relational (infant-caregiver) features of infants with regulatory disturbances. **Methods:** We compared the clinical and symptomatic features of referred infants (167) with 30 non-referred infants who were identified through a community survey (of 340 infants) who were identified as having feeding difficulties. In both samples we examine the presence of a "regulatory disorder" as well as the nature of the parent infant relationship in both groups. **Results:** In the referred group there is a high prevalence (over 60%) of regulatory disorder. In this group there was a prevalence of about 40% of relationship disorders. In the "feeding disturbance sample" we found also a high prevalence (80%) of regulatory disorders (both of the undersensitive and oversensitive types). Surprisingly, in this sample there was a very low prevalence of relationship disturbances between infant and primary caregiver. **Conclusion:** A distinctive feature of referred infants appears to be the perception by clinicians of problems in the parent infant relationship. This also seems to be a marker of how the parents cope with the unusual

sensitivities and demands of their infant. This has implications for clinical practice.

S-036-168   Topic: 39, 23
Characteristics of clinical-referred infants and parents: Implications for evaluation and treatment strategies in infant mental health

Mirelle Keren, Geha Mental Health Center, Infant Mental Health Unit, Petah-Tiqva, Israel, ofkeren@internet-zahav.net
Sam Tyano; Ruth Feldman

Objective: To characterize the infants and their parents who have been referred from the community for various reasons, to insert the implications of the findings into our evaluation and treatment approach, and to standardize our routine clinical work and create an on-going data base for determining treatments outcomes. **Methods:** Parent-infant feeding and play interactions of referred and matched non-referred dyads were videotaped and assessed clinically. The videotaped interactions were coded by independent coders. Clinicians made diagnoses based on the DC0-3 classification. **Results:** The comparison of referred parent-infants dyads interactions with non-referred ones showed significantly less optimal play and feeding interactions, regardless of the reasons for referral. The feeding situation elicited more negative interactive behaviors than the play situation, regardless of diagnoses. The distribution of DC 0-3 diagnoses of 414 infants and parents showed that 25% had no diagnosis on any of the 4 axes, 29.5% of the infants had both a Primary and a Relational diagnosis, and only 5.6% had a diagnosis on each of the 4 axes. Less than half (45%) of the infants received a Primary diagnosis, and 52% had a relational diagnosis. Mothers of feeding disordered infants showed less affectionate, proprioceptive, and unintentional touch. The infants in turn showed less affectionate touch, more negative touch, and more rejection and withdrawal from mother's touch. **Conclusion:** These findings had significant implications for our clinical work, such as the validation of the training we gave community nurses, the usefulness of the routine combined use of categorical and dimensional tools in a clinical setting, and the importance of the feeding interaction evaluation regardless of the reason for referral. These studies, added to our basic theoretical approach of integrating the nosological classification DC 0-3 with psychodynamic concepts, recently led us to the construction of a computerized clinical chart for infants ("PRINCE") that enables on-going data base and follow-up statistics.

S-036-169   Topic: 24, 40
Communicative-linguistic and behavioral profile in children with regulatory and multisystem developmental disorders

S. Maestro, Universita di Pisa, IRCCS Stella Maris, Pisa, Italy
A. Chilosi; A. Cesari; C. Pecini; L. Pfanner

Objective: To define diagnostic boundaries among 3 different clinic categories (RD, MSDD, and LT), by studying their psycholinguistic and behavioral profiles. **Methods:** Three groups of 15 children, aged between 20 and 36 months, diagnosed as RD or MSDD or LT, respectively, and selected among the children referred to our Division, were compared in relationship, linguistic and behavioural profile using specific instruments (see text).Each subject received a neurological and functional evaluation in order to make a diagnosis and to exclude an organic pathology. Linguistic evaluation was based on parental interview procedures, for collecting information on gestures repertoire and vocabulary size (MacArthur Inventory), and on direct observation, to evaluate the level of expressive and receptive grammar, with free speech samples and a Test of Early Verbal Comprehension (EVC). The parents of the children of each group were asked to compile the Child Behavior Checklist (1½–5 years) to evaluate the children behavioral profile. **Results:** Statistically significant difference was found as follows: 1) among the 3 groups at the receptive vocabulary and communicative gestures analysis; 2) between RD and MSDD groups and between the LT and MSDD ones, but not between the RD and LT ones, at spontaneous speech evaluation; 3) no significant difference was obtained at EVC test; 4) the CBCL differentiated significantly the 3 groups on the basis of Internalizing area and the Withdrawn subscale; 5) the discriminative analysis showed that receptive vocabulary and Withdrawn subscale predicted significantly the apparteneance to the 3 groups. **Conclusion:** The 3 clinical categories present different both communicative-linguistic and behavioral profiles.

S-037 Topic: 13, 70

SSRI in the treatment of depression in children and adolescents – a cause for concern? (Part I)

Track: Therapy and intervention

Chairperson: Jörg M. Fegert, Universität Ulm
Kinder- und Jugendpsychiatrie, Ulm, Germany,
joerg.fegert@medizin.uni-ulm.de
Laurence Greenhill, New York State Psychiatric Unit,
New York, NY, USA, larrylgreenhill@cs.com

SSRI in the treatment of depression in children and adolescents – a cause for concern?
(A two part symposium) – Part one
Jörg M. Fegert, Universität Ulm,
Kinder- und Jugendpsychiatrie, Ulm, Germany,
joerg.fegert@medizin.uni-ulm.de

In June 2003 the British regulatory agency issued a warning concerning the use of Paroxetine for the treatment of depression in children. In the course of the year the FDA informed about the risk assessment concerning 10 novel antidepressants. The British agency contraindicated Paroxetine and recommended contraindications for children for further SSRIs. The manufacturer of Venlafaxine issued a letter of warnings to doctors and pronounced a label upgrade. After an FDA Hearing on February 2nd 2004 the FDA asked for more control of these patients (adults or children) which are treated with SSRIs (especially at the beginning of treatment and at any change of dosage). Until now the public was not informed about the scientific results of a number of studies involving more than 4.000 children in placebo controlled trials with SSRIs. The double symposium with four lectures in the first part and the panel discussion in the second part, will inform finishing about this ongoing issue. The results of the panel discussion will be summarized by S. Kutcher and H. Remschmidt in practical recommendations for the treatment of depression in children and adolescents. These four lectures focus on different aspects, such as pharmacoepidemiology of SSRI use, pharmacodynamic, suicide risk and pharmacokinetics, as well as the results of published studies in children.

S-037-170 Topic: 13

SSRI use in children and adolescents in Europe and the United States: Cause for concern?
Jörg M. Fegert, Universität Ulm,
Kinder- und Jugendpsychiatrie, Ulm, Germany,
joerg.fegert@medizin.uni-ulm.de
K. Jahnsen; L. T. W. de Jong-van den Berg; J. M. Zito

Objective: The assessment report of the MHRA, June 4th 2003, reviewed three randomized clinical trials for the treatment of 7–18 year old depressed youths (n=748). Based on this report, paroxetine was contraindicated in the United Kingdom, other regulatory agencies announced warnings or have not yet reacted. The patent holder of venlafaxine announced a label upgrade for venlafaxine. The presentation gives a short summary about these developments and examines the variation in SSRI utilisation in youths from an international perspective and proposes strategies to clarify the issues. **Methods:** A cross-sectional analysis of administrative claims or records from three countries (United States, Netherlands and Germany) was undertaken. US data (n=125,383) were derived from a large Medicaid state program in a specific youth eligibility group most comparable to the European cohorts. Dutch data represent youth from the northern Netherlands captured in a pharmacy database (n=72,750), German data were derived from mainly middle income based single insurance program (n=334,520). **Results:** Total antidepressant prevalence was 3-fold greater in Dutch than in German youths (0.54% vs 0.16%) and 10-fold greater for the S-CHIP Medicaid-German comparison (1.6–0.16%). The SSRI subclass was 2,5 greater in US vs Dutch youths and 17 fold greater in US vs German youths. The difference is in part explained by the greater use of TCAs in German youths. Paroxetine accounted for approximately one-third of the SSRI use in Dutch and US youths but only 17% in Germany. **Conclusion:** SSRI warnings on use for depressed youths may be interpreted differently by country. Overall more than 4.000 children and adolescents have been included in clinical trials with SSRIs. Modern evidence-based child psychiatry is only possible if this database is published. If not, the SSRI debacle will likely lead to a credibility crisis for child and adolescent psychiatry.

S-037-171 Topic: 13

Selective serotonin reuptake inhibitors for the treatment of depression in 4100 children and adolescents
Laurence Greenhill, New York State, Psychiatric Unit,
New York, NY, USA, larrylgreenhill@cs.com
Kelly Posner; Anne Skrobala; Pablo Goldberg; Lisa Kotler

Objective: To review current United States Federal guidelines for the use of antidepressants in children and adolescents. **Methods:** 4100 children and adolescents in 4 published and 16 unpublished of selective serotonin reuptake inhibitors (SSRIs) treated for depression in pharmaceutical company randomized clinical trials have been evaluated by regulatory bodies in Europe and in the United States. **Results:** (1) Eight antidepressants were reviewed by the US FDA, including citalopram, sertraline, fluvoxamine, mirtazapine, nefazadone, paroxetine, sertraline, and venlafaxine and warnings issued about adverse events, including suicidal behavior, akithisia, and manic switching. (2) Only fluoxetine was found to have efficacy in the treatment of depression in children and adolescents. (3) Evaluation of safety data was hampered by inconsistent classification of adverse events. As a result, the data will be blinded and sent a panel of experts for blind review using pre-established criteria for what constitutes a suicidal event. (5) Wyeth pharmaceuticals has voluntarily included warnings in the label of venlafaxine against its use in children, and has stated it will no longer seek indications for psycho-pharmacological agents in this age range. **Conclusion:** Poor classification of safety events in the 20 trials require further classification by blinded experts for determination of adverse events. However, the enforced warnings have negatively impacted future research in pediatric psycho-pharmacology by the private pharmaceutical industry.

S-037-172   Topic: 13
The relevance of pharmacokinetic studies of antidepressants

Robert Findling, University Hospitals of Cleveland, Cleveland, OH, USA, robert.findling@uhhs.com

It is known that pharmacokinetics parameters of pharmacological agents may differ between children, adolescents, and adults. Until recently, pharmacokinetic studies of antidepressants in children and adolescents were not commonly performed. This may have been due to the impression that the intensive sampling strategies that are oftentimes a key component of this area of work might not be feasible in depressed young people. However, data from such studies can provide important information about how to develop evidence-based dosing strategies for psychotropic agents in children and adolescents. Thus, in the absence of such data, potentially important information about how to most rationally dose psychoactive drugs is not available when designing randomized, placebo-controlled efficacy trials. At present, there are published papers regarding the pharmacokinetics of several newer antidepressants in young people. These papers include data pertaining to first- and multiple-dose pharmacokinetics and describe the biodisposition of fluoxetine, sertraline, paroxetine, and nefazodone in children and adolescents. Review of these pharmacokinetics studies indicate that this area of research can provide important, clinically relevant information about how these agents might be most rationally administered to young people. The clinical and scientific relevance of these studies will be discussed. Based on the results of published papers, studies that examine antidepressant biodisposition can be developed and successfully completed in depressed children and adolescents. This avenue of work can provide the information necessary to develop evidence-based dosing strategies for antidepressants that could be employed within the context of randomized clinical trials.

S-037-173   Topic: 13
Antidepressant medication treatment and suicide risk in adolescents

Jan Buitelaar, University Medical Center, Psychiatry & Adolescent, Nijmegen, Netherlands, jb@psy.umcn.nl

Objective: There is both ongoing discussion about risks of increased suicidal thoughts associated with SSRI treatment of pediatric depression, as appreciation that increasing antidepressant medication treatment for adolescents may be linked to corresponding declines in suicide rates. **Methods:** This presentation will review evidence in support of the latter possibility that antidepressants prevent youth suicide. **Results:** Pharmaco-epidemiological studies (e.g. Olsson et al., Arch General Psychiatry, 2003) document a relationship between regional changes in antidepressant medication treatment and changes in suicide in adolescents from 1990 to 2000. **Conclusion:** This suggests that early recognition of pediatric depression and appropriate medication treatment may have preventive effects on adolescents suicide. The results of pediatric studies on the relationship between suicide risk and medication treatment will be compared to similar data in adults.

S-038   Topic: 84
Improving access and quality of care for Attention Deficit Hyperactivity Disorder (ADHD):
International public health perspectives
Track: ADHD

Chairperson: Regina Bussing,
University of Florida Dept. of Psychiatry, Gainesville, FL, USA, rbussing@psychiatry.ufl.edu

Improving access and quality of care for Attention Deficit Hyperactivity Disorder:
International public health perspectives

Regina Bussing, University of Florida, Dept. of Psychiatry, Gainesville, FL, USA, rbussing@psychiatry.ufl.edu

In many international communities Attention Deficit Hyperactivity Disorder (ADHD) is a child psychiatric disorder with significant public health implications, because it is common, has significant adverse effects on affected children, carries considerable risk for future development, and because it is potentially treatable. Prevalence estimates vary by country, with some suggesting that this reflects differences in diagnostic schemes more than true differences in child behavior or cross-cultural differences in professional perception. Rates of ADHD identification and intervention vary considerably by country, as does the role of primary care providers, schools, and parents in this process. This symposium brings together researchers from five countries with different health care systems, and their presentations will focus on unique challenges to improving access and quality of care for ADHD from a public health perspective. Dr. Bussing presents data from the United States addressing gender differences in access to ADHD interventions in the medical and school sectors from a longitudinal cohort study. Drs. Sayal presents data from the United Kingdom examining the pathways to care through primary care by focusing on parents' role as gatekeepers to specialist services for ADHD. Dr. Mitchell summarizes an Australian research effort to improve general practitioners' skills in diagnosing and managing ADHD, developed in response to limited numbers of mental health specialist resources and restrictions imposed on generalists' stimulant prescription in many parts of the country. Dr. Huss presents findings from a large European observational study, focusing on the effects of ADHD treatment on health system use. Dr. Gillberg will present data from his research in Sweden. A panel discussion followed by audience dialogue serves to highlight universal access issues in ADHD care as well as steps for improvement unique to specific health systems.

S-038-174 Topic: 84, 3

Pathways to treatment for girls with Attention Deficit Hyperactivity Disorder (ADHD): What drives inequitable access?

Regina Bussing, University of Florida, Dept. of Psychiatry, Gainesville, FL, USA, rbussing@psychiatry.ufl.edu

Objective: Community-based studies in the United States reported that girls might be significantly less likely to receive ADHD treatment than boys, even when controlling for symptom severity and comorbidity. Further research is needed to identify what determines pathways to care for girls with ADHD. **Methods:** Data are from an observational longitudinal cohort study of youth initially identified as high risk for ADHD during elementary school years. ADHD treatment is assessed over four time points and role of gender is examined as predictor of interventions, against the backdrop of three theoretical frameworks, Andersen's Behavioral Model, Kleinman's Explanatory Models, and Pescosolido's Network Episode Model. **Results:** Using Andersen's approach to adjust for other factors known to influence access to care, male gender emerged as a potent predictor of ADHD treatment (Odds Ratio OR 2.5; p < 0.0001). Parental explanatory models varied only minimally by gender, such that mothers were more likely to attribute ADHD symptoms to stressful life events for their daughters (OR 2.1; p < 0.05) and to genetic influences for their sons (OR 2.6; p < 0.01). No gender differences were ascertained for worries, preferred treatments and desired outcomes. Parents reported fewer help-seeking steps for girls than boys, with more reliance on family members or school professionals for advice than on health care professionals. Interventions for girls were more commonly provided through the lay care or school system than the health system for girls, while the latter was the leading source of intervention for boys. **Conclusion:** Cultural gender stereotypes shared by parents, school and health professionals and embedded in network transactions appear to influence pathways to ADHD care in the United States, beyond clinical need, and lower access to treatment for girls. Gender disparities in access to care for ADHD warrant further study to define the underlying mechanisms and to develop corrective measures.

S-038-175 Topic: 84, 3

Pathways to care in children at risk of Attention Deficit Hyperactivity Disorder (ADHD)

Kapil Sayal, Institute of Psychiatry, Dept. of Child Psychiatry, London, United Kingdom, k.sayal@iop.kcl.ac.uk

Objective: For children at risk of ADHD, to quantify the filters in the help-seeking pathway through primary care and to investigate factors influencing progress through each filter. **Methods:** An epidemiological study of 5–11 year olds in UK primary care. Pervasive hyperactivity (n = 127) was identified using parent and teacher SDQs. Parental interview informed about clinical factors and parental attitudes towards behaviour and services. Using logistic regression analysis, children who passed each filter (parental perception of problem, primary care attendance and general practitioner (GP) recognition of disorder) were compared with those who had not. **Results:** The strongest predictor of parental perception of problems was the actual and potential financial impact on either parent's work. Non-financial effects on the parent's working ability were also important. Primary care attendance was only associated with parental perception of the behaviour as problematic. However, GP recognition was related to both parent and child factors – parental request for referral and conduct problems. GP non-recognition was the main barrier in the pathway to care; following recognition most children were referred. **Conclusion:** The identification of barriers to help-seeking could reduce inequities in access to services. The effects of child behaviour problems on perceptions of carers are multi-dimensional. The impact of hyperactivity on families' finances is substantial. As most children at risk of ADHD attend primary care this provides an opportunity for recognition of those with a disorder and to enable access to effective treatment. Parents can be regarded as the main gatekeepers for access to specialist services. The recognition filter is particularly important since most recognised children do go on to be referred. This contrasts with adult psychiatric disorders where the referral filter is relatively impermeable.

S-038-176 Topic: 84, 19

Improving General Practitioner's ability to diagnose and manage Attention Deficit Hyperactivity Disorder in Australia

Geoffrey Mitchell, University of Queensland, School of Medicine, Herston, Australia, g.mitchell@sph.uq.edu.au

The prevalence of ADHD in Australian school aged children is 7.8%, with 1–2% of children on stimulant therapy. In most jurisdictions, General Practitioners (GPs) are not legally allowed to prescribe stimulants, which leads to an overload of scarce mental health resources. This presentation reports on two research initiatives that aim to make primary care management of ADHD more practicable. A survey of 399 GPs showed most would not attempt a formal diagnosis, but would refer on to specialist paediatricians or child psychiatrists. They expressed the need for means of assisting them in this task. We have developed and are currently planning validation of a diagnostic workbook that assists GPs in gathering the collateral information required for diagnosis. It also guides practitioners in the identification of the positive diagnostic features of the condition, as well as alternative diagnoses to be considered. We have also developed a method of testing the efficacy of stimulant therapy in children with established ADHD and on stable medication regimes, where the efficacy of treatment is in doubt. Individual Medication Effectiveness Tests (IMETs) are within-patient double blind, crossover, placebo controlled trial of stimulants vs placebo, or one stimulant vs another stimulant. These trials were carried out nation-wide by patient's primary physicians (GPs and paediatricians), and supervised centrally by phone. Seventy-four patients out of 90 who started completed 3 pairs of treatment periods. 29 were clear responders to the drug being tested against placebo, 28 were non-responders, and 12 were possible responders. 4 did better on dexamphetamine than methylphenidate, and 1 on methylphenidate than dexamphetamine (results of another one were unclear). Clinically useful information assisted decision-making for all participants. Medication management changed immediately after the IMET for 29 (39%). 39 (53%) stayed on the same medication, no data for 6 patients (8%). These two complementary pieces of research are developing methodologies to allow GPs to have the confidence to manage ADHD at a primary care level.

S-038-177 Topic: 84, 15
Stimulant treatment of ADHD: Effects on health system

Michael Huss, Charite Berlin,
Kinder- und Jugendpsychiatrie, Berlin, Germany,
michael.huss@charite.de
Barbara Högl; Renate Grimmlinger

Objective: Attention-Deficit-Hyperactivity Disorder (ADHD) has a substantial economic impact on health care systems. Stimulant treatment of children with ADHD is known to positive influence primary symptoms of ADHD as well as peer relations and the climate in the family. However, little is known about long-term medication effects on the use of health care and the educational systems. This large naturalistic European study focused on the effect of stimulant treatment on the developmental pathway of ADHD children with respect to academic achievement and health care use. **Methods:** Parental reports on the development of 2.022 children diagnosed with ADHD by paediatricians or child and adolescent psychiatrists with ADHD were gathered in Germany (n = 1664) and Austria (n = 358). 81% of the participants are boys. Mean age was 13.1 years (SD 4.7 years). Using chi-square statistics, stimulant treatment was related to global parameters of health care use and academic achievement. **Results:** The number of participants treated with stimulants significantly differed between Germany (79%) and Austria (52%) (Chi-Sqr 77, df = 1, p < 0.001) even though main symptoms of ADHD were more pronounced in the Austrian sample. As expected, severity of symptoms predicted the probability of stimulant treatment. In the German sample, stimulant treatment was the strongest predictor of school continuation without repeating classes. With respect to direct economic indices of health care use no effect was found for stimulant treatment. However, including indirect health care costs – especially long-term costs of substance use disorders – stimulant treatment seems to be associated with a better economic outcome. **Conclusion:** In contrast to controversies in public opinion, this naturalistic study indicates strong empirical support for academic benefits and lower health care costs in children with ADHD treated with stimulants.

S-039 Topic: 10, 47
Family assessment
in clinical and cross-cultural perspectives

Track: Therapy and intervention

Chairperson: Karl Christoph Käppler, Universität Zürich
Kinder- und Jugendpsychiatrie, Zürich, Switzerland,
kaeppler@kjpd.unizh.ch

Family assessment in clinical and cross-cultural perspectives

Karl Christoph Käppler, Universität Zürich,
Kinder- und Jugendpsychiatrie, Zürich, Switzerland,
kaeppler@kjpd.unizh.ch

The consensus referring to the relevance of family relations in developmental processes of individuals contrasts with the amount of empirical research already accomplished. This is true especially for studies including clinical and cross-cultural perspectives. The situation refers also to a lack of appropriate assessment instruments on family relations which are applicable as well for clinical as research purposes. Thus, in the symposium different approaches of family assessment procedures will be presented and findings from different clinical and trans-cultural studies are reported. The session will end with a reflection of future perspectives of family assessment and its different approaches.

S-039-178 Topic: 23
Quality of life in families of children with and without psychiatric disorders

Fritz Mattejat, Universitätsklinik Marburg,
Kinder- und Jugendpsychiatrie, Marburg, Germany,
mattejat@med.uni-marburg.de
Helmut Remschmidt

Objective: Research on quality of life aspects was neglected for a long time, especially in the field of child and adolescent psychiatry. This is due to the lack of adequate theoretical concepts as well as the lack of research instruments which are appropriate for the application in children and their families. **Methods:** For this reason the Inventory for the Assessment of the Quality of Life in Children and Adolescents (ILC, Mattejat & Remschmidt et al., 1998) was developed. It allows to differentiate various aspects of quality of life (in school, family, peer group, clinic etc.) and it is able to assess the quality of life from different perspectives (the child/adolescent itself, parents, therapist). In a recent study with the ILC two samples of families, one with children/adolescents suffering from psychiatric disorder and a non-clinical sample, were compared. **Results:** Results indicate remarkable differences of the two samples in relation to various quality of life dimensions. Thus, study findings support a strong association between quality of life and mental health status in children. **Conclusion:** As a consequence, quality of life aspects should be given more attention in intervention with these children and their families and should also be considered in treatment evaluation.

S-039-179 Topic: 48
Family cohesion and quality of life in Brazilian children

Maycoln M.L. Teodoro, Freiburg, Germany,
mlmteodoro@compuserve.de
Karl Christoph Käppler; Marimilia Rodrigues Lambertucci;
Sylvia Hiromi Oswald

Family cohesion can be seen as an important factor for the formation of family structures and for the mental healthy status of their members. However, there is a lack of empirical research about family cohesion and its relation to quality of life. The current study investigated both concepts in a sample of 47 middle-class Brazilian children (age 6–10, mean = 8.13, sd = 2.21). For each dimension two different instruments were applied: for the assessment of cohesion we used the Familiogram (Teodoro & Käppler, 2003), which is based on Moreno's Sociogram and modern network approaches from sociology, and the Family-System-Test (Gehring, 1998). For quality of life aspects the Inventory for the Assessment of the Quality of Life in Children and Adolescents (IQLC, Mattejat & Remschmidt et al., 1998) and the Quality of Life Evaluations Scale (AU-QUEI, Assumpção et al., 2000) were applicated. The sample was divided in three groups (low, middle and high quality of life) according to percentiles from IQLC and AUQUEI. Results did not show any influences by age or sex. Multivariate analyses revealed that children with high quality of life present higher scores of family cohesion than children with low quality of life according both instruments. Subsequent linear regressions analyses with different family sub-systems showed that cohesion among siblings is an important predictor for quality of life. Thus, the results of this study provide empirical support for a significant association between family relations and quality of life in children's own perspective.

S-039-180   Topic: 3, 52
Children living in poverty: A intervention program against violence in Brazilian families

Janine M. Dagnoni, Belo Horizonte, Brazil,
jmdagnoni@hotmail.com
M. I. Pinheiro; C. T. Heleno; R. Rothe-Neves; V. G. Haase;
A. Del Prette; Karl Christoph Käppler

Objective: Domestic violence is affecting more and more families and seems to become a serious social problem. Frequently intra-familiar violence is related to little knowledge of parents about strategies to deal with inappropriate behaviors of their children. Thus, a lot of parents are used to rely on coercion and aggression attempting to resolve intra-familiar conflicts. Using this perspective a parental training program (Barkley, 1997) was adapted for groups of parents of poor families in Belo Horizonte, the third largest city in Brazil. **Methods:** The program consists of eight steps which can be realized on average in ten sessions (with two week intervals). During the meetings the family relations, their influence on the behavior of the children and the parents themselves are discussed. The program emphasizes forms of interactions which are based on the understanding of the functional meaning of problems in the family context. At the same time the sessions offer the opportunity for a training in discriminating situations, giving sufficient attention, reinforce adequate behavior of the children by using motivational strategies helping to enhance socially competent behavior and to reduce socially not desirable ways of (inter-)acting. **Results:** In the ongoing project we attended 55 parents of lower social class families in several groups. The results of a preliminary evaluation (based on questionnaires) already show a significant decrease of problematic interactions in the parent-child relation from the viewpoint of the parents. **Conclusion:** Finally some future perspectives of dealing with violence phenomena in families are going to be discussed.

S-039-181   Topic: 45, 37
Family assessment in different cultural contexts – a comparison study in Brazil and Germany

Marimilia Rodrigues Lambertucci,
Universidade de Minas Gerais, Dept. of Psychology,
Belo Horizonte, Brazil, lambertuccimr@yahoo.com.br
J. L. Rodrigues; P. M. Freitas; C. A. P. Lourenco; H. C. W.
Carvalho; Maycoln M. L. Teodoro; Karl Christoph Käppler

Objective: The consensus referring to the relevance of family assessment contrasts with the amount of empirical research actually been done. This holds even more for studies including a cross-cultural perspective. The aim of the present study was to investigate basic dimensions of family structures in culturally different countries. **Methods:** Two recently developed devices in family assessment were applied. The FAST, in the tradition of sculpture techniques, consists of wooden figures which symbolize the family members and allow analysis of the two basic dimensions

of cohesion and power/hierarchy in family relations. Subjective representations of the family should be given three times by the participant: in normal daily life, during a conflict and as an ideal constellation of the family. The Family- Identification-Test (FIT) allows to describe different self-concepts (real, ideal ...) and concepts from others (parents, peers ...) by sorting 12 cards with attributes derived from common personality dimensions (intro-, extra-version; emotional stability/lability ...). The correlations between these concepts indicate identification patterns (i.e. "I'm like my mother", "I want to be like my father" ...). 400 Brazilian and 180 German children of both sexes varying between 8 and 18 years participated in the study. **Results:** The results show discrepancies in identification patterns between the two samples indicating a lower level of identification with the parents in the Brazilian group. In this group, however, the level of identification with persons in the social network outside the family (like best friend or teacher) is stronger compared to family members (also siblings). **Conclusion:** The findings will be discussed in terms of the significance and future development of family psychology and assessment.

S-039-182   Topic: 47, 84
Changes of family relations during treatment in ADHD children

Karl Christoph Käppler, Universität Zürich,
Kinder- und Jugendpsychiatrie, Zürich, Switzerland,
kaeppler@kjpd.unizh.ch
J. Baumeister; M. Weisenhorn; S. Stadelmann;
Maycoln M. L. Teodoro; S. H. Oswald; H. Ruder

Objective: Children with externalizing behaviors like ADHD (Attention Deficit Hyperactivity Disorder) can be seen as a good example for the involvement of the family context in individual development. In a specialized clinic for young ADHD patients and their parents we investigated the family relations during treatment using the Family-Identification-Test (FIT, Remschmidt & Mattejat, 1999) and the Family-System-Test (FAST, Gehring, 1998). **Methods:** With the FIT different self-concepts (real, ideal ...) and concepts of significant others (parents, siblings ...) can be described by sorting 12 cards with attributes derived from common personality dimensions (e.g. intro-/extraversion ...). The similarities between these concepts indicate identification patterns (i.e. "I am like my mother", "I want to be like my father" ...). The FAST, in the tradition of sculpture techniques, consists of wooden figures which symbolize the family members and allow analysis of the two basic dimensions of cohesion and power/hierarchy in family relations. The treatment process is sequentially structured: the patient and a family member enter the clinic three times for a one/two week period during 18 months. Each time the family assessment were applicated with the child and at least one parent. **Results:** From a sample of families (N=46) longitudinal data are available. The results demonstrate significant changes in some family variables which indicate improvement over time. **Conclusion:** The study demonstrates that family assessment procedures are able to reflect dynamic changes during treatment and can be useful in clinical practice with children and their families.

S-040   Topic: 81
Child and adolescent psychiatry interventions in the disability with particular regard to the mental retardation

Chairperson: Ernesto Caffo, University of Modena Dept. of Neuroscience, Modena, Italy, caffo@unimo.it

Child and adolescent psychiatry interventions in the disability with particular regard to the mental retardation

Ernesto Caffo, University of Modena, Dept. of Neuroscience, Modena, Italy, caffo@unimo.it

Our work describes the pertinence of the ICF – International Classification of Functioning, Disability and Health – in the description of the Mental Retardation state and underlines, furthermore, the limits of its application in child's field – incapacity for checking up the evolutional dimension – of body function and structure, activities and participation – that is so strong in this phase of life. Also it provides clinical exemplifications about how the Child and Adolescent Psychiatrist can operate with selective and different ways on every decisive factor for health state – applying medical and psychiatric knowledge for the treatment of the associated disorders; prescribing treatment plans fit to specific needs; revealing scientific knowledge to the families and the Community –. Moreover our work explains the differences between medical and social models of Disability according to the view of 'Independent Living' movement and claims a predominant role of the social model in the comprehension of Mental Retardation condition during childhood. At last it describes the family role in the promotion of the mental health in children with Disability and with Mental Retardation and shows the Community's role and underlines the importance of collaboration with others disciplines and sectors according to the perspective suggested by the World Health Organization.

S-040-183   Topic: 81
The use of ICF (International classification of functioning, disability and health) in mental retardation and its application limits in child psychiatry field

Myron Belfer, Harvard Medical School, Dept. of Social Medicine, Boston, MA, USA, myron-belfer@hms.harvard.edu

The ICF (International Classification of Functioning, Disability and Health) is an important document that embraces a number of concepts useful for child psychiatry. However, it is little recognized in the professional community of child psychiatry and thus an opportunity is lost for it to influence the lives of those children and adolescents cared for by child psychiatrists and their colleagues. In essence the ICF embraces a rights framework and urges the full participation of those with a wide range of disabilities including mental disabilities. ICF is not a classification of people, but rather a classification of health characteristics in the context of an individual's life. Thus, it is the interaction of environment with the individual's characteristics that are identified and addressed by the ICF: An illustration of the use and implications of the ICF will come from a discussion of autism.

S-040-184   Topic: 81, 24
Developmental psychopathology and mental retardation: Which indications can be derived for the assistance?

Ciro Ruggerini, University of Modena e Reggio Emilia, Modena, Italy, ruggerini.ciro@unimore.it Stefania Vicini; Ernesto Caffo

Objective: This report summarizes a part of the studies conducted by our Department on the variations in the quality of the adaptation of the people with Mental Retardation during their lifetime; it points out a conceptual frame (the Developmental Psychopathology) which can give meaning to whole the data as well indications for the organization of the assistance. **Methods:** a) survey on the adult disabled person: 483 people (age 15–65); in 70% of the cases there is a presence of factors interfering with the quality of life of biological or environmental nature; b) study of single life histories: 2 people with Mild MR (age 40–60); variations in the quality of life are possible at any phase of their cycle of life; 9 people with Moderate or Severe MR (age 18–44) residents; each history has 2 to 5 moments with strong discontinuity of the quality of life; c) study of the effects of the introduction of guide-lines in the clinical practice: 28 patients (age 15–46) afferent in the psychiatric clinic (admittance or ambulatory); frequent modification of the classification of the MR – 20 cases out of 28 –; frequent modification of the Dual Diagnosis – confirmed only in 13 cases out of 33 – with improvement of the therapeutic drug's efficacy; d) study on the rationalization of the psychotropic drug's use; 50 subjects with Severe and Profound MR residents (age 15–52); in a five-year period a part of the subjects has stopped the assumption of neuroleptics – 9 cases out of 30 and/or of benzodiazepines – 7 cases on 16 –; e) study of 10 "critical cases" followed by a Territorial Service of Child and Adolescent Psychiatry (age 4–18); it is possible to specify the factors - partly modifiable which make the assistance critical. **Conclusion:** The MR is an existential condition in which the quality of the adaptation is strongly conditioned, in every age, by the balance between the factors of vulnerability and protection; the data of the research indicate medical, psycho-educational and social nature of these factors as well as the mechanism through which they acts. Psychiatry can contribute to the activation of factors of protection at different levels: cultural – diffusion of concepts that underline the possibility of development in every age of the life –; technical the use of diagnostic devices suitable for the individualization of the Dual Diagnosis –; organizational – realization of assistance treatment that continues, in coherent way, in the various phases of the life cycle.

S-040-186   Topic: 81
The necessity to change the child and adolescent psychiatrist's role in the care of patients with mental retardation

Enrico Pupulin, University of Modena e, Reggio Emilia, Modena, Italy, penrico@aol.com

According with the OMS global report on "Innovative care for chronic conditions" and the rehabilitation based on the community, there is the need to change the Child and Adolescent's Psychiatrist role concerning patients with Mental Retardation. Although in order to have the best approach to this kind of problems it is claimed the importance of the Community's role and it is hopeful that there should be in the future the collaboration with others disciplines and sectors according to parents will.

S-040-187   Topic: 2
The role of child psychiatrists: Clinicians and/or mediators?
Antonio Guidi, Italy

The goal of child psychiatry is not only providing diagnosis, support and care to children and adolescents who find themselves in difficult situations but also activating networks between family, school, hospital and local agencies. This latter role is particularly carried on in the interventions on disability. In this field, even if family and school played a fundamental role, all agencies are involved. The child psychiatrist plays, inside his team, the role of mediator. Along with the difficult role of finding the right diagnosis and rehabilitation, often complicated by the "ambiguity" of the syndrome, the child and adolescent psychiatrist has to promote effective actions to remove prejudices and stigma strongly connected to mental retardation. This means to activate a complex cultural action, often through autonomous and personal means. This presentation wants to underline and discuss the critical points which characterize this route.

S-041   Topic: 39, 24
WAIMH Symposium on Infant Psychopathology
Chairperson: Massimo Ammaniti, Univ. Roma La Sapienza Psicologia Dinamica e Clinica, Rome, Italy, maammani@tin.it

WAIMH Symposium on Infant Psychopathology
Massimo Ammaniti, Univ. Roma La Sapienza, Psicologia Dinamica e Clinica, Rome, Italy, maammani@tin.it

The topic of the Symposium deals with the structuring influence of parents-infant interactions not only in the normative infant development but also in the risk and psychopathological development. In the Symposium the different presentations will give an articulated picture of the research in this fields.

S-041-188   Topic: 39, 24, 48
Mother-infant emotional resonance
Massimo Ammaniti, Univ. Roma La Sapienza, Psicologia Dinamica e Clinica, Rome, Italy, maammani@tin.it

Objective: In the last years the emotional communication (Tronick) has received an increasing value in the clinical field (Kouth; Modell) and in the infant research with as evidenced the central role of emotional exchange between mother and infant in the first year of life. **Methods:** More recently the neurobiological research has given a further support to these observations through the discovery of mirror neurons, which have a great importance in imitation and emotional resonance. **Results:** This evidence has a central importance in the development of the child especially in the first year of life but also in maternal risk situations. **Conclusion:** In maternal risk situations it can be evidenced a difficulty in mirroring and containing the infant's emotional expressions of distress.

S-041-189   Topic: 39, 24, 48
The effect of a primary care intervention on mother-infant interaction
Kaija Puura, Tampere University Hospital, Dept. of Child Psychiatry, Tampere, Finland, kaija.puura@pshp.fi
Tuula Tamminen; Mirjami Mäntymaa; Ilona Luoma

Objective: To evaluate the effect of a primary care intervention on mother-infant interaction. **Methods:** 165 healthy mother-infant dyads were asked to participate in a comparative, prospective study. For the study 15 well-baby clinic nurses, trained in relationship skills and in supporting early parent-infant interaction, recruited mothers to form the Intervention Group (n = 93). Twelve nurses without additional training recruited mothers for the Comparison Group (n = 72). The mother-infant dyads were assessed at two months with the HOME observation method and a 5 minute period of their interaction was videotaped. The Intervention Group nurses then focused on supporting positive early mother-infant interaction during the follow-up period of two years, while the Comparison Group worked as they usually would. Outcome assessment to all mother-infant dyads was done at 24 months. **Results:** Compared to the Comparison Group the Intervention Group mothers were initially significantly less responsive to their infants (Mann-Whitney, p = 0.02), and had lower total scores in the HOME (Mann-Whitney, p = 0.01). No differences were found between the Groups in the videotaped interaction analysed with the Global Rating Scale Method. In the outcome assessment no differences were found between Intervention and Comparison Groups in any of the HOME scores. In the Intervention Group 80% of mothers who initially had low total scores in the HOME, scored higher in the outcome assessment. In the Comparison Group 40% of mothers who initially had low total scores scored higher in the outcome assessment. No significant differences were found in the analyses of 5 minute videotaped interaction. **Conclusion:** The intervention helped mothers initially poor in maintaining positive mother-infant interaction to become more responsive. In this study short observation periods did not spot mothers with good interaction skills but poor ability to maintain positive interaction with the infant.

S-041-190   Topic: 39, 24, 48
Parental capacities for triadic relationships during pregnancy: Early predictors of children's behavioral and representational functioning at preschool age
Kai von Klitzing, Universität Basel, Kinder- und Jugendpsychiatrie, Basel, Switzerland, kai.vonklitzing@unibas.ch

Objective: There is a lack of longitudinal research linking the qualities of early family relationships with psychosocial strengths and psychotpathological symptoms of the children. This paper elaborates the concept of the parental capacity for triadic relationships (father–mother–child) and presents a longitudinal study which links parental triadic capacities, assessed before the birth of the child, with the development of behavioral and representational systems in the child until preschool age. **Methods:** 80 parental couples were given an intensive psychodynamic interview during their first pregnancy, to assess how they anticipated their future parenthood and their relationships as threesomes (mother–father–child). **Results:** The triadic capacity was defined as the capacity of mothers and fathers to anticipate their family relationships their family relationships without excluding either themselves or their partners from the relationship with the infant. **Conclusion:** Three and five years later, the representational and behavioral functioning of their children were assessed in depth, using parent interviews (RABI), play observations (FEAS), child narrative interviews (MSSB), and behavior ratings.

S-041-191 Topic: 39, 24, 48
Specifying the role of touch in infant feeding disorders: Maternal, child and environmental correlates

Mirelle Keren, Geha Mental Health Center, Infant Mental Health Unit, Petah-Tiqva, Israel, ofkeren@internet-zahav.net
Ruth Feldman; Orna Rosvald; Sam Tyano

Objective: To specify the role of touch in infant feeding disorder. **Methods:** Children (9–34 months) diagnosed with feeding disorders (FD: n = 20), other primary disorders (OD: n = 27) and case-matched controls (MC: n = 47) were observed in mother-child play and feeding sessions and the home environment was assessed. Microanalysis detected touch patterns, response to partner's touch, and proximity position at play. Relational behaviors were coded during feeding. **Results:** Compared to OD and MC, mothers of FD showed less affectionate, proprioceptive, and unintentional touch. FD children showed less affectionate touch, more negative touch, and more rejection and withdrawal from mother's touch. Mothers responded instrumentally or negatively to child touch and positioned children more often out of arms' reach (p < 0.05). FD children exhibited more withdrawal during feeding (p < 0.001) and the home environment was less optimal (p < 0.05). Feeding efficacy was predicted by mother-child touch, reduced maternal depression and intrusiveness, and lower child withdrawal and difficult temperament (R2 = 0.45, p < 0.001). **Conclusion:** Proximity and touch are especially disturbed in cases feeding disorder, suggesting fundamental difficulties of attachment. Mothers provide less touch that supports growth and children demonstrate signs of touch aversion. Touch patterns may serve as risk indicators of potential growth failure. Key Words: Feeding Disorders, DC 0-3, Touch, Mother-Infant Relationship, HOME.

S-042 Topic: 57
EFCAP Symposium: Diagnosis and treatment

Chairperson: Hans-Ludwig Kröber,
Charite Berlin,
Inst. für forens. Psychiatrie, Berlin, Germany,
hans-ludwig.kroeber@charite.de

Diagnosis and treatment

Hans-Ludwig Kröber, Charite Berlin,
Inst. für forens. Psychiatrie, Berlin, Germany,
hans-ludwig.kroeber@charite.de

Diagnosis and treatment of juvenile delinquency and several aspects of antisocial behaviour will be shown and elaborated from various perspectives. Especially the forensic assessment and treatment for juvenile sex offenders with normal intelligence and learning disabilities will be described. The results of an epidemiological study on antisocial behaviour of youth and some gender differences will be presented. On the basis of a case study, interesting aspects of a fire setting female patient will be interpreted.

Priority is given to practical issues and the translation of scientifically insights into practice.

S-042-192 Topic: 57, 96
Forensic treatment of a female pyromanic/fire setter

A. Stöver, Germany, P. Proske; Rainer Semmelbeck;
Oliver Bilke

Objective: The patient grew up with her two younger siblings and her mother. The unsteadiness of her mother brought about an early undertaking of responsibility for her siblings that led to growing tensions between family members. With her puberty the first apparent problems outside her family occurred – leading to school changes, repetition of classes and drug abuse. She became victim to several sexual abuses by adolescents. This fact and three suicide attempts in 2002/2003 resulted in outpatient treatment in adolescent psychiatry. The 18 assaults occurred between September 2002 and March 2003. **Methods:** The cognitive-behavioural and problem-solving therapy is planned specific to the disorder and pathology. When assuming a developing emotionally unstable personality disorder the main goals of treatment are the self-perception of emotions and self-regulation as well as the interpersonal behaviour – using parts of M. Linehans manuals. A further integral part of daily work and treatment of the patient is the experience of constant pedagogic and therapeutic relations. The explicit therapy of the chronic post-traumatic stress disorder is not yet the intention of the patient. Elements of trauma therapy would be possible for the future. In regard to a pharmacological support the patient feels very ambivalent, so that the current setting includes only sedative pharmacotherapy on demand. **Conclusion:** The successful treatment of this patient necessitates a long-termed planning that has to include the further clarification and settlement of offences. Currently no direct correlation of psychiatric disorders and offences are being observed, so that the previous therapy strategy is unchanged. The case of a 17 year old female patient who is being treated in a psychiatric clinic since April 2003 for fire setting and violence against property.

S-042-193 Topic: 85, 41
Sick girls – bad boys. Gender differences in antisocial behaviour of youth

Ulrich Preuss, Universitätsklinik Bern,
Kinder- und Jugendpsychiatrie, Bern, Switzerland,
ulrich.preuss@kjp.unibe.ch
Marc Walther; Daniel Gutschner; Matthias Schmelzle;
Monika Egli-Alge

Objective: To review current literature on gender related differences of antisocial behaviour in underage individuals in youth. **Methods:** Based on a medline and psylit and psy-index search studies were compiled to give information about the current body of knowledge in the forensic domain of gender differences. **Results:** The available literature on gender differences is restricted. A small number of study approaches are responsible for a larger number of studies, e.g. the Dunedin longitudinal study on conduct disorder, delinquency and violence. It is evident that the majority of delinquency is seen in young men while girls do not show such a high number of offences as boys. In substance related offences, girls do not differ. Boys in the delinquent behaviour and especially if girls are in intimate relationship to older and social men, they show more overall delinquent behaviour. The etiology of gender differences in delinquent behaviour is open. There exist a number of hypotheses but no unifying theory is settled now. **Conclusion:** From our findings we can conclude that antisocial behaviour in youth has less impact on lifetime course of women in contrast to men. Further research is needed to solve a number of questions for example the increase of delinquency in girls in the last decade etc. Especially research on protective factors for delinquency would probably offer some approaches to prevention of antisocial behaviour in underage men.

S-042-194 Topic: 11
Working with mentally disabled juvenile sex offenders in Switzerland:
First experiences and further developments
Monika Egli-Alge, forio, Weinfelden, Switzerland,
monika.egli-alge@forio.ch
Matthias Schmelzle; Ulrich Preuss

Objective: To describe a current treatment program for working with sexually abusive male youth who are mentally disabled in Switzerland. We present and describe the first results of our pilot project. **Methods:** Based on several already existing programs from the Netherlands and UK (Scotland), we portray the developments and adaptations of the important parameters for Switzerland, we present the conceptual backgrounds, based on the theories of the actual knowledge of sexually abusive youth. The special approach, that is needed for working with mentally disabled youth in the issue of educational theories also will be shown. Further, there is given an overview of the disorders of these juveniles and the indications. Also, we gain an insight into our practical work and the scientifically evaluation of the pilot project. **Conclusion:** Sexually abusive youth with mental handicap have very especial needs. The common treatment programs, based on cognitive-behavioural, delict-oriented and group-psychotherapeutic parameters are not suitable for this kind of abusers. They need more education and a very basic training in their sexual knowledge, relationship and about boundaries. The persons who look after them and the foster-care-institutions have to be included in the treatment process as much as possible. The main issue of this work is to prevent additional abuse.

S-042-195 Topic: 57
The adolescent sex offender assessment park – useful applications in German speaking countries
Richard Beckett, United Kingdom
Constanze Gerhold; Matthias Schmelzle; Monika Egli-Alge; Lieselotte Türkmen-Barta; Ulrich Preuss

Objective: To describe a current research project, founded by Richard Beckett in UK for the assessment of juvenile sexoffenders. The Adolescent Sexoffender Assessment Pack – ASAP – will be described, also its psychometric construction and the current use in some European Countries as Switzerland, Germany and Austria. **Methods:** The prediction of sexual abusing behaviour is quite difficult and object of this international research project. Because of the little number of recorded sexual abusing juveniles in several countries, it is necessary to promote an international cooperation. The ASAP is used in the named countries since some years and now adapted and improved. For the measurements of treatment outcome, the ASAP is a useful

instrument. In this study with 11–12 questionnaires personality-profiles of the juvenile sex offenders are established, for example: self-esteem, emotional loneliness, anger management, general empathy and also delictoriented marks as attitudes to children and sex, cognitive distortions, sexual deviancy. The questionnaires are partial known and validated, partial new developed and revised in the frame of this project on N=479 juvenile sex offenders at the age of 12 to 18 years and standardized at the norm-control-group. **Results:** We will present first results of the running study, using the ASAP in the named countries, focusing the personality structures of the juvenile sex offenders. A cluster analysis showed some effects and especial factors of the personality and typology of the offenders. Also some risk-factors and determinations can be described. Aim of the study is the classification and the finding of reliable criteria to assess the risk of reoffending and to judge the need of treatment. The random sample did not distinguish between the norm-control-group in many characteristics. The cluster-analysis showed some interesting results, that will be shown in this symposia. **Conclusion:** It is a high need of instruments to measure treatment attempts and effects of the treatment of juvenile sex offenders and to assess their risk of reoffending. First of all, treatment-needs must be identified, before the treatment-programs can be developed further. The ASAP-Study is a very skilful instrument and gives us new insight in the personality-profile of juvenile sex offenders.

S-043 Topic: 76, 24
Gender Identity, development and vicissitudes
Chairperson: Colette Chiland, Université René Descartes, Paris, France, cchiland@wanadoo.fr

Gender Identity, development and vicissitudes
Colette Chiland, Université René Descartes, Paris, France, cchiland@wanadoo.fr

The subject of this symposium, which will be held in English, is the current state of knowledge on Gender Identity, its development and vicissitudes. Heino Meyer-Bahlburg (New York) will present a communication on "Gender and Genitals: The intersex Controversy". Domenico Di Ceglie (London) will present a communication on "Current views and controversies on the treatment of Gender Identity Disorders in children and adolescents". Colette Chiland (Paris) will present a communication on the development of Gender Identity and lead the discussion between the speakers and the floor.

S-043-196 Topic: 76, 24
Gender and genitals: The intersex controversy
Heino Meyer-Bahlburg, Columbia University, Dept. of Psychiatry, New York, NY, USA, meyerb@childpsych.columbia.edu

Objective: To discuss recent research on intersexuality in response to the ongoing controversy about the psychosocial management of intersex patients, which, along with recent advances in the behavioral sciences, contributes to an improved understanding of gender development in normative and atypical conditions. **Methods:** Research on gender development has three major foci: (1) normative gender development and its mechanisms of social learning and self-socialization; (2) the description, diagnosis, and course of gender identity disorder in somatically normal individuals; and (3) gender assignment, gender outcome, and the role of biological factors in intersex individuals. Although there is surprisingly little overlap among investigators, the same type of gender measures can be used for the assessment of individuals in the three categories, and it is highly likely that variations of the same fundamental mechanisms of gender development are involved. **Results:** Prenatal hormones, especially prenatal androgens rather than prenatal estrogens, have a marked influence on gender-differentiated behavior in humans. A contribution of sex-specific genes seems likely, but is not proven. There is growing evidence for structural sex differences in the human brain, although their specific links to systemic sex hormones and to behavioral outcomes are yet to be established. Gender identity seems to be much less directly influenced by biological factors than gender-differentiated behavior. Patient-initiated gender change varies very much with the specific intersex syndrome. Clinical observations suggest additional cognitive factor supporting gender change. **Conclusion:** The data available are not yet sufficient for an evidence-based resolution of all controversial issues in the psychosocial management of intersexuality.

S-043-197   Topic: 76, 24
Current views on the management of gender identity disorder in children and adolescents

Domenico Di Ceglie, Tavistock & Portman NHS Trust, London, United Kingdom, gidu@tavi-port.nhs.uk

In this presentation I describe a model of management of gender identity in children and adolescents, which is based on a staged and flexible approach. In this model the presence of the gender identity disorder is recognised but this is not considered as a primary therapeutic objective of the psychological and social interventions. Stage 1 of the process for children and adolescents involves the therapeutic exploration of the nature of their "atypical gender identity organization", as well as to alleviate the associated psychological and social difficulties that these children and adolescents often present. The therapeutic aims in this phase of the work will be described. Physical interventions (Stage 2 and 3) may start in late adolescence when the evolution of the gender identity disorder is towards transsexualism and it is clinically appropriate. Stage 2 includes wholly reversible interventions. These involve the use of hypothalamic blockers that suppress the production of oestrogen and testosterone. Stage 3 includes partial reversible interventions, such as hormonal treatment that masculinizes or feminizes the body. Stage 4, to be considered in adulthood (after the age of 18), includes irreversible interventions such as surgical procedures. Clinical vignette will be used to illustrate this model. The paper puts forward the view that these interventions are best carried out within an integrated, comprehensive, multi-disciplinary assessment and treatment program. The involvement in this process of the family and social network, such as the school, will also be considered. The value of this model of management will be discussed with special reference to the crucial function of engaging this group of children, teenagers and their families with the service and provide a containing framework for, at times, painful and unbearable experiences, particularly during adolescence. Clinical vignettes will be used to illustrate this model.

S-044   Topic: 78
Eating and feeding disorders/Obesity III

Track: Eating disorders

Chairperson: Ulrike Lehmkuhl, Charité, Klinik für Psychiatrie, Psychosomatik & Psychotherapie, Berlin, Germany, ulrike.lehmkuhl@charite.de

S-044-198   Topic: 78, 41
EDI 2 profile: Comparison between depressed and not depressed anorexic patients

Orlando Uccellini, Azienda Ospedaliera S. Gerardo, Neuropsichiatria Infantile, Monza, Italy, uccelliniorla@libero.it
Mario Bertolini; Francesca Neri; Delia Albanese; Raffaella Bertola

Objective: The aim of this study is to compare the eating disorder's inventory (EDI 2) profile of depressed anorexia nervosa (AN) patients with the EDI 2 profile of not depressed AN patients in an adolescent sample. **Methods:** After the admission, inpatient meeting DSM IV criteria for Anorexia Nervosa completed the Eating Disorders Inventory-2 and were also rated with diagnostic semi-structured interview Kiddie-Sads-Lifetimes – section for mood disorders. The sample was subdivided in two groups considering the association with Major Depressive Episode: a subgroup of 33 subject with an associated Major Depressive Episode, and a subgroup of 32 subject without associated depressive disorder. We compared by Two-tailed t test analysis the EDI scores of the two subgroup. The clinical sample of 65 adolescent anorexic inpatient ranged in age between 10 and 17 years, with a mean age of 14.7 (SD = 1.99). **Results:** In the depressed AN patients the global EDI2 score was significantly higher than in non-depressed patients (p < 0.05): An higher score in profile was observed for ten out of the eleven subscale scores. In particular there was a statistically significant difference in four subscales score: "bulimia" (p < 0.002), "body dissatisfaction" (p < 0.001), "feeling of inefficiency" (p < 0.1), "interoceptive awareness" (p < 0.02). **Conclusion:** The present results suggested a clearly difference in psychopathological and behavioural traits assessed with the EDI 2 between the depressed AN adolescent patient and the non depressed AN patient in adolescence. These findings raise many questions about the connection between depression and psychological features in AN: there is a premorbid personality difference between the two groups? Or is the onset of an associated depressive disorder that influence the psychological characteristic in AN? Or is different kind of psychological functioning that is linked to depression and to some EDI 2 assessed characteristics?

S-044-199   Topic: 78
Psychological and physical changes during recovery in adolescents with Anorexia Nervosa (AN)

Maartje Snoek, University Medical Center, Child & Adolescent Psychiatry, Utrecht, Netherlands, m.snoek@psych.azu.nl
Annemarie van Elburg; Martien Kas; Herman van Engeland

Objective: Anorexia Nervosa (AN) is a disorder with psychological and physical symptoms, a high morbidity and mortality rate and a protracted course. Adolescents have the highest risk for developing AN and are studied the least. Studying the recovery process will augment our knowledge of the pathophysiological and psychological changes. **Methods:** 60 female adolescents, mean age 16.7 years, diagnosed with AN according to DSM IV were included in a study looking at changes during recovery. The physical recovery process was defined complete if weight gain resulted in the resumption of a regular menstrual cycle. Psychological changes during recovery were monitored. **Results:** Data on psychological changes were collected through weekly self and expert ratings using the Profile of Mood States, a visual analog scale. Data on physical recovery included weight, body composition, activity levels and bloodsamples to determine hormone levels. 24 patients showed physical recovery within one year, another 18 showed weight recovery only. Psychological recovery varied over the groups. **Conclusion:** Psychological recovery shows a dissociation from physical recovery. This longitudinal study shows differences in recovery profile that influence outcome and may reflect genetic variation.

S-044-200   Topic: 78, 95
Results of a clinical study on comorbid anxiety during the acute phase of Anorexia Nervosa (AN)

Ulrike Margarete Elisabeth Schulze, Universitätsklinikum Ulm, Kinder- und Jugendpsychiatrie, Ulm, Germany, Silke Calame; Ferdinand Keller; Jörg M. Fegert; Andreas Warnke

Objective: Long-time studies of anorexia reveal a high percentage of anxiety disorders independent of eating disorder outcome. Except for the co-occurence of social phobia, little is known about comorbid anxiety symptoms during the acute phase of illness. **Methods:** We carried out a clinical study on a group of 29 inpatients (mean age 14.54 years, SD±1.89). Using standardized interviews, we assessed eating disorder severity (ANIS, EDI, FEV) and comorbid anxiety (STAI, SPAI-C) symptoms. Statistical analysis was performed using the SPSS and SAS statistical programs. **Results:** Mean BMI (body mass index) was 14.26 kg/m^2 (±1.50), the duration of hospital treatment varied between 14 and 202 days (mean 84.93±44.35). Correlations between trait anxiety/social phobia and anxiety/severity of eating disorder – but not with the initial BMI – were found. **Conclusion:** To achieve an effective treatment of anorexia nervosa, should be attended to the co-occurrence of anxiety and eating disorder psychopathology.

S-044-201   Topic: 78, 30
The influence of hunger states on emotional ratings of visual food stimuli in Anorexia Nervosa (AN) and healthy controls

Stephanie Santel, Universität Magdeburg, Kinder- und Jugendpsychiatrie, Magdeburg, Germany, stephanie.santel@medizin.uni-magdeburg.de Kerstin Krauel; Michael Rotte; Thomas F. Münte; Lioba Baving

Objective: The study investigates the influence of hunger state on perception and emotional ratings of visual food stimuli in young female patients with anorexia nervosa and healthy control subjects. Ratings were expected to be mostly positive in the healthy group and mostly negative in the anorexic group. Because of a general fear of food in anorexia nervosa, it was expected that the state of hunger has less of an influence on the ratings of the anorexic subjects

than on that of controls. fMRI data obtained during the task is expected to show involvement of emotional centres only in a hungry state for controls and irrespective of satiety state for anorexic patients. **Methods:** During fMRI, subjects were presented with pictures of food as the experimental condition and of neutral objects (tools) and fixation cross as control stimuli. Subjects were instructed to rate the stimuli as either pleasant, neutral or unpleasant. To investigate the influence of hunger state on emotional ratings, two separate sessions were performed. **Results:** As expected, opposite response patterns were observed in the two groups with control subjects rating most of the food stimuli as pleasant whereas anorexic subjects rated them as mostly negative. However, in both groups these response patterns were more pronounced when subjects were hungry than when they were satiated, i.e. both groups rated food more neutral when satiated. fMRI data will be presented and discussed. **Conclusion:** These data indicate that despite opposite rating patterns, both healthy controls and anorexic patients tend to rate food more neutral when satiated. Food is thus perceived as less aversive by anorexic patients when they have just eaten to satiety.

S-044-202   Topic: 78, 32
Psychoneuroendocrinological aspects of Anorexia Nervosa in adolescents during recovery

Annemarie van Elburg, University Medical Center, Child & Adolescent Psychiatry, Utrecht, Netherlands, aelburg@azu.nl Maartje Snoek; Martien Kas; Herman van Engeland

Objective: Anorexia Nervosa (AN) is a disorder with psychological and physical symptoms, a high morbidity and mortality rate and a protracted course. Adolescents have the highest risk for developing AN and are studied the least. Studying the recovery process will augment our knowledge of the pathophysiological changes. Weight loss results in changes in leptin, the hypothalamus-pituitary-adrenal (HPA)-axis, the hypothalamus-pituitary-gonadal (HPG)-axis and in several other feedback loops and target organs. **Methods:** 60 female adolescents, mean age 16.7 years, diagnosed with AN according to DSM IV were included in a study looking at changes during recovery. The recovery process was defined complete if weight gain resulted in the resumption of a regular menstrual cycle. **Results:** Data were collected on weight, body composition and several somatic parameters. Biweekly blood samples and ratings on mood changes and activity levels completed the data collection. **Conclusion:** Outcome groups showed significant differences in age, weight gain and activity levels over time, initial leptin levels, body composition, but no differences in duration of illness, length of study, comorbidity or the diagnostic subtype of anorexia nervosa. Weight gain did not differ significantly between the recovered group and a second group that gained weight without a restart of the menstrual cycle, but leptin, HPG hormones and activity levels did differ between these groups.

S-044-203   Topic: 78, 3
Eating disorders prevention programme-pilot study

Irena Namyslowska, Inst. of Psychiatry-Neurology, Dept. Adolescent & Psychiatry, Warsaw, Poland, namyslow@ipin.edu.pl

Objective: Recent research has suggested that school-based programmes of prevention of eating disorders obtained ambiguous results. The aim of our work was to establish the efficacy of the eating disorders prevention programme for schoolgirls of secondary schools. **Methods:** Subjects in the experimental groups received 8 sessions of practice with various tasks, while the control group did not participate in sessions of psychoeducation. Overall, we examined 109 adolescents participating in sessions and 117 adolescents in the control group. Participants were examined at the beginning of the programme, after the operation and 6 months later. Assessment was made with EDI, EAT-26. **Results:** Assessment before and after the study phase showed that participants in the experimental groups had not made significantly more improvement than the control group. It was also shown that in the two subgroups (girls from technical college and girls from college) there were significant differences in the pre-test, post-test and follow-up results. **Conclusion:** Similarities that were obtained through the research suggest the necessity of examining other possible relationships between chosen variables. Analysis of participants' feedback information emphasizes that the changes the programme brought appeared feasibly in the social functioning area (with peers, parents relations). It is not excluded that it is too late eating disorder prophylaxis in the phase of personal development, as some researchers argue. Differences in results between schoolgirls from college and from technical college suggest some differences in risk and protective factors. It seems important to verify this.

S-045   Topic: 83
Autism spectrum disorders: Current perspectives on etiology, diagnostics and treatment

Track: Pervasive developmental disorders (PDD)

Chairperson: Fritz Poustka, Universität Frankfurt Kinder- und Jugendpsychiatrie, Frankfurt, Germany, poustka@em.uni-frankfurt.de
Sven Bölte, J.W.Goethe-University, Child & Adolescent Psychiatry, Frankfurt, Germany, boelte@em.uni-frankfurt.de

Autism spectrum disorders: Current perspectives on etiology, diagnostics and treatment

Fritz Poustka, Universität Frankfurt, Kinder- und Jugendpsychiatrie, Frankfurt, Germany, poustka@em.uni-frankfurt.de

In this symposium, scientists from Israel, Finland and Germany report on their current research efforts in autism spectrum disorders, covering a broad array of topical issues. The first contribution, gives an overview on the search for susceptibility variants in the molecular genetics of autism, followed by a presentation of a controlled study on the broader cognitive phenotype in parents of affected individuals. Speakers three and four will focus on auditory ERPs and factor analytic studies in Asperger's syndrome. The symposium is completed by work on the neurobiologically evaluation of a computer-based program to teach emotion recognition and the retrospective evaluation of the Mifne intervention program.

S-045-204   Topic: 83, 30
The broader cognitive phenotype of autism: How specific are local processing and executive dysfunction?

Sven Bölte, J.W. Goethe-University, Child & Adolescent Psychiatry, Frankfurt, Germany, boelte@em.uni-frankfurt.de
Fritz Poustka

Objective: To examine the specificity of local processing style and executive dysfunction as components of the broader cognitive phenotype of autism in parents. **Methods:** The sample included 62 parents of subjects with an autism spectrum disorder, 36 parents of individuals with early onset schizophrenia and 30 parents of people with mental disabilities. Data on four executive function tests and two scales indicative of weak central coherence were collected in all participants and performance compared between groups. **Results:** Average performance on the Embedded Figures Test was superior in parents of people with autism, compared to both control groups and normative data. In addition, mothers and fathers of children with autism and schizophrenia performed equally poor on the Trail Making Test B. **Conclusion:** Our findings imply that an enhanced visual disembedding capacity could be a core characteristic of the broader cognitive phenotype of autism in close relatives, showing sufficient specificity for the disorder. Circumscribed deficits in set-shifting and cognitive flexibility maybe also be noteworthy aspects of the extended cognitive phenotype in autism parents, but of rather limited specificity.

S-045-205   Topic: 83, 35
The evaluation of a computer-based emotion recognition training using FMRI

Sabine Feineis-Matthews, Uniklinik Frankfurt, Kinder- und Jugendpsychiatrie, Frankfurt, Germany, feineis-matthews@em.uni-frankfurt.de
Sven Bölte; D. Hubl; D. Prvulovic; Fritz Poustka; T. Dierks

Objective: It is likely that autism spectrum disorders are associated with impairments in facial affect recognition. In this functional MRI-study, we examined the neurobiological correlates of the effects of a computer-based program to teach emotion processing called Frankfurt Test and Training of Facial Affect (FEFA). **Methods:** 10 adolescent and adult individuals with higher functioning autism were included. Five of them were intensively trained in basic emotion detection over a period of five weeks, while the remainder did not receive any comparable intervention. Two facial affect recognition measures on the behavioral level as well as blood oxygen level-dependent (BOLD) signal changes in the fusiform gyrus and other cortical regions known to be involved in visual processing of faces were assessed at baseline and post training. **Results:** Compared to the control group, the sample of trained subjects with autism showed marked improvements on both behavioral measures, which were accompanied by higher BOLD signals in the right medial occipital gyrus and superior parietal lobule. **Conclusion:** Findings indicate that gains in facial affect recognition in autism are associated with higher activation in some cerebral regions being part of a compensatory facial processing network, not necessarily with an increase of activation in the fusiform face area.

S-045-206   Topic: 78, 28

Molecular genetic analysis of autism –
The search for susceptibility variants

Sabine Klauck, DKFZ, Molecular Genome Analysis,
Heidelberg, Germany, s.klauck@dkfz.de

Methods: In order to identify predisposing genes for autism currently 317 patients from 257 families have been collected throughout Germany and Austria, while 165 complete trios are available for association studies. In addition, the International Molecular Genetics Study of Autism Consortium (IMGSAC) has collected to date 290 families with more than one affected child or relative. Based on the results of the IMGSAC genome screen in 152 affected sibling pairs (ASP) indicating principal loci on chromosomes 2q, 7q, 16p and 17q, further analysis of the expanded IMGSAC family collection including 219 ASPs provided continued support for linkage on chromosome 7q, generating a multipoint MLS of 2.44 between markers D7S530 and D7S640 at ~133 cM. Candidate genes with a function in brain or brain development within 7q21–q33 are being systematically screened for autism relevant mutations or variants with DHPLC and sequencing followed by association studies with known or newly identified SNPs. Furthermore, we started a proteomic approach by antibody profiling of plasma probes from more than 70 autistic patients to investigate the possible influence of immune reactions in the disease. **Results:** To date several gene variants or associations have been identified in the German and/or IMGSAC sample with a possible role in the etiology of autism. However, replication in other independent samples is warranted, in order to clarify the role of these genes in autism.

S-045-207   Topic: 83, 37

Social and communicative abilities in boys and girls:
A factor analytic study of the Asperger syndrome
screening questionnaire

Irma Moilanen, University of Oulu, Dept. of Child
Psychiatry, Oulu, Finland, irma.moilanen@oulu.fi
M. Mattila; J. Laurila; K. Jussila; A. Pyper; S. L. Linna;
Hanna Ebeling; D. Pauls

Objective: Symptoms of child psychiatric disorders often differ between boys and girls, probably due to girls' better social and communicative abilities. This might be especially true for Asperger Syndrome (AS). The aim was to compare the high functioning Autism Spectrum Screening Questionnaire (ASSQ) in boys versus girls in general population and in AS. **Methods:** The population study group (PSG) is made up of all 4382 children with age 8, from the Northern Ostrobothnia Hospital District area. The clinical sample (CS) consists of all AS-children from PSG, enriched by AS outpatients, aged 7-10 (23 boys and 8 girls), from the Child Psychiatric Clinic of Oulu University Hospital, diagnosed by the Autism Diagnostic Interview-Revised and the Autism Diagnostic Observation Schedule-Generic. All subjects, having IQ 50, were rated on the ASSQ by parents and PSG children also by teachers. **Results:** The factor analysis of the PSG produced four factors on the teachers' ASSQ: 1) social reciprocal interaction, 2) nonverbal communication, 3) stereotypes, 4) verbal communication, which were used to form sum variables. In PSG, boys scored higher on teachers' ASSQ in all factors, while in CS, AS girls did not differ from AS boys in any. **Conclusion:**

Factor analysis distinguished two key symptom areas of AS as own factors: social reciprocal interaction and stereotypes, however separating the aspects of communicative abnormalities to the second and fourth factor. Also worth noticing is that girls have better social skills than boys in general, which can make their symptoms of AS more difficult to notice, probably leading to lower numbers of girls with AS.

S-045-208   Topic: 83, 36

Auditory ERPs in the study of Asperger syndrome

Pirjo Korpilahti, University of Oulu, Finnish, Saami and
Logopedics, Oulu, Finland, pirjo.korpilahti@oulu.fi
Soile Loukusa; Eira Jansson-Verkasalo

Objective: Children diagnosed as having Asperger Syndrome (AS) have problems related with auditory perception and social interaction. They also have difficulties to understand emotional messages and prosodic features of the speech. We studied, whether the auditory deficit in AS represents a primary disorder of auditory perception, or are the defects specifically related to prosodic features of the speech. **Methods:** Auditory event related potentials (ERPs), especially the mismatch negativity (MMN), were recorded with pure tones and emotionally loaded utterances as stimuli. Automatic detection of fundamental tones and emotional prosody was studied in 20 children with Asperger Syndrome. AS children were diagnosed clinically, and with ADI-R and ADOS. Our study belongs to a larger research project: A Genetic Study of Asperger's Syndrome in Northern Finland. Results were compared with 20 normally developed children, and also with the ERP data of the parents of the both groups. By doing this, we wanted to get information of the familial disposition, and whether the phenotype is common for children and their parents. Neurophysiological data was compared with the language skills in naming and in auditory associations. **Results:** MMN peak latencies were longer in AS children than in healthy controls, especially at the right hemisphere. RH dysfunction was also encountered in fathers of the AS childen when compared to the fathers of the controls. We did not find differences in ERP results between the mothers of the two groups. Based on the timing of the peak MMN values, we suggest that in AS children the detection of emotional prosody is based on different auditory features than in controls. **Conclusion:** Emotions are loaded in the lowest frequencies of the human voice. We found that children with AS have difficulties in automatic detection of low sound frequencies (F0) and the intonation of one word utterances. ERP data reflected defects of central auditory perception both at the primary level, and more specifically in detection of emotional prosody of the speech.

S-045-209   Topic: 83, 19

A retrospective evaluation of an intensive method
of treatment for children with Pervasive Development
Disorder (PDD)

Alan Apter, Schneider Childrens Medical,
Dept. of Psychiatry, Petah Tikva, Israel, eapter@clalit.org.il

Objective: This study is a preliminary evaluation of the effectiveness of a novel intensive therapy program in young children with pervasive developmental disorder (PDD). **Methods:** Twenty-three children treated between 1997 and 1999 at the Mifne Institute in Israel were retrospectively assessed. Videos taken before and after three weeks of intensive treatment at the institute and after another six months of continued treatment at patient's homes were rated blindly by trained personnel using the Childhood Autism Rating Scale (CARS) and the Social Behavior Rating Scale (SBRS). **Results:** Children showed improvement on almost all items of both scales with differences for some items reaching statistical significance. Total scores on both scales improved significantly after three weeks and after six months. Patients with more severe symptoms at baseline showed greater improvement than the milder cases. **Conclusion:** Despite the small number of patients and the retrospective design used in the study, these preliminary results are promising.

S-046   Topic: 78
Current research venues in eating disorders
Track: Eating disorders

Chairperson: Johannes Hebebrand, Universitätsklinik Essen Kinder- und Jugendpsychiatrie, Essen, Germany, johannes.hebebrand@uni-duisburg-essen.de Beate Herpertz-Dahlmann, RWTH Aachen Kinder- u. Jugendpsychiatrie, Aachen, Germany, bherpertz-dahlmann@ukaachen.de

Current research venues in eating disorders

Johannes Hebebrand, Universitätsklinik Essen, Kinder- und Jugendpsychiatrie, Essen, Germany, johannes.hebebrand@uni-duisburg-essen.de

Current research venues in eating disorders encompass a variety of methodological approaches to address pertinent questions related to etiological, endocrinological, psychopathological and developmental issues. In our symposium we will begin by contrasting genetically and non-genetically orientated etiological research. Formal genetic research has indicated substantial heritability of anorexia and bulimia nervosa; both association and linkage studies have been performed. Linkage of bulimia nervosa has been detected to chromosome 10p suggesting that a gene(s) in this region might predispose to both this eating disorder and obesity. An involvement of melanocortin-4 receptor gene mutations in binge eating disorder is viewed controversially. Based on a discordant sib-pair approach personality characteristics such as perfectionism and negative self-evaluation, missing friends, life-events and teasing experiences have been shown to be of major influence. Hypoleptinemia in the acute stage of anorexia nervosa underlies amenorrhea and potentially contributes to the hyperactivity observed in a substantial subgroup of patients. Possibly, hyperleptinemia achieved upon refeeding is a risk factor for renewed weight loss. Neuroimaging studies provide insight into the regional responses to distinct cues relevant in eating disorders. Thus, in response to food images, both currently eating disordered and recovered patients activate the ventromedial prefrontal cortex significantly more than healthy controls. Furthermore, patients with bulimia nervosa show a lack of lateral prefrontal involvement in response to food compared to healthy women or women with anorexia nervosa. Psychopathological studies of patients recovered from eating disorders indicate that these score significantly higher than controls on measures of anxiety, depression, obsessions or compulsions, as well as harm avoidance and persistence. These symptoms, which had previously also been detected premorbidly in eating disordered patients, may reflect a temperament that creates a susceptibility to the development of these disor-

ders. Finally, comparisons between adult eating disordered patients and controls indicate that the patients are characterized by a high rate of childhood neuropsychiatric disorders; preliminary evidence indicates that the highest rates apply to patients with severe eating disorders.

S-046-210   Topic: 78, 28
Genetic dissection of eating disorders

Anke Hinney, Universitätsklinik Marburg, Kinder- und Jugendpsychiatrie, Marburg, Germany, anke.hinney@med.uni-marburg.de Anne-Kathrin Wermter; Susann Friedel; Frank Geller; Helmut Schäfer; Helmut Remschmidt; Johannes Hebebrand

Objective: Formal (twin and family) genetic studies have shown a major role of genetic factors in eating disorders. Currently, the number of genetic analyses pertaining to eating disorders is increasing. Psychopathological features and extremely low body weight are inseparable in anorexia nervosa (AN), so that AN might be considered as an extreme weight condition. In patients with bulimia nervosa (BN) BMI is premorbidly often increased. The manifestation of AN and BN is predominantly in puberty. The prevalence of both is considerably higher in females. A candidate gene approach considers these clinical observations. Genome wide scans for AN and BN have recently been performed. The chromosomal region that seems to be relevant for BN had previously been detected in genome scans pertaining to obesity. Currently, the gene for the melanocortin-4 receptor (MC4R) is regarded as one of the most relevant 'obesity genes'. Binge eating disorder (BED) has been reported to be associated with mutations in the MC4R. **Methods:** Screen for mutations by SSCP, dHPLC and PCR based specific mutation detection assays in up to 3,435 individuals comprising patients with AN, BN or BED; underweight or normal weight students and extremely obese children and adolescents to perform association studies. The parents of a subgroup of these were additionally screened in order to perform transmission disequilibrium tests. **Results:** For AN, none of the rare positive association results had been unequivocally confirmed in independent study groups. Mutations in the MC4R have a major gene effect on the development of obesity in 2–4% of extremely obese individuals. A haplo-insufficiency mutation in the MC4R was detected in a patient with BN. Hence, genes relevant for obesity seem to be involved in BN. We did not find MC4R mutations in patients with BED. **Conclusion:** Major genes involved in body weight regulation have been detected; one of them involved in BN indirectly via the predisposition to obesity.

S-046-211   Topic: 78, 28
Risk factors for Anorexia Nervosa (AN):
Results from retrospective discordant sister-pair studies

Andreas Karwautz, Universitätsklinikum Wien, Abt. Neuropsychiatrie, Wien, Austria, andreas.karwautz@univie.ac.at Gudrun Wagner; Maria Haidvogl; Fernando Fernandez-Aranda; Joanna Holliday; Janet Linda Treasure

Objective: To study sister pairs discordant for an eating disorder history allows a perfect matching and control for and over several cultural and familial factors shared by siblings and allows to study non-shared individual specific risk factors which are aetiologically highly relevant for the development of anorexia nervosa (AN). **Methods:** We will present evidence for risk factors from studies on anorexia nervosa using this discordant sister-pair design. The main instrument in use was a modified form of the "Oxford Risk Factor Interview for Eating Disorders" (developed by Chris Fairburn, UK) lasting for about 4 hours each. Within the European multi-centre study on "Factors in healthy eating" we have interviewed in person 128 patients suffering from AN and also their "healthy" sisters derived from three European centres (Vienna, Barcelona, London). **Results:** Data on environmental risk factors, precursors such as childhood behaviour problems, family relationships, and personality traits will be presented. We found mainly risk factors from the personal domain to be responsible for the development of AN restricting sub-type and from the personal and dieting domains being responsible for the development of AN-BP. Childhood characteristics, parental problems and disruptive events contributed to the development of both AN-R and AN-BP (stepwise logistic regression results). **Conclusion:** In particular, personality characteristics as perfectionism and negative self-evaluation, missing friends, life-events and teasing experiences are of major influence. These will have to be emphasized in prevention programs and should be explained within aetiological models to the patients.

S-046-212   Topic: 78

Leptin's role in Anorexia Nervosa (AN): A biological and clinical perspective

Kristian Holtkamp, Techn. Universität Aachen, Kinder- und Jugendpsychiatrie, Aachen, Germany, kholtkamp@ukaachen.de
Johannes Hebebrand; C. Mika; M. Heer; Beate Herpertz-Dahlmann

Objective: Low leptin levels are an endocrinological hallmark of acute anorexia nervosa (AN); a sub-threshold leptin secretion in adipocytes as a consequence of a reduced energy intake is presumed to be the major trigger of the adaptation of an organism to semi-starvation. **Methods:** We will present two own studies, demonstrating leptins' possible role in physical activity of AN as well as possible clinical consequences of changes of leptin concentration during the re-feeding process. **Results:** The results of the first study suggest that similar to semi-starvation induced hyperactivity (SIH) in rats hypoleptinemia may be one factor underlying the excessive physical activity often found in patients with AN. The results od the second study demonstrate that high serum leptin levels at discharge from inpatient treatment may indicate a risk for renewed weight loss and an unfavorable 1 year outcome in AN. **Conclusion:** Our results may have potential implications for the understanding and treatment of excessive physical activity in acute AN. We hypothesize that elevated leptin levels may be an important factor underlying the difficulties of maintaining the target-weight in AN patients after re-feeding.

S-046-213   Topic: 78, 35

Functional neuroimaging of symptom provocation in eating disorders

Rudolf Uher, Institute of Psychiatry, Eating Disorders Unit, PO59, London, United Kingdom, r.uher@iop.kcl.ac.uk

Objective: Our investigation has been conducted to explore the functional neural correlates of symptoms in women with anorexia and bulimia nervosa. Furthermore, the state

(in)dependence of brain reactivity to relevant stimuli was investigated by including recovered subjects and comparing them with the currently ill patients. **Methods:** Functional magnetic resonance with blood oxygen level dependent contrast was used to map the brain responses to images of high-caloric food, female bodies and generally aversive scenes in 16 women with anorexia nervosa, 10 with bulimia nervosa, 9 women long-term recovered from anorexia nervosa and 19 age-matched healthy control women. Whole brain functional data was analysed using non-parametric tests at the voxel and cluster level. **Results:** In response to food images, both current patients and recovered women activated the ventromedial prefrontal cortex significantly more than healthy controls. Furthermore, patients with bulimia nervosa showed a lack of lateral prefrontal involvement in response to food compared to healthy women or women with anorexia nervosa. Women recovered from anorexia nervosa activated more lateral and apical prefrontal cortices than currently ill patients. In response to female bodies, patients with eating disorders showed less activity in the ventral occipitotemporal cortices than healthy controls. The aversion ratings of body stimuli correlated positively with activity in several brain regions, including the medial apical prefrontal cortex and the inerior medial temporal lobe. There were no between group differences in brain responses to the aversive emotional images. **Conclusion:** Ventromedial prefrontal reactivity to food images in eating disorders corresponds to similar activations during symptom provocation in obsessive-compulsive disorder and addictions. The lateral prefrontal involvement in food processing should be evaluated as a predictive factor or mediator of recovery.

S-046-214   Topic: 78, 80

Personality characteristics after long-term recovery from an eating disorder

Angela Wagner, Univ. Pittsburgh Medical Center, Dept. of Psychiatry, Pittsburgh, USA, wagnera@upmc.edu
Nicole Barbarich; Shannan E. Henry; Ursula Bailer; Guido Frank; Walter H Kaye

Objective: Previous studies of personality characteristics in subjects with eating disorders primarily have focused on subjects who are acutely ill showing that negative mood states and obsessionality are common among these. However, few studies have investigated whether such symptoms persist after recovery from anorexia (AN) and bulimia (BN) nervosa. If these symptoms persist after recovery, it is possible that these are trait rather than state disturbances resulting from the illness itself. The goal of the present study was to examine the relationship, after recovery, between personality characterisitics and diagnoses of AN including subtypes and BN. **Methods:** Around 60 young female adults who were long-term recovered (>1 year no binging, purging, or restricting behaviors, normal weight, and menstrual cycles, not on medication) from AN or BN or AN and BN together were assessed and compared to 40 matched healthy controls. Assessments included core eating disorder symptoms on the Yale-Brown-Cornell Eating Disorder Scale, the Spielberger State-Trait Anxiety Inventory, the Beck Depression Inventory, the Yale-Brown Obsessive Compulsive Scale, and the Temperament and Character Inventory. **Results:** Women recovered with all types of eating disorders scored significantly higher than NC on measures of anxiety, depression, obsessions or compulsions, as well as harm avoidance and persistence. Interestingly, the eating disorder subgroups had similar scores for these measures. **Conclusion:** These data confirm and extend studies showing that core eating disorder symptoms, personality traits indicative of anxiety, depression, and obsessionality persist following long-term recovery. These symptoms, which other studies suggest are present premorbidly, may reflect a temperament that creates a susceptibility to the development of AN and/or BN.

S-046-215   Topic: 78

Childhood onset neuropsychiatric disorders in adult eating disorder patients: A controlled pilot study

Elisabet Wentz, University of Göteborg, Child & Adolescent Psychiatry, Göteborg, Sweden, ewn@medfak.gu.se
J. Hubert Lacey; Glenn Waller; Maria Rastam; Jeremy Turk; Christopher Gillberg

Objective: Controlled study of the prevalence of childhood onset neuropsychiatric disorders (COND) in a group of severe eating disorder (ED) patients. **Methods:** A group of 30 female anorexia nervosa (AN) (n = 21) and bulimia nervosa (BN) (n = 9) patients, all recruited from a specialist hospital clinic, was compared with an age- and sex-matched group of 30 healthy comparison cases tapping into COND (ADHD, autism spectrum disorders (ASD) (including Asperger's disorder) and Tourette syndrome/chronic tic disorders). All 60 subjects were also interviewed regarding personality disorders (PDs) and dissociation. **Results:** Fifty-three percent of the eating disorder (ED) group had at least one COND. Twenty-three percent of the ED patients had an ASD, 17% had ADHD, and 27% had Tourette syndrome/chronic tic disorder. ASD and ADHD occurred only among AN patients. In the comparison group there were only 2 cases with any kind of COND (both chronic tic disorders). All but two in the ED group compared to 3 comparison cases were assigned at least one diagnosis of PD. The most common PDs in the ED group were avoidant PD, depressive PD and paranoid PD. There was an almost complete overlap between ASD and schizoid PD. **Conclusion:** These preliminary data suggest that COND may be highly overrepresented in patients with severe ED. The occurrence of COND must be taken into consideration in the treatment of ED patients.

S-047   Topic: 3

Determinants of service use in four European countries

Track: Therapy and intervention

Chairperson: Frank C. Verhulst, Erasmus MC-Sophia, Child & Adolescent Psychiatry, Rotterdam, Netherlands, m.engel@erasmusmc.nl

Determinants of service use in children and adolescents: A view from four European countries

Frank C. Verhulst, Erasmus MC-Sophia, Child & Adolescent Psychiatry, Rotterdam, Netherlands, m.engel@erasmusmc.nl

Although a considerable number of children in the community meet criteria for psychiatric disorders, few receive professional or informal help. Previous studies uncovered several determinants of the help-seeking process, but these findings have never been integrated into one overarching model. This study aims to combine existing theories and findings to formulate and test a model describing the process of help-seeking for child psychopathology in profes-

sional and informal service settings. By means of structural equation modelling, associations between several help-seeking stages, and the influence of child, family and context characteristics upon these stages were investigated in a sample of 246 Dutch children (4–11 years), who were selected for having emotional or behavioural problems. Although the Dutch GP is supposed to be gatekeeper in the provision of mental health care, his role in help-seeking.

S-047-216   Topic: 22

Help-seeking for child psychopathology: Pathways to informal and professional services

Marieke Zwaanswijk, NIVEL, Utrecht, Netherlands, m.zwaanswijk@nivel.nl
Peter Verhaak; Jozien Bensing; Jan van der Ende; Frank Verhulst

Objective: Although a considerable number of children in the community meet criteria for psychiatric disorders, few receive professional or informal help. Previous studies uncovered several determinants of the help-seeking process, but these findings have never been integrated into one overarching model. This study aims to combine existing theories and findings to formulate and test a model describing the process of help-seeking for child psychopathology in professional and informal service settings. **Methods:** By means of structural equation modelling, associations between several help-seeking stages, and the influence of child, family and context characteristics upon these stages were investigated in a sample of 246 Dutch children (4–11 years), who were selected for having emotional or behavioural problems. **Results:** Although the Dutch GP is supposed to be gatekeeper in the provision of mental health care, his role in help-seeking for child psychopathology is limited. A more influential role is played by school personnel, both in increasing parents' awareness of the need to seek help, as well as in the provision of and the referral for help. Various family characteristics were also shown to influence service need, informal or professional help-seeking. The influence of child characteristics on the help-seeking process is limited. **Conclusion:** Interventions aimed at increasing child mental health service use should focus on improving school personnel's abilities to detect and help children with psychopathology and to increase parents' awareness of the need to seek help. Future research concerning the role of GPs in the help-seeking process may provide suggestions on how to strengthen their role as gatekeepers.

S-047-217   Topic: 2, 25

Have there been changes in child mental health service use? A 10-year comparison from Finland

Andre Sourander, Turku Universital Hospital, Turku, Finland, andsou@utu.fi
Paivi Santalahti

Objective: To study child mental health service utilization at two time points, in 1989 and in 1999. **Methods:** Two cross-sectional representative samples of 8-year-old children were compared from southern Finland. The 1989 sample consisted of 985 children of whom 95% participated, and the sample 1999 of 962 children of whom 86% participated. Information was gathered from parents and teachers using Rutter's Questionnaires and other related determinants of service use, and from children using the Child Depression

Inventory. The sampling, procedure and methods were similar at both time-points. **Results:** In 1989, 2.3% and in 1999, 5.3% of 8-year-old children had used child mental health services. The increase in service use among girls was fourfold. A significantly higher proportion of screen-positive children had been referred in 1999 than 10 years earlier. Parental evaluations of child psychopathology and teacher evaluations of child's overall impairment were the strongest determinants for referral at both time points. When attitudes towards services were studied, parents preferred to seek help for their children's problems from teachers, school nurses and school psychologists rather than from specialized child psychiatric services. **Conclusion:** The present study shows that the threshold for child mental health service utilization has decreased. However, substantial unmet needs for service use still exist. It is important to develop child psychiatric services, which are as close to the child's living environment as possible to further decrease the threshold for seeking help and to promote early detection and intervention.

S-047-218   Topic: 2, 25

Services for children with psychiatric disorder: Who is seen and by whom?

Tamsin Ford, Institute of Psychiatry, Child & Adolescent Psychiatry, London, United Kingdom, t.ford@iop.kcl.ac.uk
Robert Goodman; Howard Meltzer

Objective: Little is known about the patterns and predictors of contact with specialist service use for childhood psychiatric disorder in Great Britain, but we anticipated that the "impact on others" would influence service contact as much or more than "impact on the child." Examining predictors of service use would identify potential targets for intervention to improve the proportion of children with psychiatric disorder receiving treatment. **Methods:** 2461 children from the British Child and Adolescent Mental Health Survey 1999 were followed up at two and three years. At each follow-up, a sub-sample of parents were interviewed in depth about contacts with services for mental health problems, based on their response to service use questions in the main survey. **Results:** Fifty seven percent of children with psychiatric disorder had contacted at least one service, 42% a specialist service and 25% used specialist mental health services. The impact on the child predicted contact with all specialist services, while the impact on others predicted mental health and special educational needs service use. The different specialist services were associated with different baseline characteristics of the child and the family. **Conclusion:** A slightly higher proportion of children with psychiatric disorder is seen by mental health and other services in Britain than has been reported by earlier, mainly American, study. However there is no room for complacency as three-quarters do not reach mental health services. The other predictors provide potential targets for screening vulnerable children.

S-047-219   Topic: 2

Who comes and who stays: Factors contributing to clinical service use in adolescents

Inge Seiffge-Krenke, Universität Mainz, Mainz, Germany, seiffge@uni-mainz.de

Objective: Several studies have demonstrated that utilization rates of mental health care begin to differ for boys and girls around mid-adolescence. Whereas in childhood more male patients utilize services, around the age of 15 girls seek mental health care more often than boys. Two studies on German samples, which analysed differences in health care-seeking behaviours and factors contributing to positive outcomes, are presented. Factors contributing to continuation and discontinuation of treatment are also investigated. **Methods:** The first study used data from a representative sample of 561 adolescents. Adolescents' attitudes and knowledge about psychotherapy and reasons for not consulting health care professionals were assessed. The second study analyzed case files of 316 adolescent patients in a German outpatient unit who where referred for diagnosis and treatment. **Results:** Although females showed a more positive attitude towards professional help in case of psychopathology, the readiness to accept help for all adolescents was dependent on other variables, such as a less sceptical attitude towards health care professionals, low fear and doubts about the efficacy of treatment and high self-disclosure. Gender and age differences were found in referral rates as well as in diagnoses and treatment offered. Older and female patients received single psychotherapy more frequently, while younger adolescents received more counselling. No differences emerged with respect to family therapy or group psychotherapy. As in other studies, the drop-out rate was quite high. **Conclusion:** Health care seeking behaviour in adolescents is an understudied area of great practical significance. Age and gender differences in health care seeking behaviour determine therapy outcome.

S-048   Topic: 7, 41

Understanding the expression of Asperger's Disorder in adolescence: A case presentation with developmental and psychodynamic perspectives

Track: Therapy and intervention

Chairperson: Richard Fritsch, George Washington University Center for Profess. Psychology, Washington, DC, USA, rfritsch@gwu.edu
Marika Cutler, W. Reed Army Medical Center Social Work Fellowship Program, Bethesda, MD, USA, cutler@millkern.com

Understanding the expression of Asperger's Disorder in adolescence: A case presentation with developmental and psychodynamic perspectives

Richard Fritsch, George Washington University, Center for Profess. Psychology, Washington, DC, USA, rfritsch@gwu.edu

Spectrum disorders such as Asperger's Disorder, Multiple Complex Developmental Disorder and Pervasive Developmental Disorder not otherwise specified have been the subject of recent of attention by child and adolescent clinicians and researchers. However, the value, efficacy and course of psychotherapeutic interventions for patients with this disorder are not well understood. This symposium will examine the theory and developmental underpinnings of an adolescent expression of Asperger's disorder and one approach to treatment. From a developmental perspective, adolescence is a period of significant stress and normal regression. Important transformations of cognitive, emotional and regulatory capacities occur. Disorders such as Asperger's, that involve deficiencies in representational capacity reverberates with the normal developmental tasks of adolescents, a period in which representation change is essential to yield particular psychopathological presentations. The complex interplay of trauma, developmental delay, inhibition and intrapsychic conflict, will be illuminated by the presentation of the stormy course of the psychodynamically informed psychotherapy of an adolescent patient who meets criteria for inclusion in the Asperger's diagnostic spectrum. The patient presented with affective turmoil, odd behaviors and bizarre preoccupations and had significant problems using representational thinking to navigate social venues. These social difficulties expressed his deficient understanding his own mental state and those of others. Moreover, narcissistic issues relating to physical deformity and abnormalities left him biologically and psychologically vulnerable from birth. Using psychoanalytic and descriptive perspectives, the case and theoretical ideas will be integrated and discussed as an example of how a broad approach to conceptualizing complex clinical problems facilitates positive treatment outcome.

S-048-220   Topic: 7, 41
Blind in the present: An adolescent's search for understanding
Marika Cutler, W. Reed Army Medical Center, Social Work Fellowship Program, Bethesda, MD, USA, cutler@millkern.com

Objective: This paper presents the stormy course of the psychodynamically informed psychotherapy of an adolescent patient with affective turmoil, odd behaviors and bizarre preoccupations. **Methods:** He met the descriptive criteria for the diagnosis of Asperger's Disorder and had significant problems using representational thinking to navigate social venues. **Results:** These social difficulties, attributed to incomplete development of "theory of mind mechanisms" were particularly expressed in its deficient understanding his own mental state and those of others. Moreover, narcissistic issues relating to physical deformity and abnormalities left him biologically and psychologically vulnerable from birth. Environmental trauma further complicated his development. **Conclusion:** The complex interplay of trauma, developmental delay, inhibition and intrapsychic conflict, as shown in this case presentation, illuminates one part of the more disturbed spectrum of psychopathology and how psychotherapy can be useful in such cases. The therapeutic starting point begins with the unfolding of his secret, inner world vis-à-vis his preoccupations. The steady growth of insight, as part of a developing theory of mind, leads first to self-awareness and eventually to an awareness of others minds. Specifically, the patient's preoccupations are given up in favor of social relatedness through therapeutic preoccupation, attunement, identification with the therapist and analysis of the transference.

S-048-221   Topic: 83
Symptomatic preoccupation in a teenaged boy
E. James Anthony, George Washington University, Medical School, Chevy Chase, MD, USA, vqanthony@aacap.org

Objective: This paper discusses case material presented in the symposium on the treatment of an adolescent with Asperger's disorder. **Methods:** At the onset of treatment, the adolescent was intensively preoccupied with odd ideas and interests, a commonly occurring symptom of the disorder. **Results:** The concept of preoccupation will be discussed from three vantagepoints: 1. Winnicott's concept of primary maternal preoccupation; 2. the type of ruminative preoccupa-

tions found in certain cases of Asperger's Disorder and 3: the therapist's preoccupation in response to the patient's persistent preoccupation. **Conclusion:** While results will vary across cases, in this patient the therapist's attentive containing and empathic preoccupation helped the patient to give up his odd and isolating preoccupations in favor of increased social activity. For this patient, an integrative treatment including medication and psychodynamic psychotherapy helped return him to a more normal developmental path in which odd preoccupations are not part of his presentation.

S-048-222   Topic: 83, 41
Adolescence and Asperger's disorder: Development, theory of mind and identity
Richard Fritsch, George Washington University, Center for Profess. Psychology, Washington, DC, USA, rfritsch@gwu.edu

Objective: Adolescence is a period of significant stress and normal regression. The tasks of giving up infantile objects, reorganizing the internal moral code to include sexuality, developing an autonomous identity and moving into genital sexual stage involve massive reorganization of the intrapsychic world. Powerful transformations of cognitive, emotional and regulatory capacities occur. Adolescence involves significant changes in the internal representations that orient the adolescent to reality. A disorder that involves deficiencies in representational capacity reverberates with the normal developmental tasks of adolescents, a period in which representation changes is essential. Theory of Mind Mechanisms (THMM) constructs have proven to be useful constructs at our current level of understanding of disorders that include impairment in representational capacity as part of the syndrome. **Conclusion:** Developmental challenges connected to cognitive developments in adolescence interact with a hypothesized TOMM deficit that lead to the particular kind of representational impairments found in certain Asperger's Disorder adolescents. Representational capacity that allows for social intelligence is dependent on the acquisition both of cognitive capacities, (the level of complexity and the kind of logical systems available) and emotional capacities, that is, the comprehension of the emotional object.

S-049   Topic: 46, 65
Historical and ethical issues
Chairperson: Per-Anders Rydelius, Karolinska Institutet Woman and Child Health, Stockholm, Sweden, per-anders.rydelius@ks.se

S-049-223   Topic: 46
The History of the IACAPAP during the Postwar Years
Rolf Castell, München, Germany, oliver.flach@psych.imed.uni-erlangen.de

Objective: Between 1948 and 1962 child-psychiatry changed from psychoanalysis to a broader point of view. The main issues dealt with psychosocial and somatic factors, prevention and epidemiology. The change was indicatetd by European child-psychiatrists in 1958. **Methods:** Investigations into the publications of 4 congresses of the IACAPAP. **Results:** In 1948 the congress was held in London. The main issue was on psychoanalytic psychotherapy with regard to aggression in the development of children, in families, in education and society. In Toronto in 1954 the presentations dealt with mother-child interaction for the first 6 years of life, for which many casereports were given. In Lisbon in 1958 happened a marked change. Although the interpretations by means of psychoanalysis of mother-child interaction of the age-group from 6 to 10 years dominated, one day was devoted to somatic causes of psychopathology. It was G. Heuyer from Paris, who iniciated this change. In Leiden (the Netherlands) in 1962 the main topic was on prevention. No pure analytical presentation was given. **Conclusion:** G. Heuyer was the main initiator for the change from psychoanalysis to an eclectic and much broader way (including behaviour therapy) to think and work about problems of children.

S-049-224   Topic: 65, 46

A psychiatric analysis of 62888 files from sterilized Swedish men and women: What can we learn from the genetic and eugenic paradigm of medical science?

Per-Anders Rydelius, Karolinska Institutet, Woman and Child Health, Stockholm, Sweden, per-anders.rydelius@ks.se

Objective: In 1997, the Swedish Government decided to make up for persons who had been sterilized according to the Swedish Acts on Sterilizations 1935–1975. A psychiatric analysis was done based on the records used for the decisions on sterilizations. The questions were: Who was sterilized?; Which were the indications? Did the principles for sterilizations change over the years? **Methods:** After a pilot-study, a sample of 2088 (everyone born on day 15th of each month of each year) of the 62888 files of sterilized persons was selected for the psychiatric analysis. The stored files consist of forms filled in by the subject him/herself, a parent, relative or authorized guardian, a doctor's certificate including hereditary, social, medical and somatic factors, IQ-tests and an evaluation of the subject's legal competence (all according to given criteria). Finally, a decision on operation by the National Board of Health. – Descriptive statistics was used. **Results:** The first Act on sterilization, influenced by Darwin's theory on evolution, was passed in 1897 in Michigan, USA (in order to sterilize delinquent youth) followed by a similar act based upon an eugenic paradigm in Indiana, USA in 1907. In 1926 such laws had been passed in 32 US States and in 1928 appeared in Alberta, Canada and one of the Swiss Cantons, in 1929 in Denmark, in 1932 in Mexico, in 1933 in Germany, in 1934 in Norway and Sweden, in 1935 in Finland and in 1937 in Latvia and Iceland etc. Acts on Sterilizations from eugenic reasons were passed in countries all over the world, but with some exceptions in Catholic Countries. The Swedish situation: 62888 persons were sterilized. The sex ratio (men:women) was 1:14. There were three indications: eugenic, social and medical reasons. 1935–1952, mentally retarded were sterilized on eugenic indications. 1953–1975, sterilizations were decided mainly upon psychiatric and medical indications giving multi-para worn out women safe contraceptives. From 1976, when sterilizations were allowed on voluntarily decisions, the number increased when men wanted to be operated upon from contraceptive reasons. **Conclusion:** In Sweden and until the 1940's the medical profession was active arguing for acts on sterilizations based upon genetic and eugenic paradigms.An eugenic paradigm existed until the 1950's when a shift to a psychiatric sociomedical paradigm took place. It seems as if the main reason for sterilizations was then to support multi-para worn-out women to have safe contraceptives.

S-049-225   Topic: 61

Antistigma Project for highschool adolescents

Milica Pejovic-Milovancevic, Institute of Mental Health, Dept. Children & Adolescents, Belgrade, Serbia and Montenegro, mpejovic@eunet.yu
Miroslav Pavlovic; Smiljka Popovic-Deusic; Olivera Aleksic

Objective: During spring 2004 we conducted the program named "The preventive antistigma program for adolescents and educators in high school". The goals were to prevent discrimination of youths with mental problems and to reduce established discrimination against those with mental health problems. We wanted to find out how active attitude in mental health promotion can change opinions toward mental health. **Methods:** Our pilot program started in one Belgrade high school (around 60 adolescents) and lasted for 7 consecutive weeks. Each session lasted for 90 minutes and was organised carefully: first 30 minutes we had small lectures about some relevant topics (what is mental health, what are the problems of mental health, etc.) and lately we had workshops where adolescents worked on their personal attitudes toward differences among people, personal problems and other. All participants obtained parental permission form, and filled out OMI (Opinion about mental illness) scale at begin of the program and at the end. **Results:** Results clearly show improvement in understanding the problems of mental health as well as attitudes towards it. **Conclusion:** Our project showed that better understanding of mental illness would help reduce the stigma that stops young people asking for help, and also contributes to better understanding those with mental health problems on the way toward social integration.

S-049-226   Topic: 65

Informed consent for adolescents treated by electroconvulsive therapy

Yuval Bloch, Shalvatal Mental Health Center, Child & Adolescent Outpatient, Hod-Hasharon, Israel, blochy@netvision.net.il
Noa Kalman; Muli Linder; Ido Luria; Yechiel Levkovitz; Gidi Ratzoni

Objective: Electroconvulsive Therapy (ECT) has gained its place as an important and legitimate tool in the treatment of severe mental disorders in adults. With adolescents its use is much more controversial, with many questions raised about informed consent, satisfaction, and long term outcome. We investigated, in persons who received ECT in adolescence, their attitudes regarding the treatment, their feelings about the informed consent procedure used, and their satisfaction with both. We compared these attitudes to those held by them about other forms of therapy including hospitalization, psycho pharmacotherapy and psychotherapy. In order to evaluate how specific these attitudes of adolescents are, an adult group treated in the past with ECT was also studied. **Methods:** We tried to contact all the patients who were treated with ECT in our center during the years 1990–2002. Thirteen adolescents and 25 adults agreed to cooperate in a semi structured interview **Results:** Most patients in both age groups considered ECT a legitimate and effective type of therapy, thought it should be used more, and were appreciative of the help it gave them. There was no correlation between satisfaction about the explanation of ECT and its' subjective efficacy. It was the least effective therapy for the adult group (p > 0.05). For the adolescent group psychotherapy was the most subjectively effective type of therapy (p > 0.05), significantly more effective than for adults (p = 0.026). **Conclusion:** Satisfaction with the explanation does not influence the subjective efficiency of therapy. Adolescents' attitudes differ from those of adults and should be studied separately. Comparison of different therapies is important in studying attitudes and satisfaction of patients.

S-050   Topic: 83

Pervasive developmental disorders I

Track: Pervasive developmental disorders (PDD)
Chairperson: Kosuke Yamazaki, Tokai University, Sagamihara Kanagawa, Japan, araki-ken@k-con.co.jp

S-050-227   Topic: 83, 37

Sensory integration in children with relation and communicating disorders

Pedro Caldeira da Silva, Hospital Dona Estefania, Unidade da Primeira Infancia, Lisboa, Portugal, pedrocs@lycos.com
Graça Santos; Filipa Martins

Objective: Sensory integration is a neurological process through which central nervous system collects, selects, organizes, associates and interprets sensory "input" in order to generate an adapted response to the environment. These responses generate new stimuli themselves. If the initial stimulus is not processed and organized in a correct way, non-adaptive motor/behavioural responses are produced by an altered feedback effect. Children who do not have adequate sensory integration abilities often show physical and emotional non-adaptive responses to the environmental stimuli. Children with relating and communicating disorders (or autistic spectrum disorders) are described as often presenting disturbances in sensory processing and modulation. The aim of this study is to identify sensory processing difficulties in children with relating and communicating disorders when compared with a group of normal children. **Methods:** 30 children aged between 3 and 10 with a diagnosis of Relating and Communicating Disorder (Multisystem Developmental Disorder – DC 0-3 or Pervasive Developmental Disorder – DSM IV) were compared with an age- and gender-matched group of 30 children with no pathology. Dunn's Sensory Profile questionnaire was filled up by parents of all children. Statistical analysis using independent samples t-test of means and Bonferroni correction was used in order to determine differences between the groups. **Results:** Statistical differences were identified in seven of nine categories of the sensory profile. **Conclusion:** The results highlight the need for an accurate assessment and intervention in the field of sensory integration in children with Relating and Communicating Disorders.

S-050-228   Topic: 83, 41

Individuals with Pervasive Developmental Disorders (PDD) diagnosed in adolescence:

Implications for clinical practice

Yen-Nan Chiu, Nat. Taiwan University Hosp., Dept. of Psychiatry, Taipei, Taiwan, philipch@ha.mc.ntu.edu.tw
Wei-Tsuen Soong; Wen-Jer Tsai; Shur-Fen Gau; Chang-Chang Tseng; Shu-Chen Su

Objective: To explore the reasons of referral and the causes of late diagnosis of individuals with pervasive developmental disorder (PDD) who seek psychiatric help for the first time in adolescence. **Methods:** The study is carried out at Children's Mental Health Center (CMHC) of National Taiwan University Hospital. The computer system of the hospital first printed out the names of those patients who visited CMHC in 1988 to January 2004, carried the diagnosis of PDD and were 12 years or older during visit. The researchers reviewed the medical records of these patients for the PDD subtype diagnosis, the age of the first diagnosis of PDD, and the causes that precipitated the referral. **Results:** 1. Fifty-one cases were confirmed to have PDD diagnosed in 12 years or older. Among them 20 were Autistic Disorder, 18 were Asperger Disorder, and the rest had diagnosis of PDDNOS or Atypical Autism. Three fifth of them had at least one comorbid neuropsychiatric diagnosis among which adjustment disorder was the most common. 2. The most common presenting problems precipitated their visits in adolescence were emotional, behavioral, academic and interpersonal problems. 3. The reasons for late diagnosis of PDD could be attributed to comorbid psychopathology, mild or atypical autistic features, high ability of compensation, and other psychosocial factors. The changing concept of PDD, the increased awareness of PDD among parents, teachers and other professionals, and sophistication of the assessment skills of mental health workers to diagnose PDD were also important to diagnose these mild atypical cases in adolescence. **Conclusion:** Comorbid psychopathology and mild atypical autistic features might hinder the early diagnosis of PDD. Mental health workers need to have adequate training to achieve early diagnosis and, therefore, to provide better service for individuals with PDD and their families.

S-050-229   Topic: 83, 32

Testosterone in autism

Jan Croonenberghs, University of Antwerp, AZ Middelheim, Antwerp, Belgium, jan.croonenberghs@ocmw.antwerpen.be
Lucas Brouw; Annick Wauters; Dirk Deboutte

Objective: Research on the biological pathophysiology of autism has found some evidence that alterations in androgenic hormones may play a role in the pathophysiology of that disorder. As a consequence we expected to find that autism is accompanied by abnormalities in the serum Testosterone concentration. **Methods:** This study examines the serum Testosterone concentration on 9 consecutive time points between 08.00 AM and 12.00 AM. 18 high- functioning male youngsters with autism (age 12–18) and 22 healthy volunteers participated in this study. ANOVA with repeated measurements were employed to check the influences of time and diagnosis and the time×diagnosis interaction during the test. **Results:** ANOVA with repeated measurements revealed a significant time effect, with a decline in the Testosterone concentration during the test (F = 21.4, df = 6/494, p = < 0.00001) and time×diagnosis interaction (F = 2.2, df = 6/494, p = 0.03) within the total group of subjects and a diagnosis effect (mean score 1.51 in autism and 1.86 in normal controls; F = 7.55, df = 1/36, p = 0.009) between both groups of subjects. **Conclusion:** There is an expected diurnal rhythm in the total group but, pending on the diagnosis this rhythm differs between both groups. Moreover the total testosterone concentration over the 9 time points is significantly lower in the autism group suggesting that a decrease of the serum Testosterone concentration may take part in the pathophysiology of autism. Perinatal Testosterone concentrations are known to play an important role in brain morphogenetic processes in general and especially in sex-dependent developmental disorders such as autism where there exists a clear predominance in boys. Further research should be directed at the study of Testosterone concentrations in umbilical cord blood and in saliva during the weeks after birth.

S-050-231 Topic: 83, 30

Visual-spatial processing in normal children and children with autism

Nicole Bruning, RWTH Aachen,
Kinder- und Jugendpsychiatrie, Aachen, Germany,
nbruning@ukaachen.de
Zina Manjaly; Kerstin Konrad; Gereon Fink;
Beate Herpertz-Dahlmann

Objective: Several studies indicate that compared to healthy children, autistic children have an advantage in performing visual-spatial search tasks like the "Embedded Figures Task". This task is commonly used to study local visual search processes, by searching for a target shape hidden in a more complex figure. A prominent theory for explaining these findings is the "theory of weak central coherence" according to which autistic individuals exhibit a deficiency in central processes responsible for combining component features into a coherent whole. Within the present study we aimed to investigate the specific neural processes underlying visual search. **Methods:** Using functional magnetic resonance imaging (fMRI) we studied 12 right-handed male autistic adolescents (diagnosed according to ICD-10) and 12 healthy controls (M = 14.65, SD = 3.17 years). While lying in the Scanner all subjects performed the Embedded Figures Task (EFT), a control task and a simple shape recognition task by using a categorial block design. All data were collected in a 1.5 T scanner. Data were analyzed with SPM2. **Results:** First data indicate an increased neural activitiy in the right temporoparietal junction, the right superior temporal gyrus, and the left cerebellum in childrem with autism. These preliminary data will be discussed in comparison to a healthy control group. **Conclusion:** Current data demonstrate task-specific activations in brain regions which have been previously implicated in functional studies of autism. The predominant right-hemispheric temporoparietal activations of the autistic group might reflect a disturbance of the normal local (left hemisphere)global (right hemisphere) balance. This is in accordance with the theory of weak central coherence.

S-050-232 Topic: 83

Differential diagnostic problems in child and adolescent psychiatry: Example of autistic spectrum disorders

Olivera Aleksic, Institute for Mental Health, Belgrade,
Serbia and Montenegro, imz@imh.org.yu
Nenad Rudic; Milica Pejovic-Milovancevic;
Smiljka Popovic-Deusic

Objective: Within the range of pervasive developmental disorders, autism, as the central syndrome is often difficult to be marked off out of the variety of developmental disorders in childhood, at the beginning of diagnostic procedures. First manifestations in children could match the initial prominent difficulties in language expression, attention deficit disorder, mental retardation with psychosis, deafness with behavioural problems, etc. We analyzed the evolution of psychopathological manifestations in children diagnosed as pervasive developmental disorders, as well as the timely evolution of established diagnosis (over the de-

cade). **Results:** On the beginning of treatment 71 children had diagnosis in the category of autistic spectrum. At the end of therapeutic process (after 5–10 years) was found: 52.11% of children got the diagnosis of autisme, 8.45% got the diagnosis of Asperger syndrome, 15.49% Mental retardation with minimal psychotic features, 7.04% early childhood psychosis, 14.08% developmental disorders of language, 2.82% Mental retardation with hypercinetic symptoms. **Conclusion:** Early working diagnosis established by child psychiatrist is generally of dynamic character and therefore could be considered as wrong by laymen or even some experts. We are discussing main reasons for these difficulties.

S-051 Topic: 13

SSRI in the treatment of depression in children and adolescents – a cause for concern? (Part II)

Track: Therapy and intervention

Chairperson: Stanley P. Kutcher, Dalhousie University,
Halifax, Nova Scotia, Canada, stan.kutcher@dal.ca

SSRI in the treatment of depression in children and adolescents – a cause for concern? Part II

Jörg M. Fegert, Universität Ulm, Kinder- und
Jugendpsychiatrie, Ulm, Germany,
joerg.fegert@medizin.uni-ulm.de

In addition to the speakers of the first part of the symposium, a panel of experts will have the opportunity to discuss the clinical consequences of the SSRI crisis. Prof. Müller-Oerlinghausen, the president of the German Drug Commission, will inform about spontaneous report systems in Europe and mention specific German cases from the German Medical Report System for adverse events. A representative from the pharmaceutical industry as well as a representative from regulatory agencies have been invited. Child psychiatrists from different countries representing their national professional societies complete the panel. Profs. Remschmidt and Kutcher will summarize the results of the panel discussion and formulate interim recommendations for the use of SSRIs at that moment. The organizers off the two SSRI-symposia are convinced that it is necessary to keep this somewhat open space for a panel discussion because at the moment of abstract submission there was a steady flow of new information in this field. For example, the FDA announced 03.22.2004 that the agency asked manufacturers to change the label of 10 antidepressants to include stronger cautions and warnings about the need to monitor patients for the worsening of depression and the emergence of suicidal thoughts, regardless of the cause of such worsening. The 10 antidepressants covered under that warning are paroxetine, bupropion, fluoxetine, sertraline, citalopram, escitalopram, venlafaxine, mirtazapine, nefazodone and fluvoxamine. The FDA is currently reviewing studies of the use of antidepressants in pediatric populations but aimed this warning at both pediatric and adult use of the drugs. In this session, the first part of this workshop will be continued by a panel discussion with the same experts as in part I.

S-052   Topic: 83, 24
Multiple complex developmental disorders:
A developmental category on the interface of Autism and Schizophrenia Spectrum Disorder
Track: Pervasive developmental disorders (PDD)

Chairperson: Rutger Jan van der Gaag, UMCN ACKJON Nijmegen Child & Adolescent Psychiatry, Nijmegen, Netherlands, rutger.jan.van.der.gaag@skjpon.nl

Multiple Complex Developmental Disorders:
A developmental category on the interface of Autism and Schizophrenia Spectrum Disorder
Rutger Jan van der Gaag, UMCN ACKJON Nijmegen, Child & Adolescent Psychiatry, Nijmegen, Netherlands, rutger.jan.van.der.gaag@skjpon.nl

Multiple Complex Developmental Disorder (McDD) is the heuristic name given by the late Donald Cohen (1940–2001) to a category of developmental psychopathology well known in clinical practice. These children/adolescents present with problems – in the development of reciprocal social relations and social sensitivity, – in the regulation of affects & cognitive problems e.g. thought disorder. In this symposium three aspects will be highlighted: – Rutger Jan van der Gaag will reflect on the usefulness of this categorical approach in the light of research on validity and outcome, but also with regard to the increasing demand for dimensional approaches in developmental psychopathology. – Lucres Jansen will present data on stress response in children with autism versus McDD, and the resemblance of the latter group to responses by individuals with schizophrenia spectrum disorders. – Bertine Lahuis & Hanna Swaab-van Barneveld discuss data on neurocognitive profiles based on a neuropsychological pilot study in children with McDD as compared to controls both within and beyond the Autistic Spectrum. Finally – Carolien Gevers will present a comprehensive treatment and guidance approach for these children and their families and teachers based on the best available evidence.

S-052-233   Topic: 83, 69
Multiple Complex Developmental Disorders (MCDD): A subcategory within Autism Spectrum Disorder (ASD) or a precursor of schizophrenia
Rutger Jan van der Gaag, UMCN ACKJON Nijmegen, Child & Adolescent Psychiatry, Nijmegen, Netherlands, rutger.jan.van.der.gaag@skjpon.nl

Objective: To introduce the concept of Multiple Complex Developmental Disorder a heuristic category on the interface of autism spectrum disorders and schizophrenia spectrum disorders. **Methods:** Review of the evidence in the literature: In 1986 the regretted late Donald Cohen proposed a heuristic category McDD for inclusion within DSM IV in order to foster studies on children frequently seen in clinical practice yet difficult to classify properly. They share the problems in the development of reciprocal social relations with children and adolescents with PDD/ASD. Yet they are also characterized by their severe problems in regulating affective states and thought disorders. In a series of studies (Towbin 1993; Van der Gaag 1995; Paul 1999) the face validity of the concept was underscored. **Conclusion:** Follow up studies has given support both to the hypothesis that McDD is comparable to Asper-

ger's a persistent condition within Autism Spectrum Disorders, but also with an incidence of psychotic episodes in more than 10% of the adult follow up cases, a sign that McDD has a risk comparable to schizotypal personality disorder vis à vis schizophrenia. In this presentation these data will be presented and critically discussed.

S-052-234   Topic: 83, 69
Differentiation between autism and Multiple Complex Developmental Disorder (MCDD) in the response to psychosocial stress: Relevance to schizophrenia
Lucres Jansen, VU Medical Center, Child Psychiatry, Duivendrecht, Netherlands, jaapenlucres@zonnet.nl
Christine C. Gispen-De Wied; Herman van Engeland

Objective: Multiple Complex Developmental Disorder (MCDD) forms a distinct group within the autistic spectrum. Unlike autistic children, part of MCDD children develops schizophrenia in adult life. Despite differences, both disorders are still characterized by abnormal reactions to their social environment. **Methods:** In the present study, MCDD children were compared to autistic children in their response to a psychosocial stressor, consisting of a public speaking task, and in their response to a physical stressor, consisting of 10 minutes of bicycle exercise. Biological responses to the stress tests were measured on heart rate and salivary cortisol. **Results:** Although both autistic and MCDD children showed decreased heart rate responses compared to normal controls, autistic children showed normal cortisol responses, while MCDD children showed decreased cortisol responses to the psychosocial stressor. The difference in cortisol response was specific for psychosocial stress, since no significant differences between groups in heart rate or cortisol responses to the physical stress test were found. **Conclusion:** The results may indicate that disturbed reactions to the social environment in autism and MCDD have different biological backgrounds. Moreover, the decreased response to stress in MCDD children resembles our previous finding of a selective impairment in the cortisol response to the same psychosocial stressor in schizophrenia. Therefore, the decreased cortisol response in MCDD may be a vulnerability factor for the development of schizophrenia that is present in MCDD children but not in autistic children. It might even be argued that MCDD children should be placed in the schizophrenic spectrum, rather than the autistic spectrum.

S-052-235   Topic: 83, 30
Discriminating MCDD subtype from PDD-NOS based on cognitive parameters
Bertine Lahuis, University Hospital Utrecht, Childpsychiatry, Utrecht, Netherlands, b.e.lahuis@azu.nl
Hanna Swaab; Jolijn Pietersen

Objective: The studies of Towbin (1993) and van der Gaag (1995) gave support to the validation of the MCDD concept. Further research on the MCDD group is focusing on finding discriminating parameters which can help define MCDD as a subtype of PDD-NOS. This might further reveal that the MCDD group may represent patients on the spectrum between autism and schizophrenia. This would be in line with the findings of the follow-up study of van der Gaag who found a high percentage of patients with MCDD who developed a diagnosis in the schizophrenia spectrum at a later age. **Methods:** In order to differentiate between patients with PDD-NOS and patients with PDD-NOS, subtype MCDD, cognitive performance on several specific tasks was evaluated. Children who were admitted at the psychiatric child clinic of the University Hospital Utrecht in the period 1998–2003 and received the diagnosis PDD-NOS or PDD-NOS, subtype MCDD are included in the present study. All had an extensive standardized psychological evaluation in the first 8 weeks of their admission. Several specific aspects of cognitive functioning in both groups will be presented, like verbal reasoning, concept formation, visual information processing and social reasoning. **Results:** The results will be presented and discussed in the light of the question whether MCDD is a relevant subtype within PDD-NOS.

S-052-236   Topic: 83, 19
A treatment guideline for children with Multiple Complex Developmental Disorders (MCDD) and their families

Carolien Gevers, AMC – de Bascule, Amsterdam, Netherlands, boergevers@planet.nl

Objective: The present presentation focuses on the treatment approach for children and adolescents with Multiple Complex Developmental Disorders. **Methods:** The programme is based on the clinical experience with these children and their families in the University Hospital of Amsterdam over the past recent years. The diagnostic classification Multiple complex Developmental Disorder (McDD) has been proposed for a sub-group of children within the pervasive developmental disorder-spectrum. McDD children prove to be less disturbed in social interaction, communication and show less stereotyped and rigid behaviour than children with autism but in contrast are found to show more thought disorders, primitive anxieties and aggression. Until now no specific treatment methods for children with McDD are available. The usual treatment methods for children with PDD-NOS, aimed at enhancing emotion recognition, social cognition and social skills prove not to be sufficient for children with McDD. **Conclusion:** In this presentation a provisional treatment modality for McDD children will be offered. In this modality elements will be used, derived from the treatment of children with anxiety disorders, children with conduct disorders and adolescents with schizophrenia.

S-053   Topic: 83, 87
Asperger's syndrome: A Pervasive Developmental Disorder (PDD) characterized by an integration deficit of cerebral functions

Track: Pervasive developmental disorders (PDD)

Chairperson: Helmut Remschmidt, Universität Marburg Kinder- und Jugendpsychiatrie, Marburg, Germany, remschm@med.uni-marburg.de
Inge Kamp-Becker, Universitätsklinik Marburg, Kinder- und Jugendpsychiatrie, Marburg, Germany, kampbeck@med.uni-marburg.de

Asperger's syndrome: A pervasive developmental disorder characterized by an integration deficit of cerebral functions

Helmut Remschmidt, Universität Marburg, Kinder- und Jugendpsychiatrie, Marburg, Germany, remschm@med.uni-marburg.de

Asperger's syndrome, described by Hans Asperger in 1944, is a pervasive developmental disorder that manifests itself at preschool age. It is characterized by qualitative impairments of social interaction, deficits in empathy, motor disturbances, and restrictive, repetitive and stereotyped patterns of behavior, interests and activities. A genetic etiology is assumed in context with brain dysfunctions and neuropsychological deficits which are mainly focussed upon non-verbal learning, even though the general intellectual level is within or above the normal range. Neuropsychological and brain imaging studies support the theory that cognitive and emotional functions as well as cerebral functions are less integrated in these individuals than in non-affected persons. This can be demonstrated by investigations of executive functions, theory-of-mind tasks and information processing tasks with regard to central coherence. Treatment must take into account the individual aspects of each case and is mainly based on behavior therapy, group training of social skills, vocational training in adaptation, and if necessary on medication. Pharmacological treatment is indicated in the presence of special symptoms such as hyperactivity, aggressive behavior, sleep disorders or depression. The papers of this symposium are focussed on diagnostic aspects (e.g. a new screening procedure) of the disorder, on neuropsychological investigations and on the long-term course.

S-053-237   Topic: 83, 37
Prospective neuropsychological study to evaluate external validity in Asperger's disorder

Helmut Remschmidt, Universität Marburg, Kinder- und Jugendpsychiatrie, Marburg, Germany, remschm@med.uni-marburg.de
Inge Kamp-Becker; Isabell Germerott

Objective: Despite its recent inclusion in DSM-IV and ICD 10, the validity of Asperger's syndrome (AS) is still controversial. AS has not been studied as extensively as childhood autism. The few available studies are difficult to compare, as they often differ with regard to diagnostic criteria. The purpose of this study is to contribute empirically based results to the current debate pertaining to the validation of Asperger's disorder. Special emphasis is placed on the distinction of AS from high-functioning autism (HFA). **Methods:** 66 autistic children and adolescents were investigated. The 'Autism-Diagnostic-Interview-R' (ADI-R) and 'Autism-Diagnostic-Observation-Schedule-Generic' (ADOS) was used as basic diagnostic methods. 39 probands received the diagnosis of Asperger's syndrome (AS), 27 received the diagnosis of high-functioning autism (HFA). The 'Vineland Adaptive Behavioral Scale' was used to assess adaptive functioning in communication, daily living skills and socialization. The neuropsychological assessment consisted of the following items: Intelligence profile, handedness, sensomotor abilities, visual-motor coordination, central coherence, visual-spatial perception, facial recognition, perception of emotions, executive functioning, social cognition ('theory of mind') and diagnostic tools to assess attention deficits. **Results:** The overall IQ as well as the verbal and performance IQ differentiated the groups: The AS group showed higher IQ-levels, but also the HFA group reveals a significantly higher verbal IQ than performance IQ. As to the other neurocognitive measures, only the social attribution task and the one-dimensional mental rotation task differentiated the groups (AS with better results). With regard to adaptive functioning (Vineland) the AS group showed better results. **Conclusion:** The AS group is less impaired than the HFA group. The IQ of the probands seems to be the most important factor to discriminate AS and HFA.

S-053-238   Topic: 83, 37
The screening and diagnosis of Asperger's syndrome
Inge Kamp-Becker, Universitätsklinik Marburg,
Kinder- und Jugendpsychiatrie, Marburg, Germany,
kampbeck@med.uni-marburg.de
Isabell Germerott; Helmut Remschmidt

Objective: Patients with Asperger's syndrome (AS) are often diagnosed later than those with childhood autism, also often other diagnoses are first assigned. There are only a few diagnostic instruments for this special PDD group: Most of the available instruments are validated for childhood autism at a low function level, so they may not identify children or adolescents with a milder variant of the disorder (without mental retardation or obvious language delays). The purpose of this study is to present a screening instrument (Marburg rating scale for Asperger's syndrome (MBAS)) and to analyse available instruments (The 'Autism-Diagnostic-Interview-R' (ADI-R) and 'Autism-Diagnostic-Observation-Schedule-Generic' (ADOS-G)) in aspects of suitability for this special autistic group. **Methods:** The psychometric properties of these instruments were investigated at a sample of 66 patients (39 with the diagnosis of AS and 27 with High-functioning Autism (HFA)), additional a control-group without autism was compared. Examinations for item difficulty, internal consistency, reliability, validity, sensitivity and specificity were made. For all instruments comparisons of means were made to differentiate AS from HFA Discriminant analysis and factor analysis were undertaken. **Results:** The MBAS is a reliable and valid instrument for screening and generating suspicion-diagnosis of AS. Results indicate substantial interrater reliability for ADI-R and ADOS-G. Comparisons of means indicated some differentiation of AS from HFA. A new algorithm with specific thresholds was developed to differentiate AS from HFA.

S-053-239   Topic: 83, 42
Adult outcomes for individuals with autism and Asperger syndrome
Patricia Howlin, St. Georges Hospital,
Community Health Sciences, London, United Kingdom

Objective: To explore long term outcomes in individuals with autism and Asperger syndrome. Three principal questions will be addressed: 1) What is the long-term prognosis for individuals diagnosed with ASD in childhood? 2) What factors in childhood appear to predict later outcome? 3) Is there a difference in outcome between high functioning individuals with autism and those with Asperger syndrome? **Methods:** a) A 20-25 year follow-up of 68 individuals initially diagnosed with autism in early childhood. Outcome was assessed in terms of cognitive, linguistic and social functioning. b) A comparative study of outcome in adult life for individuals with a diagnosis of autism and

those with a diagnosis of Asperger syndrome matched on variables such as age, sex, language and IQ. **Results:** Early IQ proved to be a relatively good prognostic indicator; no individual with a childhood IQ below 70 was rated as having a good outcome in adulthood. However, above IQ 70, outcome was very variable and other factors, including severity of ritualistic behaviours, onset of psychiatric problems and accessibility of adequate support systems also appeared to play an important role. No differences in outcome were found between individuals with a diagnosis of autism and those with a diagnosis of Asperger syndrome when IQ was controlled. **Conclusion:** Long term outcome in autism is highly variable. Although factors such as IQ are important, other variables, such as the severity of ritualistic behaviours, the development of additional problems in adulthood, or lack of appropriate support systems may all play a crucial role. Developing adequate support networks in adulthood is now a major challenge.

S-054   Topic: 3, 4
The role of helplines in child and adolescent mental health: Effectiveness and perspectives
Track: Therapy and intervention
Chairperson: Ernesto Caffo, University of Modena,
Dept. of Neuroscience, Modena, Italy, caffo@unimo.it
Annie Gaudière, Allo Enfance Maltraitée, Paris, France,
secdir@allo119.gouv.fr

The role of helplines in child and adolescent mental health: Effectiveness and perspectives
Ernesto Caffo, University of Modena, Dept. of Neuroscience, Modena, Italy, caffo@unimo.it

Given the high proportion of children and adolescents who do not receive any care for their mental health problems, telephone and Internet might represent an accessible and "acceptable" medium for care and/or the entry point into the mental health system. Clinical and research literature suggest that telephone and on line counseling/therapy can be used to provide help and support for those individuals whose access to services is limited by geographical/physical and emotional barriers. Positive features include anonymity and accessibility, which is also supported by the recent explosion in the use of mobile phone and Internet among adolescents and children. Compared to face-to-face counseling, telephone and web counseling (or therapy) are immediately accessible, allow anonymity and give a sense of control. These strengths are believed to make counseling possible for some who would not otherwise seek or receive help, as children and adolescents. A child, as a subject of rights, during the development carries a wide range of needs and requirements that first have to be known and understood – therefore "listened to" and then to be adequately satisfied. Listening is therefore a way of promoting well-being and health in children, as stated by the Convention on the Rights of the Child (1989, art. 12) and recognized by the European Parliament (in a document of November 25, 1996). There is much debate in the literature about the need of seeking for high quality methods to evaluate telephone and web services. It is clear that many more efforts have to be spend in researching this field in order to define standards and best practices and to develop effective training course for telephone/web counselors. In front of a widespread diffusion, only in the last few years there have been an increasing interest in theoretical aspects of telephone and web consultation, their application fields, their positive effects and limits, competencies required and quality issues. It is remarkable how research on telephone/Internet counseling is still limited. Little evidence exists to support its effectiveness for certain circumscribed problems, such as smoking cessation or youth suicide prevention. Anyway, research has not been adequately extended to evaluate its efficacy for general mental health concerns and, in particular, for children mental health (prevention and intervention). In order to guarantee all children to receive an effective answer and professional service, both public and private organizations are requested to offer a service according to basic quality requirements. But how defining the "effectiveness" of an helpline? Does it deal with the number of case referrals or with a reduction of risk factors for maladjustment or psychopathology?

S-054-240   Topic: 2
Adolescent psychopathology and helplines
Philippe Jeammet, Université Paris VI, Psychiatrie de l'Enfant, Paris, France, philippe.jeammet@imm.fr

Developmental disorders are based on individual vulnerabilities that most often will only be expressed and organised as pathological behaviours according to social context, events, and encounters. Detecting the potential for them before the appearance of any disorder in the patient presupposes a theory of personality development not based on symptomatic and behavioural manifestations alone. In the same way, treating these disorders does not mean merely reducing them to their most patent manifestations, it is also means preventing both their organisation into a stable behaviour and the risks of future disorganisation. It also means preventing damage to self-image and self-esteem in these subjects due to disorders which marginalize them, sabotaging their potential and compromising their future. This evolution challenges current approaches and interventions as to what constitutes the most effective means of bringing about change in children and adolescents. Beyond the theoretical approach, what is taking shape is a theory of the psychical care of children and adolescents. According to this introduction, helplines might be used to provide help and support for those children and adolescents who are in difficulties, in emergency (e.g. suicide attempts) and whose access to services is limited by geographical, physical and emotional barriers. Compared to face-to-face counseling, telephone counseling (or therapy) is immediately accessible, allows anonymity and gives a sense of control. These strengths are believed to make treatment and care possible for some who would not otherwise seek or receive help.

S-054-241   Topic: 2
Emergency lines and the mental health system
Barbara Forresi, University of Modena, and Reggio Emilia, Modena, Italy, forresi.barbara@unimore.it
G. Lepri; Ernesto Caffo

Objective: The author will illustrate rationale, ongoing process and evaluation procedures of the Italian public emergency line (114) that Telefono Azzurro has been assigned to manage since January 2004. Delivering a quality service is a major challenge helplines must face nowadays. It is further more important in case of emergency situations concerning children and adolescents (runaways, child abuse and neglect, family violence, attempted suicide, car accidents, etc.): a detailed assessment of needs, risk and protective factors is needed, as well as a prompt activation of local services. Much research show that an effective care of children and adolescents in emergency situations (preventing psychopathological outcomes such as post-traumatic disorders) is possible if adopting a multidisciplinary and multiagency approach: it implies collaboration among different professionals/specific agencies (Health and Social Services, Court, Law Enforcement) and a comparison between different languages and methods of intervention. Since the end of March 2003 Italian government entrust Telefono Azzurro with a new public emergency helpline (114). From May 2004 the service is definitely provided in three representative regions in Italy: Lombardia, Veneto and Sicily. **Methods:** Since a systematic and sensitive follow up is necessary to guarantee an effective intervention, a proper data collection methodology has been brought up to allow the follow up. The evaluation of the 114 effectiveness (and, at the same time, of the local network) will be brought on through a case study methodology. A second step will be a quantitative analysis on cases reported to 114 during the period January–May 2004. **Results:** In addition to define a more detailed overview on violence and abuse in childhood and adolescence in Italy, we expect that the service will be useful to: defining best practices of intervention in emergency situations; improving and possibly spreading a multidisciplinary and multiagencies model to face emergency situations; defining operators' competencies and performance indicators (referring to "European Helpline Operators Competencies', European Daphne Project 1999); preventing short, medium and long term psychopathological outcomes. **Conclusion:** First suggestions on preliminary data and ongoing processes will be presented.

S-054-242   Topic: 51
"Allô Enfance Maltraitée":
The role of helplines in child maltreatment
Soumaila Laval, France

Allô Enfance Maltraitée is a free 24 hour phone number, whose aims are helping children and adolescents in situations of abuse, protecting children in danger and preventing developmental maladjustment and psychopathology. Counsellors provide immediate and caring support, information and, if necessary, referral to local community or social service agency. Allô Enfance Maltraitée is also involved in epidemiological studies on child maltreatment. The helpline is composed by professionals: psychologists, lawyers, social workers. Four competences are necessary to become a telephone counsellor: relational skills; knowledge of maltreatment-related pathologies; knowledge of local services; use of social networks. A telephone counsellor listens to children and adolescents, evaluates the described situation, intervenes in order to help the caller, giving psychological support or information about local structures. A team of coordinators represents the interface between 119 and local agencies. Within the context of the Daphne project – promoted by the European Commission for the Protection of Women and Children – Snatem, in collaboration with other European helplines (Telefono Azzurro, NSPCC, etc.) contributed to the development of a European child helpline network. This project got many important results: the European Chart of Telephone Hotlines – easily adaptable to different countries – the definition of quality indicators and the development of a training guide for telephone counsellors.

S-055   Topic: 39, 48
Infant Psychiatry: Diagnostic and therapeutic pathways
Chairperson: Andreas Wiefel, Charite Berlin Kinder- und Jugendpsychiatrie, Berlin, Germany, andreas.wiefel@charite.de
Kai von Klitzing, Universität Basel Kinder- und Jugendpsychiatrie, Basel, Switzerland, kai.vonklitzing@unibas.ch

Infant Psychiatry: Diagnostic and therapeutic pathways
Andreas Wiefel, Charite Berlin, Kinder- und Jugendpsychiatrie, Berlin, Germany, andreas.wiefel@charite.de

In the field of infant psychiatry several international groups are dealing with different categorical classification systems and dimensional assessment as an approach to infant psychopathology. In this symposium empirical data and clinical experience on these issues are presented. Wiefel et al. examined a heterogenous clinical group with infant psychiatric disorders and measured the quality of the relationship in videotaped interaction with the "Emotional Availability Scales". They compared the ratings with clinical findings. Dunitz-Scheer et al. describe their intervention program for tube weaning in 207 children with a mean age of 29 months. Cordeiro and Caldeira will contribute with a clinical case of severe interaction and regulatory disorder in a 6 month follow up. Tyano et al. report on their experience in an Israel infant mental health center. Muratori et al. describe a clinical sample of children under five with emotional disorder. They give a definition of severity and present their therapeutic procedure. Maldonado-Duran et al. validated DC 0–3 diagnosis in 200 infants age 0–3. Finally von Klitzing et al. report about 200 patients and their data about temperament qualities, depressive feelings of the parents and relational problems in the families. They present an interdisciplinary approach.

S-055-243   Topic: 39
Emotional availability in infant psychiatry
Andreas Wiefel, Charite Berlin, Kinder- und Jugendpsychiatrie, Berlin, Germany, andreas.wiefel@charite.de
Z. Biringen; Karl Titze; K. Lenz; C. Seither; B. Witte; Ulrike Lehmkuhl

Objective: This study contributes to the understanding of the connection between parent-infant-relationship quality and infant psychopathology. Emotional availability (EA) is a key variable in this domain. We expected different EA between diagnostic groups and to find lowest EA in cases with high extent of recommended intervention independent from diagnostic groups. **Methods:** We describe an ongoing sample of infants age 0–3 and their parents referred for infant psychiatric disorder to our "Baby-Consultation". At the moment, from more than 100 referrals data of 68 mother-child dyads are completed. Based on DC 0–3 axis I we created six different clinical groups (regulation-, feeding-, attachment-, externalizing-, other- and "no" disorders). We assessed relationship quality with the "Emotional Availability Scales" (EAS) based on videotaped interaction. The extent of recommended intervention was deter-

mined by clinical expert rating and allocated into three groups. Statistical analyses were controlled for age, gender and SES. **Results:** Significant lowest EA-ratings were found in dyads with feeding disorders particularly in contrast to regulation disorders which showed the best results (p < 0.001). The extent of the recommended interventions was highest in dyads with low EA (p < 0.001). **Conclusion:** Diagnosis of relationship-quality, as measured with EAS, proved to be a leading dimension in diagnostic process of infant psychopathology. Our results in feeding disorders indicate that quality of relationship determines severity of infant psychiatric disorders. The EAS could be helpful in developing screening tools for grading relationship disturbances and the extent of interventions.

S-055-244   Topic: 39
Weaning of the feeling tube in early infancy
Marguerite Dunitz-Scheer, Universitätskinderklinik Graz, Graz, Austria, marguerite.dunitz@klinikum-graz.at
Markus Wilken; Alexandra Krasnovsky; Peter Scheer

Prolonged tube feeding is often compromised by the medical and psychological complications. Tube weaning after long-lasting tube feeding depends on therapeutic counselling. But therapeutic concepts for tube weaning are rarely developed and seldom evaluated. Therapeutic Program:We present an home based and impatient tube weaning program.The program is interdisciplinary and focus on self regulated of feeding. The program based on psychodynamic psychotherapy assumptions. Evaluation: 207 children between 6 mon. and 7.7 years (M = 29.7 mon.) of age were involved in the intervention program. Medical and psycho-social factors suggested to influence tube weaning and the beginning of nutritional intake after termination of tube feeding were recorded. All important areas of development are described by multiaxial ZTT-DC: 0–3. Results: After intervention 96.3% of the whole sample were totally oral fed. Age at tube weaning, duration of tube feeding and medical reason for tube feeding did not influence therapy success. Conclusions: The home based intervention for weaning tube feeding is an effective intervention program. Further evaluation has to be done.

S-055-245   Topic: 48
A clinical case of severe interaction disorder
Maria Cordeiro, Hospital de Dona Estefania, Lisbon, Portugal, mjgoncalves@hdestefania.min-saude.pt

S-055-246   Topic: 40, 86
Emotional disorders in under five children
Filippo Muratori, Division of Child Neurology an, Pisa, Italy, filippo.muratori@inpe.unipi.it
S. Maestro; B. Felloni; A. Cesari

Across multiple epidemiological studies, approximately 10% to 15% of preschool children have mild to moderate behavioral and emotional problems. Longitudinal studies demonstrate that many early childhood behavioral and emotional difficulties occur at age 3 with adult psychopathology. Early diagnosis of these problems is paramount. Objective of this study is to examine how the Diagnostic Classification of Mental Health and Developmental Disorders of Infancy and Early Childhood (DC 0–3) primary diagnoses, Parent-Infant Relationship Global Assessment

Scale (PIR-GAS), and Child Behavior Checklist (CBCL/1.5–5) externalizing and internalizing symptoms augment the DSM-IV informations and can guide treatment. Method: 64 children aged 18 to 52 months, who presented with emotional disorder to an early childhood psychiatry clinic, were diagnosed, using DC 0–3, as affected by regulatory disorders or disorders of affect. Statistical analysis were used to compare these two groups of children on PIR-GAS and CBCL scores. DSM-oriented scales were also considered. The attended major results are 1) a clinical description of young children with emotional disorders, 2) a definition of severity of these behavioral and emotional problems, and 3) an improvement in therapeutic procedure for young children.

S-055-247   Topic: 39, 37

Empirical validation of a child symptom checklist for the zero to three diagnostic classification system

Martin Maldonado-Duran, Family Service and Guidance, Child Psychiatry, Topeka, USA, maldo2000mor@aol.com
Charles Millhuff; Linda Helmig; Peter Fonagy;
Chris Moody; Jim Fultz

Objective: The purpose of this study was to empirically test a child symptom checklist (ECAP) in predicting diagnoses made according to the Zero to Three Diagnostic Classification of infant emotional/behavioral disturbances. Methods: Data on symptoms exhibited by 167 children aged 0–3 years who were seen at an infant mental health clinic were reanalyzed to determine the extent to which different diagnostic categories could be distinguished from one another on the basis of symptom clusters. Results: Through a statistical technique called a classification tree, symptoms clustered in a way that was able to predict children's diagnoses based on their severity of symptoms in several areas of symptoms/functioning: communication difficulties, anxiety, unusual sensitivities, sleep difficulties, motor problems, anger, and excessive crying/irritability. The model produced sensitivity of 71% and cross-validation sensitivity of 59%. Conclusion: The diagnostic classification tree provides preliminary validation for several diagnostic categories, including disorders of relating and communicating (autistic spectrum), adjustment disorder (a mild and transient disturbance) and for regulatory disturbances (particularly motorically disorganized and hypersensitive types). Implications for clinical use and validity of the classification are discussed.

S-055-248   Topic: 4, 39

Assessment of temperament, psychopathology and parental depression within an interdisciplinary early intervention program for infants with regulatory disorders

Kai von Klitzing, Universität Basel,
Kinder- und Jugendpsychiatrie, Basel, Switzerland,
kai.vonklitzing@unibas.ch
René Glanzmann; Nathalie Lutz-Latil; Agnes van Wyl

Objective: Some years ago, we have created an interdisciplinary clinical program for infants with regulatory, feeding, and sleep disorders. The parents and children are assessed and treated by an interdisciplinary team of pediatricians, child psychiatrist, and nurses. Methods: In the symposium we will present the data of the first 180 patients of this clinical program. The diagnostic assessments were documented by the DC 0–3 system, additionally the parents complete questionnaires concerning the infant's temperament (ICQ) and their own depressive feelings (EPDS). Results: We found high numbers of infants' difficult temperament characteristics, depressive feelings (mostly in mothers but also in fathers), and relational problems in the families. Additionally, a few infants had biological risk factors. In most cases, short interventions (2–5 sessions) were sufficient to improve the infants' and the families' regulatory and relational competencies. Conclusion: The diagnostic procedures, treatment options and difficulties in the interdisciplinary work will be discussed.

S-055-249   Topic: 40

Infant psychiatry in Israel

Sam Tyano, Geha Mental Health Center, Petah Tiqva, Israel, styano@post.tau.ac.il
Mirelle Keren

Objective: To describe the phases of the process of implementation of a new field in Israeli child psychiatry, i.e., Infant psychiatry. Methods: Conceptualisation of the theoretical concepts that underlied the successive steps of the implementation of a network of Infant Psychiatry. Results: 7 units of infant mental health (multidisciplinary teams) have been implemented in the community across the country, while in parallel a two-years academic training program has been set up at the Tel-Aviv university medical school. A computerized multilingual clinical chart for Infants has been created in order to collect comparative data, within the country as well as outside of it. As part of the basic conceptualization of these units, research projects have been inserted into the clinical work. A change can be observed in the referral sources along time: it started with well-baby clinics nurses, then self referrals, pediatricians, social workers, and last come adult psychiatrists, child psychiatrists and adoption services. Conclusion: The process of implementing a new field within child psychiatry specifically, and in medecine in general, is interesting in itself, because it is the result of the interplay between accumulation of knowledge in the specific domain, motivational factors of the specific persons involved, and availability of resources at the specific period of time.

S-056   Topic: 2

The WHO-task force on child and adolescent mental health in Europe: Risks and challenges of psychosocial development

Track: Therapy and intervention
Chairperson: Franz Resch, Universität Heidelberg
Kinder- und Jugendpsychiatrie, Heidelberg, Germany,
franz_resch@med.uni-heidelberg.de

The WHO-task force on child and adolescent mental health in Europe: Risks and challenges of psychosocial development

Franz Resch, Universität Heidelberg, Kinder- und Jugendpsychiatrie, Heidelberg, Germany,
franz_resch@med.uni-heidelberg.de

Mental health problems of children and adolescent represent a key area of concern in recent WHO mental health programmes. Psychosocial risks in countries of transition, changes of social processes with differential impact on girls and boys and a virtual absence of specific policies facing the basic needs of children and adolescents in Europe have became a major challenge for mental health professionals. Advocacy as an essential part of health policy requires a set of knowledge, support and interdisciplinary dialogue to raise awareness of these important issues.

S-056-250   Topic: 2, 45
Analysis of obstacles for implementation of best practices in child mental health services in Central and Eastern Europe
Dainius Puras, Vilnius University, Centre of Child Psychiatry, Vilnius, Lithuania, dainius.puras@mf.vu.lt

Objective: There is a growing concern about poor mental health of children in former communist countries of Eastern and Central Europe and lack of adequate and effective response from governmental agencies in the field of child mental health. Analysis of obstacles for effective child mental health policies in Lithuania was performed. **Methods:** Analysis of mental health scene in the Republic of Lithuania was performed with the help of "Country profile" – a new instrument (Jenkins R. et al.) which has been designed to gather and enhance the use of qualitative and quantitative data from relevant country expertise about mental health issues. Special emphasis was made on context, resources, processes and outcomes. **Results:** Analysis revealed basic cluster of obstacles for development and implementation of effective child mental health policies: 1. Poor governance and low level of cooperation between different governmental agencies. 2. Further medicalization (after several decades of ideologically based biomedical reductionism in Soviet psychiatry) of social aspects of public mental health problems, as a result of transition of mental health services to new health insurance schemes based on narrow biomedical paradigm and lack of traditions of teamwork and effective psychosocial interventions. 3. High level of stigmatization of vulnerable groups (including families, children and youth at risk of social pathology) among general population. 4. Absence of evidence-based child mental health policy. In this situation of "vicious circle" development of effective modern public mental health approaches (involvement of families and communities) is often ignored by authorities, and priority in allocation of limited resources is given to traditional system based on the "historical" principles of social exclusion and institutionalization. **Conclusion:** Attitudes of general population, politicians and professionals, based on stigma, learned helplessness, paternalism and lack of political will, are major obstacles for development and implementation of modern child mental health policies. Lack of funding for effective child and family mental health interventions appears to be just a secondary negative outcome of prevailing attitudes. This conclusion challenges the traditional view which emphasizes lack of financial resources in former communist countries as basic obstacle for development of modern mental health services. The process of enlargement of European Union should be used more effectively for introducing best public health and social inclusion practices in the field of child mental health services in the countries of Eastern and Central Europe.

S-056-251   Topic: 66
Children's rights
Amaia Hervás, Hospital Mutua de Terrassa, Child & Adolescent Men. Health, Terrassa, Spain, 32989ahz@comb.es

Children and adolescents have the right to be protected and parents, teachers, judges, politicians and society in general have the duty to fulfil the children and adolescents rights. Every country independent of the level of political stability or level of socio-economic development must protect their children against abandonment, abuse and exploitation. A children act worked together by all professionals in care of children and in the best interest of the child should be developed in each country. Children have basic and essential rights to be emotionally, physically, educationally and sexually looked after what must address issues such as parenting competence, child custody and family law. More specific issues are those related to mental health services are those related to consent to treatment, confidentiality, ethics of what must be or not adequate in the care of mentally disturbed children, clinical responsibility sometimes against children wishes (risk versus responsibility). Ethics are especially relevant to the more vulnerable children and adolescents such as the ones with cognitive delay. The development of research has also brought up issues in relation to the protection of children involved in research studies. Clinical trials, community research, genetics and neuroimaging studies has opened the need for common protocols to defend the ethics and rights of the children. Relevant to the training of all professionals working with children must be the learning of ethics in their clinical and research practices.

S-056-252   Topic: 3, 63
The European Early Promotion Project (EEPP): A training programme for primary health care professionals
John Tsiantis, Aghia Sophia Hospital, Child & Adolescent Psychiatry, Athens, Greece, itsiantis@cc.uoa.gr
T. Dragonas; H. Davis; Kaija Puura; Tuula Tamminen; V. Ispanovic; A. Paradisiotou

Objective: The European Early Promotion Project constitutes of longitudinal and multicultural study aiming to develop intervention procedures that can be used by Primary Health Care Professionals (PHCPs) in order to promote early psychosocial health of children. **Methods:** A group of PHCPs participated in an intense training programme, with the goal of further developing their skills in identifying factors that can jeopardize early psychosocial development and intervene accordingly. The participating PHCPs conducted home visits in a sample of pregnant women, from the 4th week before birth until the child was 24 months old. The PHCPs' home contacts were arranged in frequency according to the families' need status. In families characterized as "in need", the PHCPs worked with the mother, under the regular supervision by experienced child health professionals. **Results:** The evaluation of the programme was based on the comparison of the work of the trained PHCPs (intervention group) with the work of an untrained group of PHCPs (control group). The evaluation process was conducted by trained and independent evaluators and was focused on: 1) the change of PHCPs knowledge and attitudes, as part of the training programme, 2) their skills in identifying factors that may jeopardize early psychosocial development and 3) the result of their intervention in the families and the child at 24 months of his/her life. **Conclusion:** Results will be presented indicating a change in PHCP's knowledge level to the expected direction and provide evidence towards the more accurate identification of family need level by the trained PHCP's. The implication of these findings for the organization of preventive services will be discussed.

S-056-253   Topic: 93, 3
Depression and suicide prevention in children and adolescents in Russia
Tatjana Dmitrieva, Center for Mental Health of Children and Adolescents, Nizhny Novgorod, Russia, tndmitr@sandy.ru

Objective: During the last ten years in Russia some of negative trends such as sharp socio-economic problems, extreme class stratification and the ideological changes have been apparent. The official statistical data demonstrated the high level of mental disorders in children. Difficult situation for children can be shown by the increased number of suicides, which rose visibly during the last ten years. About 25% depressive children also show conduct disorder that increased markedly. This is important to identify and help such children and adolescents as soon as possible. **Methods:** There were investigated all school children aged from 11 to 15 years in three ordinary schools of Nizhny Novgorod by special instrument (Depression Scale of Balashova). **Results:** High frequency of depressive disorders was found. The ways to help these children and their families in the multidisciplinary way are discussed. **Conclusion:** Psychiatric health services should be used as accessible and non-stigmatizing for children. Connection of child psychiatrists and school specialists could be very helpful because school is a significant area for depression/suicide prevention and mental health promotion. Early identification of affective and conduct disorders in children and qualified help is an important way to prevent suicidality.

S-056-254   Topic: 43, 45
Child and adolescent mental health in post conflict countries
Mimoza Shanini, USA.
Lynne Jones; A. Uka; A. Rrustemi

Objective: To describe week and strong points that have been taken in consideration on setting up a new service on Child and Adolescent Mental Health (CAMHS) in Kosova. **Methods:** Data were collected from different researches done in Kosova during last five years. **Results:** a) Kosova lacked adequate public health data on the child and adolescent mental health needs prior to the conflict. On such situation it was very important to analyze the nature of social interchanges and other very important aspects as economical, political that interferes on setting services, especially on child and adolescent mental health. A comprehensive, culturally appropriate child and adolescent mental health service is needed to address a wide range of problems b) The service should be developed through local actors, and build on already established local infrastructure. Services can also play an educational role in stigma. c) Developing the Mental Health Services about the resilience and other copying family mechanisms as a unique model of mental health service organization in the region, today present the official policy and basic orientation of the reforms in mental health. d) The Education and support for other health professionals

and NGO-s was essential part of the service. **Conclusion:** Based in the work done in Kosova after the war ended we think the development of a sustainable, community based child and adolescent mental health service has to be in congruence with the whole system of care.

S-056-255   Topic: 43, 68
Risk taking behaviour, alcohol and drugs in adolescents
Anne-Liis von Knorring, University Hospital Uppsala, Child & Adolescent Psychiatry, Uppsala, Sweden, anne-liis.von_knorring@bupinst.uu.se

Objective: The ethiology of alcohol and drug abuse is multidimensional. Early onset with antisocial and disruptive behaviour is highly genetic, often called type 2 alcoholism. **Results:** Type 2 alcohol abuse/dependence is mostly combined with abuse of other "street" drugs. Very often the onset of drug abuse is preceeded by oppositional defiant and conduct disorder with or without ADHD. Personality traits related to type 2 alcoholism is sensation seeking behaviour (Zuckerman) or novelty seeking behaviour (Cloninger) or monotony avoidance (Karoliska scales of personality, KSP; Schalling). Type 2 alcoholism is also associated with low momoamine oxidase activity in platelets, a marker of low seronergic turnover. MAO activity in platelets is highly genetic. **Conclusion:** It seems plausible that low serotonergic turnover is genetic and one of the factors underlying sensation seeking behaviour and early onset drug abuse. This is supported by the finding of low 5-HIAA in CSF of conduct disordered boys found by Kruesi et al.

S-056-256   Topic: 2
A frame work for organisation and content of child mental health
Dirk Deboutte, Jansen-Cilag, Antwerp, Belgium, dirk.deboutte@zna.be

Objective: To develop elements for a framework for organisation and content of child and adolescent mental health. **Methods:** A large study of the literature was done about the different theories and models for organisation of child and adolescent mental health and for description and definition of the content. **Results:** A framework is developed based on the fundaments of human and child rights, the principles of evidence based care, the factors influencing mental health of children and the aetiology of psychiatric disorders of children. **Conclusion:** In policy and practice of organising mental health for children and adolescents, it is very important to make a distinction between 'care for mental health' and 'mental health care'.

S-057   Topic: 78
Eating and feeding disorders/Obesity I
Track: Eating disorders
Chairperson: Alan Apter, Schneider Childrens Medical Dept. of Psychiatry, Petah Tikva, Israel, eapter@clalit.org.il

S-057-257   Topic: 78, 95
Eating disorders

Alan Apter, Schneider Childrens Medical Dept. of Psychiatry, Petah Tikva, Israel, eapter@clalit.org.il

Objective: To assess the influence of comorbidity and personality on the symptoms and severity of Anorexia Nervosa in adolescents. **Methods:** 94 adolescent girls with AN were assessed. Comorbidity was measured with the Structured Clinical Interview for Diagnosis, and personality was assessed with the Cloninger's Tridimensional Personality Questionnaire. Symptoms severity was measured with the Eating Disorders Examination, the Eating Disorders Inventory-2, Body Mass Index (worst ever), number of hospitalizations, duration of symptoms prior to hospitalization, and the Beck Depression Inventory. **Results:** Patients who suffered from any comorbid psychiatric illness (OCD, depression, anxiety, substance use) showed more severe symptomatology, and showed a specific pattern on the TPQ. **Conclusion:** Comorbidity needs to be carefully assessed in the evaluation of patients with AN, and is a confounding variable in any research performed in this area.

S-057-258   Topic: 78, 56
Quality of life among Moroccan adolescents with obesity

Souraya Dorhmi, CPU Ibn Rushd, Dept. of Psychiatry, Casablanca, Morocco, sourayadorhmi@yahoo.fr
Mohamed Agoub; Driss Moussaoui; Omar Battas

Objective: The obesity has a significant impact on the psychosocial status and the quality of life. Physical and psychosocial functioning are negatively impacted by overweight. The aim of the present study was to investigate the psychological profile of Moroccan adolescents with obesity and to determine its impact on their quality of life and their self-esteem. **Methods:** Participants (50 adolescents with obesity and 50 controls of normal weight) completed the Rathus Assertiveness Schedule and the SF-36 health Survey to assess respectively the self-esteem and the quality of life. **Results:** Results showed lower self-esteem in obese adolescent and a deterioration in the majority of SF-36 domains. **Conclusion:** Quality of life and psychological approach of obese adolescent should be included in the global management of these patients in developing countries.

S-057-259   Topic: 78, 10
Good outcome of early-onset Anorexia Nervosa (AN) after systematic treatment integrating family therapy and treatment to restore physical health

Inger Halvorsen, Sykehuset Buskerud, HF, BUPA, Nesbru, Norway, inger.halvorsen@r-bup.no
Anne Andersen; Sonja Heyerdahl

Objective: The aim of the study was to investigate the intermediate to longterm outcome of the eating disorder (ED), other psychiatric problems and psychosocial functioning of childhood and adolescent onset Anorexia Nervosa (AN) in a representative county-sample. **Methods:** The project is a follow-up study 3.5–14.5 (mean 8.8) years after treatment start. Subjects: Fifty-one of 55 female patients under 18 years with a DSM-IV AN-diagnosis referred to treatment in Buskerud County during the period 1986–1998. Mean age at treatment start was 14.9±SD 1.8 years,

mean BMI 15.1±SD 1.5. All received family therapy integrated with treatment to restore physical health. Thirty-one (61%) were hospitalised in the paediatric ward. Twenty-five siblings were used as a control-group and 34 mothers/27 fathers as informants on psychosocial functioning. At follow-up personal interview, measurement of weight/height and questionnaires to the former patients, siblings and parents were used. Instruments: EDE, EDI, MINI, Y-BOCS, S-GAF, Achenbach's YASR/BCL. **Results:** Forty-two (82%) had no ED at follow-up, 1 had AN, 1 had Bulimia Nervosa and 7 had EDNOS. There was no mortality. Attitudes to eating and body weight were relaxed for 23 (61%) and somewhat strainful for 15 (39%) of those without ED at follow-up. Twenty (41%) had one or more other axis-1-psychiatric diagnoses at follow up. Depression and anxiety disorders were frequent. The S-GAF ratings were very good (>80) for 26 (53%) on the functioning-scale and for 19 (39%) on the symptom-scale. Questionnaire-results reported by both parents and the former patients were in agreement with interview-results. Compared with the siblings, the former patients were high on internalizing problems (YASR/BCL). The cross-informant agreement between self-reported and parent-reported problems was high. **Conclusion:** The outcome of the eating disorder was good. However, in accordance with other studies, many subjects had other psychiatric problems at follow-up. The former AN-patients had more internalizing problems than their siblings.

S-057-260   Topic: 78, 43
A cross-cultural study of risk and protective factors for eating and weight disorders in youth living in France and North America

Martine Flament, University of Ottawa, Inst. Mental Health Research, Ottawa, ON, Canada, mflament@rohcg.on.ca
Denise Baillot; Michele La Roche; Claudia Furino; Annick Buchholtz; Gary Goldfield; Katherine Henderson

Objective: A wide range of personal, familial and societal factors have been shown to contribute to the onset of eating and weight disorders in adolescence. This study aims at comparing cultural and environmental factors involved in the development of healthy or unhealthy body image, eating practices, and body weight in youth living in France and North America, while controlling for the individual and family factors that have been shown in previous research to contribute to the development of eating and weight disturbances. **Methods:** Several lycées in France, and high schools in the United States (grades 9–12) have been approached, in order to obtain, in both countries, a wide and unselected sample of youth, varied in geographic and socio-demographic distribution (N=1500 subjects per country). Validated and reliable self-report questionnaires have been selected to measure a variey of constructs, including body image, emotional regulation, coping, interpersonal functioning, family functioning, societal pressures, eating beliefs and behaviours. The questionnaire package is individually filled by students in the course of normal class time, under supervision. **Results:** At this time, the survey has been successfully completed by 600 students in France, and 752 in the United States. Preliminary results will be presented. **Conclusion:** Even though obesity and the eating disorders are more and more prevalent in industrialized countries, and have been shown to be largely culturally determined, very few studies have compared weight preoccupations, body image and healthy or disordered eating between Western countries, in relation to prevailing societal and environmental influences. Findings from the study are expected to advance knowledge about the interplay of individual, environmental and societal factors that contribute to the development of body satisfaction or dissatisfaction, healthy or unhealthy eating, and weight status in adolescence. The international perspective should permit identification of both common and divergent risk/protective factors across varying cultures.

S-057-261 Topic: 78, 10
Psychoeducation for parents of adolescents with eating disorders

Ulrich Hagenah, RWTH Aachen, Kinder- und Jugendpsychiatrie, Aachen, Germany, uhagenah@ukaachen.de
Varinja Blume; Marlene Flacke-Redanz; Beate Herpertz-Dahlmann

Objective: Psychoeducation is a well-established component of cognitive-behavioral therapy in adult patients with eating disorders. Our department has offered a group model of psychoeducation to parents of adolescents with eating disorders. **Methods:** A group model of psychoeducation has been offered by our department for the past four years to parents of $n = 136$ adolescents with anorexia or bulimia nervosa. For a subgroup a self-constructed questionnaire concerning eating disorder psychopathology and family coping abilities was administered at the starting point. A second questionnaire was administered after the last session to estimate parents agreement with the psychoeducation program. **Results:** More mothers ($n = 130$) than fathers ($n = 88$) participated. After the psychoeducation program parent reports ($n = 100$) demonstrated high levels of agreement according to the relevance for a better understanding of treatment modalities (85%) and coping with the illness (88%). **Conclusion:** Preliminary data indicate that parents, according to their own report, appreciate this means of support to help them to cope with their child's illness.

S-057-262 Topic: 78, 1
Obesity – A big problem in the United States: Are we exporting it? Can it be 'reduced'?

Angelique A. Sallas, Chicago, IL, USA, drsallas@aol.com

Obesity among the young in the United States is on its way to reaching epidemic proportions. One out of every four children is overweight; Type 2 diabetes diagnosed in children is on the increase; and, 85% of children diagnosed with Type 2 diabetes are obese. The emotional and physical health issues associated with obesity could overwhelm the health care system The question arises: How did we get from food, which is fuel, necessary to the survival and health of all organisms from single cells to humans, to obesity as a health problem of epidemic proportions? Both the problem and solution are multi-faceted. They involve genetic, physiological, environmental, behavioral, psychological, socioeconomic and cultural factors. This paper will focus, in particular, on the problem of obesity in America from the perspectives of culture and behavior. The following questions will be addressed: Are we exporting this problem? What are the trends in other countries? What can be learned from an examination of

the underpinnings of the problem in the United States about factors that could help guide the development of strategies to curb or prevent obesity and its concomitant physical and psychological/emotional problems from becoming world-wide problems of epidemic proportions?

S-058 Topic: 63
Experience of teaching child and adolescent psychiatry and psychotherapy in developing countries

Chairperson: Hubertus Adam, UKE Hamburg-Eppendorf Kinder- und Jugendpsychiatrie, Hamburg, Germany, adam@uke.uni-hamburg.de
Joachim Walter, Luisenklinik, Bad Dürrheim, Germany, drjoachimwalter@web.de

Experience of teaching child and adolescent psychiatry and psychotherapy in developing countries

Hubertus Adam, UKE Hamburg-Eppendorf, Kinder- und Jugendpsychiatrie, Hamburg, Germany, adam@uke.uni-hamburg.de

While countries of the so-called "First World" have well established Child and Adolescent Psychiatry and Psychotherapy (CAPP) Programmes, there remains a paucity of teaching programmes in many countries of Asia, Latin America and Africa where even basic services remain unavailable. Where rudimentary services are functional, teaching and training is often limited to the area of prevention or to psychotherapeutic responses to social trauma. The arena of transcultural and intercultural teaching offers new insights to both lecturers and trainees. This symposium will examine the experience of CAPP trainers and trainees coming from the developing countries of Mozambique (Boia Efraime), Kosovo (Aferdita Uka), South Africa (Umesh Bawa) and Iraq (Fakhri Khalik). Discussion regarding the appropriateness of issues of culture, their interrelatedness to contextual approaches to CAPP and the experience of indigenous knowledge systems in CAPP interventions will be shared and explored.

S-058-263 Topic: 63
Training in child psychotherapy in Mocambique

Boia Ephraime jr., Mozambique, Joachim Walter

During the years 2000–2004 a complete CAPP curriculum including 220 hours of seminars and lectures, case discussions and supervision, as well as psychoanalytic didactic analysis in a group setting was conducted by local monitors and lecturers from Germany, Portugal and Brazil. The experience of the concrete use of education in Mozambique, sustainability of projects, intra- and transcultural issues, as well as the lessons to be learnt for the planning and implementation of similar curricular projects will be shared.

S-058-264 Topic: 63
Training in child psychotherapy in Kosovo

Aferdita Goci-Uka, Children for Tomorrow, Frankfurt, Germany,
Susanne Schlüter-Müller

During the years 2000–2004 a psychotherapeutic training of co-therapists was run in Kosovo for psychoeducational teams including nurses, translators, and drivers. Cooperating with the University of Pristhina, supervision was provided for child and adolescent psychiatrists in training and treatment structures were established. The experiences that will be discussed include issues of treatment and the development of new structures for child psychiatry within a traumatised, post-war society.

S-058-265   Topic: 63
Training in child psychotherapy in South Africa
Umesh Bawa, University of the Western Cape Town, Cape Town, South Africa
Hubertus Adam

Since 1999 the Children in Crisis Project in the township of Langa, Cape Town provides psychotherapeutic services for psychically traumatised children. In co-operation with the University of the Western Cape as well as the University of Stellenbosch, a training has already been established for project personnel, and a full CAPP curriculum for psychologists in the public and private domain is envisaged. Experiences will be discussed regarding training in post-apartheid times, as well as curriculum issues confronting indigenous Xhosa speakers. Of crucial importance will be the exploration of the challenges facing Western psychology when confronted with local expertise.

S-058-266   Topic: 63
Training in child psychotherapy in Near and Middle East
Fakhri Khalik, Darmstädter Kinderkliniken, Abt. Psychosomatik, Darmstadt, Germany, fakhrikhalik@aol.com
Nima Forouher

Training in child psychotherapy in Near and Middle East: In 2003 a group of Iraqi Child Psychiatrists living in German exile collaborated to offer psychotherapeutic support for children of Iraq. It is intended to run curricula for psychologists and paediatricians in Iraq and in Germany. Experiences will be discussed regarding the development of services and teaching under severe security conditions, as well as the challenge to integrate different cultural approaches in providing psychotherapeutic support to war traumatised children.

S-059   Topic: 83
Biology of autism: Current research and future perspectives of the research in Japan
Track: Pervasive developmental disorders (PDD)
Chairperson: Per-Anders Rydelius, Karolinska Institutet Woman and Child Health, Stockholm, Sweden, per-anders.rydelius@ks.se
Kosuke Yamazaki, Tokai University, Sagamihara Kanagawa, Japan, araki-ken@k-con.co.jp

Biology of autism: Current research and future perspectives of the research in Japan
Per-Anders Rydelius, Karolinska Institutet, Woman and Child Health, Stockholm, Sweden, per-anders.rydelius@ks.se

It is known the prevalence of autism spectrum disorders is steadily increasing in recent years in United States. The similar trend is noted in Japan as well, now getting a matter of newspaper's concern. As well known, concordance of autism in monozygotic twins is very high, which implies heavy involvement of genetic factors. However it may be unlikely the genetic factors are the sole contributor to the recent increase of autistic disorders. Here we intend to overview current biological research of autism in Japan, with focus on molecular genetics, environmental factors as well as clinical neuroimaging studies.

S-059-267   Topic: 83, 90
Animal model of autism:
Possible implication of thyroid hormone
Miyuki Sadamatsu, Shiga University, Dept. of Psychiatry, Otsu, Japan, sadamatu@belle.shiga-med.ac.jp

Objective: Thyroid hormone is essential for mammalian brain development, but the mechanisms are poorly understood. It is well known that maternal hypothyroidism can lead to neurological deficits in the offspring. We have reported that rat pups exposed to antithyroid agent, propylthiouracil (PTU) via maternal milk exhibit hyperactivity, spatial learning impairment and hypersensitivity to sound that develops seizures after matured. Since a dose of PTU is weak (0.02%), those rats display only a mild hypothyroidism, and recovered thyroid function after weaning, despite they show lifelong deficits in behavior. These behavioral abnormalities are thought to resemble those observed in human autistic patients, but conventional laboratory investigations so far failed to reveal any specific pathology after matured. Recently, knockout mice lacking of thyroid hormone receptors (TRKO) have been suggested to show behavioral abnormalities and auditory deficit. **Methods:** In this study, we studied the development of cerebellum and several other brain regions in PTU rat pups and TRKO (a,β) with use of immunohistochemical and TUNEL methods. **Results:** Hyperactivity was obvious in PTU rat pups and TRKOa. Using TUNEL method, time course of apoptosis in the cerebellum was delayed in PTU rats and TRKOa. Furthermore, expressions of several gene families like fibroblast growth factor (FGF), Wnt1, Pax6, known as essential in formation and maintenance of isthmic organization, were also delayed in the cerebellum of PTU rats. **Conclusion:** It is thus suggested that developmental hormone deficit may provoke derangement of gene expressions in the cerebellum and related structures, which in turn provides the basis of lifelong behavioral abnormalities, and also that these structural abnormalities are only manifested in some critical period.

S-059-268   Topic: 83, 28
Molecular genetics of autism:
Basic and clinical perspectives
Eiji Nanba, Tottori University, Center for Bioscience and Tech, Yonago, Japan, enanba@grape.med.tottori-u.ac.jp

Autism is considered to be most strongly genetically influenced by the family and twin studies. The inheritance mode is complex and more than 20 genetic loci on human chromosomes may contribute. Genomic imprinting, which is an epigenetic mechanism and recently focused in psychiatry disease, may play an important role. Although huge genetic studies have been reported, no contributing gene has yet been identified definitely. We have been performing genetic studies of Japanese autism from several viewpoints. First, we picked up candidate genes mainly related to early embryonic brain, neruotransmitter and the single gene disorders manifested by autism. The several genes including HOX, Gastrin-releasing peptide receptor, serotonin transporter, FMR1, and NF-1 were analyzed. GXAlu polymorphism in intron 27 of NF-1 gene, a susceptibility gene for Neurofibromatosis-1 was analyzed and the allele frequencies were different between autism and control. The unique variations of HOXA1 gene were found in the study. Furthermore, the functional abnormalities of the variations were observed by the expression using COS cells. Second, the study of (the entire) imprinting genes related to the psychiatric diseases including autism has been performed. The novel genes were found recently and the several imprinting genes have been analyzed in autism. Finally, the future approach using DNA microarray technology will be discussed. The genetic background may be unique in Japanese autism.

S-059-269   Topic: 83

Structural and functional neuroimaging of autism and Asperger's syndrome

*Nobumasa Kato, Graduate School of Medicine,
Dept. of Neuropsychiatry, Tokyo, Japan
Kiyoto Kasai*

Objective: We used multimodal neuroimaging to understand pathophysiology of pervasive developmental disorders (PDDs) including autism and Asperger's disorder. **Methods:** 1) Structural magnetic resonance imaging (MRI): Voxel-based morphometry (VBM) was applied to a monozygotic twin pair concordant for Asperger's disorder. 2) Event-related potentials (ERPs): Visual attention system was evaluated in patients with autism and control subjects using ERPs. 3) Magnetoencephalography (MEG): Auditory mismatch negativity in response to change in phonemes was evaluated in patients with autism and control subjects using MEG. 4) Near-infrared spectroscopy (NIRS): Prefrontal activity during verbal fluency test was measured in patients with PDDs and control subjects. 5) Functional MRI: Illusion and prepulse inhibition tasks were used to evaluate altered neural network in autism. **Results:** 1) The single subject analysis using VBM revealed that both twins had markedly smaller amygdala volume than healthy subjects. 2) ERPs related to visual attention were significantly different between autism and control subjects. 3) The latency of mismatch negativity was significantly prolonged in autism patients compared with normal controls. 4) Prefrontal activity was significantly decreased in patients with PDDs compared with normal controls. 5) Different neural networks from control subjects were activated in autistic subjects in accomplishing the tasks. **Conclusion:** These converging results suggest that PDDs including autistic and Asperger's disorder are associated with structural and functional abnormalities in the cortical regions including the frontotemporal neocortex and the limbic system.

S-059-270   Topic: 42, 35

Life-histories of severely autistic persons from the 1930's until today

*Per-Anders Rydelius, Karolinska Institutet, Woman and
Child Health, Stockholm, Sweden, per-anders.rydelius@ks.se
Kosuke Yamazaki; Nobumasa Kato; Miyuki Sadamatsu;
Eiji Nanba*

Objective: Until the 1930s, Swedish children suffering from Dementia Infantilis or Dementia Praecocissima, were mainly cared for in asylums and mental hospitals. From 1935, when regular treatment was still based mainly upon genetics, race biology and eugenics, an alternative treatment was introduced. The patients were offered "a meaningful treatment and a decent life" using the anthroposophical form of curative education. Until today these programs have been in progress for almost 70 years and several hundred patients have been treated. **Methods:** Case histories: A man, born in 1923, was admitted at age 12 and still lives at the same place. In 1929, at the age of 6 he was given the diagnosis of Dementia Praecox. He fulfilled the DSM-criteria for Infantile Autism as a child and those for Childhood Onset Pervasive Developmental Disorder later on. He has never developed a communicative language. For his whole life, he has had stereotyped behavior, rituals and anxiety paroxysms.Despite this, he has taken part in all the daily activities at the treatment home and benefited from this. When he became 67, the age of retirement in Sweden, he obviously was aware of his 'new status' and adjusted himself and his habits to gentler activities. A girl born in 1950 was admitted at the age of 4 years. Her status fulfilled DSM-criteria for Infantile Autism. She started to speak at age 6 years, successively improved and could attend normal school. Her behaviour seemed to normalize to the extent that she could graduated from senior high school and was later married, having an occupation, but no children. A mentally retarded boy, born in 1981, with the DSM diagnosis of Infantile Autism was admitted at the age of 9 years. Today, at the age of 23, he still has no language. From unsuccessful efforts to use speech therapy, the use of pictograms etc., and as characteristics indicated a true "concrete behavior", photos, "true pictures of his real world", have been used for communication. This has been very successful. His severe panic attacks have been mastered. **Results:** From the long experiences you may say that the majority of the patients entering the programs is having lifelong handicaps and is in need of a 24-hour supportive program. Some have developed rather well and need only day care as adults. A very few can handle their life situation as adults, with only limited support in one case an almost complete remission seems to have taken place. From experience, the staff has learnt to assess prognosis from language development. An early onset of language and a short period of an 'autistic echo-speech' indicate capacity for development.

S-060   Topic: 24, 84

Developmental Psychopathology:
Lessons from longitudinal studies

*Chairperson: Hans-Christoph Steinhausen, ZKJP Universität
Zürich Kinder- und Jugendpsychiatrie, Zürich, Switzerland,
steinh@kjpd.unizh.ch
Frank C. Verhulst, Erasmus MC-Sophia, Child & Adolescent
Psychiatry, Rotterdam, Netherlands, m.engel@erasmusmc.nl*

Developmental Psychopathology:
Lessons from longitudinal studies

*Hans-Christoph Steinhausen, ZKJP Universität Zürich,
Kinder- und Jugendpsychiatrie, Zürich, Switzerland,
steinh@kjpd.unizh.ch*

Longitudinal studies are essential for the understanding of the development of psychopathology. They answer questions concerning origins and prognosis of psychopathology across a wide age range, the relevance of various sorts of risks and protective factors for later psychopathology, and even the efficacy of interventions. Findings from longitudinal studies may also lead to a more effective planning of prevention. The objective of this symposium is to provide an overview of some recent European longitudinal studies which have been based on large epidemiological samples and have addressed important questions in developmental psychopathology Frank Verhulst and his coworkers from the Netherlands will report on the developmental trajectories of various problem behaviours from childhood to adulthood. His study is based on a large epidemiological sample that has been followed up for 14 year. The outcome includes a wide variety of psychiatric diagnoses with a special emphasis on antisocial behaviour. Based on another epidemiological study in the community Laucht and Schmidt from Germany address the question whether or not maternal smoking during pregnancy represents an independent risk factor for later development of attention-deficit-hyperactivity disorder in childhood. Based on the same cohort Esser and his colleagues from Germany studied the interplay of risk and protective factors for child psychiatric disorders. The issue of early mother-child interaction is particularly stressed in this contribution. Finally, Steinhausen and Winkler Metzke from Switzerland report on the stability of externalizing problems in another community based longitudinal study. The poor outcome of the early onset of externalizing problems has been cross-validated in this study.

S-060-271 Topic: 24, 42
Child-adult continuities and discontinuities of psychopathology
Frank C. Verhulst, Erasmus MC-Sophia, Child & Adolescent Psychiatry, Rotterdam, Netherlands, m.engel@erasmusmc.nl

Although more and more research confirms that child and adolescent psychopathology tends to be persistent, little is known about the individual developmental trajectories of various problem behaviors that children and adolescents follow across time into adulthood. In this presentation findings from a 14-year follow-up of a sample of children originally aged 14- to 16 years from the general population will be shown. Parental information obtained via the Child Behavior Checklist was collected with 2-year time intervals across an 8-year period. Six years later this sample was interviewed with a standardized psychiatric interview (CIDI). Also, standardized information on antisocial behaviors was collected. We used multilevel growth curve analyses to estimate trajectories of problem behaviors across the first 8-year interval. Associations between these trajectories and DSM diagnoses and antisocial behaviors assessed at the last measurement were determined. The results showed that trajectories of childhood/adolescent problem behaviors could be distinguished that were associated with specific outcomes in adulthood.

S-060-272 Topic: 84, 43
Maternal smoking during pregnancy: Risk factor for ADHD in the offspring?
Martin H. Schmidt, Zentralinstitut für Seelische Gesundheit, Mannheim, Germany, schmidt@zi-mannheim.de
Manfred Laucht

Objective: To examine the specifity of the association between maternal smoking during pregnancy and child behaviour problems. **Methods:** In a prospective longitudinal study of a birth cohort of 362 children at risk parental tobacco use, cognitive and social-emotional outcome and characteristics of family environment were assessed. **Results:** About a quarter of mothers reported regular tobacco use during pregnancy. Children in this group exhibited enhanced rates of ADHS. This association held even after adjustment for a number of covariates. **Conclusion:** The findings suggest that maternal smoking during pregnancy may represent an independent risk factor for ADHS in the offspring.

S-060-273 Topic: 43
Risk and protective factors for child psychiatric disorders
Günter Esser, Universität Potsdam, Inst. Klinische Psychologie, Potsdam, Germany, gesser@rz.uni-potsdam.de
Martin H. Schmidt; Manfred Laucht

Objective: The development of children who have been exposed to early stressors is characterized by high variability. Which are the determining factors of children who remain at risk and which overcome adversity? **Methods:** Data will be presented from the Mannheim Study of Risk Children, a prospective longitudinal study following a cohort of 362 children from birth into school age with assessments at 3 months, 2, 4 1/2, 8, and 11 years. Organic and psychosocial risk factors were varied in a two-factoral design. **Results:** The results up to the age of eight years indicate that developmental outcome of very low birthweight infants and of children of postnatally depressed mothers varies as a function of early mother-child interaction quality. **Conclusion:** These findings stress the importance of mother-child-interaction in the development of children at risk.

S-060-274 Topic: 24, 84
Developmental psychopathology of externalizing problems
Hans-Christoph Steinhausen, ZKJP Universität Zürich, Kinder- und Jugendpsychiatrie, Zürich, Switzerland, steinh@kjpd.unizh.ch
C. Winkler Metzke

Objective: To examine the stability and outcome of externalizing problems (EP) in a large community sample of adolescents. **Methods:** In a prospective longitudinal study (N = 624) high-risk subjects with EP and matched controls were studied at mean ages of 13, 16, and 20 years. Stability of EP, prediction of EP by a large series of psychosocial variables, and course of early onset and persistent EP vs. late onset of EP were studied. **Results:** Stability of EP across the three times of assessment was high. Antecedent aggression was the strongest predictor of EP in late adolescence and young adulthood. Early onset and persistent EP in contrast to late onset EP was associated with higher rates of substance abuse and more behavioural and emotional problems in young adulthood. **Conclusion:** This large community based longitudinal study provides further evidence of the high stability of externalizing problems and particularly for the early onset type.

S-061 Topic: 83
Pervasive developmental disorders III
Track: Pervasive developmental disorders (PDD)

Chairperson: Herman van Engeland, University Medical
Center Child & Adolescent Psychiatry, Utrecht, Netherlands,
h.vanengeland@azu.nl
Barry Nurcombe, University of Queensland,
Dept. of Psychiatry, Brisbane, Australia,
bnurcombe@psychiatry.uq.edu.au

S-061-275 Topic: 83, 37
Early screening for Autism Spectrum Disorders

Sophie Willemsen-Swinkels, UMC St Radboud Nijmegen,
Dept. of Psychiatry, Nijmegen, Netherlands,
sophie.willemsen@skjpon.nl
Claudine Dietz; Emma Van Daalen; Anne Claire Beernink;
Herman van Engeland; Jan Buitelaar

Objective: The objective was to investigate the efficacy and efficiency of very early screening for Autism Spectrum Disorders in the general population (ASD). **Methods:** Two large screening studies were performed in the Dutch population. In the first study over 30,000 parents were interviewed with a four question pre-screen. 317 pre-screen positive children were given the full Early Screening for Autistic Traits (ESAT) Questionnaire. In the second study the pre-screen phase was skipped and over 6000 parents of 14-month old children completed the ESAT questionnaire. In both studies, follow up measurements of screen positive children were performed at around 42 months. **Results:** Results indicated that it is possible to identify children with ASD already at 14 months of age. Positive predictive power markedly improved with age. A second factor that markedly improved with age was parental compliance to clinical assessment. The results of both studies combined suggested a positive predictive value of 0.34 and a specificity of 0.99 for identifying ASD in the general population. False screen positives included children with language disorders, mental retardation and/or marked hyperactivity. Data will be presented on stability and positive predictive power of individual screening items and screening algorithms. **Conclusion:** Screening on a population level for delays or disturbances in social development by means of parent response items is feasible and useful already at preschool age. Screening instruments such as the ESAT can be used for signalling the need for further evaluation.

S-061-276 Topic: 83, 84
Attention difficulties in children with Asperger Syndrome

Oliver Vidojevic, Institute for Mental Health, Child
Protection Center, Belgrade, Serbia and Montenegro,
olivido@ptt.yu
Ivona Milacic

Objective: Asperger syndrome (AS) is a term used to mark a subgroup of autism with no delay in language or cognitive delopment. Research reveal language and cognitive impairments in AS (uneven profile of abilities on Wechsler intelligence scales, pragmatic deficits). Objective of this study is to examine flexibility of attention of children with AS. Children N=12 with AS aged 7–16 yrs (11 males, 1 female). All children had IQ in normal range. **Methods:** Trial Making Test (TMT-A, TMT-B) was used to measure attention flexibility. **Conclusion:** Prolonged response time on TMT-A point to motor slowing and on TMT-B which examines working memory and shifting of cognitive set (executive functions) point to the deficit in reasoning.

S-061-277 Topic: 83
Investigation of the association of an IQ measurement with information processing in Asperger's Disorder

Rael Strous, Beer Yaakov Men. Health Center, Dept. of
Psychiatry, Beer Yaakov, Israel, raels@post.tau.ac.il
Roni Hegesh; Simion Kertzman; Z. Ben-Nahum;
Moshe Kotler

Objective: Although Asperger's Disorder (AD) is characterized by deficits in social interaction in the presence of normal intelligence, performance on the IQ subtest of the Digit Symbol Substitution Test (DSST) is poor. The objective of this study was therefore to determine among children with AS whether any association exists between the DSST and more elementary cognitive function as expressed in information processing. **Methods:** 30 male patients suffering from AD (DSM-IV criteria), were investigated (mean age 17.6±11.9 years). The control group consisted of 48 healthy subjects (mean age: 15.3±1.5 years, p=0.48). A computerized neuro-cognitive battery ("CogScan") was administered and included 15 subtests: Finger Tapping Test (FTT), Inspection time, Motion Perception Test, Simple Reaction Time, Choice Reaction Time, Immediate and Delayed Memory for Pictures, Words and Faces, Time-accuracy tradeoff test, Stroop test, DSST, and Continuous Performance test. Statistical analysis was performed using linear regression (DSST score used as dependent variable, other test results served as independent variables). **Results:** The regression equation for the AD group included: Time-accuracy tradeoff test score (beta=0.44; p=0.005), FTT score (beta=0.32; p=0.016), and Choice reaction time score (beta=0.32; p=0.030). Multiple R for the equation was R=0.862 (p=0.030). The regression equation for the healthy subjects included: Choice reaction time score (beta=0.41; p=0.003), and Stroop test score (beta=0.33; p=0.014). Multiple R for the equation was R=0.615 (p=0.014). **Conclusion:** Children with AD were significantly impaired in DSST. Deficits in DSST performance in the AD group were associated with impairments in information processing as reflected in motor speed and output. In healthy children DSST performance was more associated with shifting of attention. Compared to healthy subjects, patients with AD appeared to make use different cognitive apparatus. Future neuroimaging paradigms are needed in order to confirm different performance in IQ/information processing tests and brain functioning in AD compared to healthy subjects.

S-061-278 Topic: 83, 92
Autism spectrum disorders and macrocephaly

Emma van Daalen, University Medical Center,
Child & Adolescent Psychiatry, Utrecht, Netherlands,
e.vandaalen@azu.nl
Sophie Willemsen-Swinkels; Jan Buitelaar;
Herman van Engeland

Objective: Testing the hypothesis that infantile macrocephaly is associated with an increased risk of developing autism spectrum disorders (Bolton et al., 2001). **Methods:** In a population-based sample of very young children with autism spectrum disorders and other child psychiatric disorders head circumference was measured frequently in the first year of life. At our department two psychiatric assessments and several head circumference follow-up measurements were conducted before the age of four years. The head circumference measurements were compared with those of population based measurements (TNO, the Netherlands, 1997). The data were analysed with multilevel modelling. **Results:** Subjects with an autism spectrum disorder showed a significant larger head circumference as compared to population based measurements in the first year of life (preliminary data). **Conclusion:** Our data suggest an overgrowth of the brain in the first year of life in the children diagnosed with an autistic spectrum disorder by the age of 42 months.

S-061-279   Topic: 83, 35
Volumetric MR imaging in very young children with autism and developmentally matched controls

Mijke Zeegers, UMC Utrecht, Dept. of Child Psychiatry, Utrecht, Netherlands, m.zeegers@azu.nl
Hilleke Hulshoff Pol; Emma van Daalen; Jan Buitelaar; Herman van Engeland

Objective: Autism is a severe developmental disorder, with an onset in early childhood. To date, most neuroimaging studies have focused on older children and adults and results have been contradictory. Recently, investigators including very young children in their samples have suggested that autism may be associated with unusual patterns of brain growth very early in development. However, these studies did not necessarily consider differences in developmental stage between groups. Therefore, the objective of the current study is to investigate early brain development in autism while controlling for chronological and developmental age. **Methods:** Children with autism or PDD-NOS were compared to children with either mental retardation or language disorder. All children were aged between two and six years at the time of scanning. All children were scanned under full anaesthesia on a Philips NT Gyroscan scanner, operating at 1.5 Tesla. High-resolution T1 weighted images were required in order to define brain structures and acquire volumetric measures. All scans were appraised by a neuroradiologist. Main outcome measures were intracranial volume, total brain volume, cerebellar and ventricular volume and grey and white matter volumes. **Results:** Preliminary results suggest that there is an increased incidence of brain anomalies in both groups. This finding will be related to volumetric measures of cortical areas. **Conclusion:** Results will be discussed in terms of aberrant early brain development in autism.

S-061-280   Topic: 83, 28
Recognizable genetic syndromes in children evaluated for Pervasive Developmental Disorder (PDD)

Charles Williams, University of Florida, Dept. of Pediatrics, Gainesville, FL, USA, willicx@peds.ufl.edu
Jessica Sank; Martha Paulk; George Schwarz; Paul Wharton

Objective: To determine the prevalence of identifiable genetic syndromes in a cohort of children evaluated for Pervasive Developmental Disorder. **Methods:** A genetics team, consisting of an experienced clinical dysmorphologist and a genetic counselor, performed clinical and laboratory evaluations on children being followed in an outpatient multidisciplinary program (Center for Autism and Related Dis-

abilities). All children had a diagnosis of some type of autism spectrum disorder. In each case, a detailed pedigree was obtained, records were reviewed, and a physical examination was performed. Where indicated, laboratory tests were obtained. Most children had at least one blood chromosome study performed but other testing was usually obtained only if clinically indicated (e.g., subtelomeric chromosome analyses, FISH 15q11.2 and FISH 22.q11.2 deletion tests, Fragile-X DNA studies, urine organic acid studies and brain MRI scans). **Results:** A total of 129 individuals were evaluated. The M:F ratio was 3.3:1 and the age range was 2–21 years. In 49, subtelomeric chromosome studies were performed and none showed a subtelomeric deletion (previously reported by us: Keller et al., Am J Med Genet, 2003). Distinct disorders were identified in 6 out of 129 (4.7%): Smith-Magenis syndrome, Bannayan-Riley-Ruvalcaba syndrome (BRRS), interstitial dup15q11.2, marker 15q11.2, and 5p14.2–15.1 (2 unrelated cases). No cases of Fragile X syndrome, Angelman syndrome, Rett syndrome, Tuberous Sclerosis, or 22q11.2 deletion (Velo-Cardio-Facial syndrome) were identified. **Conclusion:** Recognizable genetic or dysmorphic syndromes are uncommon in children undergoing follow-up in a clinic for autism spectrum conditions. While Fragile X syndrome, Rett syndrome, Angelman syndrome and Tuberous Sclerosis have historically been associated with autism-like features, these conditions were either not suspected clinically by our evaluation, of if suspected, were not diagnosed by specific genetic testing.

S-062   Topic: 24
Developmental psychopathology

Chairperson: Peter Riedesser, UKE Hamburg-Eppendorf Abt. Psychiatrie, Hamburg, Germany, riedesser@uke.uni-hamburg.de

S-062-281   Topic: 24, 10
Crises in adolescence: Developmental psychopathology and family functioning

Marija Raleva, Clinic of Psychiatry, Child & Adolescent Psychiatry, Skopje, Republic of Macedonia, mraleva@yahoo.com
Kamka Paketchieva; Angelina Filipovska

Objective: The main objective in this study was to perform individual psychological analysis of the adolescents in crisis, as well as contextual analysis of the individual, family and social level of functioning of the adolescents in crisis and their families. **Methods:** The sample consists of 92 adolescents and their families. Individual level of functioning has been assessed by: CBCL, (Achenbach & Edelbrock, 1983); MMPI-201; Profile Index of Emotions (PIE, Plutchnik & Kellerman, 1974), The Life Style Index (LSI, Kellerman, 1986). The family level of functioning has been assessed by: Family genogram (McGoldrick & Gersons, 1985); Darlington Family Interview Schedule, (DFIS, 1991); FACES III, Family Communication Scale, Family Satisfaction Scale (Olson et al., 1985). The social level of family functioning has been assessed by Family Eco Map (Attenaeve, 1976; Hartman, 1983). **Results:** Adolescents in crisis can be divided mainly into 3 subgroups: a subgroup with externalizing dominant symptoms, a subgroup with internalizing dominant symptoms and a subgroup with mixed (externalizing and internalizing) symptoms. All these groups of adolescents are equipped with slightly different defensive structure. All of them belong to 3 different subgroups regarding the dominant type of family triangle: triangulation with peers, with one of the parents, with school. The results of the family level of functioning have shown that families tend to group in two extreme parts of the dysfunctional range of family cohesion: enmeshment, related to the internalizing adolescent symptomatology and disengagement, related to the externalizing symptomatology. In regard to adaptability dimension, they also tend to group in the extreme levels chaotic range. The connection of the families with other social systems shows that these families have significantly low levels of social cohesion and poor social support network. **Conclusion:** This finding significantly differs from Olson's research findings, not only due to culture-specific features of the families represented in this study, but also to prolonged stress exposition at suprasystemic level.This reflects the way of adaptation to the frequently changeable suprasystem and also acts as a risk factor in further crisis.

S-062-282   Topic: 24
Parental representation and outcomes of prematurity: A socio-emotional and neurodevelopmental approach
Carole Müller Nix, Unité de Développement CHUV, Division de Néonatologie, Lausanne, Switzerland, carole.muller-nix@inst.hospvd.ch
Margarita Forcada Guex

This work is part of a prospective longitudinal study entitled "Parental representation and outcomes of prematurity: a socio-emotional and neurodevelopmental approach". Using some of this data, we explored parents' subjective experiences and their relationships with medical staff. Semi-structured videotaped interviews (CLIP, Meyer 1993) were made at 42 weeks post-conception, and at 6 and 18 months (corrected age), with a population of 70 preterm and 30 full term parents. For the parents, having a premature baby appears to be a very stressful experience, with a direct effect on their view of themselves as parents. Most premature babies stay in the NICU for months. During this long hospital stay, the parents' relationship with their infant depends on a number of factors: the infant's health, the uncertainty of the outcome, as well as on their subjective experience. In particular, the investment into their role as parents, is challenged by the constant reference to the medical team and result in wide and complex range of feelings. Most parents have high praise for the skills, and support given by the medical team. However, parents may have difficulty affirming their position as parents, becoming either too dependant, or on the contrary too much in competition with the medical team. For example, parents may express feelings of being excluded or deprived of their parental role. Between these two extremes, it appears that a certain differentiation of the parental role as opposed to that of the medical team, is essential to the confidence and security of their relationship with their child at discharge. In light of this need for differentiation, occasional disagreements that emerge between parents and the NICU staff, are perhaps a significant part of this process. In this video presentation, we will see parent interviews which clearly illustrate the aforementioned difficulties, and ambivalent feelings.

S-062-283   Topic: 43
Hopelessness as a risk factor for coronary heart disease, and its relationship with some other psychological and physiological risk factors
Abdel-Mohsen Daigham, Faculty of Arts, Dept. of Psychology, Elminia, Egypt, mdaigham@yahoo.com

Objective: Helplessness is the belief that there is nothing that anyone can do to improve a bad situation (such as being diagnosed with an illness). In many ways, then, helplessness is a belief that control over the situation outcomes is impossible. Feelings of hopelessness, loss of libido, and increased irritability, has been proposed as a risk indicator for the onset of coronary heart disease (CHD). (Cole, et. al, 1999). Over recent years, the role of depressive symptoms like hopelessness in the development of CHD has received increasing attention. A number of studies conducted in community samples have demonstrated a prospective relationship between depression, or depressive symptoms, and CHD (e.g., Anda et al. 1993; Arrmonaa et al. 1994; Barefoot & Schrool, 1996). **Methods:** This study examined the relationship between hopeless and the psychological risk factors (e.g., type A behavior, hostility, aggression, anger, competition) and physiological risk factor for coronary heart disease (blood pressure, heart rate). The following measures were used in the study: A/psychological measurements: (Beck hopelessness scale BHS; Beck, Weissman, Lester & Trexler, 1974, transelated by Daigham); (Type A behavior pattern inventory TABP); Daigham, 2000; (The relaxation inventory Crist R., et. al, 1989, translated by Daigham). B) Physiological measurements (blood pressure & Heart rate). Participants were 70 people (Egyptian sample 35 men, 35 women), 40 people non patients (control group) 30 people patients with coronary heart disease, their aged ranged from 21 to 59). The mean age for total group 32.64 and S.D 12.42. the patients with coronary heart disease were selected randomly from minia university hospital, Heart Department. All the subjects (patients & non patients) were assessed the physiological measurement and the psychological measurement. **Results:** 1) correlation results: shows significant relation between hopeless and global type A behavior, hostility, anger and systolic blood pressure, 2) the regression results show significant effects for hopeless on systolic blood pressure, on another hand the regression results show significant effects for type A behavior on systolic blood pressure, 3) the T test results show significant difference between patients with CHD and control group in type A, blood pressure, hostility, anger. **Conclusion:** Hopelessness is a risk factor for coronary heart disease.

S-062-284   Topic: 24, 41
Psychiatric symptoms and disorders in low birth weight adolescents
Marit S. Indredavik, Norwegian Univ. Science Techn., Dept. of Neuroscience, Trondheim, Norway, marit.s.indredavik@medisin.ntnu.no
Torstein Vik; Sonja Heyerdahl; Siri Kulseng; Ann-Mari Brubakk

Objective: Evaluate the prevalence of psychiatric symptoms and disorders in low birth weight adolescents. **Methods:** A population based follow-up study of 56 very low birth weight adolescents (VLBW: birth weight < 1500 g), 60 term small for gestational age (SGA: birth weight < 10th percentile) and 83 term controls (birth weight >10th percentile) at 14 years of age. Outcome measures: Schedule for Affective Disorders and Schizophrenia for School Aged Children, ADHD-Rating Scale IV, Autism Spectrum Screening Questionnaire, Achenbach System of Empirically Based Assessment (Youth Self Report, Child Behavior Check List, Teacher Report Form), Strengths and Difficulties Questionnaire (self-, mother-, father- and teacher-report). **Results:** VLBW adolescents had more psychiatric symptoms than controls, especially attention deficit, anxiety symptoms, thought problems and reduced social skills. They had higher prevalence of psychiatric disorders than controls, particularly anxiety disorders. Although 25% of the VLBW adolescents had attention problems, ADHD was diagnosed in only 7%. The term SGA group had more attention, emotional, thought and conduct problems than controls, however, the prevalence of psychiatric disorders was not significantly increased. Results remained essentially the same when adolescents with low estimated IQ were excluded, and persisted after controlling for possible confounders. **Conclusion:** The VLBW adolescents had increased prevalence of psychiatric symptoms and disorders, especially within the domains of anxiety, attention deficit and social/relational problems. They may need mental health services during the years of growth. The term SGA adolescents had modest attention deficit, emotional and behavioural problems, without increased prevalence of psychiatric disorders.

S-062-285   Topic: 42, 30
Gender differences in the cognitive functioning of children born very preterm

Marion Cuddy, Institute of Psychiatry, Dept. of Psychology P077, London, United Kingdom, sphamcc@iop.kcl.ac.uk
Matthew Allin; Katharine Riley; Brigitte Vollmer; John Wyatt; Robin Murray

Objective: It is estimated that 5–8% of babies in Europe are born preterm (<37 weeks gestational age). Follow-up studies of preterm children have found high rates of neuro-developmental disorders and of more subtle cognitive, behavioural, and neurological abnormalities. Children born preterm are more likely than their full-term peers to require special help at school, and although most have IQ scores in the normal range, as a group they tend to score significantly lower than full-term controls. Gender has been identified as a significant predictor of outcome in preterm children. To begin with, premature birth and other obstetric complications are more common in boys. Males are also more likely to experience neonatal complications after preterm birth. In measures of IQ, preterm girls tend to perform better than boys even after similar perinatal events. **Methods:** The present study examined gender differences in the cognitive functioning of very preterm children (born <33 weeks gestation). 441 very preterm girls and 499 very preterm boys were assessed at the age of 8 years using the WISC-R. **Results:** There were no gender differences in mean Full-Scale IQ scores, or in the Verbal and Performance index scores. However, girls performed significantly better than boys in the Picture Arrangement and Coding subtests of the WISC-R. **Conclusion:** Although one might have expected girls to perform better than boys in measures of language rather than spatial ability, the findings are consistent with those of other research groups that girls fare better after preterm birth. It has been suggested that asynchronous maturational rates

between the genders may be responsible for this female advantage, as there is a lag of 1.2–2.5 weeks in pulmonary and cerebral maturation in boys. Perhaps the more advanced development of the female brain during gestation enhances its resilience to the adverse neuro-developmental consequences of prematurity.

S-062-286   Topic: 37, 70
Motor activity in depressed school-aged children and their healthy peers

Mika Soininen, Helsinki University, Dept. of Child Psychiatry, Helsinki, Finland, mika.soininen@hus.fi
E. Juulia Paavonen; Mika Fjällberg; Juha Salmi; Almqvist Fredrik; Eeva T. Aronen

Objective: Depression is a common psychiatric disorder in children. Diagnosing depression in children is difficult and many cases are left without proper treatment. Motor activity is reported to change in depression. Actigraphy is an easy, noninvasive method to study children's motor activity. The aim of this study was to compare motor activity in two groups: Depressed children 9–13 yrs and their healthy peers. **Methods:** A belt-worn actigraph was used to detect motor activity in 23 depressed children and in 23 controls. The diagnosis was based on the K-SADS-PL interview. A mean CDI for the patients was 22 (range 12–37) and the mean T for the maternal CBCL was 65 (49–82) for patients and 49 (33–66) for the controls. **Results:** The mean diurnal activity was significantly lower in cases (199.29, SD 24.97) than in controls (219.61, SD 20.39), sig. 0.004. Same pattern was observed in activity median and diurnal activity SD-parameters. The sleep parameters (sleep efficiency, %sleep) were lower in control group compared to cases. In K-SADS-PL
-interview 22/23 patients reported some sleep problems and 12/23 had sleeping problems of clinical level. **Conclusion:** Activity is altered in childhood depression. More study is needed to define possible sub-groups. Sleep parameters were more favorable in cases. Supportive data using polysomnography and actigraphs simultaneously is needed.

S-063   Topic: 26
Epidemiology

Chairperson: John Fayyad, St. George Hospital Psychiatry and Psychology, Beirut, Lebanon, jfayyad@inco.com.lb

S-063-287   Topic: 26
Patterns and prevalences of psychiatric disorder syndromes – A person-centered approach

Olaf Reis, Universität Rostock, Medizin. Fakultät, Rostock, Germany, olaf.reis@med.uni-rostock.de
Stephanie P. Bohne; Susanne Kraenz

Objective: The aim of the study is to investigate whether the factorial structure of the Youth Self Report form (YSR) of the Child Behavior Checklist (Achenbach, 1991) proves robust using an empirical person-centered approach. **Methods:** A non-clinical sample of 390 subjects aged 12–19 years representing the student population of four different schools of a middle-sized German town was analyzed. The two-step cluster-analysis conducted separately for girls (n=237) and boys (n=153) revealed patterns (types) that were different to the second-order factorial structure of the YSR with regards to the gender of the participants. **Results:** The scree-plot of the clustering process suggested a 2 or 3-Cluster solution for boys and a 3 or 4 cluster-solution for girls. The 3-cluster solution for girls converged for an internalizing (n=15), an externalizing (n=49), and a non-clinical type (n=172) almost resembling the second-order structure of the YSR. For boys, the 3-cluster solution indicated a highly disturbed type (n=10), a deviant type (n=41) and a non-clinical type (n=102). This solution was not improved by adding a fourth type of psychiatric disorder syndrome. The highly disturbed type differed from the deviant type by showing very high levels of aggressive and dissocial behavior. All other scales of the YSR did not differentiate between the highly disturbed and the deviant type. **Conclusion:** We conclude that self-descriptions of girls come closer to the second-order structure suggested by the YSR, compared to the self-descriptions of boys. Advantages and limitations of an empirical person-centered approach in child and adolescent psychiatry are discussed.

S-063-288 Topic: 25, 45
National mental health survey in Korean children and adolescents

Dong-Hyun Ahn, Hanyang University Hospital, Dept. of Psychiatry, Seoul, Republic of Korea, ahndh@hanyang.ac.kr
Tae-Ho Kim; Jun-Ho Choi; Yun-Young Kim

Objective: The purpose of this nationwide survey was to identify the status of mental health of children and adolescents for effective implementation of a community-based children and adolescents mental health system in Korea. **Methods:** A-group (N=1.478; 8 sites) used Child Behavior Checklist-Korean version (K-CBCL) for screening children's problem and B-group (N=1.113; 6 sites) surveyed children's problem with Child Problem Behavior Screening Questionnaire (CPBSQ, Ahn et al., 2003) in first step and K-CBCL in second step. Teacher's reports concerning children's mental health in elementary school were obtained in 14 sites in Korea. The efficacy of CPBSQ was evaluated by comparing the two groups. **Results:** The rate of total problems in K-CBCL was 2.91% in A group and 8.72% in B group respectively; internalizing problems and externalizing problems were 3.06% and 2.85% in A group; 8.67% and 7.46% in B group. In B-group, CPBSQ could screen 35% high-risk pupils in the general population in first step, so it's right rate the rate of B group was three times higher than the that of A group. In the survey of teacher's need, 5.6% of elementary school children had some psychiatric problems in the teacher's report. We found the CPBSQ was efficient for screening children's problems in large-scale epidemiological research. But only a small group (13%) of children with behavior problems had been referred to psychiatrists by the teachers. Most important problems of school children reported by teachers were 'difficulty in concentration and distractable', 'poor skill in peer relationship', and 'angry easily and lose temper'. **Conclusion:** In this study at least 2.91% to 5.6% children in elementary school had some mental health problems. School teachers were unwilling to refer the identified children to the mental health services. Attention Deficit Hyperactivity Disorder (ADHD), Oppositional Defiant Disorder, and Social Skill Problems (probably due to Anxiety Disorder) were most striking psychiatric problems of elementary school pupils in Korea.

S-063-289 Topic: 26
Mental health problems of adolescents in Croatia – parents' and youth reports

Ivan Begovac, Psychological Medicine, Zagreb, Croatia,
ivan.begovac@zg.htnet.hr
Milena Skocic; Vlasta Rudan; Oleg Filipovic

Objective: The aim of this study was the comparison of parents' reports and youth reports on emotional and behavioural problems. **Methods:** Achenbach's Child Behaviour Check List (CBCL) and Youth Self Report (YSR) were administered to school aged children between 11–18 comprising a non-referred sample (N=790) drawn from the whole country. **Results:** Youth rated higher scores to the Internalizing and Externalizing scales and the Total Problems scale in both sexes (p<0.001). **Conclusion:** Those were the first data on the YSR in Croatia. We confirmed a higher number of reports of emotional and behavioural problems by adolescents, what makes Croatian data consistent with other international studies. In the presentation the implications of the results and their comparison with the previous findings in Croatia, as well as comparisons to other countries will be discussed.

S-063-290 Topic: 26, 86
Emotional and behavioral problems among children and adolescents in Poland –
a normative study of the CBCL, TRF and YSR

Tomasz Wolanczyk, Medical University of Warsaw,
Dept. of Child Psychiatry, Warszawa, Poland,
twolancz@amwaw.edu.pl
Anita Brynska; Stanislaw Wojtowicz; Artur Kolakowski

Objective: The aim of the study was to investigate psychometric properties of Child Behavior Checklist (CBCL), Youth Self Report (YSR) and Teacher's Report Form (TRF) in Polish normative sample and to provide preliminary data of emotional and behavioral problems among polish children and adolescents. **Methods:** The epidemiological school-based sample consist of 3122 pupils aged 7 to 19. Procedure: proportional random sampling of 132 schools in 17 regions of Poland followed by random sampling of one class per grade per. The sample is representative with respect to ethnicity, region and urban/rural residence. The clinical sample consists of 305 patients, aged 6–19 with final ICD-10 psychiatric (chapter F) diagnosis from different Polish child and adolescent psychiatry departments. Polish Version of three standardized questionnaires CBCL, YSR and TRF were prepared and administered to parents, teachers and pupils. **Results:** All 3 Polish versions of Achenbach's questionnaires have satisfactory psychometric properties. There were significant, but weak correlations between reports of various respondents. Highest correlations were observed between parental and self-reports. Effect analyses revealed sex and age effects on emotional and behavioral problems in children and adolescents. The mean results in Total Problem Score of emotional and behavioral problems were in CBCL and TRF in higher range, but in YSR in medium range of results of several international studies using this questionnaires. **Conclusion:** This study supports previous findings from studies using CBCL – similarities in emotional behavioral problems outweigh differences in cross-cultural studies.

S-064 Topic: 3
Treatment issues
Track: Therapy and intervention
Chairperson: Salvador Celia, Instituto Leo Kanner Ltoa
Child Psychiatry, Porto Alegre, Brazil, sahc@terra.com.br

S-064-291 Topic: 11
Psychotherapy and Autism
Cisca Aerts, Doorwerth, Netherlands,
c.aerts@leokannerhuis.nl

Psychotherapy for people with Autistic Spectrum Disorder is not a matter of course. When it is undertaken, it usually involves behavioral therapy or cognitive therapy. Despite this, many people with ASD remain struggling with their disability. They cannot communicate their feelings of powerlessness, their wishes or their desires. In addition, feelings of jealousy, shame, insult and so on are often difficult to discuss in a verbal therapy. This workshop will include an overview of current literature concerning ASD and psychotherapy. The emphasis, however, will be on short and long term Guided Affective Imagery Psychotherapy (KIP by Hanscarl Leuner) for adolescence with ASD, who have normal to high intelligence. Indications and contra-indications for this type of therapy will be discussed, as well as the conditions necessary for cooperation with the patient and his environment. I will discuss the role of various abilities, such as imagination, observation of pictures, recognition of emotions, ability to process traumatic experiences and transference and countertransference in the therapy. I believe that Guided Affective Imagery Psychotherapy (KIP) gives us an excellent tool for helping people with ASD (as well as their therapist and environment) to reveal and understand their perception of the environment.

S-064-292 Topic: 11
Crisis therapy with a two year old boy:
A big and a little one is gone
Elisabeth Cleve, Erica Foundation, Stockholm, Sweden,
elisabeth.cleve@ericastiftelsen.se

This is a story from inside the child psychotherapist's room. Victor, who is two and a half years old has lost his mother and younger brother in a car accident. He is 'sunny' and 'happy' and doesn't cry. Victor is a child in deep crisis and comes for a crisis therapy. In this seminar we will follow Victor for his fifteen treatment sessions. He shows through play and activities how he is followed and piloted through his grief. The healing by play therapy is depicted in words and pictures out of the perspective of both patient and therapist. The crisis therapy will work as the first link into a new future. In spite of the tragic reasons for the meetings, 'A Big and a Little One is Gone' is a documentary story which brings both hope and courage.

S-064-293 Topic: 19
Attention-Interaction-Therapy (AIT)
in the treatment of autistic children
Hellmut Hartmann, Institut für Autismusforschung,
Roskow, Germany, dr.hellmut.hartmann@t-online.de

The effectiveness of Attention-Interaction-Therapy (AIT) in the treatment of autistic children was examined in comparison with Behaviour Therapy (BT) and with a combination of both therapies. For half a year parents of seven autistic children were instructed every second week in the therapy of their own child. They had to carry out half an hour of therapy on every weekday including a daily documentation. The children were randomized and given therapy in an AIT-group (N=4) and a BT-group (N=3). After the middle of the therapy project alternating treatment of both therapies was given to all children in the same frequency while changing the therapies irregularily. The effectiveness of individual objectives was controlled in single-case-studies (AB design and multiple-baseline-design). The effectiveness of AIT could be verified according to our hypothesis. The effect of BT was lower in the individual objectives. When progress in therapy was not sufficient a combination of both therapies was more effective than only AIT or BT.

S-064-294 Topic: 84, 17
Facial expression and visual attention in children with ADHD as a tool: Fritz Jansen's video assisted procedure for the determination of the individual stimulant dose
Hans-Jürgen Kühle, Giessen, Germany,
hans.kuehle@t-online.de
Fridjof Heidorn; Solveigh Zeyer

Objective: The purposes are to demonstrate an observational procedure for the evaluation of involuntary short term behavioral signs characteristic for AD/HD and its use for stimulant dose determination. In a former study we had shown that these signs appeared significantly more frequent in children with AD/HD than in normals. First results of validation studies are presented. **Methods:** In order to determine the optimal stimulant dose, we record patients playing cards 75 min after the intake of methylphenidate, augmenting the single dose every day for 2.5 mg. We sampled in a randomized sequence two minutes of the recordings without methylphenidate, 5 mg and 2.5 mg below as well as above the optimal dose and the optimal dose of the last 25 patients who had received at least 5 recordings. 15 patients of the control group of the former study were included also in random sequence. Two raters were trained with material from other patients. Moreover, the correct solutions of 2 minutes of oral arithmetic exercises were counted. Statistic Tests: T-test for independent and dependent samples. **Results:** Preliminary results show that visual attention loss decreased in U-form-function to its lowest level at the optimal dose and reincreased with higher methylphenidate levels. Oversized smile as a marker of the changes in facial expression without medication was significantly more frequent than in the historical controls and was reduced significantly at the optimal dose. The number of correctly calculated tasks showed an inverted U-form-function. It increased significantly to the optimal dose and decreased significantly when the optimal dose was exceeded. **Conclusion:** The procedure is independent of parents' and educators' attitudes toward the child and offers a direct view on patient's selfregulation. The procedure is a new approach for the evaluation of treatment effects and dosage finding for stimulant drugs. It is deserving further study.

S-065　Topic: 17

ESCAP Symposium: Pharmacotherapy in children and adolescents in Europe

Track: Therapy and intervention

Chairperson: Ernesto Caffo, University of Modena, Dept. of Neuroscience, Modena, Italy, caffo@unimo.it

ESCAP symposium: Pharmacotherapy in children and adolescents in Europe

Ernesto Caffo, University of Modena, Dept. of Neuroscience, Modena, Italy, caffo@unimo.it

Antidepressants, especially selective serotonin reuptake inhibitors and venlafaxine, have been used increasingly as first line treatment for depression in children. The safety of prescribing antidepressants to children (including adolescents) has been the subject of increasing concern in the community and the medical profession, leading to recommendations against their use from government and industry. Investigators' conclusions on the efficacy of newer antidepressants in childhood depression have exaggerated their benefits. Improvement in control groups is strong and additional benefit from drugs is of doubtful clinical significance. Adverse effects have been downplayed. Published data suggest a favourable risk-benefit profile for some SSRIs; however, addition of unpublished data indicates that risks could outweigh benefits of these drugs (except fluoxetine) to treat depression in children and young people. Non-publication of trials, for whatever reason, or the omission of important data from published trials, can lead to erroneous recommendations for treatment. A more critical approach to ensuring the validity of published data and a greater openness and transparency with respect to all intervention studies are needed.

S-065-295　Topic: 17, 65

Ethical challenges in paediatric pharmacotherapy

Joaquin Fuentes, Policlinica Gipuzkoa, Child & Adolescent Psychiatry, San Sebastian, Spain, jfuentes@servitel.es

Objective: To review and discuss the ethical considerations involved in using psychotropic medication in the treatment of children and adolescents with psychiatric disorders. **Methods:** An exhaustive literature search on this area was complemented with the review of practice algorithms and quality oriented pharmacotherapy systems currently used in Europe. **Results:** Ethical issues were identified both for research and for clinical practice. Thus, at the research level, issues of concern related to scientific merit of research designs, safety and efficacy of the drugs, informed consent, assessment of risks and benefits and integrity of researchers. At the clinical level, diverse areas need to be considered such as accepted decision trees, predefined procedures of good practice and accountability, off-label prescription, generic versus trade name preparations, and groups at a special risk. A local model from Spain, designed to safeguard some of these ethical principles in the administration of psychotropic medication in highly vulnerable patients, was identified. This model is characterized by lower usage of medication, a sensible approach to human rights and external, independent audit. **Conclusion:** The increasing use of psychotropic medication in the paediatric population needs to be accompanied by a careful consideration to ethical aspects in research, practice and training. Fortunately, there are progressively more and bet-ter guiding resources available and easily accessible. Ethical principles and standards in relationship to patients, colleagues, clinical settings and broader society, should be clarified and enforced, not only in the field of pharmacotherapy but in general, by our international child and adolescent psychiatric organizations.

S-065-296　Topic: 12, 69

Antipsychotic treatment

Eberhard Schulz, Universität Freiburg, Kinder- und Jugendpsychiatrie, Freiburg, Germany, schulz@psyallg.ukl.uni-freiburg.de
Christian Fleischhaker; Philip Heiser; Klaus Hennighausen; Beate Herpertz-Dahlmann; Kristian Holtkamp; Claudia Mehler-Wex; Andreas Warnke; Helmut Remschmidt

Objective: Preliminary data derived from clinical studies with small sample sizes suggest that efficacy and safety of psychotropic drugs may be different in children and adolescents as compared to adults. Various issues about neuroleptic drugs used by children and adolescents increase the need for systematic clinical research. Some of the key issues in children and adolescents are set below: – Efficacy and safety cannot always be assumed from adult data. – Children and adolescents have different pharmacokinetics and dynamics to adults and therefore have particular vulnerability to side effects and Adverse Drug Reactions (ADRs). Due to specific ethical considerations drug metabolism data in children and adolescents are very sparse at the time of registration. Lack of kinetics data may lead to under or over-dosing in some age groups: under-dosing may result in lack of benefit and non-response; over-dosing may result in an increase of side effects. – Children and adolescents are growing and may therefore be susceptible to certain side effects, as well as delayed ADRs not seen in adults. **Methods:** In our ongoing prospective multicentre study involving inpatients from four clinical sites, the Dosage Record and Treatment Emergent Scale (DOTES) was applied for recording of side effects of neuroleptic drugs. **Results:** Our data show that atypical neuroleptics olanzapine and risperidone are used in a wide range of indication in clinical treatment. Side effects are relatively common in the treatment of children and adolescents with both typical and atypical neuroleptics. This is true of the first week of treatment, as well as for maintenance therapy. **Conclusion:** In the light of these findings, drug-safety issues and clinical implications will be discussed.

S-065-297　Topic: 13, 70

Antidepressants, mania and suicide in children and adolescents: Are epidemic, continental, iatrogenic or fashion explanations most useful?

Andrés Martin, Yale Child Study Center, New Haven, CT, USA, andres.martin@yale.edu

Objective: The prevalence of psychotropic drug use in children and adolescents has steadily risen during the past decade. Despite a growing evidence base for the efficacy and short-term safety of selective serotonin reuptake inhibitor (SSRI) antidepressants in major depression, anxiety disorders, and obsessive compulsive disorder, concerns have resurfaced during recent years regarding their potential association to serious behavioural adverse effects, including suicidality and manic induction. **Methods:** Published literature on pediatric clinical trials using antidepressants will be critically reviewed, with particular attention to evidence based medicine (EBM) measures of efficacy (e.g. effect size [ES], number needed to treat [NNT]) and safety (e.g. number needed to harm [NNT]). Various viewpoints around the 2003 controversial reports from the British regulatory agency regarding suicidality associated with paroxetine will be examined, and results from a recently published pharma-coepidemiology study (Martin et al: Age-effects on anti-depressant associated manic conversion, Archives of Pediatrics and Adolescent Medicine, August 2004) will be contextualized and incorporated into the discussion. **Results:** While preliminary, findings suggest a strong inverse effect of age on antidepressant-associated manic conversion that peaks in the neurobiologically vulnerable peri-pubertal epoch. Although clinical trial data are still being reanalyzed at this time and results not yet final, it appears that initial concerns around SSRIs and suicidality may arguably have been excessive and unwarranted. Nevertheless, they have been productive in helping the field better realize that: a) Efficacy data for the SSRIs in this population may not be as robust as originally thought; b) In light of their alleged innocuous side effect profile, clinicians' decisions to prescribe SSRIs may have reached unacceptably low thresholds; and c) The 'file cabinet bias' (of negative clinical trials going unpublished, particularly if industry-sponsored) has become an urgent clinical and ethical issue for the field to address. **Conclusion:** These controversies will be synthesized by using epidemic (rising prevalence rates), continental (American vs. European), iatrogenic (medication-induced behavioural complications), and fashion (how much of the juvenile bipolar 'epidemic' is a social construct?) complementary explanations.

S-065-298   Topic: 84
Pharmacotherapy of ADHD

Anne-Liis von Knorring, University Hospital Uppsala, Child & Adolescent Psychiatry, Uppsala, Sweden, anne-liis.von_knorring@bupinst.uu.se

Objective: The use of ADHD/Hyperkinetic disorder diagnosis has been more and more accepted in Europe. Treatment studies have been carried out for several decades. **Methods:** A search of publications in scientific journals and books. **Results:** Treatment with central stimulants (CS) in more than two hundred controlled studies have been shown to be effective. It reduces the core symptoms of inattention, hyperactivity and impulsivity. The MTA study has shown that methylphenidate relieves the core symptoms more than behaviour therapy. If other symptoms i.e. aggressiveness and discipline problems are apparent is combination therapy effective. Long acting formulations that are effective during the whole day have been introduced during the last years. TCA's can be effective if the child has depressive symptoms combined with ADHD. However, the TCA treatment does not relieve inattention and hyperactivity as well as CS and the side effects are also more dangerous. Other new drugs with less abuse potential are in pipeline. Atomotexine has been introduced in USA, but not yet in Europe. **Conclusion:** Treatment with central stimulants especially methylphenidate is the first choice if problems of ADHD are prominent.

S-066   Topic: 85, 25
Risk and protective factors for antisocial behavior

Chairperson: Mary Schwab-Stone, Yale University School of Medicine, New Haven, CT, USA, mary.schwab-stone@yale.edu

S-066-299   Topic: 57, 70
Anger and social adjustment in Russian male juvenile delinquents with and without depression

Denis G. Sukhodolsky, Yale University, Yale Child Study Center, New Haven, CT, USA, Vladislav Ruchkin

Objective: Depression is a common psychiatric disorder, frequently observed in adolescents from the general population and in juvenile detainee populations. Although sad mood and social withdrawal are among the core symptoms of the disorder, individuals with depression also frequently report increased irritability and impairments in major areas of functioning. These associated problems may contribute to the developmental trajectories of delinquent behavior. This study examines anger experience and social functioning in Russian male delinquents with and without depression. **Methods:** Study group included 370 delinquents (age = 16.3(0.83)). Diagnoses were assigned using the K-SADS-PL, a semi-structured diagnostic interview. Anger was evaluated using the Aggression Questionnaire and the Multidimensional Anger Inventory. Social functioning was evaluated using the Social Problems scale of the YSR and the Interpersonal Relations scale of the BASC. **Results:** Fourty two participants (11.4%) met diagnostic criteria for depression. Depressed adolescents reported greater levels of general anger ($p < 0.01$), anger intensity ($p < 0.05$), and hostility ($p < 0.001$). Similarly, depression conferred greater levels of perceived social problems ($p < 0.05$) and lower levels of interpersonal competencies ($p < 0.01$). Despite these differences in anger, delinquents with and without depression did not differ on prospective and retrospective self-reports of aggressive behavior. **Conclusion:** This study extends research on depression and its associated characteristics to juvenile delinquents from a cultural background outside North America and Western Europe. The rates of depression in the Russian sample were consistent with those in other countries. However, clinically depressed delinquents presented with higher levels of anger and lower social adjustment than their non-depressed counterparts. Although traditionally anger is targeted as part of aggression-reduction interventions, excessive anger should be an independent focus of clinical attention in adolescents with conduct problems and depression. By contrast, interpersonal competences and ability to establish friendships with non-delinquent peers may be an important protective factor in juvenile delinquency.

S-066-300   Topic: 25, 44
Victimization by violence and antisocial behaviour and depression in 14–16 year old adolescents: A community study

Riittakerttu Kaltiala-Heino, Tampere University Hospital, Pitkäniemi, Finland, riittakerttu.kaltiala-heino@pshp.fi Robert Vermeiren; Matti Rimpelä

Objective: To examine the relationship between victimization by violence and antisocial behavior and depression in a large cohort of Finnish adolescents. **Methods:** In the School Health Promotion Study, 51,811 Finnish 14–16 year old adolescents were surveyed about a range of behaviors and symptoms including experiences of violent victimization, depressive symptoms, and non-violent antisocial behavior. Victimization was assessed through items about having been threatened with violence while being robbed, other threats of violence, and being beaten. The time frame was the preceding 12 months. Depressive symptoms were assessed with the Beck Depression Inventory. The following non-violent antisocial behaviors were assessed: graffiti, vandalism, shoplifting, and truancy. The respondent's own aggressive behavior was queried, including: starting fights and having beaten someone up. Logistic regression analyses were performed to assess the association between victimization and the two outcomes, controlling for 1) the adolescent's own violent behavior, and 2) violent behavior and socio-demographic background. **Results:** Both depressive symptoms and antisocial behavior were related to the degree of victimization experienced. When the respondent's own aggressive behavior was controlled for, in boys, both depression and antisocial behavior were related to victimization. Girls with the highest levels of victimization reported fewer depressive symptoms and antisocial behaviors than those with lesser degree of victimization, while the levels were still higher than in non-victimized girls. **Conclusion:** In Finland, a country with low levels of violence exposure, victimization by violence was demonstrated to be a risk factor for adolescent antisocial behavior, as well as depression. Implications for public health will be discussed.

S-066-301   Topic: 85, 25
Severe antisocial behavior in youths:
The role of psychopathic personality
Henrik Andershed, Orebro University, Orebro, Sweden, henrik.andershed@bsr.oru.se

Objective: Psychopathy or psychopathic personality, a constellation of (1) grandiose, manipulative, (2) callous, unemotional, and (3) impulsive, irresponsible traits, has been related to severe antisocial behavior in previous research. This presentation presents research investigating the potential importance of the psychopathic personality in the development of antisocial behavior. **Methods:** Data on youths as well as adult offenders are presented. **Results:** Findings show that the developmental pathway, etiology, type of comorbid problems, as well as degree of problem behavior are different for antisocial individuals with psychopathic personality as compared to those without this personality constellation. **Conclusion:** It is concluded that this research is in support for psychopathic personality as an important construct for understanding severe antisocial behavior in youths. Implications for prevention and treatment are briefly discussed. Keywords: antisocial behavior, psychopathy, personality.

S-066-302   Topic: 24, 25
Social support and spirituality as protective factors
for violence exposed youth
Mary Schwab-Stone, Yale University, School of Medicine, New Haven, CT, USA, mary.schwab-stone@yale.edu
Vladislav Ruchkin; Deborah O'Donnell; Michelle Pearce

Objective: To examine forms of social support and spiritual beliefs as potential protective factors for antisocial behavior and other adverse psychopathological outcomes in youth exposed to community violence. **Methods:** The Social and Health Assessment (SAHA) is a survey to assess problem behaviors, psychiatric symptoms, and risk conditions in adolescents from the general population. It has been administered to a large community sample in the

U.S. 8 times between 1992 and 2002. Data from two waves, 1996 and 1998 (N = 2600), were examined using structural equation modeling to assess the potentially protective role of various forms of social support in buffering youth at risk with respect to psychopathology and poor coping skills because of exposure to community violence. In a companion study, cohorts from the same general population who were surveyed in 2000 and 2001 (N = 1703) were utilized to examine the potential protective effects of parent involvement and religiousness with respect to the development of conduct problems in violence exposed youth. **Results:** The multidimensional conceptualization of childhood resilience was supported by findings from the first study in which parent and school support factors were positively associated with better outcomes, while peer support was associated with negative outcomes in specific behavioral domains. Religiousness, over and above parental involvement, had some protective effect with respect to risk for conduct problems. **Conclusion:** Findings from this work have implications for the prevention of conduct problems and for policies that address the needs of youth exposed to community violence.

S-067   Topic: 7, 41
ISAPP Symposium: Diagnostic considerations
and psychodynamic treatment of severely disturbed
adolescents
Track: Therapy and intervention
Chairperson: Annette Streeck-Fischer, NLKH Tiefenbrunn Psychotherapie von Kindern, Rosdorf, Germany, annette.streeck@t-online.de
Peter Riedesser, UKE Hamburg-Eppendorf, Abt. Psychiatrie, Hamburg, Germany, riedesser@uke.uni-hamburg.de

Diagnostic considerations and psychodynamic
treatment of severely disturbed adolescents
Peter Riedesser, UKE Hamburg-Eppendorf, Abt. Psychiatrie, Hamburg, Germany, riedesser@uke.uni-hamburg.de

ISAPP Symposium Adolescents with personality and behaviour disorders show complex psychopathological, neuropsychological and neurobiological abnormalities. Findings of brain and attachment research as well as advancements in psychodynamic concepts lead to modifications in the understanding and treatment of these adolescents. Thus, it seems important to assess the multiple and complex disorders of these adolescents to adjust and design the different modalities of developmentally oriented psychotherapy. Special attention is given to severely traumatized adolescents who need basic supporting and containing functions to overcome their pathological coping. Case reports give insight into different approaches of psychodynamic psychotherapy.

S-067-303   Topic: 83, 41
Adolescents with MCDD in diagnostics
and psychotherapy
Annette Streeck-Fischer, NLKH Tiefenbrunn, Psychotherapie von Kindern, Rosdorf, Germany, annette.streeck@t-online.de

Objective: Adolescents with pronounced personality and behavioral disorders (F6), particularly of the narcissistic, emotionally unstable and dissocial type (classification should only be made with appropriate caution) usually show multiple and complex disturbances which stem from chronic early traumatizations. Various authors (i.e. Debellis 1999) have demonstrated the complexity of such disorders by means of neuropsychological and neuroanatomical findings. **Methods:** 20 patients (male and female adolescents from 16 to 19 years old) are examined by different neuropsychological tests and sensomotoric diagnostics. **Results:** The adolescents evaluated by standardised interviews get 3 or more diagnosis and show various disorders, e.g. a characteristic dissoziation in the cognitive capacities, multiple attention deficits, tactile and haptic perceptions problems, problems of the vestibulare system. **Conclusion:** On the basis of these findings from adolescents with such disorders who underwent in-patient psychiatric/psychotherapeutic therapy the consequences of the diagnosis and treatment are described and discussed. The recommendation of Cohen, Towbin and Lincoln indicates that it may be reasonable to assume that these patients have a multiple complex developmental disorder (MCDD) and should be treated accordingly. The various modalities of treatment (psychodynamic psychotherapy, body-oriented therapy, training of study techniques, medications) are demonstrated using a case description.

S-067-304   Topic: 7, 41
Is reference to psychoanalytical theory still relevant as an approach to personality and conduct disorders in adolescence?

Philippe Jeammet, Université Paris VI, Psychiatrie de l'Enfant, Paris, France, philippe.jeammet@imm.fr

Objective: Personality and conduct disorders pointedly raise the question of how they should be defined and delimited. They are frequently associated with each other and are distributed along a psychopathological and clinical spectrum extending from normality to severe pathology. It is their noisiness and the unpleasantness they cause to the individual and, even more, to his entourage, that has led them to be characterized as disorders. The majority of them go unrecognized, not hindering, perhaps even helping, the success of those who have them. The pathological character of their manifestation thus depends largely upon social context, which often, insidiously and implicitly, becomes main nosiographical determinant. Anti-social conducts, narcissistic pathology, addictive conducts, borderline states, to name only the principle disorders, are based on individual vulnerabilities that most often will only be expressed and organized as pathological behaviors according to social context, events, and encounters. **Methods:** These are the pathologies of today, for they are in keeping with the social evolution of our times. Detecting the potential for them before the appearance of any disorder in the patient presupposes a theory of personality development not based on symptomatic and behavioral manifestations alone. In the same way, treating these disorders does not mean merely reducing them to their most patent manifestations, it is also means preventing both their organization into a stable behavior and the risks of future disorganization. It also means preventing darnage to self-image and self-esteem in these subjects due to these disorders which marginalize them, sabotaging their potential and compromising their future. **Results:** Psychoanalysis is, for the moment, the sole overall theory of personality development that allows for this approach. It emphasizes the importance of psychical functioning as an intermediary of the parents and an essential tool in the elaboration of con-

flicts, the containment of emotion and the protection of the subject and his potential. But this current psychopathology of conduct and personality disorders challenges psychoanalysis and causes it to evolve. The emphasis is shifted from a pathology of conflicts, fostered by a repressive society, to a pathology of connections, lirnits and dependence fostered by a permissive society. The drive-related issue of aggression and sexuality can no longer be considered as anything other than part of a dialectic with the issues of identity and lirnits and of the fear of being engulfed or abandoned by cathected persons. Defects in narcissism, such as the importance of insecure early relations in these subjects, are crucial to understanding these pathologies. The threat to narcissism generated by the cathexis of persons helps give belief phenomena and control mechanisms a decisive role in regulating interpersonal relations, self-esteem, and narcissistic equilibrium. **Conclusion:** This evolution also calls into question classical models for psychoanalytic treatment and even for psychoanalytical psychotherapy, and challenges psychoanalytical theory as to what constitutes the most fundamental data and the most effective means of bringing about change in these subjects. Beyond the psychoanalytical approach proper, what is taking shape is a theory of the psychical care of adolescents.

S-067-305   Topic: 80, 4
Inpatient treatment of adolescents with borderline personality disorder

Dieter Bürgin, Universitätsklinik Basel, Kinder- u. Jugendpsychiatrie, Basel, Switzerland, dieter.buergin@unibas.ch

Objective: Personality disorders are characterized by a long lasting and pervasive pattern of disturbances, creating suffering or restrictions in school, at work, in the family or with peers. Behaviour and self experience differ markedly from the usual way in the given socio-cultural environment. It has for a long time been discussed if personality disorders do already exist before or at the beginning of adolescence. But in the last 20 years, there is growing evidence for a real existence of personality disturbances in children and adolescents. DSM IV and ICD 10 make a distinction between personality traits and personality disorders. Because the nature of bonding is a long lasting personality feature, we often find transgenerational stability in personality disorders. Naturally, this structural disorder expresses itself during the different developmental phases in different forms. Thus, the phenotype of a personality disorder may be quite variable, but the main structure at the bottom remains stable. **Methods:** Impaired adaptation manifests itself mostly in situations with poor structure, intensive stress or necessity of major change (e.g. any form of (developmental) transition, need to perform on demand, rivalry etc.). Different ego-functions, interpersonal relationships and the self representation are impaired in adolescents with borderline disorders. Especially reality testing is not fully developed. We find a splitting in the self- and object-representations, a very common use of projections with the attempt to dominate the other, urging him or her to identify with these projections. **Results:** Thus the interpersonal relationships are primitive and partially distorted. Secondary thought processes are infiltrated by primary process activities and phantasies are easily expressed. (Ajuriaguerra J., 1982). Impulse regulation is disturbed, and there is no integration of aggressive and libidinal tendencies, what is mostly followed by a chaotic intrapsychic organisation. This, because aggressive impulses destroy the coherence of the self representation. All impulses are directly expressed, whether through the body (leading to psychosomatic manifestations), by acting out (what brings difficulties in the external word with it) or by phantasy activities which can not really be differentiated from facts of external reality. Anxieties have a special character and intensity: annihilation, intrusion, fractionation or fusion. All activities of regulation, coping, adaptation or defence are very intensive, rigid and archaic (on the psychotic pole) or fragile, labile and fluctuating on the neurotic pole. The symbolic function is impaired in its development. The usually used symbols are like blocked or bizarre or there can be seen a flight in an over-symbolisation. Stable selective secondary identifications are lacking. In most cases global primary identifications are found. In the unhomogeneous self representation compensatory structures, e.g. in form of a false self, are built up, which manifest themselves in polymorphous ways, i.e. in form of pseudo adaptations, in suddenly arising and unbound anxieties or in developmental retardation (Diatkine R., 1969). A quick change in the level of ego-functions underlines this polymorphism and makes it difficult to estimate, which level of ego-organisation dominates in which context (Ekstein R., 1973). **Conclusion:** In a case vignette of an inpatient treatment of an adolescent patient, some of these points are elaborated.

S-067-306 Topic: 4, 73
Some issues in the inpatient treatment of traumatized adolescents

John Tsiantis, Aghia Sophia Hospital, Child & Adolescent Psychiatry, Athens, Greece, itsiantis@cc.uoa.gr

Objective: In this presentation observations from the inpatient care of traumatized adolescents will be presented and discussed. **Methods:** An attempt will be made to present some basic issues of transference and countertransference phenomena observed during the inpatient treatment of traumatized adolescents exemplified by 1–2 brief vignettes: The function of the inpatient unit as a holding place will also be presented. **Results:** The importance of the unit – represented by the network of relationships among the staff, by the operating limits of the unit and its rules – is to provide the traumatized adolescents with a holding environment and function as an adequate mother, giving the adolescent's therapist and the adolescent himself the space and scope to explore the adolescent's conflicts and the roots of his difficulties, fears and expectations. **Conclusion:** The aim will be to assist the adolescents to themselves and discern the continuity in their lives, rather than continuing to repeat traumatic relationships.

S-068 Topic: 37
Methods of clinical investigation (interviews, tests)

Chairperson: Patricia Howlin, St. Georges Hospital Community Health Sciences, London, United Kingdom

S-068-307 Topic: 37
Evaluation of the self-reported SDQ in a clinical setting: II. Can clinical status be predicted by self-ratings?

Andreas Becker, Universität Göttingen, Kinder- und Jugendpsychiatrie, Göttingen, Germany, abecker4@gwdg.de Nicola Hagenberg; Matthias Berking; Veit Roessner; Tobias Banaschewski; Aribert Rothenberger

Objective: In order to further evaluate the German self-reported Strengths and Difficulties Questionnaire (SDQ) in a clinical setting, the present study compared SDQ self-ratings and corresponding YSR scores with respect to their ability to detect presence of any psychiatric disorder and subgroups of patients with more specific clinical diagnoses. **Methods:** SDQ self-reports were collected from 214 in- and outpatients (81 girls and 133 boys) aged 11 to 17 years who were seen at the Department of Child and Adolescent Psychiatry of the University of Göttingen. Results obtained with the self-rated questionnaires were compared with the clinical diagnostic classification. **Results:** SDQ self-reports demonstrated similar predictive qualities as comparable but longer YSR scales. The self-rated version of the SDQ proved to be useful and valid at distinguishing between clinically defined cases and non-cases and in detecting various subcategories of psychiatric disorders within this clinical sample. **Conclusion:** The self-rated version of the SDQ was shown to be a valid method for detecting presence of psychiatric disorders in children and adolescents. At a more specific level, SDQ subscales were able to predict different diagnostical subgroups.

S-068-308 Topic: 37
Health of the Nation Outcome Scales for Children and Adolescents (HoNOSCA).
Inter-rater reliability in a clinical setting

Ketil Hanssen-Bauer, Regional Centre East and South, Child & Adolescent Psychiatry, Oslo, Norway, ketil. hanssen-bauer@r-bup.no Odd Aalen; Sonja Heyerdahl

Objective: There is an increasing demand that the outcome of interventions provided by child and adolescent mental health services (CAMHS) be evaluated. Several broad clinical rating scales have been developed to measure outcome. In order to enable routine clinical use of these scales, investigation of their psychometric properties is necessary. The aim of this study was to assess the inter-rater reliability (IRR) of the Health of the Nation Outcome Scales for Children and Adolescents (HoNOSCA), when used in a clinical setting. Further, we wished to compare the IRR of the HoNOSCA with the Children's Global Assessment Scale (CGAS) and the Global Assessment of Psychosocial Disability (GAPD, Axis 6 in "Multiaxial classification of child and adolescent psychiatric disorders", WHO, 1996). **Methods:** HoNOSCA, CGAS and GAPD were implemented in nine Norwegian outpatient CAMHS. After a short training session all clinicians were asked to assess 10 out of 20 written vignettes. 170 clinicians used HoNOSCA, but were randomized to rate either vignettes no 1–10 or no 11–20 and to also use either CGAS or GAPD. Intraclass correlation coefficient (ICC) was used to estimate IRR. **Results:** The ICC for the HoNOSCA total score was 0.80 (CI=0.70–0.90), for the CGAS it was 0.60 (CI=0.45–0.76) and for the GAPD it was 0.59 (CI=0.43–0.75). **Conclusion:** The HoNOSCA total score can be used with high inter-rater reliability by clinicians working in CAMHS. The ICC was higher than for the CGAS and the GAPD.

S-068-309   Topic: 37
Psychopathological self assessments of patients and pupils

Jürgen Junglas, Rheinische Kliniken, Kinder- und Jugendpsychiatrie, Bonn, Germany, j.junglas@lvr.de

Objective: Are pupils less disturbed than patients of a psychiatric clinic? Can children and adolescents themselves assess if they deviant from normal feelings and behaviour? Is there any difference between paper-pencil and monitor presentation **Methods:** 666 youth, 224 pupils and 442 patients, age 12 to 17 years, answered the SAPa,cs (self assessements psychopathology adolescents, cardinal symptoms, Junglas 1999) in a paper-pencil (N=377) and a computermonitor-form (N=289), in 2002 to 2003; (men 283, women 381). The SAPa,cs included 555 items in 19 psychopathological scales. The SAPa,cs based on the AMDP and the CASCAP-D. All items could be answered with: 0=never, 1=seldom, 2=often, 3=always. **Results:** Mean average value comparison (t-test) shows significant differences between pupils and patients in all scales, apart from eating, perception, obsession, aggression and sexuality. In the most scales pupils shows higher mean average value than patients, except: depression, aggression and social behaviour. Between male and female we saw signifikant differences in eating, formal thinking, anxiety, depression and social behaviour. Depression and sexuality shows a significant age-effect. Factor analysis shows two distinct factors. **Conclusion:** Psychopathological self assessment with SAPa,cs shows similar values in the population of pupils and (in- and out-)patients. The case definition is not concordant with the self-evaluations of the youths. Maybe, psychopathological burden is overestimated as central symptom of youth in clinical treatment.

S-068-310   Topic: 37
Development of Child Problem Behavior Screening Questionnaire (CPBSQ)

Dong-Hyun Ahn, Hanyang University Hospital, Dept. of Psychiatry, Seoul, Republic of Korea, ahndh@hanyang.ac.kr
Yoon-Seok Huh; Jun-Ho Choi; Yun Young Kim; Kyung-Ja Oh

Objective: The purpose of this study was to develop a screening questionnaire to assess children's emotional and behavioral problems for epidemiological research. **Methods:** The second to fourth grade pupils (N=970) of the two elementary schools in Seoul, Korea, participated in this study. Parents and teachers of children completed a questionnaire, and parents completed the Child Behavior Checklist-Korean version (K-CBCL). The reliability and validity of the questionnaire was evaluated by comparison with the K-CBCL and by performing the factor analysis, t-test, and correlation analysis **Results:** Internal Consistency of CPBSQ was relatively good(Cronbach's alpha: parent=0.846, teacher=0.834). The result of factor analysis showed that CPBSQ has a four-factor structure: externalizing problems, internalizing problems, physical health problem, and cognitive problems. In the parent's and teacher's CPBSQ, total variance of the four factors was 37.8% and 43.8%, respectively. There were significant correlations between subscales of parent's CPBSQ and K-CBCL. CPBSQ effectively distinguished children with psychiatric or developmental problems from the general population group **Conclusion:** The results showed that the questionnaire developed in this study (CPBSQ) is effective in identifying the children's psychiatric or developmental problems and

that it is a useful and promising screening tool of children's problem behaviors for large-scale epidemiological research.

S-068-311   Topic: 37
The screen for child anxiety related emotional disorders scale: Chinese version reliability and validity

Linyan Su, Mental Health Institute, Dept. of Child Psychiatry, Changsha, China, sulinyan@sina.com
Kai Wang; Yan Zhu; Linyan Su

Objective: To examine the Reliability and the Validity of the Screen for Child Anxiety Related Emotional Disorders (SCARED) in Chinese children. **Methods:** Subjects were 1559 children in grades 3 to 9 (774 boys and 785 girls, mean age=11.79±0.11 years, all Han people) at 12 primary school and 11 junior high school in 12 cities of China. The 41-item version of the SCARED (Birmaher et al., 1999) was completed by children and their parents. One hundred and thirty nine children from Changsha city completed the Children's Self-concept Scale (PHCSS), and their parents completed the Child Behavior Checklist (CBCL) additionally. Meanwhile ninety outpatients who diagnosed anxiety disorders based on DSM-IV from three clinics of cities were evaluated. **Results:** The mean SCARED total score of school children was 15.00±10.25. It was less than the scores of South African and Dutch children significantly. Significant gender and age differences were found. The girls exhibited higher levels of all scores except school phobia subscale than boys. Scores of children aged 13-16 years were higher than those of 8–12 years,only separation anxiety subscale were less than 8–12 years children. Reliability: The child and parent versions of the SCARED have moderate parent-child agreement (r=0.49–0.59). The test-retest reliability 2 weeks after the initial screening were 0.51~0.82, 12 weeks were 0.29–0.69; split-half r=0.89 and Cronbach a=0.43–0.90. Validity: - Significant correlations were found between the SCARED scores and anxiety subscale of PHCSS (r=−0.51~0.74); and the somatic-complaints, anxious/depresses, and thought problems subscale and internalizing scale of CBCL (r=0.30~0.44). The scores of children with anxiety disorders were higher than that of school subjects. **Conclusion:** Although SCARED in Chinese children somewhat deviated from Western countries, it was found to have acceptable psychometrics properties, and seem to be useful for assessing childhood anxiety syndromes in China.

S-068-312   Topic: 37, 49
The development and factor structure of the Assessment Checklist for Children (ACC): A rating scale of psychiatric problems specific to children in foster care

Michael Tarren-Sweeney, University of Newcastle, Medical Practice, Callaghan, Australia, michael.tarrensweeney@newcastle.edu.au
Philip Hazell

Objective: Children in foster and kinship care manifest a range of mental health problems not adequately measured by existing survey instruments. These include self-injury and suicidal behaviour, sexual behaviour, dissociation and trauma-related anxiety, interpersonal behaviour suggestive of attachment disturbance and attachment insecurity, and unusual food behaviour (gorging, hoarding, etc). The Assessment Checklist for Children (ACC) was developed to measure such problems in a prospective epidemiological study of the mental health of children in long-term care. **Methods:** The ACC was developed systematically over several years using both inductive and deductive strategies. Development and validation components included a clinician survey, literature review, analysis of assessment reports and foster parent focus group. A screening instrument for low self-esteem was developed separately, and embedded within the instrument. **Results:** Item content validity was endorsed by clinicians and foster carers. Parallel data for the ACC and the Child Behavior Checklist (CBCL) were obtained for 412 children in long-term care. Principal components factor analyses (Promax rotation) of clinical items yielded 10 clinical scales. The 10-factor model explained 49% of the score variance, with scale internal consistency ranging from 0.70 to 0.96. The hypothesised clinical constructs were largely reflected in the empirically-derived scales. Three types of disturbances in interpersonal behaviour were identified: 'Pseudomature', 'Nonreciprocal' and 'Indiscriminate'. Other clinical scales were labelled 'sexual behaviour', 'insecure', 'anxious-distrustful', 'abnormal pain response', 'food maintenance', 'self-injury', and 'suicide discourse'. The factor analysis of self-esteem items yielded two distinct factors, namely 'negative self-image', and 'low confidence'. **Conclusion:** Comprehensive survey estimates of the mental health of children in care may be obtained from administering the ACC in parallel with the CBCL. The ACC offers opportunities to examine the phenomenology of psychiatric disturbance among children in care. Further validation and reliability studies need to be conducted.

S-069   Topic: 78
Eating and feeding disorders/Obesity II

Track: Eating disorders

Chairperson: Hans-Christoph Steinhausen, ZKJP Universität Zürich Kinder- und Jugendpsychiatrie, Zürich, Switzerland, steinh@kjpd.unizh.ch

S-069-313   Topic: 78, 19
Treatment strategies for identical twins concordant for Anorexia Nervosa. A case report and review of treatment possibilities

D. M. Leiblum, Uni. Medical Hospital Utrecht, Child & Adolescent Psychiatry, Utrecht, Netherlands, dleiblum@zonnet.nl
Annemarie van Elburg; Herman van Engeland

Objective: Anorexia Nervosa (AN) is a complicated disorder accompanied by several treatment dilemmas. The literature on the treatment of identical twins concordant for AN is scarce, which makes finding an effective treatment approach quite difficult. We report on the treatment of a pair of identical monozygotic female adolescent twins concordant for AN in an inpatient setting and on the difficulties and dilemmas which occurred. **Methods:** Semi structured interviews and videotaping were used to document the unique presentation of AN in a twin adolescent pair, aged 15 years, and approach to their inpatient treatment is described. Diagnosis with AN was made according to the DSM IV criteria using the Eating Disorder Examination (EDE). Besides AN they showed co morbid depression, learning disorder and numerous somatic complaints that needed to be evaluated. Complete psychological and physical assessment was performed before and during admission. Extensive review of the literature on treatment strategies specifically for identical twins, including counselling various international experts in the field of eating disorders was undertaken. **Results:** After intensive evaluation it was concluded that the psychopathological development of the twins evolved shortly after birth as a result of prematurity and several neonatal complications followed by overprotective parental involvement and a symbiotic, almost folie à deux like relationship between the twins. Treatment started in our eating disorder unit after a period of nasogastric tube feeding in a paediatric hospital and included individual, group and family therapy. Data on physical recovery including weight, body composition and blood levels all show progressive recovery. Psychological development is still threatened. **Conclusion:** The treatment of identical monozygotic twins concordant for AN brings forward unique challenging treatment strategies. The complexity is mainly a result of the special psychological development and interpersonal relationship which exists between twins and their relatives.

S-069-314   Topic: 78, 23
The "Weekly Balance" – Self reflection and assessment of experiences during therapy of anorectic inpatients

Renate Kühl, Universität Kiel, Kinder- und Jugendpsychiatrie, Kiel, Germany, ch.haase@kiju-psych. uni-kiel.de
Christian Haase; Cornelia Nötzel

Objective: Anorectic patients produce weekly written reports of situations, in which they describe experiences of dependence and independence during the preceding week. **Methods:** The "Weekly Balance" is a method with open questions in reference to the three dimensions of locus of control (Levenson 1972). Each patient has to describe a situation of internal and external control as well as a situation, in which good or bad things happened by chance. Afterwards the patients have to describe their feelings during the special situations and the importance of the event. The "Weekly Balance" is evaluated using the method of structural-contents-analysis (Mayring 1995). First results of a group of 30 anorectic inpatients are reported: **Results:** Changes in the written reports and their relation to outcome of therapy and to prognostic criteria will be described. Already at the beginning of inpatient psychotherapy successfully treated patients can be distinguished from unsuccessful inpatients. **Conclusion:** The results of the "Weekly Balance" are relevant for the indication, evaluation and prognosis of inpatient treatment.

S-069-315   Topic: 78, 95
Psychiatric comorbidity in anorectic and bulimic eating disorders

Ernst Pfeiffer, Charité Universitätsmedizin B, Kinder- und Jugendpsychiatrie, Berlin, Germany, ernst.pfeiffer@charite.de
Klaus Lenz; Ulrike Lehmkuhl

Objective: To assess prospectively psychiatric comorbidity following the first contact with anorectic and bulimic patients. **Methods:** All patients referred at our university hospital since the begin of 2002, who got diagnosis of typical anorexia nervosa F50.00/.01 (both types restrictive type

AN-R or binge/purging type AN-BP) or typical bulimia nervosa F50.2 (BN), were asked to participate in this on-going prospective study. In addition to a series of other instruments participants were assessed with the structured interview CIDI. For statistical analysis chi-square test was used comparing the AN-R-group with the AN-BP/BN-group. **Results:** 80 patients (78 female, 2 male; age 12 to 17 years) fulfilled clinical diagnostic ICD-10 criteria of AN or BN. 62 agreed to participate in the study, to date 47 are interviewed with CIDI; of these 25 had AN-R (mean age x =14.7), 14 had AN-BP (x = 15.8), 8 had BN (x = 16.8). Overall 36 patients (76.6%) had an additional psychiatric disorder using DSM-IV criteria. Significant differences were found between the AN-R-group (64.0%, affective disorders dominating) and the AN-BP/BN-group (90.9%, affective disorders and substance use disorders dominating). Only low rates (14.9%) were found using ICD-10 criteria. **Conclusion:** This study demonstrates high rates of early psychiatric comorbidity in eating disorders especially in the active forms AN-BP/BN. However, the level of comorbidity is highly influenced by the diagnostic system applied in the study.

S-069-316   Topic: 78, 4

Day care treatment for adolescent Anorexia Nervosa (AN)

Agneta Rosling, Academical Hospital, Child & Adolescent Psychiatry, Uppsala, Sweden, agneta.rosling@bupinst.uu.se

Objective: To evaluate the preliminary effects of a new, five-step, day care programme. **Methods:** The Eating disorder unit in the Dept of Child and Adolescent Psychiatry, Uppsala University Hospital, provides the only specialised treatment facility for eating disorders in the county. A revised treatment program, based on cognitive behavioural therapy, was introduced in January 2002. The treatment is in a day care setting with a multidisciplinary team including adolescent psychiatrist, paediatrician, family therapist and specialised nursing staff. Treatment includes motivational sessions, mealtime support followed by bed rest, and scheduled sessions with the nursing staff for problem solving as well as parental support and training. Medication with SSRI and/or olanzapin is used for depression, OCD and severe anxiety. After medical and psychiatric assessment, patients with considerable weight loss are offered the five-step program. The steps are, 1st stop weight loss, by eating ordinary foods and rest, 2nd establish continuous weight gain by adding high energy drinks, 3rd involves reintroduction to school, 4th handling anxiety in difficult situations and 5th is relapse prevention. Patients and parents must accept the rules of the program, which must be adhered to both at the unit and at home. For each step the patient signs a contract, if the terms of the contract are broken the program is discontinued. The family is then offered a restart after one week. **Results:** 1. Since May 2002 no patient has required inpatient care at either paediatric, psychiatric or other types of specialised treatment facilities. 2. Nasogastric tube feeding has not been required since September 2002. 3. The professional team has been able to assess and treat a larger number of patients. At present there is no waiting list for new patients. **Conclusion:** The framework of the program has already shown advantages, and a prolonged follow-up is designed to evaluate the treatment effects when more patients have completed the program.

S-069-317   Topic: 78, 3

The prevention of eating disturbances and body image dissatisfaction: The impact of a self-esteem enhancement program

Marianne Poller, Curtin University of Technolog, School of Psychology, Perth, Australia, m.poller@exchange.curtin.edu.au
Clare Roberts; Donna Cross; Robert Kane

Objective: Eating disorders are a complex, multidimensional disorder and are characterised by clinically significant disturbances in body image and eating behaviours. To date, eating disorder and body image dissatisfaction prevention programs have met with limited success and are plagued with methodological limitations. Typically interventions that involve information-giving strategies on the signs, prevalence and physical and psychological consequences of eating disorders increase knowledge with no corresponding change in target attitudes or behaviours. The present study developed and evaluated the effectiveness of a school based eating disturbance and body dissatisfaction prevention program. Self-esteem has been identified as both a risk and protective factor, is able to address a number of risk factor domains and has attained some success in the prevention literature. Thus, a program was developed using Harter's (1987) model of the determinants of self-worth. This model has been theoretically, empirically and phenomenologically validated and provides a framework in which strategies can be developed to enhance self-esteem. **Methods:** Two hundred and sixty-eight year seven students from five independent schools in Perth, Western Australia were randomised into control and intervention groups. Comprehensive self-report impact and process data was collected from the student, teacher and parent cohort at baseline, post-test and 6-month follow-up. Effectiveness of the program was evaluated comparing intervention and control groups on a number of outcome variables including measures of self-esteem, body image and eating disturbance. **Results:** At post-test, intervention participants showed significantly more symptoms of eating disorders than did controls. However this iatrogenic effects was not maintained at follow-up. Among high-risk students, at both post-test and follow-up, intervention participants showed significantly more symptoms of eating disorders than did controls. **Conclusion:** The implications of these data for universal school-based intervention programs in this area are examined.

S-070   Topic: 59, 25

Moving images and culture into developing brains and minds: A developmental neuroscience perspective on films for and about children

Chairperson: J. Gerald Young, New York University Dept. of Psychiatry, New York, NY, USA, jerry.young@nyu.edu

Moving images and culture into developing brains and minds: A developmental neuroscience perspective on films for and about children

J. Gerald Young, New York University, Dept. of Psychiatry, New York, NY, USA, jerry.young@nyu.edu

Children's films often reflect great poetic imagination, but typically are characterized by a lack of knowledge about children and their development, and about the basis for the beneficial or detrimental effects of the content of the film. Nevertheless, filmmakers act as educators for and about children, even if they often do so in a manner that might not be preferred if given knowledgeable deliberation. (Film clips) It is crucial for the well-being of children that the various elements of children's films be examined in order to determine what they are transmitting to and about children. Emerging developmental neuroscience knowledge provides a useful perspective for understanding the structure and meanings of films for and about children. Comparisons of films across cultures indicate the varied adaptive solutions to the developmental changes occurring during childhood and adolescence. Accurate conceptualization of interacting genetic influences and the effects of childhood experiences on the development of neural circuits helps us to better appreciate the potential effects of media on the development of children. Attention to selected features of brain development that generate adaptive platforms crucial to the child's evolving development illuminates the processes through which the young child's experiences, mediated by his family and culture, shape the development of his brain and mind. Examples are synaptogenesis and other developmental processes; neural mechanisms related to memory formation and consolidation; neural mechanisms underlying expanded attachment activities and enabling the development of emotional language; and the neural processes enabling imitation learning and interactive alignment in conversational dialogues. Is there evidence that these brain functions are activated in a significant manner by media experiences? Intersubject synchronization of cortical activity during natural viewing of a film indicates the uniformity of immediate effects across individuals for many cortical functions, (Film clip) while research describing the long-term effects of violent media experiences during childhood on behavior years later suggests the stability of these effects. (Film clips) The brain's openness to experience with the actual, specific environment of the infant is masterfully adaptive and controlled, as in the earliest months of life when it is restricted and focused on certain repetitive experiences. Brain mechanisms for attachment functions enable vital regulation of infant experiential learning, particularly favoring those experiences 'selected' by the mother. This facilitates the mother's regulation of infant state, motivation, and attention to predictive stimuli, but also acts to create a reliable, standard reference system for learning because attachment mechanisms nourish the mother's wish to hold the baby, orienting the infant toward the mother's face and voice – standardizing a broad range of contextual details that the infant can attend to or ignore, molding the infant's brain through the formation of memories that can influence him for the remainder of his life, and enabling the vital understanding of emotional language that will guide his or her adaptation. As the child grows older, her attachments are broadly extended beyond the mother, eventually encompassing the rituals and symbols embedded in media experiences. Moreover, the varieties of emotional language during childhood and adolescence can be observed and studied in films. (Film clips) The representation of culture in the child's brain, and the transmission of culture across generations, generate adaptive behaviors that we observe and experience daily. Crosscultural comparisons of films provide useful examples of both the stability and the variability of cultural solutions to specific developmental challenges for children and adolescents. (Film clips)

S-070-318   Topic: 59

The influence of films on children: Film theory, film criticism and film narratives

Simone Klabin, Rio de Janeiro, Brazil,
simone.klabin@verizon.net

Objective: (1) To survey and compare the strategies, methods, and results of selected previous research attempts to examine the effects of children's films on children, and on adult perceptions of children in films, and (2) to examine conventional film narrative structures and film criticism in order to specify leading influences on the production of children's films and to consider how films are likely to have significant effects on developing children, beneficial or detrimental. **Methods:** Research reports were reviewed in order to provide a perspective on current knowledge about the effects of viewing films on children and on adult conceptions of children. In addition, descriptions of 1) film history and criticism, 2) cultural and ideological influences on film content, and 3) the socioeconomic foundations of film production for and about children, were examined in order to determine the dominant perspectives influencing the production of children's films and the understanding of their effects on children and on adult perceptions of children in films. Clips from films paradigmatic of each of these influences were sought as examples providing specific content features, broad or detailed, that can be examined for potential influences on children. **Results:** Most examinations of children's films are from the perspective of film theory and criticism, not their effects on a child's emotions or behavior. Moreover, films conventionally are produced and analyzed in relation to commercial and artistic purposes and values, and more likely reflect the sentiments of individuals who lack the training necessary to understand fully the effects of children's films on children. As disputes continue about the nature of children's films and their effects on children, ambiguity about the interpretation of findings and the lack of adequate data have diminished the impact of heightened concerns and the increasingly effective exploration of film effects. Film clips vividly demonstrate the effects of all of these varied influences, and strongly suggest the potential for specific effects of explicit and implicit filmmaking decisions on the developing child. Selected film clips are utilized as examples that emphasize a) how such filmmaking decisions can alter the meaning of a standard film sequence, and b) how artistic purposes can have unintended effects on a child's experience and understanding of a film. **Conclusion:** Systematic research on the effects of children's films on children is in very early stages. Commercial purposes dominate film narratives, and cultural influences on artistic preferences and techniques are abundant. The art of cinema is the composite result of many contributing forces, colored by the use of multiple interacting theoretical and technical influences that may have great artistic value for adults but alter the meaning of the film for children in complex ways that adults commonly ignore. If filmmakers, parents, and professionals working with families are to make knowledgeable decisions about the effects on children of the structure and content of children's films, a framework for assessing these influences is needed while we await the results of systematic research.

S-070-319   Topic: 59, 25

Understanding the effects of media experiences on children by using a model for memory formation in the developing brain

J. Gerald Young, New York University, Dept. of Psychiatry, New York, NY, USA, jerry.young@nyu.edu

Objective: To develop a conceptual framework for guiding our understanding of the effects of children's films on children, utilizing current developmental neuroscience knowledge to build a model with a replicable structure and categories for analyzing a film. **Methods:** Neuroscience research reports were reviewed in order to identify neural functions likely to be essential to the experiences of children or adults while observing a film. The major concepts from these reports were then examined in relation to possible roles in a cohesive model of brain functions activated during a film experience, generating an integrated model of functional effects on the developing brain. This model was studied in relation to prior research findings, as well as film theory, film criticism, and cultural influences. Relevant film clips were subsequently selected to demonstrate how media influences might generate functional effects, and to enable further scrutiny of the framework. **Results:** When children experience a film, specific brain functions are activated, including some that can evoke memories of the experience. This process of memory formation in the developing brain is conceptualized in relation to its contributing elements, examples of which are attention, emotion, motivation, and adaptive, problem-solving thoughts. Film clips can be used for identification and assessment of how film events stimulate these elements, as well as for comparison of their capacity to elicit these elements when viewed (a) by children as opposed to adults; (b) at different developmental ages; (c) by different cultures; (d) in relation to prior research findings or to film theories and techniques. The generation of memories of film experiences can be illuminated by examining the specificity of learning mechanisms during initial, early, and later phases of learning and using film clips to indicate how the film events selected can be hypothesized to be experienced at these different phases of learning. Initial learning (roughly the preschool years) is characterized by experience-responsive neural processes that sculpt patterns of brain (especially cortical) responsiveness to specific environmental interactions, (e.g., synaptogenesis, pruning and elimination of neural processes, and the activity of neurons capable of perceptual-motor coupling), with a strong emphasis on sensory-perceptual, motor, and social learning. Models for the experience-responsive effects of synaptogenesis are presented in relation to the formation of primary memory prototypes. Synaptogenesis is described as a process of brain development with a capacity to provide experience-responsive guidance of the specification of function within neocortical areas during infancy that profoundly influences major sectors of memory-guided adaptive development, such as spoken/written language, emotional language, and social cognition. Early learning (generally, middle childhood and adolescence) and later learning (adult) are also described. **Conclusion:** Using a model for memory formation in the developing brain, including initial, early, and later phases of brain learning processes, a structure and categories for film analysis can be developed, and the effects of specific features of film episodes on a child's experiential development can be assessed and understood. Similarly, the influences of cultural differences or of alternative artistic film techniques on a child's film experiences and potential memories can be examined.

S-070-320   Topic: 59

Pathways to the enduring effects of films in children: Themes of love and violence

Diana Kaplan, New York, NY, USA

Objective: To describe the interaction of a child's experiences when viewing a film with his memories, and how this interaction determines his responses and evokes new memory formation (the enduring effects of a film), by identifying reflections of initial learning and early learning in the content of films (e.g., themes of love and violence). **Methods:** Mother-infant attachment behaviors were utilized as an example of initial learning, and as images that will evoke memories of these themes in a child viewing a film, while sequences of violent behavior, and a child's repetitive observation of violent films, were selected as an example of early learning. Films were surveyed for images related to each of these themes, and assessed for the intensity and consistency of their representation as pathways to the generation of enduring memories of the film experience in the child. **Results:** Images of consequential experiential features encountered in films rekindle internal responses (e.g., emotions, motivation, thoughts) in a child in a manner definitively different than neutral images. Knowledge of the development of the brain and mind permits prediction of which images will be significant, and film clips demonstrate the power of these evocative images. A first series of film clips was selected in relation to the mother-infant attachment paradigm. Unique features of this situation are described, as are its functions as an adaptive platform, nurturing multiple types of adaptation. Film clips show how this initial learning resonates across childhood as related, modified images, and elicit responses in a child viewer that are variants of the original, shaped by the intervening experiential memory chain. This situation is a rich source of images and themes in films. A second series of film clips was selected in relation to their depiction of themes of violence. Strong evidence that repeated viewing of violent images increases a child's propensity to violent behavior as a late adolescent or young adult is reviewed. Characteristics of film violence that might contribute to this outcome are presented in film clips and discussed in relation to elements characteristic of the early learning phase, such as repetition, practice, and habit formation. **Conclusion:** Images related to examples of the initial and early phases of learning, such as mother-infant attachment behaviors and violent activities, are readily identifiable and very common in films. The manner in which the film presents related images resonating with these themes, and evokes associated emotions and thoughts, can be traced, and their enduring effects on a child's memories can be understood.

S-070-321   Topic: 59, 30

Film techniques and neural mechanisms underlying the enduring effects of a film experience

J. Gerald Young, New York University, Dept. of Psychiatry, New York, NY, USA, jerry.young@nyu.edu

Objective: To identify neural mechanisms underlying the enduring effects of a child's film experience, by examining component influences during the interaction of a child's film experiences with his memories as they evoke new memory formation. **Methods:** Intersubject synchronization of cortical activity in primary and secondary visual and auditory areas, and also in association cortices, has recently been demonstrated to be evoked while freely viewing a film. Yet, other cortical areas fail to show a synchronous response, presumably reflecting later, post-perceptual components of the response to film stimuli that would indicate the diversity of experiences (and memories) among individuals viewing the film (e.g., emotional memories, cognitive responses, motivating symbols). The experiential memories of an individual at the core of this diversity reflect emerging adaptive preferences, and two vital neural mechanisms for learning adaptive behaviors during childhood are examined as examples. The first is the process of learning emotional language within the first 18 months of life, and the second neural mechanism is the representation and transmission of culture, and representations of these two mechanisms in film clips are examined. Both are assessed in relation to the child's film experience. **Results:** What will be remembered are those film experiences most related to the child's current developmental challenges, as these challenges interact with the child's memories of related earlier experiences and residual primary memory prototypes, especially those with continuing, intense associated emotions and conflict. These memory chains are recognizable as individual variations of enduring childhood themes, developmental lines of observable behavior like moving toward increasing self-regulation of aggressive impulses or the gradual transition from egocentricity to companionship that are reflective of the constituent memory chains; the child's responses to challenges are shaped by his unique old and continuing interactive experiences within his family, both memory chains and actual interactions. A film experience exerts a Apull@ on a memory or memory chain insofar as it contains features that are sufficiently similar to the memory template. It is the filmmaker's ability to present images that reflect these prototypical memory chains (developmental lines), yet not too obviously and with the right dose of novelty to disguise what the child is responding to, that propels the film narrative forward. Two of the most useful guides to adaptive success are emotional language and cultural symbols and rituals. Characteristics of emotional language are reviewed, and their correspondence to parallel characteristics of spoken-written language is described. In a related sector of research, the manner in which culture and cultural symbols are represented in the brain, and transmitted to subsequent generations, has begun to be clarified and is reviewed in the context of examples in film clips. **Conclusion:** The neural mechanisms of cultural representation and transmission, and of emerging emotional language, are the foundation for the social, political, and commercial guidance of children. As adults, active in any of these functions, we are creating, selecting, and transmitting culture and shaping emotional language anew for our children. We are moving images into the brains and minds of our children, and our responsibility to them compels us to increase our efforts to understand this process and its effects on the development of children.

S-071 Topic: 78, 28

Psychopathological and molecular genetic study of eating disorders – Studies based by a grant of the German-Israelic-Foundation (GIF)

Track: Eating disorders

Chairperson: Fritz Poustka, Universität Frankfurt Kinder- und Jugendpsychiatrie, Frankfurt, Germany, poustka@em.uni-frankfurt.de
Alan Apter, Schneider Childrens Medical Dept. of Psychiatry, Petah Tikva, Israel, eapter@clalit.org.il

Psychopathological and molecular genetic study of eating disorders – Studies based by a grant of the German-Israelic-Foundation (GIF)

Fritz Poustka, Universität Frankfurt, Kinder- und Jugendpsychiatrie, Frankfurt, Germany, poustka@em.uni-frankfurt.de

The course of eating disorders is very often unfavourable. Chronic course is a frequent complication and normalization occurs in less than half of cases. The etiology remains unresolved, supposing a multifactorial etiology, thus involving hereditary, other biological factors, as well as personality state and traits in origin and maintenance of these disorders. This symposium focuses on the psychopathology of patients with eating disorders and their relatives, focusing on the comorbid psychiatric disorders, metabolic alterations in the brain, and differences between anorexia and bulimia nervosa. Possibly the metabolic changes are predictors in the outcome. The role of neurotransmitters in the regulation of appetite and consequences of feeding is generally accepted. The molecular genetic studies presented in this symposium investigated the allelic distribution of polymorphisms in relevant candidate genes of the serotonergic and other systems as MAO-A, COMT and ARVCF genes. They found significant interactions between serotonin polymorphisms and personality traits as well as a transmission distortion of the COMT and ARVCF loci.

S-071-322 Topic: 78, 95

Influence of comorbidity and personality on symptoms and severity of Anorexia Nervosa

Alan Apter, Schneider Childrens Medical,
Dept. of Psychiatry, Petah Tikva, Israel, eapter@clalit.org.il
Shani Leor

Objective: To assess the influence of comorbidity and personality on the symptoms and severity of Anorexia Nervosa in adolescents. **Methods:** 94 adolescent girls with AN were assessed. Comorbidity was measured with the Structured Clinical Interview for Diagnosis, and personality was assessed with the Cloninger's Tridimensional Personality Questionnaire. Symptoms severity was measured with the Eating Disorders Examination, the Eating Disorders Inventory-2, Body Mass Index (worst ever), number of hospitalizations, duration of symptoms prior to hospitalization, and the Beck Depression Inventory. **Results:** Patients who suffered from any comorbid psychiatric illness (OCD, depression, anxiety, substance use) showed more severe symptomatology, and showed a specific pattern on the TPQ. **Conclusion:** Comorbidity needs to be carefully assessed in the evaluation of patients with AN, and is a confounding variable in any research performed in this area.

S-071-323 Topic: 78

Relatives of adolescents with eating disorders

Lars Wöckel, Universität Frankfurt, Kinder- und Jugendpsychiatrie, Frankfurt, Germany, woeckel@em.uni-frankfurt.de
Gerd Lehmkuhl; Martin Schmidt; Fritz Poustka

Objective: The distribution of eating disorders and other psychiatric disorders among relatives of offsprings with eating disorders in comparison to control groups has been rarely studied extensively and should allow some insights into possible formal genetic associations. **Methods:** Treated female probands with anorexia nervosa (AN) or bulimia (BN) and their relatives were recruited consecutively. Control groups were adolescents with a depressive disorder (DEPR) and their relatives and a matched normal control group using structured interviews and questionnaires (DIGS, FIGS, Strober Interview, GCDI, BDI, Eat26, EDES, and for abnormal psychosocial situations). Blood was also collected from nuclear families and transmitted to DNA and cell lines. 105 probands with AN (mean 16.5 yrs, mean BMI 15.6) were included; and 20 with BN, 26 with depression, and 31 normal controls (BMI 19.7, 21.7, 20.3 resp.), and first and second-degree relatives: 510 (AN), 168 (BN), 104 (DEPR), 314 (CONTR). **Results:** Relatives (r) of probands with an eating disorder (rEAT) compared with rDEPR displayed only to a small extent more AN, but less depression, anxiety disorder and less psychiatric disorders with onset in childhood; rEAT:rCONT > AN and substance abuse; rAN:rBN had less frequent AN, DEPR/anxiety (AX); rAN:rBN < AN, DEPR, or AX; rAN:rDEPR > AN, but less AX, or disorders with onset in childhood; rAN: rCONT > AN; rBN:rDEPR > AN, < DEPR; and rBN:rCONTR > AN, substance abuse, DEPR, AX. **Conclusion:** Relatives of eating disordered offsprings showed some expected differences comparing esp. BN and AN with control groups. Thus, formal heredity seems to bear some uncertain evidence.

S-071-324   Topic: 78, 35
1H-MR-spectroscopic differences between anorexia and bulimia nervosa

Lars Wöckel, Universität Frankfurt, Kinder- und Jugendpsychiatrie, Frankfurt, Germany, woeckel@em. uni-frankfurt.de
Regina Möckel; Fritz Poustka; Martin Schmidt

Objective: The aim of this study is to investigate metabolic alterations with 1H-MR-spectroscopy in the brain of patients with eating disorders. This is the first study which examinates spectroscopic differences between anorexia and bulimia nervosa and follow-ups. **Methods:** 37 anorectic and 8 bulimic female patients and 17 healthy female controls were examined by localized single voxel 1H-MR-spectroscopy (Magnetom Vision; Siemens; 1H-STEAM-spectra, TE = 50 ms, TR = 1.5 s, voxel $2 \times 2 \times 2$ cm) in two different localizations (thalamus and parietal-occipital region). The investigations were performed at the time of admission and in 26 anorectic and 6 bulimic patients in follow-up visits. **Results:** At admission a significant increase of choline/(phospho)creatine (cho/(p)cr) was observed in the white matter of patients compared to controls. The increase is more significant in anorectics (< 0.001) than in bulimics (< 0.05). Furthermore we found a significant decrease (< 0.05) of inositol/(phospho)creatine (ino/(p)cr) in the thalamus of anorectics. On the contrary ino/(p)cr is significantly (< 0.05) increased in bulimia in the white matter. The follow-up revealed reversibility in most of the changes. **Conclusion:** The nutritional state influences the cerebral metabolism which can be demonstrated by 1H-MR-spectroscopy. This concerns the choline resp. the inositol containing compounds. Specifity and extent of disturbation of the cerebral metabolism reflects a different pathophysiology in eating disorders. Brain choline and inositol levels are changed in affective disorders too. Further studies have to be made to investigate a possible correlation between nutrition, affect and cerebral metabolites.

S-071-325   Topic: 78, 28
Molecular genetic study of Anorexia Nervosa: Personality traits as endophenotypes

Shani Leor, University of Tel Aviv,
Feinberg Child Study Center, Tel Aviv, Israel; Leor Frisch

Objective: Family and twin studies indicate a significant genetic contribution to anorexia nervosa (AN), whereas data from pharmacological and clinical studies suggest a possible dysfunction of the serotonergic (5-HT) pathways in AN. These pathways play a role in physiological, behavioral, and personality features characteristic of AN. The objective is to investigate a possible association between AN and genes encoding various components of the 5-HT pathways. **Methods:** The sample presented is from an binational, multi-center, family-based association study. In Israel, 85 trios (AN proband + parents) were screened and characterized to include psychiatric diagnosis, eating attitudes, BMI (body mass index), and number of other phenotypic measures. Blood samples were collected and the trios were genotyped to determine the allelic distribution of polymorphisms in relevant candidate genes: TPH, MAO-A, 5-HTT, 5-HT2AR, 5-HT2CR. Statistical analysis was conducted in two levels, qualitative and quantitative: (1) using the Transmission Disequilibrium Test (TDT) to establish an association between AN and 5-HT polymorphisms; (2) using ANOVAs in search of quantitative trait loci (QTLs) influencing behavioral and personality traits which may play a role in the genetic vulnerability to AN. **Results:** TDT analysis show no significant association with AN for any of the candidate genes. However, MANOVAs for associations between genes and personality traits (typical of AN) revealed several significant effects and interactions. **Conclusion:** These preliminary results suggest that 5-HT polymorphisms may play a role in the genetic predisposition to AN through their associations with personality features which in turn mediate the susceptibility for AN.

S-071-326   Topic: 78
Molecular genetic study of eating disorders in German and Israelic patient samples

Sabine Klauck, DKFZ, Molecular Genome Analysis, Heidelberg, Germany, s.klauck@dkfz.de
Amos Frisch; Martin H. Schmidt; Gerd Lehmkuhl; Alan Apter; Abraham Weizman; Fritz Poustka

Objective: The eating disorders anorexia nervosa (AN) and bulimia nervosa (BN) are severe and disabling psychiatric conditions. AN is characterized by profound weight loss of at least 15%, body image disturbance and an intense fear of becoming obese. Onset of AN is mostly in the mid-teenage years with prevalence estimates from 10-100/10,000 in the population. There is a significant genetic component based on family and twin studies with a heritability of 75-80% for AN and 45-55% for BN. More than one susceptibility gene is expected for both AN and BN. **Methods:** Clinical sites in Germany and Israel are recruiting participants for the project to identify susceptibility genes for AN. Currently 90 index patients and 86 family trios have been recruited throughout Germany and 99 index patients and 85 family trios throughout Israel. The trios have been subgrouped into restricting type (rAN) and purging type (pAN). Patients with the pAN additionally show occasional episodes of impulsive eating followed by purging in contrast to the rAN patients, who show only limiting food intake. **Results:** Family-based association studies have been performed with markers relevant for several candidate neurotransmitter system genes, but most markers tested did not reveal a clear candidate. Based on a preliminary positive association of the COMT gene in Israeli and German families, this gene and the ARVCF gene, in its immediate vicinity in the candidate chromosomal region of 22q11.2 have been further investigated. Seven polymorphisms in COMT and ARVCF have been genotyped in 51 German rAN and 66 Israeli rAN families. Several single markers and haplotype analyses at the COMT and ARVCF loci revealed significant transmission distortion by TDT in the Israeli rAN sample but only a tendency towards transmission distortion in the German rAN sample. **Conclusion:** These positive results warrant further association studies and variant screening of genes from the genomic region 22q11.2.

S-072 Topic: 51
Treatment
Chairperson: Inger Helene Vandvik,
Rikshospitalet Nat. Hospital Child & Adolescent Psychiatry,
Oslo, Norway, i.h.vandvik@medisin.uio.no

S-072-327 Topic: 51
Experience of integrative treatment in children and adolescents in Nizhny
Andrey Zanozin, Centre for Mental Health of,
Children and Adolescents, Nizhnj Novgorod, Russia,
tndmitr@sandy.ru
Tatjana Dmitrieva

The incidence of psychiatric disorders in children and adolescent significantly increased over the last 10 years in Russia. The diagnostic structure of cases has been stable over the past ten years. The most widespread problems are the non-psychotic disorders with 66%. The high prevalence of non psychotic disorders demands an urgent development of the psychotherapeutic services and integrative treatment. This was one of the reasons to establish a Centre for mental health of children and adolescents in Nizhny Novgorod several years ago. The four years of experience of the Centre showed the big need for psychotherapy and the effectiveness of multidisciplinary approach for examination and treatment of young patients. About 3% of the whole child population of Nizhny Novgorod (more then eight thousand) children were examined and treated in our Centre, among them about eight hundred children aged up to 4 years. The most important therapeutic methods used in the Centre are psychotherapy and psychological training with minimal use of medication. The very important part of our work is training and the post graduate education in the field of the child and adolescent psychiatry, psychotherapy and medical psychology.

S-072-328 Topic: 88, 11
Hypnotherapy in treatment resistant nocturnal enuresis
Inger Helene Vandvik, Rikshospitalet Nat. Hospital,
Child & Adolescent Psychiatry, Oslo, Norway,
i.h.vandvik@medisin.uio.no

Objective: Nocturnal enuresis represents a practical, social or emotional problem. The present study illustrates the advantage of using hypnosis as a therapy in chronic cases. Twelve boys, median age 12 years (range 8–16), eight with primary nocturnal enuresis and four with primary nocturnal and diurnal enuresis, reported at referral median of 0 (range 0–3) dry nights per week. All patients had a family history of enuresis and had used enuresis alarm and Desmopressin; while 50% used Imipramin. Eight had been referred to psychological or child and adolescent psychiatric services for treatment. **Methods:** All patients had undergone a somatic assessment by a paediatrician, a paediatric surgeon, or an urologist. After a preliminary assessment of patient motivation, they underwent hypnotherapy with a median six sessions (range 2–8), followed by median one month with self-hypnosis exercises. **Results:** At follow-up after three months and one year, nine of 12 patients had respectively 6–7/7, and 7/7 dry nights per week. Three patients had nocturnal enuresis at follow-up; two of them were referred to a paediatric surgeon for their overactive urine bladder, and one was referred to his local psychiatric clinic because of ongoing family conflicts. **Conclusion:** Hypnotherapy had lasting effects for boys with chronic and complex forms of nocturnal enuresis. We suggest that hypnotherapy should be included in the therapeutic guidelines.

S-072-329 Topic: 76
Important gender identity disorder in a young boy: Between fascination, adaptation and position taking
Sylvie Jamart, Clin. Universitaires St. Luc, Dept. de
Pédopsychiatrie, Bruxelles, Belgium, sylvie_jamart@yahoo.fr
Jean-Yves Hayez

Objective: Starting from a clinical situation about a gender identity disorder related to early transsexualism, we are going to describe the ethical, cultural and sociological difficulties of a therapeutic position taking. **Methods:** Description of the clinical situation of a seven-year-old boy manifesting symptoms of a »child on the way to becoming "transsexual" in a particular family dynamic. **Results:** We will discuss the complexity of therapeutic choices according to the family culture, sociological pressures and ethical values. **Conclusion:** We will explain the difficulties of such pathologies for the family and individual follow-up.

S-072-330 Topic: 53, 52
The impact of early intensive intervention in children and adolescent victims of suicide bombing attacks on prognosis
Agnes Leor, Tel-Aviv Medical Center, Child Psychiatry, Tel-Aviv, Israel, agnesleo@netvision.net.il

Objective: Literature shows high rate of chronic psychic morbidity in child and adolescent after traumatic event: 20% to 67% of full Post Traumatic Stress Disorder (PTSD), high occurrence of sub-threshold PTSD symptoms and strong influence of trauma on the developing personality. The purpose of our research was to evaluate the impact of early intensive intervention on the clinical course of Acute Stress Disorder (ASR) in children and adolescents. **Methods:** Subjects: Group 1: 10 victims of suicide bombing attack (aged 2.5–17) who got the early intervention. Group 2: 11 adolescents (15–17) victims of SBA and did not get any treatment. Intervention: Treatment start at ER: social support. The essentials of intervention were 1) holding, support, orientation, cognitive and behavioral advises, respect of need to ventilate as well as the opposite need and respect the need to repress. 2) Intensiveness: session every day to three times a week during 10 days to 3 months according to specific case. 3) Full involvement of family in treatment. Assessment: 1) Structured Clinical Interview for Axis 1 DSMIV Disorders: SCID(DSMIV). 2) Child Behavior Checklist/2–4 (Achenbach): CBCL/2–4. 3) Child Behavior Checklist/4–18 (Achenbach): CBCL/4–18. Data analysis: Association between treatment and PTSD diagnose was performed using chi-square tests. Associations between treatment and CBCL data were performed using t-tests. **Results:** SCID: PTSD in treated group: 10%; PTSD in non-treated group: 37%. CBCL: significant higher scores in non-treated group. **Conclusion:** Our preliminary results showed that early intensive supportive cognitive behavioral intervention, completed by family support is effective in preventing and lowering mental and developmental morbidity including PTSD of children and adolescents after suicide bombing attack.

S-072-331   Topic: 79
Predictors for parental behaviour in atopic and healthy children

Maria Elisabeth Ahle, Universität Potsdam, Potsdam, Germany, mahle@rz.uni-potsdam.de
Jörg M. Fegert; Günter Esser

Objective: This report describes parental beliefs of child misbehaviour as perceived by parents with healthy children and those suffering from chronic atopic disease. **Methods:** A sample of 647 parents with preschool children who participated in a multicentric allergy study (MAS 90) was examined. 79 children of these parents were suffering from the chronic disease atopic eczema and/or asthma. This sample was compared with a control group of parents (n=90) whose children were healthy. The parents were screened with a new questionnaire, which measures the parental locus of control concerning child noncompliance. We examined 'parental attitude' and 'parental behaviour' towards child misbehaviour. **Results:** Parents with high fatalistic and external locus of control felt more helpless regarding child noncompliance than parents with high internal locus of control. A theoretical process model with structural equation analysis is proposed to explore the influence of the examined variables on child-rearing. The strongest effect was that of fatalistic locus of control influencing the evaluation of the child as difficult or unproblematic. A two-group model revealed significant differences between parents of ill and healthy children: 'fatalistic locus of control' and the emotions of 'guilt', 'worry' and 'feelings of responsibility' seem to play a crucial role for parents of ill children.

S-072-332   Topic: 23, 92
Absence of acute stress symptomatology in pediatric elective surgery

Galit Ben Amitay, Tel Aviv, Israel, dbecker@post.tau.ac.il
Irene Kosov; Ahuva Reiss; Roni Hegesh; Moses Tamar

Objective: The emotional consequences of elective surgery in children are not enough evaluated. A descriptive study was designed purposed to rate the prevalence and severity of Post traumatic stress disorder, Anxiety and Depression in children after elective surgery, and to survey the correlation to psychological parameters in their parents. **Methods:** The sample consisted of children who were consecutive admitted to elective surgery in a general hospital. Patients aged 7 to 18 years were eligible. Forty subjects: 21 males, 19 females, age ranged from 6.5 to 17.5 years, mean –13.05 years (SD=2.7) completed the first phase of the

study (admission day). Surgery interventions included: Orthopedics (Scoliosis, Osteomyelitis, Bone cysts, CP; General Surgery (Herniotomy, Pilonidal sinus, Varicocele, Sympathectomy); Otorhinolaryngology (Adenoidectomy, Tonsillectomy). Thirty-nine (96%) patients completed the second phase of the study in one month follow up. The sample was rated for socio-demographic data; medical history; child past trauma; KIDDIE SADS. PTSD was evaluated by CPTS-RI; Anxiety by RCMAS; Depression by CDI; the family was assessed by Olson Scale. The parents were rated for anxiety by Spielberger and for depression by Beck and past trauma. After one month follow up children and parents were interviewed (meeting or phone) and rated by: Child anxiety scale; Child depression scale; Child PTSD scale. **Results:** PTSD was diagnosed in one child only (4%), unrelated to the severity of the physical injury but to a previous exposure to trauma. Subjects of the study didn't score high for post trauma symptomatology, depression, and anxiety. No correlation was found between the rate of anxiety and depression of the children and their respective parents. **Conclusion:** In the sample of children after elective surgery in spite of the exposure to physical threat, no symptoms of acute stress depression or anxiety were observed.

S-073   Topic: 83
Pervasive developmental disorders II
Track: Pervasive developmental disorders (PDD)
Chairperson: Bernard Golse, Hôpital Necker Dept. of Pédopsychiatrie, Paris, France, bernard.golse@wanadoo.fr

S-073-333   Topic: 83, 77
Insomnia in children with Asperger Syndrome or high-functioning autism:
Associated behavioural characteristics

Hans Smedje, Uppsala University Hospital, Child & Adolescent Psychiatry, Uppsala, Sweden, hans.smedje@bupinst.uu.se
Hiie Allik; Jan-Olov Larsson

Objective: To investigate relationships between insomnia and impairments in social interaction, communication and behaviour in schoolchildren with Asperger Syndrome (AS) or high-functioning autism (HFA). **Methods:** Thirty-two 8-12 year old children with AS or HFA were investigated by use of parental reports to a sleep questionnaire and to the high-functioning autism screening questionnaire (ASSQ). Difficulties in falling asleep at least three nights per week and/or a sleep latency of at least 30 minutes was used to define "insomnia". The ASSQ, a 27-item checklist for completion by lay informants, was used to assess the extent of AS- and HFA-related symptoms and impairments in each of the participants. ASSQ results between children with and without insomnia were compared by use chi-square tests (single items), and by use of the Mann-Whitney test (total ASSQ score). A significance level of 0.05 was applied. **Results:** Twelve out of 32 children with AS/HFA suffered from insomnia. There were significant relationships between insomnia and the following ASSQ-items: "compulsory repetitions of certain actions or thoughts"; "lack of common sense"; "unusual postures"; "lives somewhat in his/her own world with restricted interests"; "idiosyncratic language"; "motor clumsiness", and "insistence on sameness. The mean total ASSQ score of the children with insomnia was significantly higher than the score of the children without insomnia; 26 vs. 18. **Conclusion:** Children with AS/HFA suffering from insomnia have increased levels of parent reported impairments in social interaction, communication and behaviour.

S-073-334   Topic: 83, 28
Regulated secretion in the neuron:
New genetic findings suggest a novel biological pathway underlying autism

Jean Steyaert, Katholieke Universiteit Leuven,
Child & Adolescent Psychiatry, Leuven, Belgium,
jean.steyaert@med.kuleuven.ac.be
Dries Castermans; John Creemers; Koenraad Devriendt

Objective: The delineation of novel candidate genes for autism is a cornerstone in understanding the biology of autism and other neurodevelopmental disorders. New techniques emerging in molecular biology can detect genes and biological pathways for autism that had previously not been associated with autism. Applying these techniques gives a broader understanding of the biology of autism. **Methods:** Positional cloning: In balanced chromosomal anomalies, e.g. reciprocal translocations, one or two genes are broken. If the anomaly is associated with a neurodevelopmental disorder, e.g. autism, the broken gene is likely to play a role in the fysiopathology of the disorder in this subject, and likely also in some other subjects with the same disorder. Positional cloning of chromosomal breakpoints is a molecular biological technique that has recently been applied in neurodevelopmental disorders, and has yielded convincing results in e.g. dyslexia (Taipale, 2003). Subjects: Chromosomal analysis was performed in more than 500 subjects with autism. In 1% of them, balanced chromosomal anomalies were detected. For positional cloning of the breakpoints, we selected the subjects with high-functioning autism, without other neurodevelopmental disorders. **Results:** Positional cloning of chromosomal breakpoints let us delineate four novel candidate genes for autism. Three of these, neurobeachin, amysin, CLIC4, participate in the same intraneuronal biological pathway: "regulated secretion". This pathway plays a role in neuronal growth and pruning. The association of neurobeachin, with autism has been replicated by another research group. Neurobeachin lies at a chromosomal locus that has repeatedly been associated with autism through linkage analysis. **Conclusion:** Positional cloning of chromosomal breakpoints allowed us to delineate a previously unsuspected biological pathway in autism: regulated secretion in the neurons. There is reasonable evidence that this novel pathway is relevant for the biology of autism in at least a sub-population of subjects.

S-073-335   Topic: 83, 91
Difficulties of diagnostic and therapeutic procedures in 9 year old boy with autistic spektrum disorder and epilepsy-3 year's observation

Marta Kaczynska-Haladyj, Neuropsychiatric National,
Health Service Lublin, Lublin, Poland,
mkaczyn@oil.lublin.pl

Objective: The aim of report to show the difficulties in diagnosis and classification of epileptic attacks in autistic spektrum disorder ASD. There is an increasing research interest in the association between autism and epilepsy in childhood. The clinical diagnosis of epilepsy in autism is complicated. **Methods:** Case report presents three years observation

of clinical course. A 9 year-old boy without pathology of prenatal and perinatal period, demonstrated from early childhood mild ASD. At the age of 6, the epilepric attacks occurred. From the beginning there was problem with classification of seizures. At next year the frequency of epileptic seizures and symptoms ADHD increased. The boy was admitted to Department of Child Psychiatry, where he was diagnosed and as participated in the comprehensive therapeutic program. **Results:** During hospitalisation complex partial seizures with impaired consciousness were registered. The neuroimaging findings CT and MR of brain were normal. The EEG recordings and Holter-EEG showed bitemporal paroxysmal discharges on the normal background activity. The boy's cognitive abilities were affected with low level of cognitive abilities with dysharmonic profiles. The use of the modifyed antiepileptic treatment valproic acid (VPA) with add-on oxcarbazepine (OCBZ) and as tailored comprehensive treatment for ASD influenced positively on improvement of psychiatric status and decrease frequency of epileptic attacks. The results of tests were presented. **Conclusion:** The primary problem in diagnosis is possibility of omitting seizures because onset is may be insidious and seizures may be mistaken for other childhood behaviours. The topographic distribution of discharges in the EEG is important in the classification of epilepsy and as use tailored antiepileptic treatment. Early correct diagnosis of epilepsy gives a chance for better quality of life.

S-073-336   Topic: 83
Clinical interview with Asperger syndrome boy

Maria Claustre Jané Ballabriga, U. Autonoma de Barcelona,
Psicologia Salut i Social, Bellaterra, Spain,
mjane@seneca.uab.es
Joaquima Judez; Empar Pelaez; Pilar Sole; Lidia Rodriguez

The aim of these videotape is to present a clinical interview with Asperger syndrome boy. The validity of Asperger syndrome continues to be the topic of considerable debate. Consistent with Asperger's original description of the condition these appear to be some important differences from autism if both conditions are strictly defined. The boy met the DSM-IV criteria for Asperger's disorder, including those with normal intelligence and absence of early speech delay. Based on work associated with PDD epidemiological study in primary care unity of Salut Mental del Parc Taulí (Sabadell, Vallès Occidental), the interview summarized information on the unique intellectual, academic, social, emotional and sensory characteristics. We believe the cognition processes of Asperger syndrome are: literality, monotropism, thinking in closed pictures and non-generalised learning non-social priorities, issues with time and motion, issues with predicting outcomes and difficulties with theory of mind (Empathy lacks and empathy gaps).

S-073-337   Topic: 83, 35
Brain volume increases in medication naive high-functioning subjects with autism, but not in their parents

Saskia Palmen, University Medical Center, Dept. of Child
Psychiatry, Utrecht, Netherlands, s.palmen@azu.nl
Hilleke Hulshoff Pol; Chantal Kemner; Hugo Schnack;
Rene Kahn; Herman van Engeland

Objective: Autism is a highly heritable, neurodevelopmental disorder associated with enlarged brain volume. As yet, it is unclear whether this enlargement is present only in young children with autism, whether it is still present during late childhood, adolescence and adulthood, and whether it is present in biological relatives of autistic subjects. Furthermore, it is unclear whether the enlargement is confined to gray and/or white matter and whether it is global or more prominent in some cortical lobes. **Methods:** Regional brain volumes of 42 medication naive autistic subjects were compared to those of 42 control subjects (2 studies were conducted, the first consisting of children aged 7–15 and the second consisting of adolescents and young adults aged 16–25). In addition, regional brain volumes of biological parents of autistic subjects (n = 19 couples) were compared to those of 20 healthy control couples. All three samples were matched on age, gender, IQ, handedness, educational level, length and weight. **Results:** The autistic subjects, both the children and the adolescents, showed a global increase in cerebral gray matter and cerebellum volume, proportional to the increase in total brain volume. The lateral and third ventricular volumes were disproportionately enlarged and remained significantly larger after correction for total brain volume. In contrast, none of the brain volumes differed significantly between the biological parents of autistic subjects and healthy control couples. **Conclusion:** Brain volume enlargement seems to be present, both in high-functioning children, adolescents, and young adults with autism. As biological parents of autistic subjects do not show brain enlargement, increased brain volumes in autism might be caused by the interaction of paternal and maternal genes, possibly with an additional effect of environmental factors, or increased brain volumes might reflect phenotypes of autism.

S-073-338   Topic: 83, 82
Language disorder and Pervasive Developmental Disorder (PDD): Pathogenetic links and outcome
Anna Fabrizi, Dipartimento di Scienze, Dept. of Neurology, Rome, Italy, anna.fabrizi@uniroma1.it
Levi Gabriel

The goal of this study is to analyze the nature of the linkages between Language Disorder and Affective- Emotional disorder among 45 Specific Language Disorder (SLD) and 45 Atypical Pervasive Developmental Disorder (APDD) children (Average age 3.6 years; IQ = 78; Average follow up 3.6 years) The typology, the distribution and the outcome of Psychiatric Disorder in SLD children and of the Language Disorder in ADPP children focus the existence of specific pathogenetic bonds between primary and selective deficits. The bonds have a different weight on the outcome forbidding a real overlap between disorders.

S-074   Topic: 2, 45
Child and adolescent psychiatry in Brazil: Research and clinical data
Track: Therapy and intervention
Chairperson: Marcos Mercadante, Mackenzie University PDD Program, Sao Paulo, Brazil, mercadante@mackenzie.com.br

Child and adolescent psychiatry in Brazil: Research and clinical data
Marcos Mercadante, Mackenzie University, PDD Program, Sao Paulo, Brazil, mercadante@mackenzie.com.br

Objective: ADHD in Brazil – Recent research and clinical findings: There is a scarcity of studies on ADHD in Brazil. This review of the literature aims to present an overview of the current status of the disorder in Brazil addressing the issue of cross-cultural validity. Epidemiological, clinical, and family data, as well as treatment findings are compared to similar studies from other countries. **Methods:** Brazilian adolescents' drug consumption increase – A reality that worries: many epidemiological researches conduced in the last fifteen years by different authors have pointed out an increase of licit an illicit drugs' consumption by Brazilian teenagers. These results will be compared with similar ones in other countries and hypothesis to explain this fact are discussed. Besides this, the main school preventions programs are analyzed, emphasizing the ones with brief intervention, which have their efficiency, evaluated. **Results:** OCD in Brazil – Recent research and clinical findings: The identification of more homogeneous subgroups of OCD patients will help in the identification of etiological factors and lead to more precise treatments strategies. This review of the literature aims to present an overview of the current efforts to identify these subgroups of OCD patients. Epidemiological, clinical, family-genetic, as well as treatment outcome studies from Brazil will be presented. These data will be compared to similar studies from other countries, addressing the issue of cross-cultural validity **Conclusion:** Autism and PDD in Brazil – Recent research and clinical findings: new techniques have been applied in the research of PDD. Strategies, such as eye-tracking, have allowed the identification of better phenotypes. This presentation will focus on the current status of research of the disorder in Brazil addressing the issue of cross-cultural validity. Epidemiological, clinical, and family data, as well as treatment findings are compared to similar studies from other countries.

S-074-339   Topic: 84
ADHD in Brazil: Recent research and clinical findings
Luis Augusto Rohde, UFRGS-HCPA-Brazil, Dept. of Psychiatry, Porto Alegre, Brazil, lrohde@terra.com.br

Objective: Several investigations have assessed different aspects of the diagnostic validity of Attention-Deficit/Hyperactivity Disorder (ADHD) worldwide, especially in the U.S. However, there is a scarcity of research findings on ADHD from other cultures like those from developing countries. Thus, this presentation aims to review recent research findings on the prevalence, symptomalogy, genetics, and treatment of ADHD in Brazil. **Methods:** We performed a systematic computerized review of the literature on ADHD in Brazil. Findings were compared to those from studies in developed countries. **Results:** We found 25 studies presenting non-duplicated research or clinical findings on ADHD prevalence, etiology, symptomatology construct, or treatment; 13 of these (52%) came from the same research center. A huge variability in the methodology of the studies was detected. The prevalence rates of ADHD (5.8% using DSM-IV criteria, 1.5% using ICD-10), the bi-dimensional factor construct (inattention and hyperactivity/impulsivity) extracted from factor analyses, the pattern of ADHD comorbidity, the family genetic data, as well as preliminary findings from a clinical trial demonstrating a similar efficacy of methylphenidate in the disorder than those from clinical trials in developed countries are presented. **Conclusion:** Although scientific research on ADHD is very scarce in Brazil, recent findings support the cross-cultural validity of ADHD in a developing country with a diverse culture.

S-074-340   Topic: 68
The question of drug use and misuse
Sergio de Paula Ramos, Mae de Deus Hospital, Chemical Dependence Unit, Porto Alegre, Brazil, serramos@terra.com.br

Objective: To show epidemiological and clinical data available in Brazil that point out the impact of drug consumption, by young people, in undeveloped countries. **Methods:** Revision of 5 national epidemiological researches on drug consumption with students between 12 and 18 years old, several criminal reports and economic consequences. Available clinical data are also discussed. **Results:** In the last 15 years, drug consumption by Brazilian teenagers has increased significantly. Tobacco experimentation raised from 23% to 52%; alcohol, from 71% to 89%; marijuana, from 3% to 28%, and cocaine, from 0,3% to 8%. These changes are related to the increase of criminality and death. From the federal government's part, there is not a policy to reduce the problem. **Conclusion:** Despite the increase of drug consumption in the last 15 years, national authorities seem not to worry with prevention.

S-074-341   Topic: 72
OCD in Brazil: Recent research and clinical findings
Maria Concecao Rosario-Campos, Bahia Federal University, Dept. of Psychiatry, Salvador, Brazil, mariacrcampos@ctmnet.com.br

Objective: Obsessive-compulsive disorder (OCD) has a bimodal age of onset and range of treatment outcomes. Although most of the studies done so far have considered the childhood and the adult forms of OCD as the same disorder, more recent data have suggested that OCD children, as well as adults with an early onset of their obsessive-compulsive (OC) symptoms, may represent a distinct subgroup. Identifying valid OCD subgroups is important not only because different subgroups may benefit from different treatment strategies but also because more homogeneous subgroups may lead to a better understanding of genetic and environmental factors involved in OCD etiology. Thus, this presentation aims to review recent research findings on early-onset OCD. **Methods:** We performed a computerized review of the literature on the prevalence, phenomenology, genetics and treatment of early-onset OCD in Brazil. Findings were then compared to those from studies in developed countries. **Results:** We found five studies presenting on the prevalence, phenomenology, neuroimaging or treatment of early-onset OCD, all generated by the same Brazilian research center. These results from theses studies were similar to the ones found by studies performed in developed countries. The presenter concludes by presenting recent data on the genetics of OCD and on the psychometrics of a new scale developed for the assessment of presence and severity of OC symptoms. **Conclusion:** Scientific research on early-onset OCD is very scarce in Brazil. Nevertheless, the findings are comparable to

studies from developed countries and indicate that early-onset OCD may represent a specific subgroup of patients.

S-074-342   Topic: 83
Autism and PDD in Brazil:
Recent research and clinical findings
Marcos Mercadante, Mackenzie University, PDD Program, Sao Paulo, Brazil, mercadante@mackenzie.com.br

Objective: Pervasive Developmental Disorders (PDD) are comprised by a group of disabling disorders, including autism (AD) and Asperger syndrome (AS). Basically, three domains are affected: social skills, communication abilities, and restricted pattern of behavior. Due to the cultural influences different presentation might be found across cultures. This presentation aims to resume the research and clinical data from a developing country. **Methods:** We performed a review in the literature on researches driven to PDD in Brazil. We also obtained information from the PDD centers and professionals' experts on the studies in developing. **Results:** We found 24 papers, only 5 in Medline. Most of all are single case reports or reviewers. One study presents molecular and cytogenetic analyses, two are focus on neuroimaging, and one explores the face recognition skill. Interestingly this study shows that Brazilian's PDD children have more difficulties in recognizing expressions of happiness and surprise. None epidemiological data can be found. In addition researches on animal model, eye-tracking technique and communicative patterns measurements are been done, according the information obtained from experts. **Conclusion:** Although the few studies done in Brazil, it is suggested that neuroanatomical and genetic data are similar to the results described in other countries, however it is tempting to consider that the consequences of the social and communication impairments in subjects living in a society with higher level of social relationship expectations are more severe in terms of personal adaptive development. To more explore this hypothesis studies have to be done.

S-074-343   Topic: 72
Pharmacological and group cognitive-behavioral treatments of childhood-onset (OCD) in Brazil:
Recent research, clinical and pathophysiological findings
Fernando Asbahr, Univ. of São Paulo Med. School, Dept. of Psychiatry, São Paulo, Brazil, frasbahr@usp.br

Objective: To compare the effectiveness of group cognitive-behavioral therapy (GCBT) and of sertraline in treatment-naive brazilian children and adolescents with obsessive-compulsive disorder (OCD). The GCBT consisted of a 12-week cognitive-behavioral protocol adapted for groups, and the sertraline treatment involved medication intake along 12 weeks. Patients were assessed before, during and after treatments and at 1, 3, 6, and 9 months following their conclusion utilizing diagnostic and symptom severity interviews, and self-report measures. Thus, this presentation aims to present recent research findings on pharmacological and psychological treatments of childhood-onset OCD in Brazil. **Methods:** Forty subjects aged between 9 and 17 years were randomized to GCBT (n=20) or to sertraline (n=20) condition. Patients were assessed before, during and after the 12-week acute treatments and at 1, 3, 6, and 9 months following their conclusion utilizing diagnostic and symptom severity interviews, and self-report measures. Findings were compared to those from studies in developed countries. **Results:** Significant improvement on OCD and secondary measures were observed along the 12-week treatments and follow-up period in both treatment conditions, with no significant differences on OCD symptom severity between groups. Treatment gains were maintained up to 9 months of follow-up, with a significant lower rate of symptom relapse in the GCBT group than in the sertraline condition. **Conclusion:** The treatment with GCBT is effective for childhood OCD, and should be considered as an alternative to individual cognitive-behavioral therapy or a medication, such as sertraline. Results support findings involving pharmacological and individual cognitive-behavioral therapy studies from developed countries.

S-075   Topic: 43
A new look at resilience
Chairperson: Michael Rutter, Institute of Psychiatry SGDP Centre, London, United Kingdom, j.wickham@iop.kcl.ac.uk

A new look at resilience
Michael Rutter, Institute of Psychiatry, SGDP Centre, London, United Kingdom, j.wickham@iop.kcl.ac.uk

After a brief introduction by the Chairman, Stephan Collishaw will present new findings on resilience in relation to a long term follow-up into mid-adult life of young people first studied in childhood/adolescence. Michael Rutter will consider the evidence on gene-environment interaction in relation to resilience, with particular reference to findings from the Dunedin (New Zealand) longitudinal study. Jana Kreppner will consider possible constraints on resilience using data from the UK study of children adopted from profoundly depriving institutions. In the fourth paper, Anne Borge will draw on a range of findings on resilience to consider the implications of resilience concepts and findings for preventive/interventive strategies. In her discussion of these four papers, Suniya Luthar will consider the concept of resilience more broadly in order to open up discussion on challenges and opportunities.

S-075-344   Topic: 43, 51
Resilience to psychopathology following childhood maltreatment: Evidence from a community sample
Stephan Collishaw, Institute of Psychiatry, MRC SGDP Centre, London, United Kingdom, s.collishaw@iop.kcl.ac.uk
Barbara Maughan; Andrew Pickles; Julie Messer; Michael Rutter

Objective: Childhood maltreatment is an important risk for adult psychiatric morbidity. However, not all maltreated children experience mental health problems as adults. Our aims were to address the extent of resilience to adult psychopathology in a representative community sample, and to explore predictors of a good prognosis. **Methods:** Data are drawn from the Isle of Wight study, a follow-up of an epidemiological sample from adolescence (age 14/15) to midlife (age 44/45). Ratings of psychiatric disorder, peer relationships and family functioning were made in adolescence; adult assessments included a lifetime psychiatric history, personality and social functioning assessments, and retrospective reports of childhood sexual and physical maltreatment. **Results:** Ten percent of individuals reported repeated and severe physical or sexual mal-

treatment in childhood. Prospective measures revealed increased rates of adolescent minor depression and peer relationship problems in this group. Rates of adult psychopathology were also elevated among maltreated individuals, and this increased risk remained controlling for childhood family adversity and parental psychopathology. A third of maltreated individuals reported no mental health problems as adults. Predictors of a good prognosis included a number of general predictors of psychopathology: family adversity, maternal psychopathology, personality style; as well as factors that were particularly important in the context of abuse: adolescent and adult relationship functioning; perceived parental care; characteristics of the abuse. **Conclusion:** These findings provide further evidence that childhood physical and sexual abuse may have a profound negative impact on adult mental health. However, the study also identified an important subgroup of "resilient" individuals, who reported no adult psychopathology over a thirty-year follow-up period. Understanding factors that promote resilience may help elucidate under what circumstances and for what reasons child maltreatment leads to psychopathology, and may inform treatment and intervention programs for children and adults who report abusive experiences.

S-075-345   Topic: 1, 3
Gene-environment interplay in resilience
Michael Rutter, Institute of Psychiatry, SGDP Centre, London, United Kingdom, j.wickham@iop.kcl.ac.uk
Avshalom Caspi; Terrie Moffitt

Objective: To consider the importance of gene-environment correlations and interactions in resilience. **Methods:** Relevant findings from both quantitative and molecular genetic research. **Results:** Attention will be drawn to the evidence of synergism between specific identified genotypes and exposure to specific measured environmental risks. The implication is that an important part of genetic effects on multifactorial disorders lies in genetic influences on individual differences in susceptibility to environmental hazards. Because the genetic effects are outcome-specific rather than stress-specific, it would seem that the genetic effects operate on pathophysiological pathways that are involved in the causation of mental disorders. Amongst other things, the findings highlight the need for research to identify the effects of psychosocial stress/disadvantage/adversity on the organism. **Conclusion:** The effective harnessing of these findings for the development of new methods of prevention/intervention will be dependent on the accurate delineations of the biological processes involved in both environmental and genetic risk/protective effects and especially the processes involved in their interplay.

S-075-346   Topic: 43, 24
Are there limits to resilience?
Findings from the Romanian study
Jana Kreppner, Institute of Psychiatry, SGDP, London, United Kingdom, jana.kreppner@iop.kcl.ac.uk

Objective: The degree of recovery from profound early deprivation following rescue from it has been the focus of an ongoing study of severely deprived children adopted from Romanian institutions into UK families. At age 6 years, children showed a remarkable potential for recovery in terms of their cognitive and social functioning (Rutter et al., 1998, O'Connor et al., 2000). However, there was a substantial minority of children who at 6 years of age presented a variety of behavioural and emotional disturbances including quasi-autistic features, disinhibited attachment, inattention/overactivity, and cognitive impairment (Rutter et al., 2001). The aims of the present paper are to investigate continuity and discontinuity in psychopathology following early deprivation. **Methods:** 165 Romanian children adopted from institutions into UK families at various ages (e.g., 0 to 42 months), were compared with 52 non-deprived within-UK adoptees who were all placed before the age of 6 months. Data were collected using a multi-reporter (e.g., parent and teacher report) and a multi-method (e.g., questionnaires, interviews, observations) strategy. **Results:** Findings will be presented on, firstly, whether or not problem behaviours observed at age 6 years persisted to age 11 years; secondly, whether or not there is a particular 'sensitive' period for recovery in terms of when children were rescued from deprivation; and, thirdly, on factors that could play a role in limiting children's resilience to early deprivation. **Conclusion:** The findings will be discussed in terms of the surprisingly persisting effects of early adverse rearing experiences on psychological development, and in terms of possible limitations to children's potential for recovery from it.

S-075-347 Topic: 43, 3
How do resilience concepts and findings aid the planning of interventions?

Anne Inger H. Borge, University of Oslo, Dept. of Psychology, Oslo, Norway, a.i.h.borge@psykologi.uio.no

Objective: For at least the last 30 years, researchers have been well aware of the need to consider both risk and protective mechanisms in relation to the psychopathological sequelae of adverse experiences. They have also appreciated that there is huge individual variation in how people respond to stress, adversity, and disadvantage. Some succumb, some appear relatively unaffected, and a few even appear strengthened as a result of coping successfully with potentially damaging experiences. Practitioners and policy makers have used findings from this considerable body of research to develop programmes designed either to prevent mental disorders or to alleviate their effects. In what ways might resilience concepts and findings either change the way we think about these preventive/interventive programmes, or make them more effective? **Methods:** In this paper I will consider several possible answers to that question. **Results:** The potentially relevant resilience features include an appreciation that: 1) experiences before, during and after exposure to stress/adversity may all be influential; 2) people are not generally resilient or vulnerable; somewhat different features may be important according to the nature of the negative experience and the type of outcome being considered; 3) coping successfully with manageable stress/challenge may be protective against major later adversities by fostering self-efficacy; 4) cognitive/affective appraisal of experiences may alter their impacts; 5) community support/cohesion may provide important protection, as may also the quality of institutions such as schools. **Conclusion:** Effective prevention is as likely to derive from population-wide interventions as in the targeted focus on high risk groups.

S-075-347A Topic: 43, 1
Discussant's commentary

Suniya Luthar, Columbia University, Clinical and Devtal Psychology, New York, NY, USA, suniya.luthar@columbia.edu

Objective: To integrate the findings from research presented in the prior four commentaries in this symposium. **Methods:** Discussions will be based on (a) data from the Isle of Wight study, a follow-up of an epidemiological sample from adolescence to midlife; (b) evidence from both quantitative and molecular genetic research on gene-environment correlations and interactions in resilience; (c) data from a study of severely deprived children adopted from Romanian institutions into UK families; and (d) applications of resilience research in prior prevention/intervention programs. **Results:** The evidence shows that serious early adversities in the form of maltreatment by caregivers or institutionalization in orphanages with poor caregiving conditions presage significant risk for psychopathology in later life, but at the same time, that good quality care by other adults can offset this high risk to some degree. It is also clear that differing types of vulnerability and protective processes including biological processes involved in both environmentally and genetically transmitted risk/protective effects – can be salient in relation to different types of negative experiences and of outcomes being considered. **Conclusion:** The importance of the early caregiving environment cannot be overstated. However, accurate delineation of the specific processes involved in moderating effects of particular risk conditions, in relation to specific outcomes, can be critical in shaping the design of effective new methods of prevention and intervention.

S-076 Topic: 84, 34
Attention Deficit Hyperactivity Disorder (ADHD): Current aspects on pharmacogenetics
Track: ADHD

Chairperson: Luis Augusto Rohde, UFRGS-HCPA-Brazil Dept. of Psychiatry, Porto Alegre, Brazil, lrohde@terra.com.br

Attention Deficit Hyperactivity Disorder (ADHD): Current aspects on pharmacogenetics

Luis Augusto Rohde, UFRGS-HCPA-Brazil, Dept. of Psychiatry, Porto Alegre, Brazil, lrohde@terra.com.br

To present recent findings on ADHD pharmacogenetics. Children and adolescents with ADHD from 6 different international centers were genotyped for polymorphisms at one or more of the following genes: dopamine D4 receptor gene (DRD4), dopamine transporter gene (DAT1), and dopamine-B-Hydroxilase gene (DBH). The response to methylphenidate (MPH) was assessed by objective scales. In addition, a quantitative trait locus (QTL) analysis to test for linkage on methylphenidate response rate in a genome-wide scan was performed in one study. An association between polymorphisms at DAT1 gene and response to MPH was detected in three samples. Although the 10/10 genotype was associated to poor response to MPH in the Brazilian sample; it was associated to a better response in the Irish sample. In the sample from Chicago, the 9/9 genotype was associated to poor response to MPH. In addition, initial results suggest that there might be an association between response to MPH and polymorphisms at DRD4 gene. ADHD children with DRD4-7R required higher doses of methylphenidate to achieve 10-point improvement in the Conners Global Index (parent/teacher) in the sample from New Jersey. Finally, a maximum Z-score of 3,52 was found on chromosome 10 in the non-parametric QTL analysis, corresponding with a LOD-score of 2,84 in a traditional Haseman-Elston analysis. Although pharmacogenetic studies of ADHD are in their infancy, these findings provide a preliminary connection between pharmacogenetics and neurobiological investigations on stimulant treatment of ADHD.

S-076-348   Topic: 84, 28
ADHD children with Dopamine reception polymorphisms have similar baseline characteristics

Stephanie Hamarman, Stanley S Lamm Institute, Brooklyn, USA, shamarman@chpnet.org
C. Ulger; J. Fossella; M. Brimacombe; J. Dermody

Objective: Genetic polymorphisms of dopamine receptors have been identified in ADHD but their frequency, relationship to presenting features, and impact on treatment remains unknown. **Methods:** 85 children with ADHD ages 7–15, (17 Hispanic, 68 African-American) confirmed by NIMH DISC-IV-P, underwent assessments of presenting features using Conners rating scales. **Results:** Dopamine transporter-1 (10,10) was identified in 51 (60%). Dopamine receptor D4- 7repeat was identified in 24 (28%). Presenting Conners Global Index were similar with/without DAT-1 (10,10) (82.8 vs 84.8; p=0.21) and with/without DRD4-7R (83.3 vs 83.4; p=0.93). Baseline emotional lability scores were similar: DAT-1 (72.6 with; 74.1 without; p=0.55) and DRD4-7R (72.4 with; 73.3 without; p=0.71). Baseline hyperactivity/impulsivity scores were similar: DAT-1 (83.2 with; 84.3 without; p=0.38) and DRD4-7R (83.5 with; 83.5 without; p=0.99). There were no differences in presenting ages or weight. Confirming our pilot report, ADHD children with DRD4-7R required higher doses of methylphenidate to achieve 10-point CGI-P/T improvement (30 mg vs 22 mg; p=0.005). There was no difference by DAT-1 status (24 mg vs 25 mg; p=0.99). **Conclusion:** Genetic polymorphisms of dopamine receptor genes are common in ADHD. Despite differences in treatment responsiveness with DRD4-7R, this study found no differences in presenting features for children with DRD4-7R or DAT-1.

S-076-349   Topic: 84, 28
Dopamine transporter genotype predicts stimulant response in children with ADHD

Mark Stein, The University of Chicago, Glencoe, USA, mstein@yoda.bsd.uchicago.edu
I. D. Waldman; C. Sarampote; A. Robb; E. H. Cook

Objective: We sought to evaluate the relationship between DAT1 3′ untranslated region Variable Number Tandem Repeats (VNTR) genotypes and response to MPH. **Methods:** Children with ADHD (n = 47), ages 5-16 (mean = 9.02), underwent a 4-week, double-blinded, crossover trial with forced weekly dosage switches. Children were genotyped for the DAT1 VNTR and evaluated on placebo and three dosage levels of OROS MPH. Parents and clinicians who were blind to genotype and medication status rated ADHD symptoms, impairment, and stimulant side effects each week. **Results:** One or 2 copies of the 10-repeat DAT1 allele as com-

pared with no copies predicted a positive response to 36 and 54 mg. of OROS MPH (Odds Ratio = 1.72 and 2.6, respectively). At the 54 mg. condition, 75% of those with one copy of the 10-repeat and 87 % of those with two copies of the 10-repeat allele displayed minimal or no impairment as compared to only 20% of those homozygous for the 9-repeat allele (2 = 6.92, df = 1, p < 0.01). **Conclusion:** Children who were homozygous for the less common 9-repeat DAT1 3′ UTR genotype displayed a different dose-response pattern and were less likely to benefit from increasing doses of stimulant medication. Further research is needed to determine the mechanisms related to poor response in patients with the 9/9 repeat genotype, and to determine if this group responds differentially to alternative treatments.

S-076-350   Topic: 84, 15
Association of the 480 bp DAT1 allele with Methylphenidate response in a sample of Irish children with ADHD

Aiveen Kirley, Trinity College, Dept. of Genetics, Ireland, aiveenkirley@hotmail.com
N. Lowe; Z. Hawi; C. Mullins; G. Daly; I. Waldman; M. Mc Carro; O'Donell; Michael Fitzgerald

Objective: Several studies have implicated the DAT1 gene as conferring susceptibility to ADHD, in particular, a VNTR situated at the 3′ untranslated region of the gene. In addition, the 10 repeat VNTR allele associated with ADHD has been reported to be associated with an over-active transporter protein (DAT). We examined the hypothesis that children possessing the variant might be particularly responsive to methylphenidate, a drug known to act by blocking the DAT. **Methods:** The association between the 10-repeat VNTR DAT1 polymorphism and retrospectively rated response to methylphenidate was assessed in a sample of 119 Irish children with ADHD. **Results:** A significant association between 10-repeat allele and response to methylphenidate was found (2 = 7.92, df = 1, p = 0.005). **Conclusion:** Our findings suggest a role for the 10-repeat allele in medication response and may predict positive clinical outcome in ADHD.

S-076-351   Topic: 84, 28
A genome-wide quantitative trait locus analysis on Methylphenidate response rate in Dutch sibpairs with Attention Deficit Hyperactivity Disorder (ADHD)

Emma van der Meulen, Harvard Medical School, Psychiatric and Neurodevelop., USA, evandermeulen_2000@yahoo.com
S. C. Bakker; D. L. Pauls; R. J. Sinke; Jan Buitelaar

Objective: This study focused on the genetic basis of methylphenidate response in a Dutch sibpair sample of ADHD patients. It was hypothesised that methylphenidate response in these patients would show linkage in a genome wide sibpair analysis. **Methods:** A group of 199 children were diagnosed with ADHD according to DSM-IV criteria, using a best estimate procedure. During the research period a subgroup of 102 of these patients had been treated with methylphenidate only. Previously, a study by our research group showed highly significant sibling correlations (r=0.563, p=0.004), and thus the likelihood of substantial genetic loading, on methylphenidate response rate. In this previous study no association with DRD4-7R or DAT1-10R risk alleles for ADHD was found. It was therefore hypothesised that other chromosomal regions would show linkage with the methylphenidate response rate. To this end quantitative trait locus (QTL) analyses were completed in Genehunter to test for linkage on methylphenidate response rate in a genome-wide scan using 400 markers with an average distance of 10 cM. **Results:** In a nonparametric QTL analysis a maximum Z-score of 2.60 was found on chromosome 7, corresponding with a LOD-score of 2.63 in a traditional Haseman-Elston analysis. Additional peaks with Z-scores of 2.74, 2.61 and 2.37 and corresponding LOD-scores of 1.95, 1.90 and 2.09 were found on chromosome 3, 5 and 9, respectively. **Conclusion:** In a genome wide QTL analysis, the threshold for significance is generally believed to correspond with $Z = 4.1$ and $LOD = 3.6$. Given the relatively small size of the current sample, the peak regions on these chromosomes still warrant further research. No evidence for linkage was found in the peak region on chromosome 15q15.1, in which our research group previously found a LOD score of 3.54 in a larger sample of 164 affected sibpairs.

S-076-352   Topic: 84, 26

Dopaminergic genes and response to methylphenidate in ADHD

Guilherme Polanczyk, Porto Alegre, Brazil,
gvp.ez@terra.com.br
C. Zeni; J.P. Genro; Tatiana Roman; Mara Hutz;
Luis Augusto Rohde

Objective: To assess the role of polymorphisms at the Dopamine Transporter Gene (DAT1) and the Dopamine-Hydroxylase gene (DH) in the response to methylphenidate (MPH) in Attention-Deficit/Hyperactivity Disorder (ADHD). **Methods:** In a first blind naturalistic study, 50 male ADHD youths were treated with MPH. In a second study with similar methodology, 150 ADHD youths received MPH. Efficacy of the medication was measured by the 10-item Conners Abbreviated Rating Scale (ABRS) (first study), or the SNAP-IV (second study) and measures of global functioning. We assessed polymorphisms at the 40 bp variable number of tandem repeats (VNTR) located in the 3′ untranslated region of DAT1 gene, the Taq I restriction site in the 5th intron and the HhaI restriction site at the promoter region of the DH gene. **Results:** In the first study, significantly higher number of youths without the 10/10 genotype (15/20) demonstrated an improvement higher than 50% in the ABRS scores with MPH, than the number of the subjects with 10/10 genotype (14/30) (one-tailed $p = 0.04$). In addition, the group without this genotype had significantly higher increase in the CGAS scores than the other group (one-tailed $p < 0.01$). In preliminary analyses of the second study (111 subjects), no effect was found in the response to MPH for any of the two polymorphisms assessed at the DH gene. Overall findings for the second study, including those for the DAT1 gene, will be presented at the symposium. **Conclusion:** Although our preliminary findings suggest a role for the DAT1 gene in the response to MPH in children with ADHD, the same was not true for the assessed polymorphisms at DH gene.

S-077   Topic: 4, 44

Ambulant child and adolescent psychiatry in Europe with social psychiatric care

Track: Therapy and intervention
Chairperson: Christa Schaff, BKJPP, Weil der Stadt,
Germany, bkjpp@dr-schaff.de

S-077-352A   Topic: 2

Ambulant child and adolescent psychiatry in Germany as a therapy network for mentally ill children and adolescents close to their family environment

Christa Schaff, BKJPP, Weil der Stadt, Germany,
bkjpp@dr-schaff.de

The number of independent operating child and adolescent psychiatrists has been constantly increasing constantly in Germany throughout the last 15 years. Today, about 500 doctors are working in independent practices, which amounts nearly to half the total of all child and adolescent psychiatrists. Parallel to this trend, it is possible to perceive a notable increase in ambulant treatment in hospitals with the appropiate facilities. This development offers new possibility fot the therapy of mentally ill children and adolescents, because treatment can begin at a younger age and in the well-known and comfortable surroundings of family and school. The ambulant child and adolescent psychiatry and psychotherapy concentrate on different focal points than the stationary treatment in clinics. Children are treated at a younger age and attention is paid to different clinical pictures. Through social-psychiatric interventions of remedial teachers, social educationists and psychologists the treatment capacity is rather big in the meantime. In cooperation with clinics and other specific institutions, a network of possibilites for the psychiatric treatment of children and adolescents is forming. In the following presentation, the actual treatment supply situation will be introduced and discussed by means of different models of ambulant and multidisciplinary therapy.

S-077-353   Topic: 1, 63

'Lamentation on a high level' – why Switzerland doesn't have sufficiently child and adolescent psychiatrists

Patrick Haemmerle, Psychiatrische Klinik, Kinder- und Jugendpsychiatrie, Fribourg, Switzerland, haemmerlep@fr.ch

Objective: To examine why Switzerland still doesn't have a sufficient number of child and adolescent psychiatrists, although according to international epidemiological data – it is the best equipped country with child and adolescent psychiatrists. **Methods:** A survey in all 21 public child and adolescent psychiatric institutions and to a major number of more than 300 private practices. **Results:** Nevertheless the relatively high number of child and adolescent psychiatrists in the country, specialists in private practice are most of the time overloaded and the child and adolescent clinics in the public sector have introduced waiting lists. The consequences for the mentally ill children and adolescents and their families shouldn't be underestimated. **Conclusion:** Currently, it is not yet possible to give precise results or conclusions from the survey but we may formulate some hypothesis: Children and adolescents in Switzerland may be psychologically more vulnerable or more ill; specialists in this country may work too slowly or not sufficiently efficient. It will be discussed what may be the influences of the demanding specialist training as well as the economical circumstances on the inadequate offer and how many child and adolescent psychiatrists a country really does need. The "case example Switzerland" should allow us to discuss possible solutions for these questions about an offer based on need.

S-077-354   Topic: 63, 45

Child and adolescent psychiatry in France

Harald Sontag, Association Francaise de, Psychiatrie, Strasbourg, France, harald.sontag@wanadoo.fr

The CAP in France is caracterized by an insufficient and too short basic formation of 1 year and a half after 3 years of adult psychiatry and the CAP is considered as an optional part of general psychiatry, and the different maters are very differents from one medecine faculty to the other one In the private praxis exists a shortage of psychiatrists (700 on 1.200 CAP, for a population of 62 Millions inhabitants) where the low fees make more and more difficult the exercice of CAP. In the hospitals, the CAP is related with universitary departments and sectorized services but also in a unsufficient number due to his new development since 30 years ago. We assist on a very high increase of the demand of care due to "new pathologies", not always concerning psychiatry, like problems of violence, acting out due to drugs, and so on. Nevertheless, CAP in France will still be a part of the adult psychiatry and its development still important.

S-077-355   Topic: 44, 45

Social psychiatric situation in Hungary

Agnes Vetro, Szeged University, Child & Adolescent Psychiatry, Szeged, Hungary, vetro@gyip.szote.u-szeged.hu
Julia Gadoros

Private praxis in child and adolescent psychiatry (CAP) almost unknown In Hungary, because the Social Security system das not appropriately reward the time spent with this time-demanding activity. All 19 counties have one CAP outpatient institute. The levels of both staffing and infrastructure differ widely within the country. The networks of child guidance clinics usually run by a teacher or psychologist. Occasionally, a child psychiatrist is also employed, so the psychiatric diagnoses should be adequate and the therapeutic work acknowledged. Each county, founded by the social department of the regional government office, organizes network of family help centers. Besides the perinatal intensive care centers, early developmental centers have also been established in many regions the country. In order to deal with the growing problems of drug abuse, regional drug centers have been established to monitor drug-addicted patients. 9 inpatient units were established over the past 45 years, but in the last 8 years 3 have already shut downs. It is clear there is a great deal still to be done in Hungary in the field of CAP. Without improvement of the present health-care system, the training of professionals, scientific research and financial help, we cannot move forwards. It is highly encouraging that the present small group of professionals is enthusiastic in their work, and we are gradually achieving developments in an increasing number of fields.

S-077-356   Topic: 4, 45

Inpatient services in child and adolescent psychiatry in Austria

Georg Spiel, Landeskrankenhaus Klagenfurt, Neurologie und Psychiatrie, Klagenfurt, Austria, georg.spiel@kabeg.at

Besides the fact, that child and adolescent (neuro)psychiatry has a long tradition in Austria, there is no structured development of outpatient facilities for children in the country. There are multiple reasons for this disastrous situation.

Child and adolescent psychiatry is in Austria still an additional medical qualification on the basis of neurology, pediatrics and psychiatry. Minimal duration for achieving this specialization is 9 years, and if one also take's into consideration the general medical training it lasts approximately 12 years before one can work independently as a practitioner in this field. There are only three departments covering the whole spectrum of child and adolescent (neuro)psychiatry in the country. Because of this the training capabilities are low with the consequence that only a few trained child and adolescent psychiatrists are prepared to serve in the community. Actually there are between 15 and 20 child psychiatrists working in private practice. Because of the fact, that child and adolescent psychiatry is an additional medical qualification in Austria, those working in private practice, treat not only children and adolescents with psychiatric problems, but work mostly in their primary fields (neurologist, pediatrics, psychiatrist). In the given situation working as a child and adolescent psychiatrist in private practice is not very appealing, because there is no specific agreement with the general insurance system. The regulations of the health system in Austria do not support the development of cooperative "Group practices" which would be the most appropriate structure for fostering mental health care system. This situation is in evident contrast to the epidemiological facts regarding psychiatric problems in children and adolescents. After discussing this general situation, the specific situation of service delivery in child and adolescent (neuro)psychiatry in Carinthia, a county in the south of Austria and the development of the system in the last 13 years will be shown with a focus on the outpatient part of the system.

S-077-357   Topic: 3, 44

A special form of social-psychiatrical assistance in German ambulant psychiatry of children and adolescents

Gotthard Roosen-Runge, Mölln, Germany, rorupraxis@aol.com

Follwing the philosophy of ICD-10-MAS-system of diagnosis and therapy of children and adolescents with psychiatric disorders multimodal, somato-psycho-social diagnoses and therapies became common in the psychiatry of children and adolescent patients. Different medical and non-medical professions and institutions have to cooperate in a "patient-parents-helper-group" to perform an individual and entire view of the patient, his disorders and the necessary measures. In Germany practicioners of psychiatry for children and adolescents can built a multiprofessional team of doctors, psychologists, social-workers, ergotherapists etc., established by a law and payed by the assurances, called "Sozial-Psychiatrische Versorgung" (SPV). These teams cooperate with the psycho-social network of the surroundings, schools, public health care, other therapists. So an assistance of the patients near to their families, schools and friends is guaranteed. Many diagnostical and therapeutical methods and strategies of neurological, individual and systemic psychotherapy, pedagogic measurers, indivdual and familiar social work will be combined for individual plans of multimodal therapy. About 60% of the psychiatric practitioners of psychiatry of children an adolescents in Germany work with this SPV. In our lecture we describe the characteristics of this kind of ambulant, social-psychiatric assistance, its theoretical basis, stuctures, rules of working and its outcome.

S-078 Topic: 52
Violence and PTSD

Chairperson: Jocelyn Hattab, Jerusalem Mental Health Center Child & Adolescent Psychiatry, Jerusalem, Israel, jocelyn@vms.huji.ac.il

S-078-358 Topic: 52, 57
Does profession predict outcome?
Some remarks concerning research in juvenile delinquency, especially juvenile sex offenders

Peter Hummel, Sächsisches Krankenhaus, Kinder- und Jugendpsychiatrie, Arnsdorf, Germany, peter.hummel@skhar.sms.sachsen.de

Objective: Research in Germany concerning juvenile sexual delinquency is mainly only done by medical professionals, i.e., by assessing case histories.In Canada, Great Britain and in the USA this research is mainly only done by psychologists, i.e., by means of psychometric assessment. The purpose of this study was to compare adolescent sex offenders with adolescent assaultive offenders by combining both assessment methods. **Methods:** Three offender groups were compared: Adolescent Sex Offenders (ASO) whose victim/s was/were female adolescent/s or adult/s, ASO-A, n=38; ASO whose victim/s was/were child/ren of both sexes, ASO-C, n=36; Adolescent Assaultive Offenders, whose victim/s was/were male adolescent/s or adult/s, n=33. All male subjects were matched as follows (to restrain confounding variables): German nationality, average intelligence, only hands-on offences, single perpetrators, age at time of the offence between 14 and 20 years. Development of the individual, his family, his sexuality (case histories) and his personality (psychometric inventories) was examined. Reclassification was done after factor analysis and subsequent discriminant analysis. **Results:** ASO-A were best predicted by the sexual development(63%), respective by individual, familial and sexual development (71%). ASO-C were best predicted by the individual development (78%), no combination was better. AAO were best predicted by familial and personality development (67%), no combination was better. **Conclusion:** Assessing defined groups of juvenile offenders with different assessment tools seem to be a helpful method to describe the profile of the respective offender group. Items of the case histories seemed to be more powerful than psychometric inventories. Limitation of the study concerns the choice of the psychometric instruments, the possibility of concealed offences not going with the respective group, and other aspects of developmental psychopathology within the respective group (e.g. impulsivity).

S-078-359 Topic: 52, 24
Level of exposure to terrorism and mental health outcomes among adolescents in Israel

Orna Braun-Lewensohn, Vrije University Brussels, Dept. of Psychology, Uccle, Belgium, orna.braun-lewensohn@vub.ac.be
Smadar Celestin-Westreich; Ingrid Ponjaert-Kristoffersen

Objective: Recent research on adolescents' responses to terrorism had inconsistent results regarding the effects of level of exposure on the psychological outcomes. Given that adolescents in Israel are at high risk of being exposed to terror attacks, this study aimed to investigate differences in mental health outcomes according to level of exposure to terror, and gender. **Methods:** The study was conducted in Israel on Sep. 2003 after three years of ongoing terror attacks. Data were gathered from 913 adolescents aged 12–18 (M=14.45, SD=1.27) evenly distributed by gender. Students attended grades 8, 9 and 11 in four different schools, representing different levels of exposure to terror attacks. Subjects completed a standardized set of self report measures among which Achenbach's Youth Self Report, Brief Symptoms Inventory and specifically designed questionnaire covering detailed demographic and exposure to terror data. **Results:** About one third of the adolescents (32.3%) reported to have been present in one or more terror attacks and almost half (48.3%) reported to know someone who was hurt. It appeared that 20.3% of the boys and 17.3% of the girls experienced clinically significant emotional and/or behavioral problems (YSR). Analogously, 23% of the boys and 29.7% of the girls experienced more psychological distress than the Israeli mean norms (BSI). Data analysis furthermore revealed significant relationships between personal exposure to a terror attack and problem behavior (YSR, $p < 0.002$) as well as psychological distress (GSI, $p < 0.008$). Knowing someone who was hurt in a terror attack also was significantly linked to emotional, behavioral problems ($p < 0.004$) and psychological distress ($p < 0.000$). **Conclusion:** These data underscore the importance of level of exposure and type of exposure to mental health symptoms. Further discussion highlights the nature and significance of these relationships within the context of a coping model.

S-078-360 Topic: 73, 52
Effects of violence-related posttraumatic stress on maternal perception of very young children and on response to videofeedback

Daniel Schechter, Columbia University, Psychiatry, NYSPI Unit 40, New York, NY, USA, dss11@columbia.edu
Charles Zeanah; Michael Myers; Michael Liebowitz; Mark Davies

Objective: This research presentation explores the hypotheses that a) maternal posttraumatic stress symptoms (PTSS) inhibit mothers' sensitive perception of their children before and after a trial parent-child intervention involving videofeedback, and b) sensitive perception predicts maternal behavior with her child. **Methods:** Forty-one referred dyads including violence-exposed mothers with significant posttraumatic stress symptoms (PTSS) and their children ages 9–50 months (mean age 32 months) participated. Dyads completed three videotaped visits: 1) Clinical interview; 2) Parent-child interaction; and 3) Clinician-assisted videofeedback session (CAVES). Maternal perception was measured at baseline via the Working Model of the Child Interview (WMCI), and continuously over three time-points via a simple rating scale. Maternal behavior was coded from video tapes using the Atypical Maternal Behavior Instrument (AMBIANCE). Two years later, data on child violence-exposure and symptomatology were obtained. Independent measures included the SCID, Posttraumatic Symptom Checklist, Reflective Functioning Scale, and Child Behavior Checklist (CBCL). **Results:** a) Baseline maternal PTSS and reflectiveness contributed as much as 20% of the variance of continuous measurement of degree of perceptual negativity and distortion (sig < 0.05). Negativity/distortion dropped significantly by the completion of CAVES; PTSS and reflectiveness accounted for 19% of the variance of responsivity to the intervention as measured by decrease of negativity/distortion (sig < 0.05). b) Distorted classification on the WMCI at baseline accounted for 13% of the variance of maternal atypical behavior on the AMBIANCE (sig < 0.05). **Conclusion:** Maternal violence-related PTSS and attachment-related reflectiveness are important predictors of maternal perception of her child as well as of response to trial parent-infant intervention. Maternal perception predicts maternal behavior and should be considered as a useful marker of risk/resilience. Preliminary violence exposure and CBCL data on children two years later will additionally be discussed.

S-078-361   Topic: 73, 53
Psychological reactions of 1–5 year-old children to a devastating earthquake: 3 years later

Wei-Tsuen Soong, Nat. Taiwan University Hosp., Dept. of Psychiatry, Taipei, Taiwan, soongwei@ntu.edu.tw

Objective: To study the PTSD symptoms, 3 months after 921 Earthquake, in children 1-5 years of age and their relation to earthquake exposure(EE) experience. The study also explored the behavioral emotional problems of these children 3 years later and their relation with EE, PTSD symptoms, parental mental health, and family stressors. **Methods:** 750 children aged 1–5 years during a devastating earthquake in middle Taiwan in 1999, the 921 Earthquake, who had various degree of EE, were enrolled as subjects after written consent obtained from a guardian. Questionnaires of EE and PTSD symptoms, 3 months after the quake, of the child were completed by a parent. Chinese Health Questionnaire (CHQ) to measure parental health, Family Inventory for Life Events (FILE) to measure family stressors, and Child Behavior Checklist (CBCL) to measure behavior emotional problems were completed by one parent or main caregiver 3 years after the 921 Earthquake. **Results:** 1. The valid sample, around 740, in the analyses varied according to the variables used. 18.3% of them had at least 1 EE experience. 2. 65 (7.89%) fulfilled PTSD criteria for young children proposed by Sherringa et al. in 1995. 3. Among PTSD symptoms, New Fears or Aggression, Reexperiencing and Arousal were more common, while Numbing was rare. 4. EE experience was significantly associated with the number of PTSD symptoms 3 months after the quake. 5. CBCL scores, measured 3 years after the quake, were marginally associated with EE experience. CBCL scores were predicted by previous PTSD symptom scores, current parental CHQ, and Intrafamily Strains and Financial Strains of the family measured with FILE. **Conclusion:** 1. A devastating earthquake will increase PTSD among young Children. 8% of 1–5 year-old children fulfilled the PTSD criteria proposed by Sherringa et al. 3 months after the 921 Earthquake. 2. PTSD predicts children's later emotional behavioral problems. Parental health and family stress are also important predictors for children's behavior emotional problems.

S-078-362   Topic: 52, 41
The response of adolescents to bullying

Deborah James, Regional Child & Family Centre, Dept. of Child Psychiatry, Drogheda, Ireland, deborah.james@nehb.ie
Maria Lawlor; Nick Sofroniou

Objective: This study explores the emotional reactions of those bullied in Second level schools In Ireland. **Methods:** Students were asked about their experiences of being bullied in school. They were then asked to consider a range of emotions and to rate on a five point scale whether they had expereinced each emotion. Factor analysis was used to explore the dimensions underlying the emotional variables. **Results:** Two distinct factors emerged which were termed sadness/anxiety and anger/frustration. Victims reported feelings of anger/frustration regardless of the frequency of the bullying. Feelings of sadness/anxiety increased with frequency of bullying. Those who experienced having rumours spread about them had significantly higher scores on both the sadness/anxiety and anger/frustration factors. Victims of exclusion had significantly higher scores on the sadness dimension. 21% felt very suicidal as a result of the bullying. **Conclusion:** This study indicates that a substantial number of students are bullied and that victimisation produced a complex emotional response. Given that these victims of bullying are at the adolescent stage of their development, feelings of anger and frustration are more likely to lead to disruption of classes, increased clashes with teachers, parents and other students, resulting in poor academic performance. The extensive feelings of sadness and anxiety are also likely to negatively affect academic performance. Schools need ongoing training and support systems to enable them to deal effectively with school bullying. Given the high level of distress and suicdal ideation caused by bullying, mental health practitioners need to be aware of all forms of bullying and to ask young people about it when they contact their services.

S-078-363   Topic: 19, 52
Issues of adolescents criminal behavior prevention

Marine Gegelashvili, Tbilisi, Georgian Republic, marinegegelashvili@hotmail.com

Objective: The difficult social and political situation in Georgia increased the number of poverty, high rate of adolescents criminalization. In the last decade prevention has moved into the forefront and become a priority in terms of policy, practice, and research. Importance of preventive interventions is a central activity for the improvement of children's mental health in Georgia. In order to collect data base for creation psycho-preventive models Organization EOC carried out the psychosocial investigation in the juvenile punitive colony. **Methods:** Rey Complex Figure Test-Recognition Trial (Neuro-psychological Methodology), Bus-Dark's questionnaire on aggression, Rocket's test on self-estimation, test on assessment of system of values and a specially worked-out social-psychological questionnaire was used. Questionnaire includes some social aspects about children and adolescents and their families, children and adolescents interpersonal feelings, their attitude to family members, friends and to the society. Also questionnaire covers some educational problems, delinquent behavior and consumption of alcohol, drugs and tobacco. **Results:** 23 juvenile offenders were investigated. Age 15-17 years. The data was proceeded by EXEL. As a result of clinical-psychological study the following peculiarities that should be considered during psycho-corrective and psycho-therapeutic activities are revealed, such as: Social-psychological warping of person is due to unstable type and tendency of anti-social behavior.Increased aggression in every sphere, affective tension. The experience gained during our work in juvenile punitive colonies enabled us to assess the whole specter of social problems and stages of their delinquent career also. The most important of them, in our opinion, is the following: the majority of these adolescents are from poor families, they experienced social-pedagogic indifference since childhood and had behavior derangement and different psycho-neurological problems but no adequate attention was paid to this. In most cases, adolescents are deprived of their choice of how to live, neither gaining any positive experience in the colony. as there is no any rehabilitation structure. The problem of sexual minorities, which were victims of sexual violence both before and after arrest, should also be mentioned. They belong to the most unprestige strata of the colony community. We studied medical documentation of adolescents and reviewed of expert psychiatric conclusions and stated different opinion in three cases. **Conclusion:** It's necessary to create rehabilitation structure furthering to these adolescents' adaptation and socialization in the society. Issues of primary and secondary prevention of adolescents criminal behavior and necessity of creation special agencies as well as Juvenile Justice System promotion in Georgia is discussed.

S-079   Topic: 34
Psychopharmacotherapy
Track: Therapy and intervention

Chairperson: Jan Buitelaar, University Medical Center Psychiatry & Adolescent, Nijmegen, Netherlands, jb@psy.umcn.nl

S-079-364   Topic: 12, 34
Prospective study of second-generation antipsychotic-induced Insulin resistance in antipsychotic-naïve children and adolescents

Christoph Correll, The Zucker Hillside Hospital, Dept. of Psychiatry Research, Glen Oaks, NY, USA, ccorrell@lij.edu Umesh Parikh; John M. Kane; Anil K. Malhotra

Objective: Second-generation antipsychotics (SGAs) have been associated with a risk for diabetes. Since prospective data in antipsychotic-naïve and pediatric patients is missing, this study aimed to assess the effect of SGAs on glucose metabolism and insulin resistance in youth independent of the confound of previous antipsychotic treatment. **Methods:** 12-week, prospective, open-label study in antipsychotic-naïve subjects, age 5–18 years with psychotic, mood and/or disruptive behavior-spectrum disorders, treated with riperidone, olanzapine or quetiapine. Comedication were not restricted. At baseline, 4 and 12 weeks, height, weight, fat mass and percentage (via impedantiometry), waist circumference, fasting glucose, insulin, prolactin, leptin and SGA levels (ensuring compliance) were measured. Insulin resistance was calculated using the homeostatic model (HOMA-IR: insulin umol glucose mmol/22.5). **Results:** In 93 antipsychotic-naïve youngsters (mean age: 14.1 ± 3.4 years, 54.8% male, 46.2% Caucasian), treated with risperidone (n=51), olanzapine (n=30) or quetiapine (n=12) for 8-13 (mean: 11.6 ± 1.7) weeks, fasting glucose (p=0.004), insulin (p=0.01) and insulin resistance (p=0.004) increased significantly. One premorbidly obese youngster (1.1%) developed diabetes on quetiapine. Medications did not differ significantly in their effect on glucose (p=0.95) and insulin (p=0.29), or on absolute and relative HOMA-IR changes (olanzapine: $0.81 \pm 1.6 = 62.2\%$; quetiapine: $0.95 \pm 2.4 = 19.1\%$; risperidone: $0.30 \pm 1.5 =$ 32.0%, p=0.31 and p=0.25, respectively). However, when analyzing changes from baseline to endpoint for each drug separately, increases in glucose reached significance only for risperidone (p=0.01), while increases in insulin and HOMA-IR remained significant only for olanzapine (p=0.02, respectively). In a logistic regression model, glucose increase was correlated with olanzapine treatment (p=0.03), mood and disruptive behavior disorders (p=0.03) and antipsychotic-naïveté (p=0.05) ($R2 = 0.09$, p < 0.001). Increases in insulin ($R2 = 0.12$, p<0.0001) and HOMA-IR ($R2 = 0.10$, p=0.0003) were correlated with divalproex co-treatment (p=0.0007 and p=0.003, respectively) and weight gain (p=0.005 and p=0.02, respectively). **Conclusion:** Increased insulin resistance in youth after three months of treatment with olanzapine, risperidone and quetiapine, a risk state for the future development of type II diabetes, is of considerable concern. Careful selection of appropriate patients for SGA treatment and routine monitoring of weight and glucose metabolism are strongly recommended in this vulnerable population.

S-079-365   Topic: 12, 34
Safety of aripiprazole in children and adolescents with psychotic, mood and disruptive behavior disorder

Christoph Correll, The Zucker Hillside Hospital, Dept. of Psychiatry Research, Glen Oaks, NY, USA, ccorrell@lij.edu Manoj Shah; Richard R. Pleak; Ronen Hizami; John M. Kane; Anil K. Malhotra

Objective: While aripiprazole, a second-generation antipsychotic (SGA) with a novel mechanism of action and possibly more favorable side effect profile compared to other SGAs, is used increasingly in child psychiatry, data is lacking regarding its risk profile in youth. This study aimed to prospectively evaluate the safety of aripiprazole in children and adolescents. **Methods:** 12-week, prospective, open-label study in subjects age 5–18 years with psychotic, mood and/or disruptive behavior-spectrum disorders. At baseline and monthly, height, weight, body mass index (BMI), fat mass and percentage (impedantiometry), waist circumference, fasting glucose, insulin, insulin resistance, prolactin, leptin and aripiprazole levels (ensuring compliance) were measured. **Results:** Of 34 youngsters (mean age: 14.1 ± 2.9 years, 61.8% male, 52.9% Caucasian, baseline BMI: 24.6 ± 5.5) started on aripiprazole (mean dose: 16.0 ± 7.5 mg/day), 12 (35.3%) discontinued treatment prematurely (lack of efficacy: 18.6%, side effects: 15.6%, non-adherence: 3.1%) and two (5.9%) were lost to follow-up. Neither weight (1.2 ± 4.1 kg, p=0.18), BMI (0.2 ± 1.4, p=0.49), fat mass (0.57 ± 3.0 kg, p=0.41), fat percentage ($2.9 \pm 10.9\%$, p=0.26), waist circumference (1.5 ± 4.2 cm, p=0.16) or leptin levels (0.77 ± 7.1 ng/mL, p=0.66) changed significantly from baseline, although 5 (20%) of the 20 youngsters completing the trial gained more than 7% of weight. The same was true for indices of glucose and lipid metabolism, including fasting glucose (0.27 ± 10.3 mg/dL, p=0.77), insulin (-0.42 ± 7.5 umol/L, p=0.81), insulin resistance (-0.15 ± 1.6, p=0.70), total cholesterol (-3.2 ± 30.9 mg/dL, p=0.66), HDL-cholesterol (0.95 ± 9.1 mg/dL, p=0.66), LDL-cholesterol (-6.4 ± 25.7 mg/dL, p=0.33), and triglycerides (5.4 ± 50.5 mg/dL, p=0.65). Conversely, prolactin decreased significantly compared to baseline (-14.9 ± 19.5 ng/mL, p<0.005). Three-month weight gain was predicted by early weight gain at 4 weeks (p<0.0001) and antipsychotic-naïveté (p=0.05), explaining 64% and 13% of the variance, respectively. **Conclusion:** Preliminary findings suggest that in youth aripiprazole has no significant effect on body composition or indices of glucose and lipid metabolism. However, data from larger samples and antipsychotic-naïve youngsters are needed to reconfirm this. Subjects with marked early weight gain should be monitored closely.

S-079-366   Topic: 16, 34

Continued Atomoxetine in pediatric patients with Attention Deficit Hyperactivity Disorder (ADHD) after 1 year of treatment

Jan Buitelaar, University Medical Center, Psychiatry & Adolescent, Nijmegen, Netherlands, jb@psy.umcn.nl
David Michelson; Marina Danckaerts; Christopher Gillberg; Alessandro Zuddas; Shuyu Zhang

Objective: We assessed the efficacy of atomoxetine in maintaining symptom response following 1 year of treatment. **Methods:** Subjects were children and adolescents with DSM-IV-defined ADHD who responded to atomoxetine acutely, completed 1 year of double-blind atomoxetine treatment, and were then randomly assigned in a double-blind fashion to continued atomoxetine or placebo substitution for 6 months. The primary outcome measure was a comparison of distribution of days to relapse following randomization. **Results:** Atomoxetine was superior to placebo in preventing relapse (p=0.008, Wilcoxon test) and in maintaining symptom response as measured by ADHD RS score (p<0.001). Among patients randomly assigned to placebo substitution, the degree of symptom return was generally to a level of severity less than that observed at study entry. **Conclusion:** After 1 year of treatment with atomoxetine, continued treatment over the ensuing 6 months was associated with superior outcomes compared with placebo substitution. However, there was considerable variability between individuals in the magnitude of symptom return after drug discontinuation, suggesting that some patients treated with atomoxetine for a year with good results may consolidate gains made during drug treatment, and could benefit from a medication-free trial to assess the need for ongoing drug treatment.

S-079-367   Topic: 16, 34

Effect of oppositional defiant disorder on risk of ADHD relapse during treatment with Atomoxetine

Philip Hazell, Hunter Mental Health Services, Dept. Child and Youth Health, Wallsend, NSW, Australia, philip.hazell@hunter.health.nsw.gov.au
P. Zeiner; Joanne Barton; M. Johnson; Shuyu Zhang; Marina Danckaerts; Tomasz Wolanczyk

Objective: A 9-month relapse prevention study to assess the efficacy of atomoxetine during long-term treatment of attention-deficit/hyperactivity disorder (ADHD) was recently completed. An exploratory subgroup analysis was conducted to better understand the effect of co-morbid oppositional defiant disorder (ODD) on risk of relapse. Overall study results have been presented elsewhere. **Methods:** Patients aged 6–15 with DSM-IV-diagnosed ADHD whose symptoms remitted during initial 12-week atomoxetine treatment were randomly assigned to 9 months of double-blind continuation therapy with atomoxetine or placebo substitution. Forty-two percent of patients taking atomoxetine and 45% of patients taking placebo had current ODD. **Results:** Atomoxetine was superior to placebo in reducing

risk of relapse (22.3% and 37.9% relapsed, respectively; hazard ratio=0.518 [0.355, 0.754]). There was an interaction between treatment and ODD status; patients with ODD received greater protective effect from atomoxetine than patients without ODD (p=0.037). For patients with both disorders, the relapse rate after 9 months of treatment was 17.1% for the atomoxetine group and 42.9% for the placebo group; for patients without ODD, the relapse rates were 25.6% (atomoxetine) and 33.8% (placebo). The difference in mean time to relapse between the drug-treated groups and placebo-treated groups was similar for patients with or without co-morbid ODD (atomoxetine: with ODD mean days [SD]=215.1 [7.4], without ODD=211.1 [7.6]; placebo: with ODD=136.2 [11.3], without ODD=151.1 [9.1]). **Conclusion:** Although this study was not designed to specifically address ODD outcome, data suggest that atomoxetine has a protective effect in all patients with ADHD and that this effect may be most pronounced in patients with comorbid ODD.

S-079-368   Topic: 14, 34

Psychopharmacological treatment with antiepileptic drugs – an overview

Frank Häßler, Universität Rostock, Kinder- und Jugendpsychiatrie, Rostock, Germany, frank.haessler@med.uni-rostock.de

Objective: The report concerns various psychiatric indications for the treatment with antiepileptic drugs. First, epilepsy as a major neurological disorder can cause a lot of difficulties, such as school problems, that may surface as psychiatric symptoms. Second, antiepileptic drugs have a history as mood stabilizers in cases of bipolar disorders, impulsivity/disruptive behavior, anxiety disorder, PTSD, bulimia and withdrawal syndrome. According to the sparse data available the use of antiepileptic drugs in children covers a wide range of symptoms if the practitioner considers the specialties of a treatment of children. **Methods:** The various antiepileptic drugs, such as carbamazepine, valproate, lamotrigine, oxcarbazepine and topiramate will be reviewed outlining the scientific evidence for their psychotropic, mood-stabilizing properties and side effects. Two examples of a Landau-Kleffner syndrome will be introduced to illustrate the complexity of epilepsy and its pharmacological treatment. Both patients were admitted to our hospital with a diagnosed mutism. Mutistic symptoms vanished when our patients were treated with lamotrigine. **Results:** Furthermore the state of the art in research about antiepileptic drugs will be reported. Only a few studies investigated the use of antiepileptic drugs so far. The majority of these studies was done with adults, used a short-term uncontrolled design. **Conclusion:** The paper argues for the use of antiepileptic drugs in psychopharmacological strategies for children and adolescents with various psychiatric disorders. Several reasons for an extended use are discussed, such as the long history, the favourable risk-benefit-ratio, and the low costs of antiepileptic drugs.

S-079-369   Topic: 16, 34
Atomoxetine in the treatment of Attention Deficit Hyperactivity Disorder (ADHD) in children and adolescents: Effects on broader efficacy

Prasad Suyash, Basingstoke, United Kingdom, suyash@lilly.com
Edmund Sonuga-Barke; Lynne Poole

Objective: To evaluate the effects of atomoxetine, a potent inhibitor of the presynaptic noradrenaline transporter, across broader areas of functioning in paediatric patients with attention-deficit/hyperactivity disorder (ADHD). **Methods:** Approximately 200 patients (aged 7–15 years) who met DSM-IV criteria for ADHD will participate in this multicentre (20 UK sites), randomised, controlled, open-label trial. Patients will receive either once-daily atomoxetine (0.5–1.8 mg/kg/day) or standard current therapy (medication or counselling) for a total of 10 weeks. Broader efficacy will primarily be assessed using the parent-rated Child Health and Illness Profile (CHIP-CE) which assesses the domains of satisfaction, comfort, risks avoidance, resilience, and achievement. Other outcome assessments will include the Family Burden of Illness Module, the Harter Self Perception Profile for children, the ADHD rating scale (ADHD RS), and the Clinical Global Impression (CGI) scale. **Results:** This study is ongoing with final data expected in 2005. The primary efficacy measure will be the total score in the CHIP-CE over 10 weeks. The primary analysis will be a repeated measures mixed model analysis. The primary treatment comparison will be change from baseline to week 10 of atomoxetine vs. standard current therapy. The secondary measures, including the Family Burden of Illness Module and the Harter Self Perception Profile, will be analysed using an analysis of covariance. This paper will explore the study design, rationale for scales, and statistical methods used in this study. **Conclusion:** Atomoxetine has established efficacy for the treatment of core symptoms of ADHD. Emerging data suggest that atomoxetine may provide additional benefit, with improvements in broader areas of functioning (including self-esteem, quality of life, and impact on family, i.e., broader efficacy). To date, the potential broader efficacy of atomoxetine has not been fully assessed in children and adolescents with ADHD

S-080   Topic: 54
Refugee children

Chairperson: Salvador Celia, Instituto Leo Kanner Ltoa Child Psychiatry, Porto Alegre, Brazil, sahc@terra.com.br

S-080-370   Topic: 54, 65
Psychiatric assessment of children and families in immigration detention in Australia – clinical and ethical issues

Sarah Mares, NSW Institute of Psychiatry, Parramatta, NSW, Australia, sarah@nswiop.nsw.edu.au
Louise Newman; Jon Jureidini; Zachary Steel

Objective: To report the issues arising in two studies, each of 10 families of 20 children, that used contrasting methodologies to assess the mental health of this detained population of asylum seekers. The 20 families of 40 children, in two remote Immigration Reception and Processing Centres in Australia, were assessed between February 2002 and 2003. The length of time in immigration detention was 12 to 32 months. **Methods:** In one study, 16 adults and 20 children (age range 11 months to 17 years) underwent comprehensive clinical assessment by allied health clinicians and child psychiatrists after referral to a Child and Adolescent Mental Health Service. The second study of 14 adults and 20 children (age range 3–19 years) used structured diagnostic interviews and standardised questionnaires administered by telephone. **Results:** Very high levels of mood and post traumatic symptoms were found in both populations. All children had at least one parent with psychiatric illness. In the clinical sample all of the 10 children over 3 years fulfilled criteria for both post-traumatic stress disorder and major depression with suicidal ideation. The majority of preschool age children were identified with developmental delay or emotional disturbance. Suicidal ideation and deliberate self harm were common including in preadolescent children.In the second sample all children and adults met diagnostic criteria for at least one psychiatric disorder and many had multiple disorders. **Conclusion:** Child and adult asylum seekers in Immigration Detention demonstrate exceptionally high levels of psychopathology, much attributable to experiences in detention. There are multiple obstacles to adequate service provision. The principles of access for all to adequate health and mental health services and the duty of health professionals to care for patients regardless of citizenship or visa status are significantly compromised by Australia's current immigration policy. The impact on involved clinicians is discussed.

S-080-372   Topic: 54, 66
Mental health professionals and Australian Immigration Policy – responding to mandatory detention of child asylum seekers

Louise Newman, NSW Institute of Psychiatry, Parramatta, BC, Australia, lnewman@nswiop.nsw.edu.au
Sarah Mares; Zachary Steel

Objective: To review the involvement of mental health professionals in the debate over detention of child asylum seekers under Australian immigration law and the effects of detention on child mental health. **Methods:** Over 2500 children have been held in arbitrary detention under Australian law, including 50 infants born in detention centres. A broad Alliance of child advocacy, health and mental health groups have conducted a review of the effects of detention and alternate models for management of child asylum seekers. **Results:** The Alliance has urged Government to revoke the policy of mandatory detention and to develop mental health services for traumatised children. Professional bodies are developing ethical guidelines for work in this area. **Conclusion:** The Policy of Mandatory Detention has raised professional concerns about the harmful effects of government policy, the need for a united professional response and ethical responsibility to advocate for human rights of asylum seekers.

S-080-373   Topic: 54, 45
Traumatized refugee children and their families: Features and limitations of a treatment concept for this highly vulnerable group of patients in a specialized psychiatric unit in Hamburg

Torsten Lucas, UKE Hamburg-Eppendorf, Kinder- und Jugendpsychiatrie, Hamburg, Germany, lucas@uke.uni-hamburg.de
Stephanie Paulus; Martin Aßhauer; Birgit Möller; Hubertus Adam; Peter Riedesser

Objective: In Germany there is a lack of empirical data on the prevalence of emotional distress and its consequences for refugee children as well as treatment concepts for this group. **Methods:** In our unit around 380 patients from a number of crisis regions received treatment since 1994. Services offered include assessment, short and long term psychotherapy, crisis-intervention as well as outpatient, day and inpatient clinics. Treatment takes place in a complex reality often characterised by many stressors such as constant fear of expulsion. Patient support is initially focussed on aspects of every-day-life to empower patients and to ensure a minimum of safety and normality. Social workers, teachers, counsellors, guardians and lawyers are contacted in the sense of networking in order to raise adequate support. The focus is then shifted to establish a psychotherapeutic setting which enables patients to reexamine coping-mechanisms adopted in situations of extreme distress. Gradually the personal as well as trauma history can be explored in more detail. Selected data are presented to characterize our patient population, based on the "Basic Documentation for Child and Adolescent Psychiatry". **Results:** BaDo-data (sociodemographic, psychopathology, diagnosis, ...) are in progress. Limitations to treatment options as a consequence of external as well as internal factors and the relevance of recent developments in trauma research for this patient population are discussed. **Conclusion:** After experiencing war and persecution related trauma living conditions in the country of refuge as well as adequate treatment are considered decisive factor for the stabilization and further development of refugee children. Presenting symptoms are often psychosomatic or psychiatric. Adequate health services need to include child psychiatric expertise as well as transcultural competence and translation.

S-080-374   Topic: 53, 54
Psychiatric symptoms of refugee children in German schools: Individual trauma and social reconstruction

Hubertus Adam, UKE Hamburg-Eppendorf, Kinder- und Jugendpsychiatrie, Hamburg, Germany, adam@uke.uni-hamburg.de
Martin Aßhauer; Peter Riedesser

Objective: Migration and flight are important issues for the German public domain. This study investigates the psychiatric symptoms of refugee children in German schools, and further examines the psychic problems and coping mechanisms of those refugee children who are not in the psychiatric care of any institution. Finally it explores the opportunities, protective factors and negative consequences of the experience of migration and flight on refugee children's development. **Methods:** The sample consists of 215 refugee children, 56% of whom were boys, from Afghanistan, Kosovo and Bosnia with a mean age of 14.8 years (SD = 2.1). The children were interviewed in 2003 at 27 schools in Hamburg by psychologists and child psychiatrists of the Outpatient Department for Refugee Children and their Families at the Child and Adolescent Psychiatry Clinic at the University of Hamburg. The psychological status was assessed with a newly developed set of questionnaires for refugee children viz. the "Scales for Children afflicted by War and Persecution" (SCWP). This instrument measures the following variables: Exposure to War Trauma, Perception of Parental Functioning, PTSD, Depression, Anxiety. Coping Strategies and Attitude to Reconciliation. **Results:** Initial results indicate that up to one third of the until now undiagnosed and untreated refugee children fulfil the potential criteria for a psychiatric diagnosis. Of importance is the finding that the presence of posttraumatic stress and depressive symptoms are excessively high. Symptoms are strongly correlated to the refugee children's experiences of violence. Furthermore, findings regarding coping mechanisms and the ability to reconcile with the former enemy will be presented. **Conclusion:** A high percentage of refugee children at school show undetected psychiatric disorders requiring urgent psychiatric treatment. Teacher awareness of the impact of these psychically traumatic difficulties and resultant psychopathology on diminishing school performance need to be increased. In order to stabilize the mental health of these children, psychiatric assessment is crucial. This would have the effect of enhancing their development as well as give them increased opportunities to receive an education in exile. The consequent benefit of this would be to enhance the quality of their contribution to the rebuilding of their own society after repatriation and return, as well as functioning like a "bridge" between the German and indigenous cultures.

S-080-375   Topic: 45, 37
Psychological evaluation and brief family therapy with refugee children

Gunilla Jarkman Björn, Linköping, Sweden, gunilla.jarkman-bjorn@lio.se
Christina Bodén; Per Gustafsson

Objective: The main purpose of this study is to achieve a deeper knowledge of children of refugee families and evaluate the efficiency of brief family therapy. In the project 27 families from Bosnia and Herzegovina participated. They were randomly assigned to two groups; one group has received three family therapy sessions while the other one served as an untreated comparison group. One criterion for inclusion was that there was a child 5–12 years old in the family. The non-intervention group has been offered family therapy at the follow-up interview. **Methods:** The two groups are interviewed both at the beginning and about half a year later. The symptoms of one of the children in the family are evaluated. Various projective psychological methods have been used. **Results:** Result of the psychological assessment in the intervention group will be presented evaluating the play method in comparison with symptom rating and war- time experiences. In the assessment of the play method 4 out of 13 were evaluated normal in all three evaluation sessions before the family therapy sessions. 10 out of 11 children who had participated in the family therapy sessions and had attended the follow-up play evaluation session were evaluated normal (p < 0.01). All but one of the children in this group were rated low on a psychiatric symptom scale. **Conclusion:** The background of refugee children is analysed from what importance the social network and experiences of actual war-situations have, in relation to their inner world, evaluated by a play method. In the psychological assessments there are signs showing that they have gone through traumatic experiences but it is not possible to pin down exactly from where the trauma originates. Other factors are influencing their inner world like parent support, network and living in a strange environment during the war situation. Brief family therapy might help to support their well-being.

S-080-376   Topic: 54, 41
Psychosocial complications of refugee adolescents

Milica Pejovic-Milovancevic, Institute of Mental Health, Dept. Children & Adolescents, Belgrade, Serbia and Montenegro, mpejovic@eunet.yu
Viola Povse Ivkic; Lazar Tenjovic; Radosavljev Jelena; Smiljka Popovic Deusic; Olivera Aleksic

Objective: One of the most difficult problems that we are facing as professionals in Belgrade is work with refugee populations, and most of all with adolescent refugees. Many NGO's, health services and government dally working on improving of living conditions of this population. Unfortunately, less attention is paid to their psychosocial problems, and this paper is aimed to analyse this particular issue. **Methods:** In one collective centre for refugees in Belgrade area is settled 124 refuges from Kosovo since 1999. They are living in ex-psychiatric hospital with their parents and relatives. We analysed 24 adolescents, currently living in that particular Centre, and compared this group (group A) with refugees form other centres (living in other facilities different form psychiatric clinic) (group B) and control group of not refuge adolescents (same age) (group C). We use standard semi structural interview and Youth self report. **Results:** Our results show that group A and group B statistically significant differ from group C in almost all domains of symptom scale of Youth Self Report. Only in depression/anxiety subscale we found statistically significant differences between group A and group B. Concerning their academic achievement, group A statistically significant differ from both other groups. **Conclusion:** We found that so called "double stress", i.e. living as a refugee and living in ex psychiatric clinic (local citizen usually call them lunatics) have great influence on their emotions and behaviour. In this paper we would present the strategies that we organized to improve their academic achievements and to overcome psychosocial problems.

S-081   Topic: 38
Qualitative research in child psychiatry 'Not everything that counts can be counted'

Chairperson: Philip Graham, London, United Kingdom, pjgraham1@aol.com

Qualitative research in child psychiatry 'Not everything that counts can be counted'

Philip Graham, London, United Kingdom, pjgraham1@aol.com

The symposium shows how rigorous qualitative research can contribute to some of the challenges of modern child psychiatry in our multi-cultural societies. While quantitative research help to answer questions of 'how many' or 'how much' qualitative research tends to focus on questions like 'how' and 'why'. This is particularly useful when exploring patients and professionals illness conceptualisations and treatment decision making and helps to understand the organisation of health care services as well as treatment experiences. H. Klasen will introduce the symposium by giving a brief overview of qualitative methodology and uses some of her own data on attitudes to disruptive behaviours to develop an analytical framework to systematise approaches in social psychiatry. Next C. Javo will report on norms and values in peer relationships among Sami and Norwegian pre-adolescents focusing on cultural variation of expressions of child aggression. J. Tan examines how qualitative methods can illuminate ethical dilemmas around competence and treatment decision making in anorexia nervosa. Similarly M. Koelch uses semi-structured qualitative methods when examining treatment consent in young mental health and paediatric patients who have been asked to participate in drug trials. A. Dias-Caneja looks at the experience of mentally ill mothers who report on how their own illness and treatment affect their parenthood. Finally J. Fegert rounds off the symposium by showing how qualitative and quantitative methods can complement each other in his study on treatment experiences and treatment decisions of child psychiatric in-patients.

S-081-377   Topic: 38, 85
Disruptive behaviours: Personal choice, illness or social disease: Using an anthropological framework to understand how attitudes may affect outcome

Henrikje Klasen, Child and Family Service, Chichester, United Kingdom, h.klasen@iop.kcl.ac.uk

Objective: This talk gives an introduction to qualitative research in child psychiatry. Using own data on attitudes of carers and professionals towards disruptive behaviours we show what type of question qualitative research seeks to answer and how this fits into a wider framework of social research in child psychiatry. **Methods:** We discuss methods used in one completed and two pilot studies of qualitative research. This includes semi-structured interviews, focus groups and qualitative feedback forms. Interviews were audiotaped and transcribed. Data was analysed using grounded theory. **Results:** Anthropologists conceptualise society as an onion like model of related hierarchies ranging from the individual, to kinship and neighbourhood, to social institutions and finally to underlying values and norms. Uncertainties about the status of disruptive behaviours pervade all these levels. Parents were often unsure when to punish behaviours and when to show compassion. They generally preferred to medicalise and label the problem while GPs and teachers tended to relate behaviours to family and societal stresses. Young people could see advantages in a diagnosis but also struggled when interpreting effects on their identity. Uncertainties exist as to which institutions should take the lead in service provision. Underlying are controversies about values such as individual choice versus biological or social determinism. Qualitative research was able to uncover some of the complexities of illness conceptualisation and their effects on clinical care. **Conclusion:** Qualitative research in child psychiatry can help exploring areas of research focussing on "how" and "why" rather than "how many". This can be particularly useful when exploring patients and professionals attitudes to disorders and their treatment. Qualitative research is a useful addition in the toolkit of research methodologies for child psychiatry. An anthropological framework can improve and systematise the analysis of social and qualitative data.

S-081-379 Topic: 65, 78
The use of qualitative methodology to study the ethical issues of competence and treatment decision-making in Anorexia Nervosa (AN)

Jacinta Tan, University of Oxford, Inst. of Health Science, Oxford, United Kingdom, jacinta.tan@nuffield.oxford.ac.uk
Tony Hope; Anne Stewart; Raymond Fitzpatrick

Objective: The aim of this presentation is to discuss the usefulness of qualitative methodology in understanding the ethical issues with respect to competence and treatment decision-making in anorexia nervosa. **Methods:** Patients with anorexia nervosa characteristically refuse or resist treatment, even though they tend to have a very good understanding of the risks of their disorder. At the same time, they are often a significant risk to health and life through their self-induced weight loss and associated behaviours. This raises ethical issues with respect to competence to make treatment decisions. This study used qualitative methodology to interview adolescent and young adult females with anorexia nervosa, and their parents. The approach taken to this research was a modified grounded theory one, designed to allow new themes to emerge from the interviews. **Results:** The analysis of the interviews raised three issues. First, the analysis of interviews with patients and parents revealed relatively little use of theoretical concepts traditionally employed by medical ethicists. Second, the participants framed their dilemmas more in terms of dynamic relationships and struggles, with an emphasis on issues such as trust, rather than as conflicts of principles as usually framed in ethics literature. Third, the psychopathology involved, young age and relative immaturity of some participants, and the participation of parents, meant that in some cases there were also conflicting accounts of the same behaviours and events. This requires the development of an analysis that would not necessarily take participants' accounts at face value. **Conclusion:** We conclude that sociological qualitative methodology has a lot to offer in terms of the empirical exploration of ethical issues; however our study shows that this can be challenging to the traditional theoretical approach to medical ethics, and may mean having to extend traditional sociological methodology beyond its usual bounds.

S-081-380 Topic: 65, 38
Information and assent of minors in clinical trials the Mac Arthur competence assessment tool for clinical research

Michael Kölch, Universitätsklinikum Ulm, Kinder- und Jugendpsychiatrie, Ulm, Germany, michael.koelch@medizin.uni-ulm.de
Jörg M. Fegert

Objective: Information of minors about clinical trials and getting their assent are basic elements for "participation". Without these prerequisites it is impossible and not ethically reasonable to conduct a trial with minors. But how should someone inform minors in the "correct way"? What are the capacities and what are minors needs in informa-

tion. In a pilot study we examined the possibility to inform minors to make them capable to give assent. **Methods:** We adapted the qualitative semi-structured interview instrument "Mac Arthur Competence Assessment Tool for Clinical Research" (MacCAT-CR) for minors. We examined two samples, one with psychiatric ill minors in "phase-III-trials" (20 minors with ADHD and ODD), and one with about 120 chronically somatic ill minors enrolled in placebo-controlled drug-studies. Interviews were conducted with parents and the minors. The answers were rated and a qualitative analysis was made. **Results:** In the psychiatric sample most of the minors were able to understand the information about the trial. They were able to appreciate the benefits and risks and the follows for every day life. Problematic was the appreciation of the primary goal of the trial, almost none of the minors seemed to be able to understand this topic completely. Age-specific aspects, disruptive aspects and aspects of intelligence need to be taken into account. In the somatic ill sample research is ongoing, so results will be presented at the congress. **Conclusion:** The MacCAT-CR is a tool to improve information about clinical trials in children. Minors receive skills of reasoning about decisions of joining or declining participation. Using this instrument information gets more transparent. Minors are more involved in the process of decision-making, so their interests of participation are better satisfied. Results point out the use of the instrument in decision making in difficult therapeutic decisions.

S-081-381 Topic: 38, 1
The views and experiences of severely mentally ill mothers: A qualitative study

Angeles Diaz-Caneja, CNW NHS Trust, Child & Adolescent Psychiatry, London, United Kingdom, adiazcaneja@hotmail.com
Sonia Johnson

Objective: Experiences and views about motherhood, services and needs for support in parenting **Methods:** Semi-strutuctured interviews were carried out wiith 22 women with schizophrenia, bipolar affective disorder or severe depression with psychotic symptoms in inner London. Interviews were transcribe, verbatim and qualitative thematic analysis was carried out. **Results:** Most participants who look after the children described motherhood as rewarding and central to their lifes. However, they described the demands associated with parenting and at the same time coping with severe mental illness as considerable and some feared would be adversely affected by their illness. Parenting responsabilities created practical impediments to engaging with mental helath services. fear of losing custody or access to children dominated interactions with mental health services and social services making most participants reluctant to disclose difficulties in parenting to professionals. Services were perceived as offering little continuing support in relation to parenting, intervening only in crisis. **Conclusion:** Little attention has been so far been paid in research and service develooopment to the fact that the majority of mentally ill women are mothers. Strategies for assessing and meeting the resulting unmet needs should be developed and evaluated

S-081-382   Topic: 66

Participation of children in treatment decisions in child and adolescent psychiatry

Jörg M. Fegert, Universität Ulm, Kinder- und Judenpsychiatrie, Ulm, Germany, joerg.fegert@medizin. uni-ulm.de
Ines Dippold; Katja Wiethoff; Ferdinand Keller

Objective: Results of qualitative and quantitative interviews with child psychiatric impatients are presented. Interviews focus on the aspect of participation in treatment decisions and an children's knowledge about child psychiatric hospital treatment. **Methods:** Based on qualitative Interviews with in child psychiatric inpatients we developed an empirical instrument for the quantitative collection of data on information and participation. A random sample of 298 patients who were admitted consecutively to two (East and West German) child psychiatric hospitals (East Germany 147 patients, West Germany 151 patients) was studied. **Results:** Qualitative interviews show that children expect to be involved in treatment decisions but they often don't know anything about child psychiatric hospitals. 16% of the minors had not been informed prior to there treatment by there physicians who admitted them. 40 % of the patients had no information about the duration of their stay in the hospital, where 73 % considered themselves sufficiently informed about the hospital rules. About 90% of the patients expressed their need for information and asked specific questions. About 20% of the patients described their stay in a psychiatric facility during the first four weeks as involuntary. The decision about their admission is experienced by about 20% as emotionally distressing. An important number of children fear to be stigmatised because of their stay in hospital. **Conclusion:** A statistical relationship between the quality of information and motivation and even perceived treatment results could be shown.

S-082   Topic: 57, 37

EFCAP Symposium: Assessment and treatment in forensic CAP

Chairperson: Robert Vermeiren, University of Antwerp Child & Adolescent Psychiatry, Antwerp, Belgium, robert@vermeiren.name

Assessment and Treatment

Sue Bailey, BSTMHT/UCLAN, Gardener Unit, Manchester, United Kingdom, ntattersall@gardener.bstmht.nhs.uk

The new mental health screen for young people that has been implemented across the Youth Justice Board in England and Wales will be presented along with a comparison with the MAYSI-2 and the Salford Needs Assessment Schedule for Adolescents (SNASA), detailing the considerations in developing and implementing the tool. A new inventory designed to screen for experienced risk factors in young people who display delinquent behaviours (The Multidimensional Clinical Screening) will be outlined with initial results presented. Finally, preliminary findings from a survey of the views of young people in secure care on physical and mental health services will be presented.

S-082-383   Topic: 57

The new mental health screen for young people in the youth justice system

Sue Bailey, BSTMHT/UCLAN, Gardener Unit, Manchester, United Kingdom, ntattersall@gardener.bstmht.nhs.uk

Objective: To compare the psychometric properties of the new Youth Justice Board screening tool with the MAYSI-2, Strengths and Difficulties Questionnaire and the gold standard mental health needs assessment (Salford Needs Assessment Schedule for Adolescents). The screener was commissioned to aide the identification of young people with, or at high risk of developing, disorders and to assist youth justice workers in the decision making process of referrals to meet mental health needs. **Methods:** A national sample of young offenders (both males and females, aged from 10–18 years) was used, sampled from a secure unit, a Young Offenders' Institute, a Secure Training Centre and a Youth Offending Team. 135 young people completed the screening tools and research interviews. **Results:** The new mental health screening tool was successfully validated against the gold standard mental health needs assessment tool and the North American MAYSI-2 tool. **Conclusion:** Screening for mental health disorders can be achieved but is only moderately effective as trade offs need to be made between sensitivity and specificity to achieve a workable screening programme. There are ethical issues around screening and what happens to those who screen positive need careful consideration.

S-082-384   Topic: 57, 52

Aggression management in an adolescent forensic service

Riittakerttu Kaltiala-Heino, Tampere University Hospital, Pitkäniemi, Finland, riittakerttu.kaltiala-heino@pshp.fi

Objective: To describe the development of a structured aggression management process and its implementation from the viewpoints of clinical utility and management challenge. **Results:** Aggression management process comprises both architechtural/technical and functional approaches, and focuses both on the unit as a whole and individually on each youth. The aggression management process includes architechtural and technical solutions, intensive and continuous staff training in de-escalating techniques and safe physical intervention to prevent violence, comprehensive guidelines for the various staff groups as to safety practices, violence risk assessment, behavioural analyses, gradually increasing external support in escalating situations, physical intervention with youth losing control, structured evaluation of escalating situations that require physical intervention, continuous monitoring of escalating situations, and continuous development of best practices. Over the first year of the Unit's functioning, a decrease in resources needed for physical intervention was observed, and an increase in the variety of non-contact de-escalation techniques. **Conclusion:** In a unit serving adolescents with most challenging behaviour and complex needs, a structured and proactive approach to escalating situations is needed in order to avoid harm and to ensure the therapeutic milieu. A structured and constantly monitored aggression management programme also decreases the risk of staff demoralisation and the risk of unnecessary coercion due to negative counter-transference. Background: The Psychiatric Treatment and Research Unit for Adolescent Intensive Care (EVA) is a tertiary level psychiatric inpatient service for adolescents with a forensic background and/or violent and non-compliant behaviour. The service started in April, 2003. Aggression management is pervasively considered in all the activities carried out in the Unit, and the aggression management process receives support from the two other main processes, namely structured assessment and individually structured treatment processes.

S-082-385   Topic: 57, 1
The multidimensional screening inventory for delinquent juveniles

Belinda Plattner, Universitätsklinik Wien, Abt. Neuropsychiatrie, Wien, Austria, bplattner@gmx.at

Objective: To present a new inventory designed in order to screen juvenile delinquents on experienced risk factors. The inventory provides a detailed insight into the life-history of these juveniles. Additionally, we are going to present the impact of experienced risk factors on psychopathology, severe and repeated offending. **Methods:** The Multidimensional Clinical Screening for delinquent juveniles is a semi-structured interview that covers the following topics: school and work history, psychiatric history, family history (psychiatric and criminological), social history, trauma, ethnical background. Psychopathology was measured with the MINI Kid. **Results:** We found that delinquent juveniles show a high amount of experienced risk factors. Risk factors seem to have an impact on repeated and severe offending and trauma-related psychopathology. We found significant differences concerning the family background in different ethnicities. **Conclusion:** The Multidimensional Clinical Screening Inventory for delinquent juveniles provides detailed understanding of background and lifestyle of juvenile offenders. This knowledge will give us a more detailed understanding of pathways into delinquency and therefore enable us to include the multidimensional bio-psycho-social model in our approaches for treatment.

S-082-386   Topic: 57, 1
A qualitative survey of the views of young people in secure care on physical and mental health needs

Nathan Whittle, Bolton, Salford & Trafford, Mental Health Trust, Manchester, United Kingdom, njwhittle@gardener.bstmht.nhs.uk

Objective: To conduct a systematic qualitative survey of the views of current service users and providers of services of physical health, mental health and substance abuse services to adolescents in the secure estate in England. This will focus on the continuity of care between custody and the community, the integration of physical health and mental health care and models of best practice, including models of interagency working. **Methods:** A sample of young people will be interviewed to examine their views about current services, what treatments they have already been offered, those they thought were most appropriate and those they considered to be most effective. Specific enquiry will be made about the continuity of care across agencies and over time. **Results:** This study is currently ongoing and some preliminary results will be presented. **Conclusion:** While there is growing evidence that adolescents in secure care have a high level of physical health, mental health and substance abuse problems, they often

fall through the gaps of conventional services. There is a strong argument for the integration of these services, but before contemplating this it is necessary to survey the views of adolescents in the secure estate.

S-083   Topic: 36, 82
Neurophysiology of Specific Language Impairment (SLI)

Chairperson: Klaus Hennighausen, Universitätsklinikum Freiburg Kinder- und Jugendpsychiatrie, Freiburg, Germany, klaus.hennighausen@klinikum.uni-freiburg.de

Neurophysiology of Specific Language Impairment (SLI)

Klaus Hennighausen, Universitätsklinikum Freiburg, Kinder- und Jugendpsychiatrie, Freiburg, Germany, klaus.hennighausen@klinikum.uni-freiburg.de

In the past years, neurophysiological methods have been proven to be a powerful tool in the investigation of developmental and language disorders in children. In this symposium, results from studies with event related brain potentials (ERP) in children with Specific Language Impairment (SLI) will be presented. Different ERPs reflecting different stages of information processing will be discussed. Experts from Finland, Germany, the USA, and Hungary will give insight into their research and present data from studies using mismatch negativity (MMN), processing negativity, P3 and late auditory evoked potentials. **Language and attention problems in SLI and ADHD children: Behavioral results and neurophysiological implications** Gregor Kohls, Verena Maas, Tanja Rinker, Swantje Zachau, Klaus Hennighausen, Gabriele Christmann, Anna Jaremkiewicz & Michael Schecker **Auditory event related brain responses as indices of language impairment** Pirjo Korpilahti & Eira Jansson-Verkasalo **Auditory perception in children with developmental language disorders: an ERP study** Waldemar v. Suchodoletz, Ruth Uwer, Ronald Albrecht & Lisa Glass **Brain activity correlates of disturbed speech perception and sentence comprehension in Specific Language Impairment** Valéria Csépe, Ferenc Honbolygó, Anett Ragó & Éva Mészáros **Lexical comparison processes in the working memory of children with SLI** Richard G. Schwartz & Valerie L. Shafer:

S-083-387   Topic: 82, 84
Language and attention problems in SLI and ADHD children: Behavioral results and neurophysiological implications

Gregor Kohls, Universität Freiburg, Neurolinguistik Labor, Freiburg, Germany, gregor.kohls@zfn-brain.uni-freiburg.de Verena Maas; Tanja Rinker; Swantje Zachau; Klaus Hennighausen; Gabriele Christmann; Anna Jaremkiewicz; Michael Schecker

Objective: Specific Language Impairment (SLI) represents one of the most common types of developmental disorders in childhood and shows increased rates of psychiatric disorders such as Attention Deficit Hyperactivity Disorder (ADHD) compared to children with normal language development. In addition to this, research has demonstrated a high prevalence of language impairment in children with ADHD. An important question concerns the underlying factor that results in both, language impairment and attention deficits. **Methods:** Preliminary data of an ongoing pilot work about 'attention and language development' will be presented. We compared 3 groups of boys between the age of 7–10 (15 children diagnosed with ADHD, 15 children diagnosed with SLI and 15 healthy boys). All groups were tested with different language development tests, tests for auditory discrimination, attention tests (e.g. Continuous Performance Test), one non-word repetition test and the Child Behavior Checklist. **Results:** The results support the expectation that children with SLI have (modality independent) attention problems (even confirmed through parent rating). Children with ADHD have language problems if the task requires attention. Both groups show difficulties in auditory discrimination. To conclude, we suggest that in both disorders a reduced attention span may be responsible for the found data. It might be assumed that limitations of attentional resources cause problems maintaining the focus of attention in both disorders. Nuerophysiological implications: Nevertheless, behavioral studies content with methodological limitations such as the ensemble acting between language processing, memory, and attention functioning. It is necessary to disentangle these three constructs as good as possible. For this, neurophysiological investigations are required. Using Mismatch Negativity (MMN) and Processing Negativity (PN/Nd) automatic and controlled attention can be examined. Memory functions could be checked by the P300 component. For higher-order language functioning, some language-dependent components such as N400 or ELAN shall be established.

S-083-388   Topic: 82, 36
Auditory event related brain responses as indices of language impairment
Pirjo Korpilahti, University of Oulu, Finnish, Saami and Logopedics, Oulu, Finland, pirjo.korpilahti@oulu.fi
Eira Jansson-Verkasalo

Objective: As deficient auditory processing have been reported in many children with specific language impairment (SLI) and in autistic disorders, the aim of this study was to refine the understanding of central auditory processing in SLI, in Asperger syndrome, and in children born preterm. We also investigated effects of music-based intensive training on electrophysiological parameters of information processing and behavioral language skills. **Methods:** Auditory event related potentials (ERPs), and especially the mismatch negativity (MMN), were recorded with NeuroScan. Pure tones, vowels, syllables, words and pseudo-words were used as stimuli. The SLI children came from two special schools in Southern Finland. Children with Asperger Syndrome and preterm born children were selected from the Northern population of Finland. Developmental data was based on hospital reports and questionnaires fulfilled by parents and teachers. Speech and language therapists tested language skills. **Results:** Longer latencies of ERPs, as well as lengthening of latencies of the early and the late MMN were found in all our research groups, representing neurologically based communication disorders in children. MMN was attenuated in SLI for the detection of differences in sound frequencies and in speech stimuli. At behavioral level, poor auditory discrimination and deviant naming skill was connected with decreased brain activation. In the intervention study training effects were found as normalized MMN amplitudes and better discrimination of consonants and naming skill. **Conclusion:** Auditory ERPs and the MMN research paradigm can be used as objective tools in the early diagnosis of language impairment. ERPs are based on a good time resolu-

tion, which makes this method very suitable in studies of language perception and sequential processing of auditory information. Training and rehabilitation experiments give further information of the clinical use of the method. Combining behavioral and neurophysiologic data increases the reliability of the studies.

S-083-389   Topic: 82, 36
Auditory perception in children with developmental language disorders: An ERP study
Waldemar von Suchodoletz, Universität München, Kinder- und Jugendpsychiatrie, München, Germany, suchodoletz@lrz.uni-muenchen.de
Ruth Uwer; Ronald Albrecht; Lisa Glass

Objective: It has been proposed that developmental language disorders are a consequence of deficits in auditory perception. The aim of this study was to determine if event related potentials provide evidence of central auditory processing deficits in language impaired children. **Methods:** The late auditory evoked potentials (LAEP), mismatch negativity (MMN) and P3 were recorded in children with developmental language disorders and in unimpaired children. The ERPs were elicited in an odd-ball paradigm by non-verbal and verbal stimuli. **Results:** The groups did not differ in amplitude, latency or distribution of the LAEP. Dipole source analysis of the LAEP showed a similar activity progression in the primary and secondary auditory cortex for language impaired and normally developed children. There were no significant differences with respect to localisation and orientation of the LAEP dipole sources. Mean MMN amplitudes were calculated to investigate the automatic auditory processing. In language impaired children attenuated MMNs were observed for speech but not for tone stimuli. No differences were found in latency or amplitude of the P3 at Pz. The global field power of the auditory evoked P3, however, was higher in children with specific language disorders than in children of the control group. **Conclusion:** The results suggest that early auditory processing in the primary and secondary auditory cortex is undisturbed in children with developmental language disorders. There is, however, evidence of a specific deficit in automatic discrimination of verbal information. In late and conscious auditory processing the overall cortical activation is found to be higher for language impaired children. Altogether the findings emphasise that early auditory processing is unimpaired whereas deficits can be found in higher auditory functions.

S-083-390   Topic: 82, 36
Brain activity correlates of disturbed speech perception and sentence comprehension in Specific Language Impairment (SLI)
Valéria Csépe, Institute for Psychology, HAS, Developmental Psychophysiology, Budapest, Hungary, csepe@cogpsyphy.hu
Ferenc Honbology; Anett Rago; Éva Mészáros

Objective: Difficulties in sentence comprehension have been taken as evidence that Specific Language Impairment (SLI) involves a grammar-specific impairment. However, there is an alternative view, that grammatical deficits in SLI are sequelae of impaired speech perception. This perceptual deficit may especially affect phonological processes relying on the phonological subsystem of working memory as well as on representational qualities of the phonological lexicon. **Methods:** In our recent studies this hypothesis was explored by using event-related brain potentials (ERPs). The mismatch negativity (MMN) evoked potential component elicited by violated local (phonemes) or global (suprasegmental cues) was measured in SLI children and in age-matched controls. The MMN to voice onset time (VOT) and stress pattern changes of bisyllabic Hungarian words were measured in passive oddball paradigm. **Results:** Our results showed that in normal controls the MMN latency was time locked both to the stressed and unstressed syllables. In SLI children abnormal or missing MMN was detected both to local and global features of spoken words. ERPs to subject-verb number agreement showed marked attenuation or lack of the P600 component in SLI, while another type of sentence violation, that is the temporal agreement of verb and adverb, did not give rise to a significant ERP difference. **Conclusion:** These results are consistent in part with behavioral data concerning syntactic deficits in SLI. The marked deficit in processing suprasegmental cues is an experimental demonstration of how a perceptual deficit could give rise to grammatical deficits in SLI.

S-083-391   Topic: 82, 30
Lexical comparison processes in the working memory of children with SLI
Richard G. Schwartz, City University of New York,
Speech and Hearing Sciences, New York, USA,
rschwartz@gc.cuny.edu
Valerie L. Shafer

Objective: Children with specific language impairments have deficits in working memory, in vocabulary, in vocabulary development, and in the phonological and semantic representations of their mental lexicons. This study employed a match-to-sample task to examine comparison processes for matching, minimal, and non-matching pairs of words or nonwords in working memory. **Methods:** Event related potentials permitted us to examine the fine-grained temporal course of these processes. By including nonwords and words, we were able to examine working memory access to the lexicon. Nine children with TLD (7.0–10.10, three female) and seven with SLI (7.1–11.2, three female) participated in the experiment. **Results:** The children with SLI showed a PN negativity similar to children with TLD. However, this negativity was later for the SLI compared to TLD group for words differing in the onset. The children with SLI also were faster at responding to words differing in the onset compared to the coda, whereas children with TLD showed no significant difference in RT for onset versus coda pairs. The children with SLI produced more response errors to pairs of words that differed for the Nonword/Real word order. The children with TLD, but not SLI, also showed a considerably larger slow positivity to pairs of words that differed compared to those that were the same. **Conclusion:** These findings will be discussed in relation to our previous findings with adults and in relation to data from some additional presentation conditions.

S-084   Topic: 52, 41
ESCAP Symposium: Management of aggressive behaviour in adolescents
Chairperson: Philippe Jeammet, Université Paris VI
Psychiatrie de l'Enfant, Paris, France,
philippe.jeammet@imm.fr

S-084-392   Topic: 4, 41
Prospective study of UK child and adolescent psychiatry inpatient treatment
Jonathan Green, Booth Hall Childrens Hospital,
Dept. of Child Psychiatry, Manchester, United Kingdom,
B. Jacobs; L. Kroll; J. Briskman; G. Dunn; J. Beecham;
C. Tobias; L. Baird

Objective: To investigate process, outcomes and economic evaluation of child and adolescent psychiatry treatment in the UK. **Methods:** A prospective longitudinal cohort study of unselected admissions (n = 150) to 8 inpatient units (4 adolescent, 4 child) across the UK, followed from preadmission to 1 yr follow up. Extensive evaluation includes research diagnosis, symptom ratings from multiple informants, global functioning (Childrens Global Assessment Scale, CGAS), structured health needs assessment, economic evaluation. **Results:** 56% boys and 46% girls of median age 13.9 yr had admissions of median 14.1 wks length (IQR 6.9–20.7). Diagnostic profiles show much comorbidity (19% have 3 DSM diagnoses). From median admission CGAS of 41 (IQR 35–55), there is a 16 point improvement to discharge and 17 point to follow up. Similar significant gains are seen on other measures of psychopathology and health needs. Predictors of CGAS gain are: 1) length of stay; 2) child alliance with the ward milieu. Admission is expensive for families and does not reduce post admission costs. **Conclusion:** These results have clinical implications. Inpatient treatment is associated with significant improvement in complex disorders independent of diagnosis. Longer lengths of stay and positive alliance improve outcome. Families may need financial support during treatment.

S-084-393   Topic: 19, 41
Multisystemic treatment of adolescents with serious behavior problems
Terje Ogden, United Kingdom,
terje.ogden@atferd.unirand.no

MST is an intensive home- and community-based intervention for youths with serious antisocial behaviour including aggressive and criminal behavior as well as drug abuse. MST has been effective at reducing out-of-home placements and producing favourable clinical outcomes in Norway as well as in the U.S. Research results and experiences from a Norwegian large scale implementation of MST and a randomized controlled outcome study (RCT) are presented. Participants in the RCT were 100 seriously antisocial youths in Norway who were randomly assigned to Multisystemic Therapy (MST) or usual Child Welfare Services (CS) treatment conditions. Data were gathered from youths, parents, and teachers pre- and post-treatment. Pre-post results showed that MST was more effective than CS at reducing youth internalising and externalising behaviours and out-of-home placements, as well as increasing youth social competence and family satisfaction with treatment.

S-084-394   Topic: 52, 34
The place of the psychotropic drugs with violent adolescents
Beat Mohler, Uster, Switzerland, beat.mohler@kjpdzh.ch

Objective: Issues of prescription, use and abuse of psychotropic medication for aggressive behaviour in adolescents are widely discussed. The presentation will give an overview on corresponding literature in this area, describe correlates of aggressive behaviour and corresponding differential diagnostic questions to be raised, and it will discuss diagnostic and treatment guidelines. **Methods:** The analysis is based on a literature review, clinical case examples, and study results from a project on experience of violence in adolescents. The population of this study included 208 youths from a randomised general population sample, 30 delinquent youths, and 45 adolescent psychiatric patients, aged between 11 and 19 years. **Results:** Aggressive behaviour in adolescents is being reported quite often. Many youth with violent behaviour report symptoms of depression or anxiety and have been exposed to violence as victims or witnesses. Analysis of the literature leads to controversial results. More specific drug treatment (neuroleptics and/or mood stabilisers, antidepressive drugs) is suggested for aggressive behaviour in psychotic or bipolar youth and posttraumatic or depressive disorders. **Conclusion:** The analysis supports that with exception of sedation in acute situations – a very careful differential diagnosis and a functional behavior analysis should precede psychopharmacotherapy specifically aimed at symptoms of aggression. Violent behaviours in adolescents occur very often in the process of specific psychiatric disorders which themselves should be the focus of interventions.

S-084-395   Topic: 52, 7
A psychodynamic approach of adolescents' aggressive behaviours. Management of the setting
Philippe Jeammet, Université Paris VI, Psychiatrie de l'Enfant, Paris, France, philippe.jeammet@imm.fr

Aggressive behaviours are one of the privileged expressions of the adolescent but also one of the most difficult to treat for the therapist. A better understanding of behaviour psychopathology can help us to work on our therapeutic answers. Those are very much linked to the quality of our relationship to those patients. Therefore, it seems essential to understand what happens in those relationships. Many adolescents are confronted with what we consider to be a true paradoxical situation when their affective dependency puts them in direct contradiction with a need to assert their autonomy. We feel that this situation, wherein the adolescent feels his very identity threatened by his relational needs, produces defensives reactions in the form of acting out and behavioural disturbances. All of adolescent behaviour pathology seems to include this dimension, which must be taken into account when setting up therapeutic measures. Indeed, the more necessary relationships are for these adolescents, the more intolerable they seem. Behaviours disturbances can then be seen as playing a role in the internal equilibrium of the adolescent and regulating the distance in his relationships with others. Violence for instance seems to allow the Self to pull itself together when threatened by a loss of identity or a loss of boundries. Even the most brutal acting out does not come about by chance. Violence always serves a purpose in the psychic economy. It seems to me to be essential in protecting the Self. It releases the Self's internal tensions which threaten to overflow, but it also allows for a control over the object by replacing it and freeing the Self of its influence. Every act of violence reinforces the boundaries between the Self and the object. Physical blows are a good example. When you strike someone, not only do you touch him but you differentiate yourself from him and are opposed to him. A blow allows for contact and yet one can

ignore one's need for contact. We can see how adolescents can soothe their depersonalization crisis through masochistic behaviour, like burning themselves with a cigarette, and how this act helps them to find themselves again. Pleasure, especially sexual pleasure can create depersonalization because one loses one's boundaries. On the contrary, pain, provided that it doesn't go too far, can re-establish boundaries, and because of this helps the subject to find himself again. The need to hang on to external reality makes this reality all the more interesting. It is thus important to organise, in external reality, a setting that is able to sustain these differentiating functions that are threatened by the adolescent process itself.

S-085   Topic: 84
Attention Deficit Hyperactivity Disorder (ADHD)
Track: ADHD
Chairperson: Michael Fitzgerald, Trinity College Dublin Child and Family Center, Dublin 10, Ireland, fitzi@iol.ie

Attention Deficit Hyperactivity Disorder (ADHD)
Michael Fitzgerald, Trinity College Dublin, Child and Family Center, Dublin 10, Ireland, fitzi@iol.ie

Kurt Cobain and Attention Deficit Hyperactivity Disorder Before Kurt Cobain completed suicide he was one of the major pop singer and musicians of the 20th century. Examination of his biography shows that he received a diagnosis of ADHD as a child and was prescribed Ritalin. Even in retrospect it is clear that this was the correct diagnosis and treatment. He also showed clear evidence of Oppositional Defiant Disorder. As he got older he engaged in very serious drug addiction and adolescent depression and completed suicide at age 27 years.

S-085-396   Topic: 84, 28
Dissecting the Attention Deficit Hyperactivity Disorder (ADHD) phenotype: Studies of sustained and spatial attention in relation to Dopamine system candidate genes
Mark Bellgrove, Trinity College Dublin, Dept. of Psychiatry, Dublin 2, Ireland, bellgrom@tcd.ie
Michael Gill; Ian H. Robertson

Objective: The application of molecular genetics to disorders such as Attention Deficit Hyperactivity Disorder (ADHD) provides an exciting means of refining complex phenotypes. Dopamine system candidate genes have proved attractive for research in ADHD given that stimulant medications, such as methylphenidate, act primarily on the dopamine system. Thus associations have been reported between ADHD and the 10-repeat allele of the Dopamine Transporter Gene (DAT1), the A2 allele of a Taq1 polymorphism of the gene encoding Dopamine Beta Hydroxylase (DBH) and also between ADHD and alleles of a number of genes encoding dopamine receptors (e.g., the 7-repeat DRD4 allele). Although the existence of an attention deficit in ADHD remains controversial within the neuropsychological literature, here we aimed to determine whether analyses of neuropsychological function, in relation to genotype, could clarify this picture. **Methods:** We report data on our ongoing genotype/phenotype studies of children and adolescents with ADHD in relation to DAT1,

DBH and COMT genotype using attentional measures as potential endophenotypes. **Results:** We report on a number of studies undertaken that indicate that the inconsistently reported phenomenon of left spatial inattention in ADHD is associated with the 10-repeat allele of the DAT1 gene, with 10-repeat homozygotes displaying left-neglect. Further, we report that sustained attention in ADHD is influenced separately by both the 10-repeat DAT1 allele and the A2 allele of the DBH polymorphism. Further, the Met allele of the COMT gene appears to be associated with poorer sustained attention and dual-task performance. **Conclusion:** We discuss our results both in terms of neuropsychological and catecholamine/frontostriatal theories of ADHD.

S-085-397   Topic: 84, 85

Is Attention Deficit Hyperactivity Disorder (ADHD) missed in children with conduct disorder?

Paul McArdle, Newcastle University, Dept. of Child Psychiatry, Newcastle, United Kingdom, mcardlep@aol.com

Objective: To review the origins of conduct disorder in childhood and adolescence. **Methods:** Two large Newcastle upon Tyne representative samples of 7–8 year olds and 11–12 year olds totalling 4,000 children obtained in the 1970s were reanalysed. Data included screen questionnaire data on all of both samples and clinical diagnosis on screen positive and a proportion of screen negative children. **Results:** The clinical diagnosis of conduct disorder was made using criteria similar to those that obtain currently. The prevalence of severe conduct disorder was similar to that in current epidemiological studies. All 7–8 year old children with severe conduct disorder scored as hyperactive according to questionnaire data. Among 11–12 year olds, the rate of comorbid hyperactivity was less. Where conduct disorder was present in the absence of hyperactivity, there was evidence of severe adversity. **Conclusion:** Prior to the dissemination of the concept of ADHD, children with disruptive behaviour disorders received the diagnosis of conduct disorder. It is clear that the majority of younger children with this diagnosis are likely to have had symptoms of hyperactivity; the significance of which was not understood at the time. It is still common practice in the UK to consider the diagnosis of conduct disorder as tending to exclude hyperactivity-related diagnoses such as attention deficit hyperactivity disorder. In fact, in most children with conduct disorder hyperactivity is likely to be also present. This is particularly likely among younger children.

S-085-398   Topic: 84, 37

A study of the diagnosis and management of symptoms of Attention Deficit Hyperactivity Disorder (ADHD) in children and adults. A computerised clinical interview schedule for ADHD in use in an Irish Clinic

Amanda Burke, Child and Family Guidance, Roscommon, Ireland, amandaburke@eircom.net

Objective: To survey the views of Consultant Psychiatrists on the frequency of symptoms of ADHD in children and adults, both with and without learning disabilities. We were interested in assessing the confidence that these mental health professionals had in making the diagnosis, the order in which they ranked diagnostic symptoms, the methods used for diagnosis and the treatments that they

found effective. **Methods:** We designed a postal questionnaire, using a series of multiple choice, open ended questions and a visual analogue scale for answers. We sent this to a total of 302 Consultant Psychiatrists working in Ireland. Responses were anonymous. **Results:** Respondents working with children were significantly more confident in diagnosing ADHD and in treating the condition, than those working with adults irrespective of whether they had a learning disability. There were also definite patterns and significant differences found in the symptoms that were ranked as diagnostic. Symptoms of ADHD were less likely to be treated if the individual had a learning disability. **Conclusion:** There is a lack of clarity among Consultant Psychiatrists in their clinical management of people with symptoms of ADHD. The second part of the presentation will focus on a computerized clinical interview schedule for ADHD in use in an Irish Clinic.

S-086   Topic: 1, 2

WPA Global program on child and mental health: Task force awareness

Track: Therapy and intervention

Chairperson: Sam Tyano, Geha Mental Health Center, Petah Tiqva, Israel, styano@post.tau.ac.il

Child mental health awareness project

Sam Tyano, Geha Mental Health Center, Petah Tiqva, Israel, styano@post.tau.ac.il

Child Mental Health is an issue which suffers from several "disorders". First of all, it is stigmatic as always are all other issues concerning psychiatry. Secondly, children are not independent to express their suffering loudly therefore they have to rely on adults to express their issues. Third, children are usually considered as non-suffering compared to the adults because they do not express this independently. WPA got a presidential project on Awareness of Child Mental Health in the world and invited IACAPAP and WHO to lead its project in most of the countries in the world. The goal of our task force is to prepare all the materials and to elaborate in different promulgation techniques in order to convey child psychiatry content to all professionals. The techniques we have recommended and the way we propose to convey this information to lay people and professionals will be presented during our symposium.

S-086-399   Topic: 63

Raising awareness of child mental health among medical students

K. Michael Hong, Cheju National Universtity, College of Medicine, Cheju, Republic of Korea, kmhong@cheju.ar.ky

Medical students are certainly a very important target group for our task force to aim to raise awareness on child mental health because it will reduce their bias and misconceptions on child mental disorders and as a result, it will improve their attitude and skills to recognize and deal with child mental health issues and problems in their medical practices after graduation. It will also increase the probability for them to choose child psychiatry as their specialty without being stigmatized. In addition, they will become a major group to provide proper information on child mental health to the patients and the public ,and to advocate children with mental health problems. Contents of child mental health in medical school curriculum should include contents related to child mental health; such as, child development, neurobiological basis and socio-cultural factors in child development and psychopathology, child rearing practices, mother-child relationship, attachment, functions of family in child development and psychopathology, children's reaction to physical illness and fatal illness, major mental disorders in childhood and adolescent period, continuity and discontinuity of child mental health into adulthood, early detection and appropriate referrals, and intervention and treatment as a primary physician. Strategies and methods of teaching of medical school curriculum are through the lectures and clinical clerkships in 1) Behavioral science, 2) Pediatric, 3) Child psychiatry, 4) Family Medicine Availability of qualified child psychiatrist faculty in medical school is critical to carry out the above described missions. However, the reality is that most countries outside of western world do not have qualified child psychiatrist at all. It is urgent and utmost important for WPA, WHO, and IACAPAP to help developing countries to secure a minimum number of child psychiatrists and other child mental health specialists. One way to accomplish this mission would be to set up Regional Child Psychiatry/child Mental Health Training Centers, one or two, in Asia, South America and Africa and provide technical and financial assistance.

S-086-400   Topic: 25
A manual for addressing awareness:
Child and adolescent mental health
Christina Hoven, Columbia University, USA

The purpose of the manual is to outline a pragmatic approach for the implementation of a campaign whose goal is to increase awareness of mental health problems in children and adolescents. This document first presents evidence as to the magnitude of these problems, giving evidence of their severity and their prevalence. A review of common disorders and resources for help then follows. The manual moves on to present other components of a campaign, describing populations that the campaign should target, from children all the way up to international organizations. Finally, the manual guides the user toward methods of implementing the campaign, from the use of print material to the use of the Internet and cell phones. Thus, the manual provides a guide, in as much detail as possible, toward implementing an effective campaign to combat a general lack of public knowledge about mental health issues relating specifically to children and adolescents.

S-086-401   Topic: 3, 25
Increase awareness about suicide preventive programmes in schools
Danuta Wasserman, NASP, Stockholm, Sweden, prof.wasserman.secretary@ipm.ki.se

Increasing youth suicide rates, especially among males, constitute a major public health problem in Europe. In the past two decades motor accident fatalities have been decreasing while suicide, especially among young males, has been increasing. Although suicides among young people aged 15–24 constitute a considerable burden on the society, the approach of initiating prevention at a very early stage of the suicidal process is scarcely applied. Intervention is much more difficult once the suicidal process has progressed beyond a certain stage. Therefore, suicide preventive programmes should be tailored in close collaboration with staff working in schools, as many children in the world attend compulsory school. The WHO's world wide initiative to prevent suicide has published a resource series, and among them a resource for teachers and other schools staff on how to prevent suicidal behaviours and strengthen mental health among pupils. Experiences from using this material will be presented.

S-087   Topic: 34
Developmental psychopharmacology –
Basic research and clinical implications
Track: Therapy and intervention
Chairperson: Eberhard Schulz, Universität Freiburg , Kinder- und Jugendpsychiatrie, Freiburg, Germany, schulz@psyallg.ukl.uni-freiburg.de

Developmental psychopharmacology –
Basic research and clinical implications
Eberhard Schulz, Universität Freiburg, Kinder- und Jugendpsychiatrie, Freiburg, Germany, schulz@psyallg.ukl.uni-freiburg.de

It is generally accepted that environmental influences during certain sensitive periods of early postnatal life have a strong impact upon later development and behavior, however, the mechanisms whereby early experience induces such long-lasting and perhaps permanent effects upon the behavior are still quite unclear. Early separation from the parents and family is a stressful, traumatic experience, which under continuing adverse socio-emotional conditions can result in a variety of cognitive and emotional disturbances. Experimental studies in non-human primates and in rodents revealed strikingly similar behavioural disturbances after different manipulations of the socio-emotional environment during early life periods. The remarkable stability of theses deprivation-induced behavioural abnormalities may reflect dysfunctions of limbic circuits. In this symposium, data derived from animal models of early environmental factors influencing brain development are presented and clinical implications are discussed.

S-087-402   Topic: 34
Emotional experiences regulate synaptic densities in the limbic system
Katharina Braun, Universität Magdeburg, Inst. für Biologie, Magdeburg, Germany, braun@ifn-magdeburg.de Jörg Bock; Carina Helmecke; Michael Gruß; Gerd Poeggel

Objective: Early brain development is constantly modified by environmental influences. Stress constitutes one aspect of these environmental influences, which present the maturing brain with experiences that will crucially and potentially adversely affect its development and functional capacities during later life periods. **Methods:** In two rodent models, laboratory rats and Octodon degus we found that early emotional experience modifies limbic synapses. **Results:** The densities of dendritic spines were quantified in the anterior cingulate cortex (ACd) and in the somatosensory (SS) cortex, in degus the hippocampus and the amygdala were also analyzed. The parentally deprived animals (PND 21) in both species showed increased spine densities in the ACd, these synaptic changes are long lasting and resistant to "resocialization". Spine development in the SS-cortex was not affected by parental separation or other emotional experiences. In the CA1 region of parentally deprived degus spine densities were increased, whereas decreased densities were observed in granule cells of the dentate gyrus. No changes were found in the amygdala at this age. Recent pharmacological experiments strongly indicate that HPA activation as well as serotonergic mechanisms are involved in these synaptic changes. **Conclusion:** Our results demonstrate that stress and parental deprivation modifies synaptic inputs in limbic areas. The observation that the late developing prefrontal cortical areas are particularly sensitive may have implications for some mental disorders such as depression and schizophrenia.

S-087-403   Topic: 34
Isolation rearing in the rat:
Persistent effects on neuronal structure and function
Charles Marsden, University of Nottingham,
Inst. of Neuroscience, Nottingham, United Kingdom,
charles.marsden@nottingham.ac.uk
S. Muchimapura; M.-C. Pardon; M. Bianchi

Objective: Social isolation is a risk factor in psychiatric disorders, such as depression, involving altered serotonergic function. We investigated the effects of rearing rats from weaning in social isolation on pre- and post-synaptic serotonergic function to identify factors important in development of neuronal systems involved in stress. **Methods:** Male Lister hooded rats were housed either singly or in groups from weaning. 2–4 weeks later behavioural (conditioned emotional response (CER), neurochemical (in vivo microdialysis), in vitro electrophysiological and immunohistochemical (c-fos, synaptophysin, ERK, MAP-2 etc) testing started. **Results:** Isolation reared compared to group reared controls showed enhanced CER with increased freezing behaviour in response to the contextual cue but decreased aversion-induced release of 5-HT in the hippocampus while the opposite occurred in the nuc. accumbens where release in response to aversion was enhanced. Restraint stress also increased 5-HT release, a response blunted in the hippocampus of the isolates. Changes in hippocampal 5-HT function appear to be presynaptic as release after PCPA administration was reduced. Expression of c-fos following restraint stress in the isolates was increased in the hippocampus compared to group reared rats together with reduced synaptophysin. While expression of MAP-2 and other makers of neuronal plasticity were reduced. **Conclusion:** These results demonstrate that isolation alters the neuronal response to stress and that serotonergic function is important for 'coping' with stress. Isolation reared rats offer an excellent model to investigate the various signalling mechanisms involved in the control of the neuronal response to stress.

S-087-404   Topic: 34
Animal models of depression: Long-term neurobehavioral effects of early life adversity in rats and monkeys
Joram Feldon, ETHZ Zürich, Behavioral Neurobiology Lab.,
Zürich, Switzerland, feldon@behav.biol.ethz.ch
Daniela Rüedi-Bettschen; Andrea C. Dettling;
Christopher R. Pryce

Objective: There is considerable evidence in mammals that the offspring's postnatal environment can exert a marked impact on its long-term development. Much of this evidence has been obtained in studies of individuals that experienced extreme forms of postnatal environment, including: daily deprivation of maternal care in rat pups; permanent or daily deprivation of maternal care in monkey infants; and parental loss, parent-child emotional or physical neglect, or parent-child emotional or physical abuse, in humans. The human epidemiological evidence is that major early life stress events can markedly increase vulnerability for developmental and adulthood psychopathology, including posttraumatic stress disorder, attention deficit hyperactivity disorder, conduct disorders, and depression. **Methods:** Prospective, controlled animal studies provide opportunity to increase understanding of the causal relationships between species-atypical early life stressors, the development of abnormal neurobiological, physiological and behavioural phenotypes, and their pharmacological responsiveness. **Results:** In rats, early deprivation in the form of 4 hours separation from dam and littermates on postnatal days 1–14 resulted in adult offspring that exhibited reduced interest in obtaining sucrose reward on a progressive ratio schedule of reinforcement (vis. anhedonia), and impaired coping ability following mild punishment (vis. helplessness). Both of these chronic behavioural effects of early deprivation were attenuated by chronic treatment with fluoxetine. Physiologically, relative to control subjects, early deprived adult rats were characterized by increased cardiophysiological reactivity and reduced plasma corticosterone reactivity to environmental adversity. In marmoset monkeys, early deprivation in the form of 0.5–2 hours separation from the parents and twin on postnatal days 2–28 caused acute stress responses in terms of adrenal cortisol and catecholamines. In infancy, physical development was retarded, basal plasma cortisol was increased, and motivation for social play was reduced. As juveniles, early deprived monkeys exhibited increased basal cardiophysiological activity and increased basal urinary catecholamine levels; behaviourally they were more impulsive than controls. Following brief social separations, early deprived juveniles were less motivated to seek social contact than were controls. As adolescents, early deprived monkeys exhibited reduced interest in obtaining sucrose reward on a progressive ratio schedule of reinforcement (vis. anhedonia) and a deficit in responding to changes in the reward-predicting properties of environmental stimuli. **Conclusion:** Therefore, the approach of investigating and comparing the long-term effects of neglect-like early adversity in rats and monkeys is yielding evidence for commonalities, both between different animal species and between animals and humans. As such, these developmental animal models can increase understanding of: environmental regulation of neurobehavioural development, the neurobiology of developmental psychopathologies, and their neuropharmacological treatment.

S-087-405   Topic: 34

In vivo release of Glutamate and GABA in the rat hippocampus after periphal and central application of secretin

Hans-Willi Clement, Uni-Krankenhaus Freiburg, Kinder-und Jugendpsychiatrie, Freiburg, Germany, clement@psyallg.ukl.uni-freiburg.de
O. Sommer; A. Pschibul; C. Rombach; M. Gerlach; Eberhard Schulz

Objective: In 1998 Horvath reported three autistic children, who showed dramatic behavioural improvement (improved eye contact, alertness, and expansion of expressive language) 5 weeks after application of secretin. Currently, several anecdotal reports and a few controlled trials with conflicting results have been published regarding the use of secretin in autism. Nevertheless only little is known about the role of secretin in the central nervous system. Aim of this study is the investigation of the effect of secretin on secretion of neurotransmitters in the rat brain. **Methods:** Experiments were undertaken in anterior hippocampus of freely moving Lewis-rats. Microdialysis technique was used to collect microdialysate each 20 min during 4 h. High Performance Liquid Chromatography (HPLC) with fluorescence detection was used to measure the amount of amino acids in microdialysate. Concentrations of the neurotransmitters were compared before and after application of secretin versus a control group. Secretin (Secrelux) was applied intraperitoneally (i.p.) or intracerebroventriculary (i.c.v.). **Results:** A significant increase of glutamate and GABA could be shown after application of secretin (8.7 µg/kg i.p.). Also the i.c.v. application of secretin (0.015 µg to 5 µg) lead to dose dependent elevations of microdialysate glutamate and GABA. Since secretin is thought to have greater benefit in young children, experiments were also performed in young (4–5 weeks) rats. In these experiments the secretin (30 kU/kg i.p.) application did not change glutamatergic neurotransmission. **Conclusion:** Our study strengthens the role of secretin as a neuromodulator affecting the glutamatergic and the GABAergic system. Furthermore, our study could support the theory of Carlsson of autism as a hypoglutamatergic disorder. Thus, the increased secretion of glutamate after application of secretin could explain the behavioural changes as seen in Horvath's study. The differences in the action of secretin in young and adult rats cannot be explained yet, but will lead to further experiments to clarify the observed differences.

S-087-406   Topic: 34

Mouse brain gene expression changes after chronic treatment with psychotropic drugs

Claudia Mehler-Wex, Universität Würzburg, Kinder- und Jugendpsychiatrie, Würzburg, Germany, mehler@kjp.uni-wuerzburg.de
S. Zeiske; E. Grünblatt; G. Gille; D. Rausch; Andreas Warnke; Manfred Gerlach

Objective: Recent data suggest that many antipsychotic drugs, in particular "atypical" neuroleptics, are associated with weight gain. The underlying mechanisms are unknown. On the other hand, psychostimulants often produce weight loss. The aim of this study was to examine changes in gene expression of the mice cortex following chronic treatment with the neuroleptics haloperidol and clozapin compared with the anorexiant drug phenylpropanolamine. **Methods:** Each 15 10–12-week-old male C57BL6-mice for 4 weeks orally received either haloperidol (1 mg/kg/day), clozapine (10 mg/kg/day) or phenylpropanolamine (3 mg/kg/day). The control group (n = 10) was given usual food pellets. After 4 weeks mice were sacrificed by decapitation. The brains were quickly removed for cortex dissection. Total RNA was isolated, treated with DNaseI and purified (RNeasyKit, Qiagen). For gene changes analysis GeneChipMicroarray (Affymetrix) was used. Confirmation of some of the gene changes found was done using quantitative real-time PCR. **Results:** Comparing the clozapine, haloperidol and stimulant treated groups with controls, microarray analysis revealed several significant differences in gene expression. With real-time PCR we confirmed an up-regulation of the glutamate transporter-mRNA gene following typical and atypical neuroleptic treatment and of tumor necrosis factor-stimulated gene 6 (TNF-6) in the haloperidol group. Cytochrome c oxidase subunit VIIc gene was down-regulated in the clozapine group. **Conclusion:** Microarrays allow parallel screening of the expression patterns and regulation of thousands of genes. The changes found in gene expression may underlie abnormal energy metabolism and body weight changes following neuroleptic therapy.

S-088   Topic: 2, 1

EMACAPAP Symposium

Chairperson: Amira Seif El-Din, University of Alexandria Faculty of Medicine, Alexandria, Egypt, amira@contact.com.eg

EMACAPAP Symposium

Amira Seif El-Din, University of Alexandria, Faculty of Medicine, Alexandria, Egypt, amira@contact.com.eg

Children in out Region constitute about 40% of the total population of this Region. Child and adolescent psychiatry in the EMACAPAP Region is a recent and new speciality, where child psychiatrists providing this services in most of the countries of the Region are very few and adult psychiatrists can provide it with more focus on drug therapy. Child mental health promotion and sometimes intervention is mainly related to the family and in some occasion the school has a role. Many of the intervention approaches applied are related to cultural issues related to family rearing. The representative countries of the Region will focus on the child mental health profile in their countries.

S-088-407   Topic: 2, 1

Mental health of children and adolescents in Lebanon: Needs, services and research

John Fayyad, St. George Hospital, Psychiatry and Psychology, Beirut, Lebanon, jfayyad@inco.com.lb

Objective: The purpose of this presentation is to describe the status of child and adolescent mental health systems of care and ongoing research efforts in Lebanon. **Results:** Data on Lebanese population demographics and encountered disorders and mental health problems in the community will be presented. Available systems of care and professionals specialized in child mental health will be described. Child mental health services as well as services for special populations (e.g. developmental disorders, juvenile delinquents, abused and neglected children, children in contested custody following divorce) and the laws pertaining to them will be discussed. Ongoing research studies in epidemiology, adolescent substance use and abuse, Attention Deficit Hyperactivity Disorder, and the impact of war on children's mental health will be highlighted. Finally, cultural factors that affect systems development will be described. **Conclusion:** There is a broad spectrum of child mental health services available in Lebanon. Research is needed on the prevalence and burden of disorders in childhood and adolescence, country specific risk and protective factors as well as barriers to care. The presentation will rely on published data and information collected from Lebanese Non Governmental Organizations.

S-088-408   Topic: 25
Child and adolescent mental health in Morocco
Nadia Kadri, Psychiatry Chu Ibn Rochd, Casablanca, Morocco, n.kadri@casanet.net.ma
Houda Hjiej Andaloussi; Khadija Chihabeddine; Driss Moussaoui

Psychiatry is a neglected specialty in medicine. Child and adolescent psychiatry is the neglected sub-specialty in psychiatry, especially in developing countries meanwhile the half population is under 18. In Morocco, and till now there are 250 psychiatrists and 6 child and adolescent psychiatrists. There is no public institution for mentally ill children. NGOs play some role to fill this emptiness. However some studies were conducted to have data concerning some of the problems such as mental retardation, school mental health, enuresis and circumcision impact on children mental health. The first study was conducted on 183 mental retarded children with the most prevalent risk factors: neonatal pathology (29%), Down Syndrome (24%) epilepsy (11%) and consanguinity (11%). As survey conducted on 500 pupils found that prevalence of school deficiency was 9.7% with the following risk factors: Lack of preschool education, long distance between school and home, Bad time-space structuration, enuresis, and psychomotor instability. Enuresis was explored through 500 children consulting a GP and pediatricians. Its prevalence was 41.4%.

S-088-409   Topic: 45
Child mental Health in Egypt
Amira Seif El-Din, University of Alexandria, Faculty of Medicine, Alexandria, Egypt, amira@contact.com.eg

The total population of Egypt is 70 millions nearly half the population are children and adolescents. Most of the health services provided to children is the physical health services. Mental health care for this sector is limited. There are different mental health problems related to different age groups where early childhood psychological problems are; physical abuse, some behavioral problems as thumb sucking, temper tantrum, nocturnal enuresis and ADHD, in addition to lack of awareness of parents of psychosocial development of children. The major problem for middle childhood and adolescent period is the great concern of parents and teachers to focus on academic competition in schools with lack of awareness on individual variation of children and to push them to get the highest score in their academic education without putting in consideration the individual differences. The common mental health problems faced at this age group are; anxiety, dissociative

disorders, depression, school drop out and acute psychosis. The care for rehabilitation of mentally handicapped children is one of the important areas where a well developed activities from governomental and non governomental organizations are working and developing community support for their families and special education for this category. Although in Egypt we have 18 faculties of Medicine but there is no degree in child psychiatry. Most of the psychiatrists working with children are adult psychiatrists with special training or interest in child psychiatry. Recently the awareness of parents toward the field of child and adolescent psychiatry started to improve which increase the demands towards mental health services.

S-088-410   Topic: 1, 26
Validity of the self-report version (SRQ) of the strengths and difficulties questionnaire (SDQ) in Yemen
Mohammed Almaqrami, Mental Health Hospital, Child & Adolescent Psychiatry, Sana'a, Yemen, almagrami@yahoo.com

Objective: The main objective of this study is to determine the validity of the Arabic version of the SRQ of SDQ in Yemen. **Methods:** Follwing translation and back-translation of the scale into Arabic language by a panel of expert, psychometric properties were assesd using 600 students from schools and 57 patients attending the mental health hospital in Sana'a city – Republic of yemen from January to April 2002. The age-range of the two groups was from 12 to 17 years old.Discrimitive validity, concurrent validity, and factorial validity were studied. **Results:** The difference between the means of the total difficulties scores in both groups was highly significant (p < 0.001). The Area Under the Curve (AUC) of the total scores and subscales' scores were ranged from 0.77 to 0.89. The chance-corrected agreements between the clinical diagnosis and the SRQ subscales' prediction were significant. The sensetivity and specificity were 72% and 55% respectively. Factor analysis yielded five dimensions of emotional symptoms, conduct disorders, hyperactivity, peer problems and prosocial items. **Conclusion:** Results of this validation study reveals that the Arabic version of the SRQ of the SDQ is valid in Yemen; and it can be a useful tool for investigating child and adolelescent behavioral and emotional problems in clinical settings.

S-089
Free communication I
Chairperson: Alexander von Gontard, Uniklinik des Saarlandes, Homburg, Germany, alexander.von.gontard@uniklinik-saarland.de

S-089-411   Topic: 73, 40
Traumatic events and its symptomatology in child and adolescent
Keizo Nagao, Sakakibara Hospital, Dept. of Psychiatry, Japan, gzb06665@nifty.ne.jp
M. Kisida; M. Okuno; E. Shindo

Objective: To examine the incidence, causes and clinical symptoms of traumatic events including PTSD in child and adolescent in Japan. **Methods:** 104 nursing students were investigated on average 20 years old. Answer was obtained in shape of one of the authors to read out the question items though the investigation was a questionnaire method. **Results:** (1) The severity of traumatic experience was as follows; a criteria of DSM-4 of PTSD is 8 (8%), strong stress experience not yet arrive at A criteria is 52 (50%), tremble trauma experience is 23(22%) and no traumatic experience is 21 (20%). (2) Traumatic events of sixty of the former two groups mainly comprise of bulling and distressed personal relationship in 24 (40%) and the loss of an intimate friend or near relatives in 18 (30%). (3) Symptoms of these two groups were compared. The self-reproach idea and depression in bulling and distressed relationship were dominant higher though there was no difference in the three main PTSD symptoms and other concomitants as somatic complaints. **Conclusion:** (1) Bulling and the loss are thought to be the maximum cause which can become traumatic experiences and PTSD at this age in our country. (2) Preventive education will be needed on these two subjects because of high frequency. (3) Treatment of bulling should be focused more on self-reproach and depression than main PTSD symptoms to encourage school attendance in clinical cases.

S-089-412   Topic: 56, 19
Quality of Life: Improvement during and after inpatient treatment
Kurt Quaschner, Universitätsklinik Marburg, Kinder- und Jugendpsychiatrie, Marburg, Germany, quaschne@med. uni-marburg.de

Objective: Research on quality of life aspects in the field of child and adolescent psychiatry has been neglected for a long time. With the development of research instruments it is now possible to investigate more specific questions. In this study one of these instruments – the Inventory for the Assessment of the Quality of Life in Children and Adolescents (ILC, Mattejat & Remschmidt et al., 1998) – was used to investigate quality of life aspects in different diagnostic groups of psychiatric inpatients. **Methods:** The Inventory for the Assessment of the Quality of Life in Children and Adolescents (ILC) was administered to a sample of psychiatric inpatients (N = 520) and parents (N = 449) during and after treatment. The inpatient sample consists of the most frequent diagnoses including schizophrenia, adjustment disorder, ADHD, Anorexia, conduct disorder, emotional and neurotic disorders. **Results:** Results indicate significant differences between diagnostic groups and changes over time. Thus, study findings support an relation between quality of life and diagnoses in psychiatric inpatients. **Conclusion:** As a consequence, quality of life aspects in psychiatric inpatients should be interpreted in regard to diagnosis and symptomatology.

S-089-413   Topic: 84, 28
Life events during pregnancy and attention problems in the offspring
*Niels Bilenberg, Odense University Hospital, Child & Adolescent Psychiatry, Odense C, Denmark, niels.bilenberg@ouh.fyns-amt.dk
Carsten Obel; Tine Brink Henriksen; Morten Hedegaard; Niels Jørgen Secher; Jørn Olsen*

Objective: Attention problems is among the most common psychiatric disorders. Animal studies suggest that stress in pregnancy cause structural changes in the fetal brain and behavioral changes in the offspring. Studies in primates suggest a specific effect of prenatal stress on attention in the offspring. The aim of the study was to investigate the association between stressful life events during pregnancy and attention problems in the offspring. **Methods:** A follow-up study from early pregnancy to the age of 9–11 years was performed in a community sample of pregnant women recruited in Aarhus, Denmark from 1989 to 1991. The 4031 Danish-speaking women provided information twice during pregnancy about life events in the first and second trimester respectively. Main outcome measure was an 'ADHD problem score', based on a selection of questions from the Child Behavior Checklist and registrered by parents when the children were 9 to 11 years of age. We used an a priori defined cut off with known relation to the diagnosis Attention-Deficit Hyperactivity Disorder (ADHD) in a similar population. **Results:** A high ADHD problem score was found in 7% of boys and 5 % of girls. Women, who reported more than one stressful life event in first as well as second trimester of pregnancy, gave birth to children with a high problem score (OR = 2.1; 95% CI 1.4–3.0). In boys a trend was found between number of life events in second trimester and a high ADHD problem score (P < 0.001). **Conclusion:** Stress in pregnancy was associated with attention problems in the offspring.

S-089-414   Topic: 41, 45
Peer rejection in children and adolescents: Recent data from a Portuguese study
António Fonseca, University of Coimbra, Faculty of Psychology, Coimbra, Portugal, acfonseca@fpce.uc.pt

Many researchers have studied, during the last decade, the association between poor peer relationship and antisocial behaviour in childhood and adolescence. In this context, particular attention has been given to the effects of peer rejection on subsequent forms of social maladjustment. This paper is aimed at presenting a review of the main findings accumulated in such studies and at pointing out some issues deserving further enquiry. In addition, we will present and discuss several data from a longitudinal study currently going on in Portugal and designed to assess the outcome of rejected children. These children were identified at the beginning of the elementary school by parents and teachers and, subsequently, assessed at different time points, throughout adolescence, in several important domains: mental health, juvenile delinquency, social skills, learning difficulties and school achievement. Several informants and instruments were used for this purpose. Results showed that rejected boys and girls have worse outcomes in any of these domains. And this negative effect of early peer rejection remained stable, even after controlling for comorbidity or associated conditions. Based on such findings, several suggestions are made for the development of preventing programs aimed at reducing the risk for later mental health problems and social maladjustment as well as for subsequent research in this field.

S-089-415   Topic: 92
Effects of parental psychosocial factors on health status of children undergoing stem cell transplantation
Isabelle Nathalie Koch, Universität Tübingen, Kinder- u. Jugendpsychiatrie, Tübingen, Germany, inkoch@med.uni-tuebingen.de

The aim of this study was to gain further understanding of the coping mechanisms mediated by parental psychosocial variables of children undergoing stem cell transplantation (SCT), a field of research which has – until now – largely been neglected. On the basis of the actual health status we focussed on the relationship between children and their primary caretaker as it was evaluated by health care personel. On the side of the child a semiprojective instrument (MacArthur Story Stem Battery – MSSB) and several questionnaires evaluating the child's perceived level of illness impairment, its intro- and extraversion (HANES), its level of anxiety (AFS) and its body schema (KBMT-K) were administered. To evaluate the level of psychosocial stress of the primary caretaker she/he was asked to fill in questionnaires pertaining to his/her perceived level of depression (BDI), amount of social support (F-SOZU) and actual health status. The health care personel was asked to rate the quality of parent-child interaction, stress level by means of the BASES-Scales. The actual health status was measured by medical parameters. Although the overall study is based on a pre-post-design we focuss on the results after SCT. By means of multiple regression analyses the most influential variables onto the actual coping of the child shall be determined.

S-089-416   Topic: 51, 52

Relationship between adult attachment styles, childhood abuse experience and violence in intimate relationships

Ieva Bite, Riga, Latvia, ieva@skalbes.lv

Objective: The aim of this current study was to examine the relationships among adult attachment styles, childhood abuse experience and physical violence between partners in intimate relationships. Methods: One-hundred-ninety-seven heterosexual male and female participants aged 25–50 completed self-report measures of violence and abuse history and adult attachment styles (secure, preoccupied, fearful and dismissive). Fifty-six (29%) respondents reported physical violence in their current intimate relationships. Results: Results indicated that experience of childhood physical, sexual or emotional abuse, and insecure adult attachment style was related to involvement in a violent partner relationship. Multiple regression analysis showed that a history of childhood physical abuse experience was the most significant predictor of being involved in a violent relationship, and a second significant predictor was preoccupied attachment style. These tendencies were important for both men and women and for both violence victims and perpetrators. Conclusion: Experience of childhood abuse and preoccupied attachment style are strongly connected with involvement in violent intimate relationships. These findings highlight the importance of attachment theory, adult attachment style and childhood history of abuse in understanding the dynamics of domestic violence.

S-090   Topic: 85

Oppositional defiant and conduct disorders

Chairperson: Phyllis Cohen, Yale Child Study Center, New Haven, CT, USA, phyllis.cohen@yale.edu

S-090-417   Topic: 85

The interplay between adverse parenting and mentalising in the 2 year outcomes of clinic referred antisocial boys

Jonathan Hill, University of Liverpool, Dept. of Psychiatry, Liverpool, United Kingdom, jonathan.hill@liverpool.ac.uk
Katrin Russell; Nichaela Broyden

Objective: To examine whether lower mentalising, evidenced in doll play assessments, is predictive of increased externalising behaviours over two years in antisocial boys. Methods: Sixty boys aged 5–8 years referred for antisocial behaviour problems were assessed using mother and teacher reports (CBCL and TRF). Standard tests of verbal IQ and story telling ability were administered, together with six scenarios from the MacArthur Story Stem Battery (MSSB), of which two portrayed conflict and two a distressed child. We developed new scales of aggression and mentalising (intentionality), and demonstrated satisfactory inter-rater reliability for the scales applied to each story stem. Intentionality reflected the extent to which the story was told in terms of characters' motives or feelings. Parenting was assessed using the self-report Alabama Parenting Questionnaire, and through detailed interviewing with parents. We traced and assessed 40 (66%) of the sample with maternal and teacher reports two years later. Results: Teacher rated externalising problems at two years were strongly predicted by an interview assessment of 'explosive parenting' (prolonged verbally abusive behaviour towards the child). On the basis of previous findings of low intentionality responses to distress stories in antisocial boys, we predicted that teacher rated externalising behaviours would be associated with lower intentionality. This was not supported. However, among those without explosive parenting (N = 28) exernalising problems were predicted by lower intentionality in response to the distress stems Scary Dog (rho = –0.49) and Burnt Hand (rho = –0.22), but in the presence of explosive parenting the correlations were in the opposite direction (rho = 0.44 and 0.62). The interaction terms between explosive parenting and intentionality with teacher rated externalising problems as the dependent variable were significant for Scary Dog (p = 0.027) and Burnt Hand (p = 0.006). Conclusion: The findings are consistent with the proposal that the same factors may confer vulnerability or resilience for persisting antisocial behaviours depending on environmental stressors.

S-090-418   Topic: 85

Aggressive and mentalising processes evidenced in the doll play of antisocial boys

Jonathan Hill, University of Liverpool, Dept. of Psychiatry, Liverpool, United Kingdom, jonathan.hill@liverpool.ac.uk
Gillian Lancaster

Objective: To examine, using responses to doll play, whether antisocial boys show evidence of both high aggression and impaired mentalising, depending on the social context. Methods: Forty one boys aged 5–8 years referred for antisocial behaviour problems were compared with 25 non-referred boys of similar age and socio-economic status. Emotional and behavioural problems were assessed from parent and teacher reports. Standard tests of verbal IQ and story telling ability were administered, together with six scenarios from the MacArthur Story Stem Battery (MSSB), of which two portrayed clear conflict and two a distressed child. We developed new scales of aggression and mentalising (intentionality). The intentionality scale assessed the extent to which the child told the story in terms of characters' motives, emotions or beliefs. We demonstrated satisfactory inter-rater reliability for the scales applied to each story stem. Ratings using these scales were made from transcripts blind to group membership. **Results:** The narratives of the referred boys had higher levels of aggression, but not lower intentionality, than controls, only in response to both conflictual story stems (Fight with a friend $p < 0.001$, Lost keys $p < 0.001$). Responses to distress story stems were characterised by lower intentionality in the antisocial group, but not increased aggression (Scary dog $p = 0.001$, Burnt hand $p < 0.001$). In logistic regression controlling for age, verbal IQ and story telling ability, only aggression predicted group membership for the conflictual stems, and only intentionality for the distress stems. **Conclusion:** If responses to doll play scenarios reflect social cognitive processes in real life interactions, the findings suggest that different processes are relevant to the responses of antisocial boys depending on the social challenge. Antisocial problems may therefore arise from the combination of social cognitive processes leading to aggression in conflictual situations, and those associated with impaired mentalising in response to distressing challenges. We propose a model linking the two, which suggests that therapeutic approaches may have to tackle both.

S-090-419   Topic: 89

Attachment relevant experiences of boys with disruptive behavior disorders

Christina Eichhorn, Universitätsklinik Ulm, Kinder- und Jugendpsychiatrie, Ulm, Germany, christina.eichhorn@medizin.uni-ulm.de
Karola Tiedtke; Ute Ziegenhain; Jörg M. Fegert

Objective: Pilot study on the relationship between disruptive behaviour disorders and attachment relevant experiences with respect to transgenerational transmission of attachment. **Methods:** 15 boys aged 8 to 12 years with diagnosis of conduct disorder (ICD-10: F91) or hyperactive conduct disorder (ICD-10: F90.1) and their mothers have been studied. Diagnosis was done with DISYPS according to DSM-IV/ICD-10 criteria. Attachment quality of boys was examined with the Separation Anxiety Test (SAT), and the Child Attachment Interview (CAI). In addition, questionnaires were utilized to assess social support and self-esteem. Attachment representation of mothers was assessed with the Adult Attachment Interview (AAI). Mothers were interviewed about attachment relevant experiences of their children. This clinical sample is compared with an already existing longitudinal-sample of 17 non-referred boys and their mothers, who were assessed in infancy with the Ainsworth strange situation, and at ages 6 and 10 with the SAT. Mothers were interviewed with the AAI. **Results:** The distribution of secure vs. insecure types of quality of attachment in the clinical sample are presented and compared to the non-clinical sample. Indices of high insecurity are analyzed with respect to the amount and/or intensity of negative attachment relevant experiences in the boys with disruptive behaviour disorders. **Conclusion:** Implications for treatment as well as applications for clinical, child welfare and home settings are discussed.

S-090-420   Topic: 85, 9

A study of 701 youths in community-based group treatment: Implications for mental health intervention and research

Ronald Feldman, Columbia University, School of Social Work, New York, NY, USA, raf1@columbia.edu

Objective: To examine the efficacy of treating antisocial youths in "integrated" community-based groups consisting primarily of prosocial peers. **Methods:** A $3 \times 3 \times 2$ factorial design was employed over the course of 8 months with 701 male subjects. Key independent variables were mode of treatment group composition (antisocial youths only vs. prosocial youths only vs. prosocial youths plus 1–2 antisocial youths), group treatment method (behavioral vs. traditional vs. minimal), and extent of therapist experience (experienced vs. inexperienced). The research employed an 8-week baseline period, systematic behavioral observations, and numerous standardized measures. **Results:** The findings demonstrate that significantly greater gains in prosocial behavior occur on the part of antisocial youths treated in integrated, or prosocial, peer groups (as opposed to antisocial youths treated in groups consisting solely of peers referred for antisocial behavior). Adverse outcomes were not found for the prosocial youths exposed to small numbers of antisocial peers over an 8-month period. **Conclusion:** Group therapists should strive to compose treatment groups for antisocial youths in ways that maximize the likelihood of prosocial behavior gains. Community-based treatment groups consisting primarily of prosocial peers constitute an especially promising venue for such interventions. The complexities and benefits of group treatment can best be studied and revealed through the use of a wide array of rigorous research methods and measures.

S-090-421   Topic: 85, 9

Community-based prosocial groups: A promising venue for treating antisocial behavior

Ronald Feldman, Columbia University, School of Social Work, New York, NY, USA, raf1@columbia.edu

Objective: Employing a highly controlled field experiment, this study examined the efficacy of treating antisocial youths in 'integrated' groups consisting primarily of prosocial peers. **Methods:** A $3 \times 3 \times 2$ factorial design was employed over the course of eight months. The key variables were mode of treatment group composition (antisocial youths only vs. prosocial youths only vs. prosocial youths plus 1–2 antisocial youths), group treatment method (behavioral group treatment vs. traditional group treatment vs. minimal group method), and extent of therapist experience (experienced vs. inexperienced). The research employed a baseline period, systematic behavioral observations by nonparticipant observers, and checklists and self-reports of child behavior and peer group integration. Analyses included proportionate behavioral profiles, arc sine transformations of proportionate behavioral scores, analyses of covariance for changes in behavior, and endpoint, dropout and survivor analyses. **Results:** Significantly greater gains in prosocial behavior occurred on the part of antisocial youths treated in 'integrated', or prosocial, peer groups (as opposed to antisocial youths treated in groups consisting solely of peers referred for antisocial behavior).

Further, prosocial youths in the integrated groups do not manifest higher levels of antisocial behavior than prosocial peers who are not exposed to antisocial peers over the course of eight months. **Conclusion:** Group therapists ought to strive increasingly to structure treatment groups in ways that maximize the likelihood of prosocial behavior gains on the part of adolescent patients. Community-based groups consisting primarily of prosocial peers constitute a particularly promising venue for such interventions.

S-091   Topic: 84
Current neurobiological research results in ADHD
Track: ADHD

Chairperson: Beate Herpertz-Dahlmann,
RWTH Aachen Kinder-u. Jugendpsychiatrie, Aachen,
Germany, bherpertz-dahlmann@ukaachen.de
Andreas Warnke, Universtitätsklinik Würzburg,
Kinder- und Jugendpsychiatrie, Würzburg, Germany,
warnke@kjp.uni-wuerzburg.de

Current neurobiological research results in ADHD
Beate Herpertz-Dahlmann, RWTH Aachen,
Kinder- und Jugendpsychiatrie, Aachen, Germany,
bherpertz-dahlmann@ukaachen.de

This symposium on neurobiological aspects of ADHD is focussed on results in experimental brain imaging. Results suggest less striatal activation (f MRI, Durston et al.) altered brain structures and mechanism (Konrad et al.), source localisation of distinct P 300 components without medation (ERP Brandeis et al., Fallgatter et al) and under stimulant medation (ERP, Warnke et al.).

S-091-422   Topic: 82, 36
Electrophysiological differences in visual information processing between dyslexic children and controls
Andreas Warnke, Universtitätsklinik Würzburg,
Kinder- und Jugendpsychiatrie, Würzburg, Germany,
warnke@kjp.uni-wuerzburg.de
Peter Scheuerpflug; V. Vetter; Ellen Plume; Jürgen Bartling;
Gerd Schulte-Körne; Helmut Remschmidt

Objective: Specific deficits of visual subsystems like the magnocellular and parvocellular systems are assumed for dyslexia. This study examined whether dyslexics compared to controls show different evoked potentials to moving stimuli based by the magnocellular system. **Methods:** We recorded the EEG of 16 dyslexic and 15 control children according to standard parameters and procedures. 2 different tests were conducted: 1. the motion-onset paradigm showed a vertical grating pattern moving with different velocities to the right or left side. 2. the coherent-motion condition showed a random-dot kinematogram with a variable percentage of dots moving coherently to the left or right side. **Results:** Data showed a significant influence of the speed/coherence to ERP-amplitudes, where as significant differences between both groups were detected only in the motion-onset condition. **Conclusion:** We developed motion-specific experiments which might suppose a changed motion detection in dyslexic children under special conditions. Detailed investigations in latency, topography and microstates are discussed.

S-091-423   Topic: 84, 35
Imaging the development of attentional networks and their dysfunction in children with Attention Deficit Hyperactivity Disorder (ADHD)
Kerstin Konrad, RWTH Aachen, Kinder- und
Jugendpsychiatrie, Aachen, Germany, kkonrad@ukaachen.de
Susanne Neufang; Charlotte Hanisch; Gereon R. Fink;
Beate Herpertz-Dahlmann

Objective: The functional development of attentional networks and their dysfunction in children with Attention Deficit/Hyperactivity Disorder (ADHD) is poorly understood. **Methods:** We used event-related functional imaging (fMRI) and a multistep strategy to investigate differences in brain activation related to three particular aspects of attention (alerting, reorienting, executive control) between 16 healthy adults, 16 healthy children and 16 treatment-naïve children with ADHD (aged 8 to 12 years), controlling for effects of task performance or morphometric differences. **Results:** While the normal development of attentional networks was characterized by immature fronto-parieto-cerebellar activation patterns, children with ADHD showed a fronto-striatal dysfunction which was performance-independent and paralleled by structural changes in the same regions. **Conclusion:** Thus, the data provide evidence for developmentally deviant, altered brain structures and mechanisms in treatment naïve ADHD children.

S-091-424   Topic: 84
Activation of striatum and cerebellum in response to expectancy violations in children with ADHD
Sarah Durston, UMC Utrecht, Child Psychiatry, Utrecht,
Netherlands, s.durston@azu.nl
Matthew C. Davidson; Nim Tottenham; Julie Spicer;
Adriana Galvan; John Horvitz; John A. Fossella;
Richard Watts; B. J. Casey

Objective: Cognitive control is dependent on our ability to predict the occurrence of events, based on previous experience. In ADHD, deficits in cognitive control have been associated with reduced activation of striatal and frontal regions. The cerebellum has also been implicated in this disorder, and it has been suggested that input from this structure may modulate activation in these regions. **Methods:** In this study we set out to examine the effect of violations of expectancy in what event occurred and when it occurred on activation of cerebellum and fronto-striatal regions in ADHD, using a rapid mixed-trial fMRI design. We manipulated the probability of events (target and non-target) within a visual detection task, and compared patterns of neural activation to unexpected events and the omission of expected events. **Results:** Our preliminary results suggest that children with ADHD show less striatal activation during violations of expectancy than subjects without ADHD, even in the absence of behavioral differences. In contrast, however, activation of the cerebellum appears similar to that in healthy children and adults for this task. These findings add to previous reports of reduced striatal activation in ADHD, but suggests that activation in the cerebellum may be less affected. **Conclusion:** One preliminary conclusion that may be drawn from these findings is that fronto-cerebellar circuits may be functioning adequately, but may not be able to modulate cognitively controlled actions through fronto-striatal circuits that have been shown to be disrupted in children with ADHD.

S-091-425   Topic: 84
Separating attention and control deficits of ADHD children through electrophysiological timing and topography

Daniel Brandeis, Universität Zürich, Kinder- und Jugendpsychiatrie, Zürich, SwitzerlandTobias Banaschewski

Objective: Deficits of attention and control in ADHD (Attention Deficit Hyperactivity Disorder) have proven difficult to separate on theoretical and empirical grounds. We examine how the increased resolution of event-related potential mapping, the use of tests separating aspects of attention and response control, and the control over comorbid disorders has improved this situation. **Methods:** Brain mapping of attention and response control in the cued continuous performance task (CPT A–X/O–X) was performed using topographic event-related potentials (ERPs). In studies with up to 148 participants, performance and ERPs of children with ADHD combined, and of ADHD children with and without comorbid ODD/CD were compared to normal controls. **Results:** Deficits of attention and/or response control were detected in all ADHD groups. Topographic recordings separated the distinct P300 components to cue, go, and no go signals, and permitted source localisation. While attention deficits dominated and preceded the response control in pure ADHD groups, response control deficits were the most prominent marker of ADHD children with comorbid ODD/CD. **Conclusion:** Timing and topography of ERPs distinguishes covert brain activation due to attention, preparation, and response control. It reveals multiple attention and regulation problems rather than isolated inhibition deficits in ADHD.

S-091-426   Topic: 84, 36
Altered response control and anterior cingulate function in ADHD

Andreas J. Fallgatter, Universität Würzburg, Psychiatrie und Psychotherapie, Würzburg, Germany, fallgatter^a@klinik.uni-wuerzburg.de
Ann-Christine Ehlis; Jürgen Seifert; W. K. Strik; Peter Scheuerpflug; K. E. Zillessen; Martin J. Herrmann

Objective: To measure deficits in allocation of attention as well as in response control and inhibition, which belong to the clinical core deficits in ADHD. These symptoms may in part be explained by a dysfunction of the anterior cingulate cortex (ACC), which is considered as an important interface between prefrontal cortex and limbic system. **Methods:** By means of a simple method (Continuous Performance Test with simultaneous 21 channel-EEG), it seems feasible to measure an electrophysiological correlate of the ACC-function termed NoGo-Anteriorisation, NGA. This ERP-measure is characterized by a high interindividual stability, a high short- and long-term test-retest reliability and is independent from age- and gender. **Results:** The NGA was diminished in 24 adult patients with personality disorders and additional hints for an ADHD during childhood as compared to age- and gendermatched healthy controls. By means of a three-dimensional source location analysis with LORETA an electrical dysfunction of the ACC in this patient group was shown. Moreover, a corresponding dysfunction of the ACC was also found in children with ADHD in comparison to healthy control children. **Conclusion:** In future studies the questions will be addressed whether this electrophysiological endopheno-type may contribute to the diagnosis of subgroups of ADHD and to the measurement of treatment effects on ACC-function.

S-092   Topic: 82
Early precursors and genetics in dyslexia
Track: Therapy and intervention

Chairperson: Gerd Schulte-Körne, Universitätsklinik Marburg Kinder- und Jugendpsychiatrie, Marburg, Germany, schulte1@med.uni-marburg.de
Heikki Lyytinen, University of Jyväskylä Child Research Center, Jyväskylä, Finland

Early precursors and genetics in dyslexia

Gerd Schulte-Körne, Universitätsklinik Marburg, Kinder- und Jugendpsychiatrie, Marburg, Germany, schulte1@med.uni-marburg.de

Dyslexia is a specific disorder in learning to read and spell in spite of adequate educational resources, normal intelligence, no obvious sensory deficits, and adequate sociocultural opportunity. Dyslexia occurs in all alphabetic orthographies, and especially spelling disorder often persists into adulthood. Although dyslexia can be diagnosed at school age the identification of early precursors is important step into early diagnosis and prevention. The Jyväskylä Longitudinal study of Dyslexia (JLD) is a follow-up study from birth to adolescence of children at risk for dyslexia and control children. A large battery of psychosocial, neuropsychological and neurophysiological measurements were applied to the children and their parents. Dyslexia tends to run in families, a finding noted for the first time at the beginning of the last century. Family studies revealed a familial aggregation of dyslexia with a familial recurrence of about 40–50%. The analysis of familial patterns suggested a higher risk for siblings and parents of a child disabled for reading and spelling independent of the child's orthography. Segregation analyses for both the clinical entities and quantitative traits have been undertaken and suggest that dyslexia generally does not segregate in a simple Mendelian fashion but needs to be interpreted as a complex genetic disease. Both linkage analyses and association studies have identified possible loci on chromosomes 1, 2, 3, 6, 15, and 18.

S-092-426A Highlights of the results from a longitudinal study of Dyslexia from birth to school age

Heikki Lyytinen, University of Jyväskylä, Child Research Center, Jyväskylä, Finland

The Jyväskylä Longitudinal study of Dyslexia (JLD) has now followed two hundred children up to school age. Half of them are at familial risk for dyslexia. About half of the at risk group have acquired reading skill late their achievements are at the level of the lowest 10% of the control group. This presentation complements the two papers which examine the predictive role of brain event-related potentials collected at an early age in the JLD and one which analyses the role of environmental factors in supporting reading-related development. Here, the role of language development is reviewed on the basis of measures taken from different ages from 2 to 7 years. It will be shown how early identification of difficulty to acquire basic reading skill is possible using relatively easily implemented measures. This introduces a challenging question how is this knowledge applied for the benefit of the children? A method for early prevention executed before school age is proposed and promising pilot results of the related operations are illustrated.

S-092-427   Topic: 82, 36

Brain event-related potentials (ERPs) to speech stimuli at birth are associated with reading skills in children with abd without familial risk for dyslexia

Tomi Guttorm, University of Jyväskylä, Department of Psychology, Jyväskylä, Finland, tomi.guttorm@psyka.jyu.fi
Paavo Leppänen; Anna-Maija Poikkeus; Kenneth M. Eklund; Paula Lyytinen; Heikki Lyytinen

Objective: To predict later language and reading skills from newborn ERPs in children with and without familial risk for dyslexia. **Methods:** ERPs to synthetic consonant-vowel syllables (/ba/, /da/, /ga/; presented equiprobably with 3910–7285 ms interstimulus intervals) were recorded from 26 newborns at risk for familial dyslexia and 23 control infants participating in the Jyväskylä Longitudinal Study of Dyslexia. Later language skills were measured at 2.5, 3.5, and 5 years of age, and early reading skills were measured at 6.5 and 7 years of age. **Results:** The correlation and regression analyses showed that the at-risk type of response pattern at birth (a slower shift in polarity from positivity to negativity in responses to/ga/at 540–630 ms, the latency identified by principal component analysis) in the right hemisphere was related to significantly poorer receptive language skills across both groups at the age of 2.5 years. The similar ERP pattern in the left hemisphere was associated with poorer verbal memory skills at the age of 5 years. Our preliminary results also show that newborn ERPs are associated with early reading skills. The responses in the left hemisphere predicted poorer reading skills at 6.5 years, and poorer reading accuracy and fluency, as well as poorer spelling skills, at 7 years of age in children with and without familial risk for dyslexia. **Conclusion:** These results indicate that newborn ERPs predict later language and reading problems, and would thus have applications in the future for the early identification of children at risk for developmental language problems. This would further facilitate well-directed interventions even before language problems are typically diagnosed.

S-092-428   Topic: 82, 42

Longitudinal associations between literacy environment, literacy interest and phonological awareness development in children with and without familial risk of Dyslexia

Minna Torppa, University of Jyväskylä, Dept. of Psychology, Jyväskylä, Finland, minna.torppa@psyka.jyu.fi
Anna-Maija Poikkeus; M.-L. Laakso; E. Leskinen; Paavo Leppänen; A. Tolvanen; Heikki Lyytinen

Objective: To examine the development and associations between home literacy environment, children's literacy interest, and phonological awareness development in children with and without familial risk of dyslexia. **Methods:** Out of 187 children, 97 had a familial background of reading difficulties (the at-risk group), and 90 children came from families without such background (the control

group). All of the families were participants of Jyväskylä Longitudinal Study of dyslexia. Parental reports of home literacy environment and children's literacy interest were collected at ages 4, 5, and 6 years and phonological awareness was assessed at ages 4.5, 5.5, and 6.5 years. We employed Latent Growth Curve (LGC) modeling, which allowed us to analyze both multivariate developmental change and individual variations. **Results:** On average, the at-risk group children manifested lower phonological awareness than the control children at every assessment time, and their parents were less active readers themselves than the control group parents. Group differences did not emerge in frequency of parent-child shared reading, access to written language, or children's literacy interest. In the at-risk group (but not in the control group), we found children's higher literacy interest and more frequent parent-child shared reading to be associated with faster development in phonological awareness. **Conclusion:** Because of their inherited vulnerability for phonological processing deficits the children with genetic risk of dyslexia may require extra support from their environment for age-appropriate development of phonological awareness.

S-092-429   Topic: 82, 28

Association analysis and candidate gene screening for the dyslexia susceptibility locus on chromosome 6p

Silvia Paracchini, University of Oxford, WTCHG, Oxford, United Kingdom, silviap@well.ox.ac.uk

Dyslexia is one of the most prevalent of childhood cognitive disorders, and is caused in large part by genetic factors. Linkage studies have identified regions of several chromosomes as containing putative quantitative trait loci (QTL) for this disorder. In particular, linkage to a locus on 6p21.3–22 has been found in at least five independent samples, including our own.We have previously shown, using multivariate linkage analysis, that the QTL on 6p21.3–23 seems to influence variability shared between reading-related measures, but not shared with measures of general intelligence (IQ), suggesting that IQ could be treated as noise, in further analysis of this specific locus. Controlling for IQ in linkage analysis we have refined the mapping of the QTL to a 5.8 Mb interval. Within this interval we selected genes, known to be brain-expressed, for association analysis using single nucleotide polymorphisms (SNPs). Initial significant associations within a sample of 89 nuclear families from the UK were followed up in additional families from the UK and Colorado. Mutation screening of the genes surrounding the associations was carried out.

S-092-430   Topic: 82, 28

Linkage analyses on chromosomal region 18p 11 in Dyslexia: Results from the German bicenter study

Gerd Schulte-Körne, Universitätsklinik Marburg, Kinder- und Jugendpsychiatrie, Marburg, Germany, schulte1@med.uni-marburg.de
J. Schumacher; Ellen Plume; I.R. König; Claudia Libertus; Heide Griesemann; A. Kleensang; A. Ziegler; Andreas Warnke; P. Propping; Helmut Remschmidt; M. Nöthen

Objective: We are performing a German bi-center study to analyze the molecular genetic background of dyslexia. Employing a single proband sib pair design, we have included

82 dyslectic children with at least one sibling and both parents in a study to replicate the previously reported chrosomome 18 linkage. In this sample, we genotyped 14 STR-markers, covering a 36 Mb interval on chromosome 18p11–q12. In addition to linkage analysis, we performed quantitative transmission disequilibrium (QTDT) analysis using 6 STR-markers within the linkage peak observed by Fisher et al. [2002]. **Results:** Using a battery of component processes as quantitative traits (word reading, spelling, phonological decoding, phoneme awareness, short term memory, rapid naming), we failed to detect NPL-scores above 1 in the single-point and multipoint linkage analyses. In parallel, we performed QTDT analysis and observed some associations between single-word reading and rapid-naming ability and STR-markers within the linkage peak observed by Fisher et al. [2002]. **Conclusion:** There are several possible explanations for our finding: First, the association results are false-positives and no QTL in this chromosomal region exists in our study population. Second, putative disease genes on chromosome 18p11 might confer a small relative risk to the development of dyslexia in the sample under study. In this case, the borderline association findings in the present study could be indicative for a genetic risk factor with small effect which, due to limited power, was not detected in our linkage analysis. Significantly larger linkage and association samples would be needed to reliably detect these effects. Dyslexia is a specific disorder in learning to read and spell in spite of adequate educational resources and normal intelligence. It affects about 5% of school-aged children, making it the most common of childhood learning disorders, and especially spelling disorder often persists into adulthood. Linkage studies have previously identified regions likely to harbour genes contributing to dyslexia, including regions on the short arm of chromosome 18 (Fisher et al. 2002).

S-093   Topic: 53, 3
Child and family focused interventions after trauma and disaster

Chairperson: James Leckman, Yale University Child Study Center, New Haven, USA, james.leckman@yale.edu

Child and family focused interventions after trauma and disaster

Ernesto Caffo, University of Modena, Dept. of Neuroscience, Modena, Italy, caffo@unimo.it

Each year millions of children are exposed to some form of extreme traumatic stressor. Traumatic events include natural disasters (e.g., tornadoes, floods, hurricanes), motor vehicle accidents, life-threatening illnesses and associated painful medical procedures (eg, severe burns, cancer, limb amputations), physical abuse, sexual assault, witnessing domestic or community violence, kidnapping, and sudden death of a parent. During times of war, violent and nonviolent trauma (e.g., lack of fuel and food) may have terrible effects on children's adjustment. The events of September 11, 2001 and March 11, 2004 and the unceasing suicidal attacks in the Middle East underscore the importance of understanding how children and adolescents react to disasters and terrorism. Mental health professionals are increasing their understanding about what factors are associated with increased risk (vulnerability) and affect how children cope with traumatic events. Most victims of trau-

matic experiences, children included, develop adaptation processes and react positively, both if they have been experiencing trauma directly or indirectly. It exists, however, a significant proportion of children who develop high levels of psychological distress after traumatic events, which interfere with child's social and family life and his/her developmental and learning processes. PTSD, anxiety and mood disorders, sleep disorders, conduct disorders, learning and attention disorders (ADHD) are the most common psychiatric problems following traumatic experiences. In terms of providing treatment, CBT emerges as the best validated therapeutic approach for children and adolescents who experienced trauma-related symptoms, particularly symptoms associated with anxiety or mood disorders. Family support also may be necessary to help the family through this difficult period. School must be also prepared and trained in how to manage negative emotions that may arise from traumatic experiences. Preventive strategies for fostering resilience should be tested in future controlled psychotherapy trials to verify their efficacy on children's protective factors.

S-093-431   Topic: 53, 21
The role of teachers in school reactivation programs after mass disaster

Leo Wolmer, Tel Aviv University, Tel Aviv, Israel, tlv_cmhc@netvision.net.il

Two weeks after the August 1999 earthquake in Turkey, Israeli mental health professionals initiated a multi-disciplinary effort to develop and implement a program of Community Reactivation for a displaced population in Adapazari. This presentation will describe the first phase of the process, which focused on the psychological reactivation of students and teachers. Baseline assessment showed that most of the teachers and the children were experiencing posttraumatic phenomena, with 32% of the children reporting severe symptomatology. The implementation of the School Reactivation Program consisted of (1) a session with the teachers with two objectives: debriefing and enhancement of motivation and commitment. (2) The presentation of the program to and training of the teachers. (3) An introductory session with the parents. (4) Nine 2-hour class meetings. The class meetings were led by the teachers and supervised weekly by mental health professionals. The program focused on issues such as loss and grief, anger, guilt and developing a vision of a better future. Children were allowed to normalize responses, share experiences, express and learn cognitive-behavioral ways to cope with inner suffering, all modelled by an imaginary friend communicating his experiences to the children through his letters. After the end of the program we observed a significant decrease in posttraumatic and dissociative symptoms, and a significant increase in symptoms of grief. Processes, results and risk factors will be discussed. Three years later, we followed-up a group of children (n=66) who participated in the program and a control group of children who experienced the earthquake and received no intervention (n=210). A significant symptomatic decrease was observed in the participating kids, who also showed a better functioning (academic, social and behavioral) compared to control kids, as reported by the teachers.

S-093-432   Topic: 53, 9
Group therapeutic interventions for children and adolescents exposed to war: Lessons learned from research

John Fayyad, St. George Hospital, Psychiatry and Psychology, Beirut, Lebanon, jfayyad@inco.com.lb

Objective: The purpose of this presentation is to review studies of group and community interventions delivered to populations of children and adolescents exposed to war trauma. **Methods:** While there are many accounts in the literature describing the implementation of various psychosocial interventions in various communities following war trauma, only a few used control groups to measure the effect of the intervention. Only studies with sufficient sample sizes and/or control groups including data from the presenter's own research group will be included in this review. **Results:** Studies on group, community and school-based interventions following war trauma suffer from methodological shortcomings more than studies of populations exposed to non-war traumatic events, probably due to the difficulties of conducting research in war environments. Control groups in war studies so far have only consisted of subjects on a waiting list which does not constitute an adequate control group for research in psychotherapy as it does not control for nonspecific therapist/group leader therapeutic effects. Data from a controlled community group treatment of war exposed children will be briefly presented and discussed. **Conclusion:** Combining results of prospective studies of war exposed children (showing that symptoms subside spontaneously in many) with those from controlled treatment studies calls into question the wisdom of mass interventions for this population with policy and planning implications. A suggested paradigm for the nature and timing of mental health interventions following war will be presented.

S-093-433   Topic: 3, 53
A community based and individual based intervention to overcome the negative consequences of warlike situation

Iyad Zaqout, GCMHP, Research Dept., Gaza, Palestinian Territories, iyadzaqout@gcmhp.net

Objective: Overcome the negative consequences of political violence on Palestinian children. **Methods:** A group (10-15) of Palestinian children will be exposed to the intervention and then their reactions analysed. **Results:** These children will be more amenable to develop a mature communicative style thus helping them to cope with the Trauma. **Conclusion:** There must be a trend in psychotherapy especially in dealing with traumatized children to overcome the revenge and frustration associated with the exposure to trauma to prevent the development of angry aggression which can be destructive to the self, the community, and the other communities.

S-093-434   Topic: 53
The effects of ongoing terrorism on children and adolescents

Esti Galili-Weisstub, Hadassa University, Medical Center, Jerusalem, Israel

This presentation deals with children's reactions to trauma as a result of terrorism. First we will present clinical material, describe a therapeutic tool used in the ER of a general hospital, and offer data regarding the prediction of PTSD based on risk factors. Then we will describe a practical, comprehensive, and flexible approach used in the treatment of traumatized minors as a result of terrorism. Finally we will discuss the psychological effects of ongoing terrorism on the psyche of the young members of our society.

S-094   Topic: 24, 28
Genetics, genomics and neurobehavioral phenotypes: Clinical implications

Chairperson: Gene Fisch, New York, NY, USA, gfisch@nshs.edu

Genetics, genomics and neurobehavioral phenotypes: Clinical implications

Gene Fisch, New York, NY, USA, gfisch@nshs.edu

Cognitive impairment or mental retardation (MR) produced by genetic mutations are often comorbid with other behavioral pathology. Typically, genetic disorders that produce MR are associated with specific cognitive-behavioral profiles, or phenotypes. We examine several genetic disorders the fragile X mutation, Williams-Beuren syndrome, velo-cardiofacial syndrome, Prader-Willi syndrome, Angelman syndrome, and, from a clinical perspective, autism to examine the cognitive-behavioral similarities and differences among these disorders, and, in some instances, the longitudinal changes in cognitive-behavioral abilities that may occur as individuals with these disorders age. Comorbid pathology and changes that occur over time have clinical implications for families, caregivers and educators. Speakers will address these issues for each of the disorders presented.

S-094-435   Topic: 24, 28
Behavioural phenotype of the Fragile-X-Syndrome

Alexander von Gontard, Uniklinik des Saarlandes, Homburg, Germany, alexander.von.gontard@uniklinik-saarland.de

Objective: To identify the specific cognitive and behavioural phenotype in boys with a fully mutated Fragile-X Syndrome, as well as effects on the family. **Methods:** 49 boys with a full mutation aged 5.7 to 16.10 years were recruited through parental self-help groups. Intelligence was examined with the K-ABC. Clinically relevant psychopathology was assessed with a structured psychiatric interview (Kinder-DIPS) and by the Child Behavior Checklist (CBCL). Social support was measured with the F-SOZU, parental stress with the QRS and parental coping with the F-COPES questionnaire. **Results:** The mean IQ-equivalents of the K-ABC were: 46.6 for the mental processing composite, 46.1 for the sequential processing, 46.4 for the simultaneous processing and 48.8 for the achievement scales. The most common DSM-IV diagnoses were ADHD (74%), followed by oppositional defiant disorder (29%), functional enuresis (27%), functional encopresis (20%), separation anxiety disorder (10%) and obsessive compulsive disorder (2%). 89% had a CBCL total score in the clinical and borderline range, 63.3% internalising and 67.3% externalising behaviour scores. Families with a FXS child had a high total stress level, influenced bith the high rate of DSM-IV diagnoses and aggressive, externalising behaviour (CBCL). Social support was inversely correlated with stress. The higher the stress was perceived, the less parents were able to cope actively, but resorted to passive forms of coping. **Conclusion:** Boys with a FXS show a specific behavioural phenotype with moderate mental retardation and a high rate of externalising behavioural disorders. Parents are highly stressed and require intense support and counselling.

S-094-436 Topic: 24, 28
The cognitive-behavioural spectrum in Chronosome 22q11 deletion and its implications for practice and management: The Leuven experience

Ann Swillen, University Hospital of Leuven, Center for Human Genetics, Leuven, Belgium, ann.swillen@uz.kuleuven.ac.be

Objective: To define and describe the cognitive-behavioural spectrum in children and adolescents with the chromosome 22q11 deletion syndrome (Velo-Cardio-Facial syndrome/DiGeorge syndrome), and the implications for practice and management. **Methods:** More than 200 persons with the del22q11 are followed up in Leuven. Intelligence, neuropsychological functions, and behaviour were assessed using standardized tests and multi-informant questionnaires. All children were observed at home and in the school setting. **Results:** There is a wide variability in the cognitive and behavioural spectrum of the del22q11 syndrome, which highlights the importance of individual assessments. However, a subgroup of children and adolescents with a 22q11 deletion have a typical cognitive and learning profile which can be indicative of a non-verbal learning disability (NVLD). Interestingly, the VIQ>PIQ discrepancies have been more observed among children and adolescents with a del22q11 than in adults with the syndrome. From preschool age on, both girls and boys with the del22q11 experience problems in the areas of social development (problems in relationships with peers, social withdrawal), attention and problem-solving. In puberty, anxieties and depressed mood are often reported by parents and teachers. **Conclusion:** Individuals with the del22q11 and their families need a holistic and multidisciplinary approach. Information, support and a coordinated care by a multidisciplinary expert-team are indispensable. An individualized educational plan for the child is required, and this should include training of both verbal (language/communication, articulation, (reading) comprehension) and non-verbal areas (motor skills, visual-spatial organization, cognitive retraining, general mathematical training, attention, and remediation of early social deficits).

S-094-437 Topic: 24, 28
Psychosis in the Prader-Willi-Syndrome: Phenomenology and behavioral characteristics during childhood

Annick Vogels, University Hospital of Leuven, Center for Human Genetics, Leuven, Belgium, annick.vogels@uz.kuleuven.ac.be

Objective: The present work gives a comprehensive overview of the occurrence of PWS in Flanders and confirms the association of PWS with psychotic disorders in the Flemish population. We give a detailed description of the psychiatric phenomenology of psychotic disorders in PWS and the natural history of these disorders in childhood. This work leads to a better understanding of the complex symptomatology and hopefully will lead to early diagnosis and treatment of these severe psychiatric manifestations. **Methods:** To estimate the prevalence, the method of counting all known PWS cases with a molecular confirmed diagnosis in a well-defined geographic region was used. In a second stage we wanted to confirm the association of psychosis with PWS and describe the phenomenology of this psychotic episodes. A group of 54 PWS persons was studied and 6 out of these 54 persons were diagnosed with psychotic disorder. The diagnosis was made on the base of personal observation and video recordings, family and carers informants, medical records and psychiatric reports. All 6 patient underwent psychiatric assessment using the operational criteria (OPCRIT) checklist for affective and psychotic illness. All 54 individuals had regular follow up over the past fifteen years. All case material of these patients was reviewed and detailed behavioural description during childhood was obtained from family members, caregivers, teachers and general practitioners. **Results:** The birth incidence in Flanders for the period 1993–2001 was 1:26.676, the minimum prevalence at 31.12.2001 was 1:76.574. Sixteen percent of the total group of PWS persons were diagnosed with psychotic episodes confirming the association of PWS with psychosis. An identifiable subtype of psychotic disorder was found characterized by early age of onset, acute onset, polymorphous and shifting symptomatology and a need for psychiatric hospitalization. The presence of precipitating stress factors and a prodromal phase with physiological symptoms was reported in all patients. Current diagnostic categories did not allow an unequivocal psychiatric diagnosis. **Conclusion:** In four of the six individuals with a history psychotic episodes, a characteristic behavioral pattern during childhood was found: they were described as active and extravert toddlers and showed autistic features during their primary school education.

S-094-438 Topic: 24, 28
Chromosome 15q11–13 and related phenotypes: Prader-Willi-Syndrome, Angelman Syndrome and autism spectrum disorders

Christine Freitag, Universitätsklinikum Saarland, Abt. Kinderpsychiatrie, Homburg, Germany, christine.freitag@uniklinik-saarland.de

Objective: We will review the phenotypic and genetic findings of the three known Chromosome 15q11–13 disorders and discuss differential diagnosis and treatment. **Methods:** Common features, such as developmental delay, are found in all three syndromes. Epilepsy, speech delay and hand flapping frequently occur in Angelman Syndrome and in Autism. Individuals with Prader-Willi-Syndrome can show a similar rigidity, compulsions, self-abuse and occasionally a superior performance regarding visuospacial abilities as individuals with autism. This leads to the hypothesis that there may be a genotype-phenotype relationship and a genetic basis for the commonalities between these disorders. **Results:** Deletions and duplications of Chromosome 15q11–13 lead to different phenotypes: a paternal deletion of a more proximal part will result in Prader-Willi-Syndrome, a maternal deletion of a slightly more distal part or a point mutation in the UBE3A gene is found in Angelman-Syndrome and maternal duplications or inverted duplications, resulting in tri- or tetrasomy, are associated with autism or autism spectrum disorders. **Conclusion:** We will discuss implications for the genetics of autism.

S-094-439   Topic: 24, 28
Longitudinal studies of cognitive-behavioral development in children and adolescents with genetic disorders

Gene Fisch, New York, NY, USA, gfisch@nshs.edu

Objective: Children with mental retardation (MR) are often thought to retain stable IQ scores as they get older, although children with Down syndrome exhibit declines in IQ scores as they age. The objective is to examine prospective longitudinal changes in cognitive ability and/or adaptive behavior levels in children with fragile X syndrome (FXS), Williams syndrome (WS) and autism (AD). **Methods:** We examined N = 54 children matched in age, ages 5–15 years, and diagnosed exclusively for the fragile X mutation (n = 18), or the ELN deletion in WS (n = 18), or clinically for AD (n = 18). To assess cognitive abilities (IQ), we administered the Stanford-Binet (4th Ed.) (SBFE). To obtain a measure of adaptive behavior (DQ), we interviewed parents using the Vineland Adaptive Behavior Scales (VABS). Children were tested initially, then retested 2 years later using both SBFE and VABS. **Results:** We find age-related and longitudinal declines in IQ and DQ in all children with FXS, most children with WS, a decline in IQ and DQ among younger children with AD, but an increase in IQ scores in older children with AD. Typically, younger children with FXS or WS test in the mild MR range, but as they age, their scores decline into the moderate MR range. Curiously, although FXS and WS appear as very different syndromes clinically, their cognitive and behavioral profiles exhibit similar strengths and weaknesses. **Conclusion:** Given our results, we suggest that cognitive and adaptive behavior in children with any genetic disorder that produces cognitive impairment be monitored continually as these children age.

S-095   Topic: 45
Research and clinical work in transcultural settings

Chairperson: Felicia Heidenreich, Médecins sans Frontières Hôpital Avicenne, Bobigny Cedex, France, felicia.heidenreich@avc.ap-hop-paris.fr

Research and clinical work in transcultural settings

Felicia Heidenreich, Médecins sans Frontières, Hôpital Avicenne, Bobigny Cedex, France, felicia.heidenreich@avc.ap-hop-paris.fr

This symposium wants to give an overview on different research projects and clinical work with children and adolescents in situations where clinician or researcher are not of the same origin as the patients. Understanding psychopathology and normal functioning in these situations demands specific tools and an approach where the different positions are constantly questioned. The topics are varied and include: 1) a study analysing attachment patterns and developmental processes in refugee children while families are waiting for political asylum in France, 2) a report on work in a MSF run children's center in central China with children in difficult circumstances, 3) a research project on bilingualism in immigrant children in Paris suburbs, 4) an overview about clinical work with children of different cultures in Brazil. What reunites these very diverse contributions is the strive to develop strategies to a better understanding of key issues in working in transcultural settings.

S-095-440   Topic: 54, 48
Child attachment strategies in families seeking refugee status: A study in French family refugee centers

Jean-François Bouville, Paris, France, jbouvil@yahoo.com
Felicia Heidenreich; Laetitia Atlanti-Duault;
Marie Rose Moro

Objective: To investigate parent-child attachment relationships in families seeking refugy status in France during their stay in family refugy centers. Parent-child relationships are impacted by important changes in family structure and the necessity to cope with disorganizing past and present events. How do children cope emotionally and continue to rely, more specifically, on their parents for emotional security? **Methods:** Child attachment patterns were assessed based on open-ended interviews with 21 children 5 to 12 years old and their parents seen separately in 4 family refugy centers, as well as simplified versions of the Attachment Story Completion Task (Bretherton, Ridgeway and Cassidy, 1990) and EDICODE (Pierrehumbert, Dieckmann, Milkovitch de Heredia, 1999). **Results:** Child attachment strategies and the nature of parent-child relationships were closely associated with child age and type of family structure. **Conclusion:** A better understanding of the different ways children "use" their parents to cope emotionally in family refugy centers could help improve intervention programs on their behalf.

S-095-441   Topic: 45
Psychotherapy with children in difficult circumstances in central China

Felicia Heidenreich, Médecins sans Frontières,
Hôpital Avicenne, Bobigny Cedex, France,
felicia.heidenreich@avc.ap-hop-paris.fr
Thierry Baubet; Robyn Osrow; Marie-Madeleine Leplomb;
Yves Marchandy

Objective: Since 2001 MSF runs a center for children in difficult circumstances who have been picked up in the streets by authorities in a middle-size chinese town. Besides shelter, food, schooling, medical care and social work provided for by a team of expatriate and chinese staff, an expatriate psychologist or psychiatrist proposes psychotherapy. Most of the children have experienced battering, violence, poverty and neglect and many of them show symptoms of deprivation, depression and trauma. **Methods:** This contribution explicits the particular setting of psychotherapy inside the center with an interpreter. Emphasis will be put on strategies of using cultural material brought up by the children in working on resilience and re-establishing family links. **Results:** Doing psychotherapeutic work in a transcultural setting in China confronts the expatriate mental health workers with cultural ways of expressing and explaining distress. He will also have to face different representations of his function and activity. All of these encounters need to be explicit and can be used as "therapeutic or paedagogical tools" both in psychotherapy and in teaching of local staff. **Conclusion:** In humanitarian mental health programs it is essential to work not only with cultural representations of disease but also question representations concerning therapeutic methods and health care professionals.

S-095-442　Topic: 45

Bilingualism in second generation immigrants in Paris suburbs

Malika Bennabi, University of Picardie, Jules Verne, Amiens, France

Can bilingualism of immigrant children be considered as a factor which obstructs educational issues, or as an element which favours cognitive development? First, we will show that, in order to understand the actual situation, we must consider the representations affecting immigrant children through representations affecting the languages of immigration. In France, unfavourable representations of certain foreign languages, in addition to the conception of bilingualism as a factor impairing cognitive development, are prevalent in the educational or health professions. Based on research on bilingualism with children and parents, (trough two approaches: cognitive study of language awareness with young bilingual children and clinical analysis of interviews with parents) we will try to show how young children may construct their development in two languages, in a context overlooked by monolinguism. We will analyse factors of immigrant bilingualism to define those favouring or, on the contrary, those obstructing the acquisition of the second language at school.

S-095-443　Topic: 48

Primary care interventions with mothers and babies at risk

Salvador Celia, Instituto Leo Kanner Ltoa, Child Psychiatry, Porto Alegre, Brazil, sahc@terra.com.br
Ricardo Halpern; Odon Monteiro

Objective: This study was design to evaluate early signs of problems in mother and child bonding, in a primary care setting in a small city in southern Brazil. **Methods:** During a immunization campain, a five itens scale with concerns about mother and child bonding was used in children from 0 to 12 months to identify possible problems in bonding. The whole group of children 580 and their mothers were evaluated. From this group all children identified as having possible problems were assigned as cases and the next child in the list without concern was assigned as control. A home visit was done and a questionnaire with sociodemografic and socioecononic questions was answered by the mothers along with the Beck Scale to identified signs of maternal depression. In order to evaluate possible associations amongs selected variables a qui square test was performed. **Results:** 98 families were visited in the second part of the study. 48 of them were assigned as having possible concerns in mother and child bonding according to the proposed scale, and 50 were controls. In those families identified as having problems we found a significant proportion of adolescent mothers, with low level of schooling. Signs of depression compared with those identified as not having problems in the first interview was significantly higher (p < 0.05). Also they breastfed their chidren less than those without problems (p < 0.05) and had a higher level of stress. The profile of family identified having problems belongs to low socioeconomic status and are migrants without roots in the comunity. **Conclusion:** This study showed that this five itens scale was able to identified early signs of problems in maternal and child bonding. Further studies should be done with a representative sample in order to verify the external validity of this scale. The use of this scale in primary care setting could give to health professional and inportant tool to prevent problems

and promote child's mental health. It is important to pay attention to this group of families compose of migrants who presented a higher level of problems. Because their mobility seeking job opportunities it is very difficult to identified and follow them to provide an adequate mental health care.

S-096　Topic: 85, 27

Aggression, conduct disorder and clinical research: New findings

Chairperson: Hans Steiner, Stanford University School of Psychiatry, Stanford, CA, USA, steiner@stanford.edu
Fritz Poustka, Universität Frankfurt Kinder- und Jugendpsychiatrie, Frankfurt, Germany, poustka@em. uni-frankfurt.de

Aggression, conduct disorder and clinical research: New findings

Hans Steiner, Stanford University, School of Psychiatry, Stanford, CA, USA, steiner@stanford.edu

This symposium will present results from three different sites, Stanford University, USA, Universitaet Wien, Oesterreich und J.W.Goethe Universitaet Frankfurt, Deutschland regarding new findings in clinical and basic research on conduct disorders. Professors Steiner and Poustka will cochair the symposium. Dr. Steiner will provide an overview of the problems with the diagnoses of conduct disorder. He will propose a subtyping on the basis of types of aggression and personality. He will then present data from 850 delinquents supporting the model. Dr. Belinda Plattner will present similar findings from a data base in Vienna, Austria. Dr. Poustka will then introduce his research team who will present new data on emotion processing (Dr. Christina Stadler) and Platelet 5 HT uptake (Dr. Irene Nowraty) in boys with conduct disorder. The symposium will conclude with a discussion by all participants of the implication of the findings for an improved diagnostic taxonomy.

S-096-444　Topic: 85, 57

Proactive and reactive aggression in subtypes of conduct disordered incarcerated delinquents

Hans Steiner, Stanford University, School of Psychiatry, Stanford, CA, USA, steiner@stanford.edu
Laura Delizonna; Abbey-Robin Durkin; Rudy Haapanen

Objective: Conduct disorder is a problematic diagnosis with great reliability but questionable validity. In order to refine this diagnostic category, we need to find valid subtypes which have implications for diagnosis, treatment and outcome. These subtypes need to be generated from ecologically valid samples. We report the performance of a promising intermediate phenotype, the subtypes of aggression, in a large sample of incarcerated juveniles. Our prediction was that proactive aggression would be found more prevalent in low restraint CD and youths not suffering from anxiety or mood disorders; while reactive aggression would be more prevalent in high distress youths and those who suffered from anxiety and mood disorders. **Methods:** We studied 850 (140 girls, mean age 16) incarcerated youths in the California Youth Authority. We conducted structured interviews (SCID, DICA) and collected standardized self report instruments (Weinberger Adjustment Inventory; Achenbach Youth Self Report; Massachussetts Youth Screening Instrument). Almost 100% of youths fulfilled criteria for conduct disorder. Excluding those who did not (6%), we conducted Analyses of variance, testing the main effects of psychopathology (clustered diagnoses of anxiety and mood) and a well validated typology based on personality traits, while controlling for gender effects. **Results:** The results confirmed our hypotheses (all p's < 0.05). Clustered diagnoses of anxiety and mood resulted in significantly higher YSR aggression scores, as did the reactive subtype on the Weinberger 4 quadrant typology. Delinquent act subscores were elevated in youths with low restraint compared to those with high restraint. Additionally, clustered diagnoses of anxiety and mood were significantly more prevalent in the reactive subtype, lending further convergent validity to our typology and findings. **Conclusion:** This study provides strong support for the subdivision of the conduct disorder diagnosis along the lines of clustered comorbidity and the constructs of Reactive/affective/Defensive (RADI) versus Planned/instrumental/Proactive/Predatory (PIPP) aggression. The sub-typing has implications for taxonomy, treatment and prognosis, as we have shown in previous studies.

S-096-445   Topic: 57
Austria's juvenile justice system:
Characteristics of programs, staff and delinquents

Belinda Plattner, Universitätsklinik Wien,
Abt. Neuropsychiatrie, Wien, Austria, bplattner@gmx.at
Susanne Bauer; Max Friedrich; Hans Steiner

Objective: To describe the Austrian Juvenile Justice System, its staffing and its occupants. To provide a contrast of the characteristics to the systems in the US and other European countries. The Austrian system has a strong tradition of early and preventive intervention which dates back to the 1930's. **Methods:** We examined crime statistics, population characteristics staffing patterns. We employed site visits and summary of clinical data in the two settings dealing with incarcerated youths. **Results:** In all of Austria, a country of some 8 million people, 79 youths are in confinement (0.000001%). 7 of these youths are girls. This contrasts quite favorably to states such as California (8500 per 36 million or 0.00022, a tenfold difference). Average age is 16, age ranges from 12–25. Ethnicity is varied, includes 28% non-Austrians from 77 different nations. At this point it is unknown what the exact rates of and types of psychopathology are in these youths. The system provides psychological assessment and mental health interventions by consultants. **Conclusion:** The efforts at early intervention and prevention seem to be successful in reducing incarceration rates in this middle European country. It is unknown as to whether this success in part is due to low rates of psychopathology, an effective national mental health system, or novel interventions. We will explore these problems in future studies.

S-096-446   Topic: 85
Neural and temperamental correlates of abnormal
emotional processing in conduct-disordered adolescents

Christina Stadler, Universität Frankfurt,
Kinder- und Jugendpsychiatrie, Frankfurt, Germany,
christina.stadler@em.uni-frankfurt.de
Philipp Sterzer; Andreas Kleinschmidt; Fritz Poustka

Objective: Aggressive behaviour may be the result of a failure of emotion regulation. Key regions normally involved in emotional processing include the amygdala, hippocampus, orbitofrontal cortex, and anterior cingulate cortex. It has been assumed that individuals with antisocial and aggressive behaviour have an abnormality in the central circuitry responsible for adaptive behavioural strategies. Especially the anterior cingulate cortex might play a crucial role in assessing the motivational content of internal and external stimuli and in regulating context-dependent behaviours (Bush et al., 2000, Davidson et al., 2000). In the present study, we tested whether neural responses evoked by affect-laden pictures in conduct-disordered adolescents differ from those in age-matched controls. Also we tested whether there are concomitant differences in temperament, behaviour control strategies and moral reasoning which might contribute to neural activity differences. **Methods:** We performed functional magnetic resonance imaging in 13 male adolescents with the DSM-IV diagnosis of antisocial conduct behavior aged 9 to 14 years and in 14 healthy age and sex-matched control subjects at 1.5 T (Siemens Vision, gradient booster, standard head coil), acquiring echoplanar images (24 slices, $3.4 \times 3.4 \times 35.0$ mm^3 voxel size, every 3 s. During scanning, subjects looked at pictures from the International Affective Picture System (IAPS) with neutral or strong negative emotional valence balanced with respect to content complexity, luminance, colors, human beings, faces, and animals. The statistical analysis was based on the contrast negative > neutral emotional valence and main effects as well as between-group differences were assessed using a random-effects analysis. Comprehensive neuropsychological evaluations were conducted to standardized procedures. Temperament was assed with with the German version of the Junior Temperament and Character Inventory (JTCI). Cognitive control strategies were assessed with the Wisconsin Card Sorting Test and the Gambling Task (Bechara et al. 1994). Moral reasoning is based on the Social Moral reasoning Test (Gibbs et al., 1992). **Results:** Conduct disordered children show a trend towards deficient moral reasoning and decision making processes and they significantly differ in temperamental factors. The group comparison for the contrast negative > neutral revealed less activity in the right ACC (x = 9, y = 33, z = 33) in patients as compared to controls. The calculated stepwise regression analysis reveal that novelty seeking is a significant predictor ($\beta = -0.43$, p < 0.01) for ACC responsivity to negative affective pictures. When correcting for anxiety and depressive symptoms, we additionally found a reduced responsiveness of the left amygdala to negative pictures in patients as compared to control subjects. **Conclusion:** The data support a crucial role of the ACC in emotional regulation: A deficient emotional and neural reactivity may be associated with a failure to use adequate cognitive strategies and to inhibit impulsive behaviour. Furthermore the results of this study provides a link between temperament factors and neural correlates of emotion processing. We suggest that a deficient activity in the ACC might be a linking factor between personality trait and behavioural outcome. Persons with high novelty seeking, a trait characterized by high impulsivity and excitability, and enormous difficulties in complying with rules, might thus be at risk for an impaired capacity to cognitively control emotional behaviour.

S-096-447   Topic: 85

Platelet 5-HT uptake in boys with conduct disorder

Irene Nowraty, Universität Frankfurt,
Kinder- und Jugendpsychiatrie, Frankfurt, Germany
Christina Stadler; Klaus Schmeck; W.E. Müller;
Fritz Poustka

Methods: In addition to the standardized assessment of general psychopathology methods assessing narrowband aggressive symptoms (Child Behaviour Checklist) and emotional reactivity to an experimentally induced provocation (Taylor's competitive reaction time task) were used in both groups. **Results:** We found a trend for a lower mean Vmax of platelet 5-HT uptake in 14 conduct-disordered boys compared to healthy controls (n = 15). If, however, 2 patients with a low degree of aggression and emotional reactivity were excluded, the difference became significant (M = 4.27, SD = 3.49 in patients and M = 8.45, SD = 4.63 in controls). A significant negative correlation was found between parent-rated aggression scores and Vmax (r = –0.41, p < 0.05, n = 29). These data suggest that dysfunction of 5-HT transport mechanisms might be associated with specific behaviour symptoms in conduct-disordered children.

S-097   Topic: 84, 58

The social context of ADHD: How do views and expectancies affect treatment, parenting and schooling?

Track: ADHD

Chairperson: Ulrich Knölker, Universität Lübeck,
Kinder- und Jugendpsychiatrie, Lübeck, Germany,
uknoelker@aol.com

The social context of ADHD: How do views and expectancies affect treatment, parenting and schooling?

Ulrich Knölker, Universität Lübeck, Kinder- und
Jugendpsychiatrie, Lübeck, Germany, uknoelker@aol.com

The papers of the international speakers try to answer some views and expectancies affecting treatment, parenting and schooling in the social context of ADHD. Ms. Klasen from London, Great Britain, will report on reviews on hyperactivity and the barriers of effective treatment, generating hypothesis through qualitative research. The Luebeck study about knowledge and attitudes towards attention deficit hyperactivity disorder (ADHD), what teachers know and expect of students with ADHD, is divided in two lectures: G. Schmid (et al.), Luebeck, Germany, will explain objectives and methods, whilst J. H. Puls (et al.), Luebeck, Germany, will submit results and conclusions of this study. L. Stevens from Utrecht, Netherlands, will be giving his thoughts on the common topic and present results with regard to (re)-contextualizing or ecologizing school in the Netherlands and the general importance to other countries.

S-097-448   Topic: 84, 58

Views on hyperactivity – barriers to effective treatment? Generating Hypotheses through qualitative research

Henrikje Klasen, Child and Family Service, Chichester,
United Kingdom, h.klasen@iop.kcl.ac.uk
Robert Goodman

Objective: Empirical evidence suggests that although hyperactivity disorders are common, serious and treatable, they often go untreated, at least in Britain. In addition the minority seen by specialist services are not usually the ones most severely affected. Treatment decisions depend not necessarily on scientific evidence, but at least partly on parents', teachers' and general practitioners' (GPs') attitudes towards hyperactivity and appropriate management. The study examines parents' and GPs' views on childhood hyperactivity in order to identify possible treatment barriers. **Methods:** Qualitative semi-structured interviews of one to two hours duration were carried out with 10 GPs, 10 teachers and 29 parents drawn from parents' groups, primary care and specialist centres. Interviews were content transcribed and analysed following the procedures of grounded theory. Coding categories were developed in the course of the analysis in order to fit informants accounts as closely as possible. **Results:** Parents were likely to conceptualise severe hyperactivity as a medical disorder requiring treatment in its own right, whereas GPs were unlikely to initiate treatment or referral unless parents were very persistent or clearly unable to cope. Parents, teachers and GPs disagreed on whether labelling a hyperactive child was enabling or disabling. While families found that the label of hyperactivity did more good than harm, teachers were often unsure and GPs typically predicted the opposite and withheld the label accordingly. Although all groups saw an association between family problems and hyperactivity parents saw this as an effect of living with a hyperactive child. By focusing on associated family stresses as a possible cause for hyperactivity GPs sometimes alienated parents. Early reassurance by GPs often left parents feeling rebuked or not taken seriously, which then stood in the way of parents turning again to health professionals when the problems persisted. Parents, teachers and GPs generally agreed that information on hyperactivity was insufficient and conflicting and that they lacked the specialist back-up they needed. **Conclusion:** Clashes between the views of parents, teachers and GPs can lead to misunderstandings, dissatisfaction and lack of patient compliance. The study particularly identifies areas where attitudes are likely to hinder access to effective treatment. Suggested hypotheses and changes should be tested in quantitative and empirical studies.

S-097-449   Topic: 84, 58

Knowledge and attitudes towards Attention Deficit Hyperactivity Disorder (ADHD): What do teachers know and expect of students with ADHD?

Objectives and methods

Gabriele Schmid, Universität Lübeck, Kinder- und
Jugenpsychiatrie, Lübeck, Germany, uknoelker@aol.com
Jan Hendrik Puls; Swantje Berndt; B. Behn; Ulrich Knölker

Objective: So far, there is only limited evidence on teachers' knowledge and attitudes towards ADHD in school children, although international guidelines and practice parameters (AACAP, 1997, DGKJP, 2003) consider teachers to be crucial in diagnosis and treatment of ADHD. Studies carried out so far indicate that teachers' expectancies strongly influence the educational outcome in children in general, but most of all in underachievers (Madon et al., 1997). Clinical experience shows that the educational background in teachers of the various school types is heterogeneous and knowledge of ADHD differs individually. The aim of this study is to exactly define differences in knowledge and attitudes in teachers of all school types within the German educational system towards ADHD and to determine positive and negative influencing factors as well as needs for further interventions in schools and teacher education. **Methods:** 2200 teachers were asked to complete anonymously a questionnaire dealing with knowledge and attitudes towards ADHD, based in parts upon the Test of knowledge about ADHD (KADD, Hepperlen et al., 2002), containing 69 items. 34 items are based upon the multiple choice method, including knowledge items as well as error-choice items designed for indirect measurement of attitudes. Additionally, items are included to measure attitudes directly as well as questions dealing with the personal and educational background and teaching experience of the participants. **Results:** Results and Conclusions are being presented in the following abstract: Knowledge and attitudes towards attention deficit hyperactivity disorder (ADHD) 2: what do teachers know and expect of students with ADHD? **Conclusion:** There is a substantial need for an increased quality in teacher education within the German educational system, especially concerning psychiatric disorders in children and adolescents, e.g. ADHD. Single-case interventions must take into account the possible bias of teachers, which will strongly moderate his or her will to cooperate in terms of school interventions.

S-097-450   Topic: 84, 58
Knowledge and attitudes towards attention deficit hyperactivity disorder (ADHD): What do teachers know and expect of students with ADHD?
Results and conclusions

Jan Hendrik Puls, Universität Lübeck, Kinder- und Jugendpsychiatrie, Lübeck, Germany, uknoelker@aol.com
Gabriele Schmid; Swantje Berndt; B. Behn; Ulrich Knölker

Objective: Objectives and Methods of this study are presented in the following abstract: Knowledge and attitudes towards attention deficit hyperactivity disorder (ADHD) 1: what do teachers know and expect of students with ADHD? Objectives and methods Schmid, G., Puls, J.H., Berndt, S., Behn, B., Knölker, U. Department of Child and Adolescent Psychiatry, University of Schleswig-Holstein, Campus Lübeck, Germany. **Methods:** First, the questionnaire underwent testing for psychometric properties in a pilot study (n = 80) and was refined and shortened on this basis. **Results:** Selected results of the complete study: Teachers' knowledge on ADHD shows to be very heterogeneous, depending on age, educational background and personal experience. Teachers' knowledge is profounder in primary schools than in higher education. Exact knowledge of ADHD strongly influences the attitudes towards students with ADHD in a positive way and determines the degree of cooperation **Conclusion:** There is a substantial need for an increased quality in teacher education within the German educational system, especially concerning psy-

chiatric disorders in children and adolescents, e.g. ADHD. Single-case interventions must take into account the possible bias of teachers, which will strongly moderate his or her will to cooperate in terms of school interventions.

S-097-451   Topic: 58
Towards another paradigm: (Re)contextualising or ecologising school

Luc Stevens, Utrecht University, Education, Bilthoven, Netherlands, luc_stevens@wxs.nl

Objective: A general concern of teachers in our schools is the lack of motivation of their pupils and concurrent behaviour problems. In particular at-risk populations seem vulnerable for the conditions that schools characterise. In this study one of these conditions, called schoolethos, is examined by interviewing teachers and children in quite a variety of primary and secondary schools. Particularly the qualities of teacher-pupil interaction got our interest. **Methods:** Qualitative semi-structured interviews of about one hour duration in case of the individual teachers (n (primary) = 71; n (secondary) = 76) and about half an hour in case of the pupils, organised in small groups of four to five (n (primary) = 392; n (secondary) = 211). Every interview was summarized and the summary was authorized by the interviewees. The summaries were analysed following the procedures of the grounded theory approach. **Results:** We tried to find a central meaning in the perspectives of both teachers and pupils (what occupies teachers and pupils most?). It is refered to structural attunement problems or problems of matching in school regarding supply and demand in the teaching learning process as well as mutual relationships in teacher pupil and in teacher-teacher relationships. There seems to be relatively little common understanding and in the eyes of the pupils the teacher seems relatively inaccessible (s/he wants to be in control whatever the circumstances). The teachers themselves seem to feel alone, they do not see each other, nor their pupils as a resource. **Conclusion:** Our school system as a highly standardized system (standardized on the dimensions of time, space, content and human relations (roles and functions) seems to be liable to a permanent tendency of disintegration because it is not truly supported by its inhabitants. A system like this cannot function as a protective factor for risk-populations of children. Considering what should be done it is suggested that the standardizations should be made undone, that pupils should be considered as full partners of their teachers, that the learning environment should be individualized or personalized and may be above all that the relationships should be restored. In short: what has been split up till now should be brought together, like teacher and pupils or needs of pupils and the answer of the curriculum or teachers as individuals. This approach can best be defined in terms of (re)contextualising or ecologising schools.

S-098   Topic: 4
Integrative approach in treatment of children and adolescents with psychiatric disorders
Track: Therapy and intervention

Chairperson: Joachim Jungmann, Klinik für Kinder- und Jugendpsychiatrie und Psychotherapie, Weinsberg, Germany, j.jungmann@klinikum-weissenhof.de

Integrative approach in treatment of children and adolescents with psychiatric disorders

Joachim Jungmann, Klinik für Kinder- und Jugendpsychiatrie und Psychotherapie, Weinsberg, Germany, j.jungmann@klinikum-weissenhof.de

4 Examples of integrative treatment of children and adolescents with psychiatric disorders are presented and discussed: A medical consiliary co-operation for the care of mentally disabled adolescents in a therapeutic community under the auspices of a youth welfare organisation in Heilbronn/Weinsberg, Germany, the treatment of patients with schizophrenia in "Psychiatric hospital for children and adolescents" in Zagreb, Croatia, an integrative approach in outpatient treatment of children and adolescents with psychiatric disorders in Nishnij Novograd, Russia, and Models of outpatient care with and without inpatient facilities in Ankara/Turkey and Hamm/Germany. In all treatment methods continuity of care can bee guaranteed.

S-098-452   Topic: 81, 22

A medical consiliary co-operation for the care of mentally disabled adolescents in a therapeutic community under the auspices of a youth welfare organisation in Germany

Joachim Jungmann, Klinik für Kinder- und Jugendpsychiatrie und Psychotherapie, Weinsberg, Germany, j.jungmann@klinikum-weissenhof.de

Objective: For 9 years the department for child and adolescent psychiatry at the Centre for Psychiatry in Weinsberg and the social pedagogic youth welfare organisation "Heimat für Heimatlose gGmbH Öhringen" have been running a joint project catering for the needs of adolescents with mental disorders. In accordance with guidelines laid down in a contract the cooperation offers to adolescents, suffering from a serious mental illness and having previously been receiving inpatient psychiatric treatment, supervision and care within a therapeutic community. Accompanied by adolescent psychiatric treatment these measures continue the socio-therapy which had been introduced earlier on at the clinic. **Methods:** An overview is given about target group, goal, about entry and selection procedures as well as dates about the care procedure. **Results:** Placing mentally disabled adolescents in a protective and pedagogically devised environment in which they can regain and stabilise the ability to run their own lives and plan their own future career independently is probably the most essential help our therapeutic community can give them. A vital part of the rehabilitation programme must be to prepare the adolescents for their working lives by taking their abilities into account. Areas dealing with social integration must therefore be linked with a supervised vocational training under professional guidance. It is essential that such a programme is individually and flexibly planned.

S-098-453   Topic: 69

The treatment of patients with schizophrenia in Psychiatric hospital for children and adolescents in Zagreb, Croatia

Zoran Juretic, Psychiatric Hospital for Children and Adolescents, Zagreb, Croatia; Nela Ercegovic

Objective: "Psychiatric hospital for children and adolescents" in Zagreb is the only institution in Croatia which treats children and adolescents with various psychiatric disorders on three levels: as out-patient, partial hospitalization (day clinic), or inpatient treatment, with the possibility of cascadic passing over from one level to another. As the authors are especially interested in treating schizophrenic patients, they will present their experience in this topic. **Methods:** Presentation of experiences especially in treating schizophrenic patients. **Results:** Discussion of dilemmas and problems in the work, of special problems with resocialization and education of those children as well as the difficulties wich arise after patients become 18 years old, because of lack of adequate departments for late adolescent and postadolescent age.

S-098-454   Topic: 4

Integrative approach in outpatient treatment of children and adolescents with psychiatric disorders in Russia

Andrey Zanozin, Centre for Mental Health of Children and Adolescents, Nizhnj Novgorod, Russia, tndmitr@sandy.ru

Objective: The incidence of psychiatric disorders in children and adolescent significantly increased over the last 10 years in Russia. The diagnostic structure of cases has been stable over the past ten years. The most widespread problems are the non psychotic disorders with 66%. The high prevalence of non psychotic disorders demands an urgent development of the psychotherapeutic services and integrative treatment. This was one of the reasons to establish Centre for mental health of children and adolescents in Nizhny Novgorod several years ago. **Methods:** Report about four years of experience of the Centre. **Results:** The big need for psychotherapy and the effectiveness of multidisciplinary approach for examination and treatment of young patients is shown. The most important therapeutic methods used in the Centre are psychotherapy and psychological training with a minimal use of medication. Despite all efforts a great problem in Russia is training and the post graduate education in the field of the child and adolescent psychiatry, psychotherapy and medical psychology. Many problems exist in the education and employment of social workers and other specialists that have to deal with mental health problems of children and adolescents. In Russia during the next 5 years a program of reorganisation of the psychiatric networks must be realised with emphasis on integrative care.

S-098-455   Topic: 3, 4

Models of outpatient care with and without inpatient facilities in Turkey

Renate Schepker, Westfälisches Institut Hamm, Kinder- und Jugendpsychiatrie, Hamm, Germany, r.schepker@wkp-lwl.org
Füsun Çuhadaroglu-Çetin

Objective: To compare approaches for outpatients in 2 differently developed systems of psychiatric care. **Methods:** Data on MAS classification in an outpatient department in Ankara, Turkey, and in Hamm, Germany, are compared (Documentations on 200 patients in Germany and 100 in Ankara out of 2003). Hamm having in- and daypatient facilities of 1 bed per 100,000 inhabitants, Ankara having the possibility of inpatient intake in the adult psychiatry wards. **Results:** (1) Inpatients in Germany and outpatients in Turkey do not differ as to main diagnosis, they do as to the GAFscore. (2) They do not differ as to possible intensity of treatment (like psychiatrist's contacts per week). Outpatients in Germany and outpatients in Turkey did differ on socioeconomic variables as percentage of divorced parents and family structure. **Conclusion:** The West can learn from the East: severity of illness has no impact in possible outpatient intervention in case the patient's family is reliable. Family based interventions are highly successful even in severe disorders. Continuity of care is given in this context. Group therapy is possible. The East can learn from the West that early interventions on severe states like psychosis, dissociative states etc. are effective in a multiprofessional team, repeated suicidal acts can be prevented. Interruption of disturbed family interactions by inpatient care can be helpful if family therapy is continued. Group therapy in a more secure setting for disorders like sexual assault is effective if transitional models are provided.

S-099   Topic: 84
Attention Deficit Hyperactivity Disorders VI
Track: ADHD

Chairperson: Kosuke Yamazaki, Tokai University, Sagamihara Kanagawa, Japan, araki-ken@k-con.co.jp

S-099-456   Topic: 84
Evidence for inattentive/hyperactive symptoms in patients with early onset Parkinson's disease

Susanne Walitza, Universitätsklinik Würzburg, Kinder- und Jugendpsychiatrie, Würzburg, Germany, walitza@kjp.uni-wuerzburg.de
G. Herhaus; S. Melfsen; Andreas Warnke; Manfred Gerlach

Objective: Attention deficit hyperactivity disorder (ADHD) and Parkinson disease (PD), one of the most common late-life neurodegenerative disorders, are both disorders with dopaminergic abnormalities in the striatum of the brain. Following the pandemic of von Economos encephalitis lethagica of the early 1900s, many older patients were left with clinical features resembling PD while in the child and adolescents symptoms resembling ADHD were reported (Economo, 1930). The aim of this ongoing study was to investigate whether PD is preceded by symptoms resembling ADHD. **Methods:** Currently, 47 early PD patients (mean age 51.6 ± 10.9 years; age at onset: 41.2 ± 11.9 years) and 23 controls (friends or affiliates of the patients mean age 45.9 ± 5.8 years) were included. Data were collected by means of two structured questionnaires. The first one, was the short form of the Wender-Utah-Rating Scale for the retrospective assessment of ADHD-symptoms (WURS-k). The second questionnaire was created by ourselves, based on DSM-IV criteria for ADHD and open questions about lifetime medications. **Results:** Descriptive analysis of the WURS-k demonstrated differences in the total score of patients and controls(patients $m=17.1$; controls $m=11.8$). The greatest difference between patients and controls has been found in the factor for inattentive/hyperactivity (patients $m=1.1$; $s=0.9$ and controls $m=0.7$; $s=0.7$). Using our own questionnaire we also found differences in the total scores for the symptoms, relevant for ADHD in childhood (patients $m=57.6$; $s=20.0$; controls $m=47.75$; $s=13.9$). **Conclusion:** These preliminary results suggest that PD may be preceded by inattentive/hyperactive symptoms and that PD and ADHD may have a common pathogenesis. Interestingly, non of the PD patients included in the study, reported the previous use of methylphenidate.

S-099-457   Topic: 84, 28
Association of 5-HT2A receptor polymorphism and Attention Deficit Hyperactivity Disorder (ADHD)

Linyan Su, Mental Health Institute, Dept. of Child Psychiatry, Changsha, China, sulinyan@sina.com
Daomeng Cheng; Xueping Gao

Objective: To investigate whether 5-HT2A receptor polymorphism is associated with attention deficit hyperactivity disorder (ADHD). **Methods:** Blood samples were taken from 58 children with ADHD diagnosed due to DSM-IV criteria and from 97 healthy controls. Case-control association analysis and polymerase chain reaction (PCR) and RFLP technique were used to test the association of the alleles of 5-HT2A receptor T102C polymorphic site and ADHD. **Results:** In ADHD children, the frequency of T102T was higher than in controls (51.7% vs. 27.8%, $p=0.003$, OR$=2.78$), and the frequency of T102C was lower than in controls (34.5% vs. 52.6%, $p=0.029$, OR$=0.47$); the frequency of 102T allele was significantly higher than that of 102C allele ($\chi^2=6.65$, $p=0.01$). **Conclusion:** The the T102T genotype might be a risk factor of ADHD, while the the T102C genotype might be a protective factor of ADHD.

S-099-459   Topic: 84, 37
Validating the ADHD Rating Scale-IV:
Parent version-investigator administered and scored (ADHD RS: J) in Japan

Kosuke Yamazaki, Tokai University, Sagamihara Kanagawa, Japan, araki-ken@k-con.co.jp
Donald Harder; Harry Laws; Yoshibumi Nakane; Kenzo Takeshita; Hiroshi Naruse

Objective: To validate ADHD RS: J, the Japanese version of ADHD Rating Scale, in Japanese population. **Methods:** 37 subjects (ADHD$=26$, non-ADHD$=11$) at 6 sites in Japan participated in the study. Two investigators who are qualified physicians in each site assessed the symptoms. The subjects visited the investigators twice, at approximately 2 to 3 weeks interval. At both visits, ADHD symptoms were assessed using investigator- and parent-rated ADHD RS J and the Clinical Global Impressions of ADHD Severity (CGI-ADHD-S), as determined by the investigator. The inter-rater reliability, face validity, internal consistency, test-retest reliability, convergent validity, and discriminant validity of this scale were investigated. **Results:** ADHD RS: J appears to have acceptable levels of face validity, inter-rater reliability, internal consistency, test-retest reliability, convergent validity, and discriminant validity. Differences between scores on the ADHD RS: J investigator- and parent-rated scales were small and not statistically, nor clinically significant. **Conclusion:** The results of this validation study support use of the ADHD RS: J as a valid and reliable tool for assessing the severity of ADHD symptoms in Japanese patients.

S-099-460   Topic: 84, 36
The study of the character of auditory P300 of Tourette's syndrome with and without Attention Deficit and Hyperactivity Disorder (ADHD) in China

Yan Zhu, Central South University, Mental Health Institute, Changsha, China, zhuyan4895025@hotmail.com

Objective: To investigate the character of auditory P300 of Tourette's syndrome (TS) with and without attention deficit and hyperactivity disorder (ADHD). **Methods:** There were 19 TS children, 15 TS+ADHD children and 20 normal controls recorded and compared by P300 in Fz, Cz, C3, C4 and Pz. **Results:** TS group CZ, PZ and TS+ADHD group PZ showed increased latencies and decreased amplitudes (Cz, C3, C4, Pz) than normal group P < 0.05; no group differences of latencies and amplitudes between TS and TS+ADHD group were found. The prevalence of abnormal P300 form, lateralization and topography of P300 peak in TS+ADHD group was significantly higher than in TS and normal group P < 0.05. The topography of P300 in TS group showed a lateralization to the right hemisphere and in the TS+ADHD group to the left. **Conclusion:** The finding suggest that TS with and without ADHD all have cognitive function deficits, there are some P300 differences between TS with and without ADHD.

S-099-461   Topic: 84, 35
Research on regional cerebral blood flow in children with and without hyperactivity-impulsivity in Attention Deficit Hyperactivity Disorder (ADHD)

Linyan Su, Mental Health Institute, Dept. of Child Psychiatry, Changsha, China, sulinyan@sina.com
Jun Liu; Yasong Du

Objective: In order to understand the characteristic of regional cerebral blood flow (rCBF) of inattentive type and combined subtype of ADHD (DSM-IV). **Methods:** rCBF was examined with single photon emission computed tomogragly in 40 child with ADHD and 11 healthy normal boys as controls. **Results:** Qualitative analysis results showed that the rate of low rCBF was significantly higher in ADHD groups (57.5%) than that in controls (9%). The low rCBF brain zones included: frontal lobe, temporal lobe, occipital lobe and thalamus. The rate of low rCBF was significantly higher in ADHD-combined subtype groups (66.7%) than that in inattentive type groups (47.3%). At the same time, the low rCBF in left brain zones in combined subtype group was 14 case, 10 case in right one, there was significantly difference between the left brain zones and the right ones. **Conclusion:** The results of the study suggest that the relation between the low rCBF in left brain zones and ADHD.

S-100   Topic: 57
EFCAP Symposium: New research on delinquency and mental health

Chairperson: John Sikorski, UCSF Dept. of Child Psychiatry, San Francisco, CA, USA, jbsikor@itsa.ucsf.edu

New research on delinquency and mental health

John Sikorski, UCSF, Dept. of Child Psychiatry, San Francisco, CA, USA, jbsikor@itsa.ucsf.edu

The prevalence of psychiatric disorders and overall mental health needs in young people has been associated with delinquent behaviours. This symposium aims to build upon the research already conducted within this field by presenting the findings of a number of new research projects in this area. A population-based study addressing the possible association between autism spectrum disorders and sexual and violent offending will be presented along with the implications that this has for the assessment and management of violent behaviours. The psychopathology of incarcerated young people in Russia will be outlined with a focus upon the impact of traumatic experiences and the relationship between cultural background and psychiatric disorders. In Holland, the psychiatric pathology of detained girls has been studied and the results of this will be presented with conclusions made regarding the assessment and interventions that should be offered to this at-risk population. Finally, the results of a cross-sectional study establishing the level of mental health need among young offenders in secure facilities and the community in England and Wales will be presented.

S-100-463   Topic: 57, 95
Psychopathology among Russian incarcerated juvenile delinquents

Vladislav Ruchkin, Yale Child Study Center, New Haven CT, USA, vladislav.ruchkin@yale.edu

Objective: To assess the prevalence of psychopathology among Russian delinquent youth, and to evaluate its relationships to the past traumatic experiences and to conduct problems with early onset. **Methods:** Psychopathology and trauma were assessed by a semi-structured psychiatric interview (K-SADS-PL) and self-reports in 430 incarcerated male juvenile delinquents. **Results:** Delinquent youth reported high levels of psychopathology, comparable to those in other Western countries. Most delinquents also reported traumatic experiences of different severity and 24% fulfilled DSM-IV criteria for PTSD. Higher levels of posttraumatic stress were accompanied by higher rates of internalizing and externalizing psychopathology. Delinquents with early-onset of conduct problems also had greater odds of having comorbid psychiatric diagnoses, especially in externalizing and anxiety disorders. **Conclusion:** Findings from different cultural backgrounds suggest that juvenile delinquents often suffer from various types of psychiatric disorders. Early onset conduct problems often intertwine with numerous traumatic experiences and higher levels of comorbidity. These youth may require additional clinical attention and rehabilitation.

S-100-464   Topic: 57
Psychiatric pathology in detained girls

Robert Vermeiren, University of Antwerp, Child & Adolescent Psychiatry, Antwerp, Belgium, robert@vermeiren.name
Sannie Hamerlynck; Lisette 't Hart; Lucres Nauta-Janssen; Theodore Doreleijers

Objective: To investigate the prevalence of trauma and psychopathology in adolescent girls in detention. **Methods:** For this purpose, a psychiatric prevalence study was conducted in three JJI's (Juvenile Justice Institution) in the Netherlands. In each of the JJI's, 70 newly detained girls were included in the study. The diagnostic instruments included parts of a semi-structured psychiatric interview (K-SADS) and self-report questionnaires (e.g. SDQ, trauma questionnaire, CPTS-RI, BDI). In addition, a telephone interview was conducted with the parents, which included the administration of the disruptive behavior disorder part of the Kiddie-SADS and the SDQ. **Results:** Preliminary analyses show that a history of severe physical and sexual trauma occurred in a large proportion of the girls, and that the majority of detained females had a psychiatric diagnosis. **Conclusion:** Many girls in detention suffer form severe psychopathology and constitute a population at risk. Therefore, a psychiatric diagnostic assessment should be conducted on a regular basis in this population, and therapeutic interventions must be available in juvenile justice institutions.

S-100-465   Topic: 57
The effectiveness of mental health provision for young people in custody and in the community
Prathiba Chitsabesan, University of Manchester,
Manchester, United Kingdom, pchitsabesan@yahoo.com

Objective: To determine the effectiveness of mental health provision for young offenders in custody and in the community across England and Wales. **Methods:** A cross sectional study of 301 young offenders using the Salford Needs Assessment Schedule for Adolescents to establish the level of mental health need in this population. 75 young offenders from the secure care sample were followed up six months later to establish the continuity of care and changes in need. A qualitative assessment of the strengths and weaknesses of different models of service provision was also conducted. **Results:** Young offenders have high levels of mental health and social needs with those in the community having significantly more than those in custody. Many of their needs were unmet and the biggest problem was in screening and identifying these needs. However, there were some examples of good practice. **Conclusion:** Many of the needs of young offenders are unmet as there are problems with screening, the transfer of documents and the static nature of assessments on referral or admission. The lack of local services and concerns regarding transfer disrupting interventions can lead to non-referral to services.

S-101   Topic: 1, 3
WPA Global program on child and mental health: Prevention in child and adolescent mental health
Chairperson: Helmut Remschmidt, Universität Marburg
Kinder- und Jugendpsychiatrie, Marburg, Germany,
remschm@med.uni-marburg.de

WPA Global program on child and mental health: Prevention in child and adolescent mental health
Helmut Remschmidt, Universität Marburg,
Kinder- und Jugendpsychiatrie, Marburg, Germany,
remschm@med.uni-marburg.de

All child and mental health workers agree with the slogan: Prevention is better than Intervention" However the existing knowledge is rarely adequately used in order to prevent adverse circumstances for children and in consequence psychopathological disorders. Paying attention to this situation a task force on prevention was formed within the WPA Global Program on Child and Mental Health. The

symposium of this task force comprises contributions on principles of preventive interventions followed by a systematic review of existing prevention programs to promote mental health in children and adolescents and by papers addressing more specific issues as prevention of suicide and school drop out. The latter topic is a world wide problem and is part of the WPA Global Program on Child and Mental Health with the application of preventive interventions in Alexandria (Egypt), Nishny Novgorod (Russia) and Porto Alegre (Brazil).

S-101-466   Topic: 3
The principles of preventive intervention
Barry Nurcombe, University of Queensland,
Dept. of Psychiatry, Brisbane, Australia,
bnurcombe@psychiatry.uq.edu.au

Methods: Critical review of literature. **Results:** Primary prevention refers to the prevention of psychiatric disorder before its onset, by the reduction of risk. Secondary prevention refers to the prevention or mitigation of psychiatric disorder after its onset. Interventions are classified according to the age-group of the target population, the scope of intervention (universal or selective), and whether intervention is aimed at moderating or mediating factors (or both). Preventive intervention should be based upon a theoretical model of causation. **Conclusion:** Practical issues concerning support, funding, implementation, and evaluation are discussed.

S-101-467   Topic: 3
Evidence based primary prevention programs for promoting mental health in children and adolescents: A systematic worldwide review
Martine Flament, University of Ottawa,
Inst. Mental Health Research, Ottawa, ON, Canada,
mflament@rohcg.on.ca
Hien Nguyen; Claudia Furino; Jovan Simeon; Cathy Cuzner;
Howard Schachter

Objective: This study is part of the World Psychiatric Association (WPA) Global Programme on Child Mental Health, an international initiative launched in 2003 in collaboration with the World Health Organization (WHO) and the IACAPAP. The objective is to conduct a systematic review of prevention programs that have been proposed worldwide to foster mental health or to prevent the occurrence of clinical psychiatric disorders in children and adolescents. We also aim to identify examples of successfully implemented programs that could be used as prototypes for future field studies. **Methods:** Several complementary search strategies are employed, including those directed at electronic databases and at representatives of organizations active in the fields of childhood and adolescent mental health and prevention. Identified bibliographic records, then retrieved reports, undergo an assessment of relevance by two independent reviewers. Based on abstracted data, the relevant programs' key components and effectiveness data are highlighted. **Results:** To date, our preliminary literature search has identified a number of programs currently implemented in many countries, including Canada, the United States, Australia, Netherlands, Belgium, Great Britain, Norway, Bosnia, and Israel. Some programs aim to reduce psychological trauma following exposure to war, violence or sexual abuse, while others promote self-esteem, interpersonal skills, pro-social behavior and other mediating factors related to healthy development. Risk factors associated with mental disorders, such as substance use, school drop-out, and school truancy, will be highlighted. **Conclusion:** The need to prevent child and adolescent psychiatric disorders are universal, but the specific priorities greatly vary from country to country. Evidence concerning program components and effectiveness will be discussed in light of the clinical-policy and research implications.

S-101-468   Topic: 93
Suicide prevention in children and adolescents

Danuta Wasserman, NASP, Stockholm, Sweden,
prof.wasserman.secretary@ipm.ki.se

Suicide is the leading cause of death in young men in Sweden, and one of the leading causes of mortality among young people worldwide. Analyses of trends in adolescent suicides for years 1979–1996 show that in 21 of the 30 studied European countries, male adolescent suicide rates increased during the study period, accompanied by far less increases or decreases in suicide rates of males 20 years or older. Female adolescent suicide rates rose less markedly than in males, with the exception of strong increases in Norway, Ireland and Ukraine. Data from the longitudinal WHO European Multicentre study on attempted suicide indicate that the rates of attempted suicide and suicide in the young co-vary. The association is strongest and significant for male adolescents and young adults. The recent increase in attempted suicide rates observed in the WHO European Multicentre study in young male subjects in several European countries has been proposed to signal a further increase in suicide rates. Furthermore, several studies have reported a shift to suicide methods with higher lethality for both genders in recent years in countries with increasing suicide rates. In suicide prevention, strategies can be directed at the general population or the health care services. Since suicide risk is high among psychiatrically ill adolescents, adequate treatment of psychiatric disorders and improved detection of psychiatric illnesses in the general population of young people is essential. Preventive measures in the health care services after a suicide attempt and early recognition of children and young people at risk in schools are other essential strategies. The initiative launched by the WHO in 1999 SUPRE (SUicide PREvention), a world wide initiative for the prevention of suicide, addresses this question by the resource material on how to prevent suicide for teachers and other school staff. This material can be adapted to local conditions and inserted in syllabuses with respect to training of both pupils and staff. Preliminary results from the intervention project in Stockholm schools show that suicide attempts can be decreased and "seeking help" behaviour of peers to suicide prone pupils can be improved. The results of the study will be presented at the meeting.

S-101-469   Topic: 58
A pilot study of school dropout in adolescents

Tatjana Dmitrieva, Center for Mental Health of Children
and Adolescents, Nizhny Novgorod, Russia,
tndmitr@sandy.ru

Objective: To examine the school dropout (SDO) rate in students of ordinary schools in a big industrial city and to estimate family, psychological and psychopathological problems of these children. **Methods:** All 11 to 15-year old school children of two ordinary schools (N = 1062) were examined. The following instruments were used: 1) Strengths and Difficulties Questionnaire (SDQ) for children, parents and teachers, 2) the General Health Questionnaire (GHQ) for children and 3) the Questionnaire for assessment of the family and school situation (for children and teachers). **Results:** 101 children with regular school absenteeism were found out (9.5% of all examined students). There were 7 among them (0.7%) with four weeks and longer continuous school dropout. These children have often had anxiety, somatoform and depressive disorders. Next school year the prevention program in one of these schools will be provided. The efficacy of this program will be assessed by comparison of SDO rates in both schools after this prevention program will have been finished. **Conclusion:** High rate of school absenteeism and associations between SDO and psychological and mental health problems were found. To reduce the amount of school absenteeism and further school and social maladjustment, a school based prevention program with emphasis on the timely and accurate identification of students at risk for school dropout is required.

S-101-470   Topic: 58, 19
A proposed comprehensive intervention
to reduce school drop out in public schools:
A pilot feasibility study

Ana Soledade Martins, Brazil,
Chirstian Kieling; Julia Comassetto; Renata Goncalves;
Silvia Oswald; Luis Augusto Rohde

Objective: The school drop out rate has been considered an important measure of the educational condition of a country and a useful indication of recent and possibly future problems. The UNICEF estimates that 121 million primary-school-age children are out of school worldwide. In Brazil, the estimations are that 95% of the children have access to school but only 59% of them finish the 8th elementary grade. This presentation aims to describe a pilot feasibility study to assess a comprehensive intervention to reduce school drop out in public schools. **Methods:** Two schools with comparable high rates of drop out were selected from poor areas in a large city in Brazil. In one of them, a comprehensive intervention is being developed along the year. This package includes: a) 2 meetings with teachers on normal child development and main child mental disorders; b) 3 meetings with parents on importance of education for the future of children; c) 6 letters to parents addressing issues related to school drop out and school environment; d) a manualized cognitive intervention on the advantages of staying at schools with adolescents of the 7th and 8th elementary grades; e) modifications of the school environment (e.g., contest of hip-hop on school drop out, activities with parents to help fixing small problems at school); f) global mental assessment and referral for children that stay out of school for 10 consecutive days and their families. In the control school, no intervention was implemented. **Results:** This is on-going project that started in March, 2004. Preliminary findings suggest a high acceptability of the intervention by school personal. Findings for the first 6 months of the intervention will be discussed during the symposium. **Conclusion:** School drop out is an extremely relevant problem in developing countries. Comprehensive interventions respecting cultural differences should be developed as preventive measures.

S-101-471   Topic: 58
School drop-out in Alexandria, Egypt
Amira Seif El-Din, University of Alexandria,
Faculty of Medicine, Alexandria, Egypt,
amira@contact.com.eg

School drop-out in Alexandria schools in average is 8% for the academic year 2003/2004 as reported by the Ministry of education. School backwardness constitute 25% of total number of students. It is one of the risk factors for school drop-out. This raised an important question to start our program as early as possible at Summer time instead to be at the start of the academic year 2004/2005, where the teachers and the parents reported that the most important reason for school drop-out is to support the family by doing some manual work. The selected school is a mixed primary school and all students at the fifth year transferred to the sixth year were included in the study (n = 253). The main goal to start early at Summer during the school summer camp is to help those students to get some skills that can help them to earn money to help their families without leaving the school as a way to prevent school drop-out. To achieve this goal a training for the school teachers (n = 35) and implementing the SDQ (teacher and student forms). A short questionnaire for the students to report the requested skills they want to practice it at the Summer Camp starting from July to mid September 2004. The aim of the summer camp is to fulfil the following objectives: – to improve the bonds between the students and their teachers – to provide the students some skills that can be useful for them in the future.

S-102   Topic: 36, 84
Neurophysiological approaches to the motor cortex of children with psychiatric illnesses
Chairperson: Johannes Buchmann, Universität Rostock,
Kinder- und Jugendpsychiatrie, Rostock, Germany,
johannes.buchmann@med.uni-rostock.de

Neurophysiological approaches to the motor cortex of children with psychiatric illnesses
Johannes Buchmann, Universität Rostock,
Kinder- und Jugendpsychiatrie, Rostock, Germany,
johannes.buchmann@med.uni-rostock.de

This symposium gives an overwiew about the basics of transcranial magnetic cortex stimulation (TMS) in children, hitherto existing findings of cortical correlates of neuromotor development in normal children and about specific motor inhibition and fazilitation deficits in children with ADHD and in children with Tic/Tourette. Motor hyperactivity in ADHD/Tic/Tourette can be understood either as a result of abnormal facilitation or of defective inhibition of motor programs. TMS and EEG (slow cortical potentials) are neurophysiological tools to study non-invasively the motor system in children. Because these neurophysiological approaches are relatively unknown in Child- and Adolescence Psychiatry, this symposium shall as well as introduce TMS and slow cortical potentials as also refer newest research findings in this area.

S-102-472   Topic: 35
Transcranial magnetic stimulation during childhood and adolescence: New insights into intracortical and corticospinal pathways and their modulation
J. Kirschner, USA

Transcranial Magnetic Stimulation (TMS) is a non-invasive method to study basic neurophysiological processes. The ease and safety of TMS has made it a popular tool to study the relationship between brain and behaviour in children and adolescents. Excitability of the corticospinal tract can be assessed by single-pulse stimulation and double-pulse stimulation, in which a second stimulus follows the first after a few milliseconds, gives insight into intracortical inhibitory and facilitating circuits. A number of studies have investigated the normal development and maturation of these measures during childhood and adolescence. First investigations also have shown alteration of cortical excitability in patients with epilepsy, movement disorders and psychiatric disorders. In addition, TMS has been used to track changes after the ingestion of neurotropic drugs (e.g. antiepileptic drugs or methylphenidate), in normal subjects and patients. The method of repetitive TMS can be used to influence cortical activity in distinctive areas of the brain. Whether or not this application might be useful in clinical practice to treat seizures or behavioural disorders is still controversial. Although our understanding of the physiological effects of TMS is still limited and needs further clarification TMS can already been considered as an important neurophysiological and neuropsychological research tool TMS. Further developments like the combination of TMS with functional neuroimaging will probably make it even more useful in research as well as in clinical practice.

S-102-473   Topic: 36, 24
Cortical correlates of neuromotor development in children
M. Garvey, NIH/NINDS, USA

This presentation will focus on the use of TMS as a method to examine neurodevelopment in healthy children. Background: Single pulse TMS provides a non-invasive, painless method of probing the motor system. This technique is of particular interest for studying maturation of the motor system and may provide insights into those developmental disabilities associated with specific delays of motor development. Neuromotor skills undergo a gradual process of maturation over the first 10 to 15 years of life. Autopsy and imaging studies provide evidence that callosal myelination and cortical neuronal development mature over this same time period. Together, these data suggest an association between maturation of the neuromotor skills and neurodevelopment of underlying brain structures. Motor evoked potential thresholds decrease with age until mid-adolescence while the motor cortex representation of intrinsic hand muscles does not appear to show a substantial increase until early adolescence, suggesting that TMS evoked membrane excitability at threshold and at supra-threshold intensities mature at different times throughout childhood. Although TMS-evoked inhibition of intrahemispheric circuits does not appear to have a clear maturation profile, inter-hemispheric inhibitory circuits show a clear developmental trajectory which appears to mirror the disappearance of developmental mirror movements. Future Directions: Although many investigators have published small case reports or case series, few have gone on to fully characterize the neurophysiology of childhood neurological disorders. Thus, the potential of TMS in children has not yet been fully explored and it may yet prove to be a useful tool in the investigation of normal development, developmental disabilities, neuropsychiatric disorders, and neurodegenerative diseases. TMS may be able to detect the presence (or absence) of neurological involvement, provide information about disease progression, and monitor response to treatment in neurological disorders. In addition, the potential for assessing medication compliance and therapeutic effect in disorders treated with neuroactive drugs has not yet been explored. TMS studies may also be helpful in characterization of different phenotypes of the same genetic disorder. However, much work remains to be done to confirm the validity of TMS as marker of disease burden or as a diagnostic tool.

S-102-474   Topic: 36, 84
Changes of cortical excitability in children with ADHD
Johannes Buchmann, Universität Rostock,
Kinder- und Jugendpsychiatrie, Rostock, Germany,
johannes.buchmann@med.uni-rostock.de
Gunther Moll

In children with attention-deficit hyperactivity disorder (ADHD), motoric hyperactivity is one of the striking phenomena. This motor hyperactivity can be understood either as a result of increased facilitation or of decreased inhibition of motor programs. Transcranial magnetic cortex stimulation (TMS) is a neurophysiological tool to study non-invasively the motor system in childhood. In ADHD could be described with TMS as well as a deficient intracortical inhibition in the motor cortex as also a deficient transcallosally mediated intercortical inhibition between the motor cortices. In ADHD children with comorbid Tic disorder were found a reduced intracortical inhibition and a shortend cortical silent period, what provide evidence for additive effects at the level of motor system excitability. On the one hand these findings could be interpreted as dysfunctions of frontocortical neuronal circuits (intracortical inhibition) or an imbalance of inhibitory and excitatory drive on the neuronal network between cortex layer III – the projection site of transcallosal motor-cortical fibers – and layer V, the origin of the pyramidal tract (intercortical inhibition). On the other hand a maturation deficite of neuronal fibers is to be discussed. Methylphenidate (MPH), an indirect Dopamine agonist, is successfully used in the treatment of ADHD children. The neurotransmitter dopamine also seems to be involved in restoring defective intra- and intercortical motor inhibition. MPH enhanced as well as the deficient intracortical inhibition as also the disturbed transcallosally mediated intercortical motor inhibition in ADHD children. In sum, TMS is an effective method to investigate cortical excitability in ADHD children and may be a useful supplementory diagnostic tool to discriminate between ADHD and normal children.

S-102-475   Topic: 36, 84
Training of slow cortical potentials in children with ADHD
Hartmut Heinrich, Universität Erlangen, Heckscher Klinik,
München, Germany, harmut.heinrich@heckscher-klinik.de

Objective: Learned self-control of slow cortical potentials (SCPs) may be clinically helpful in neuropsychiatric disorders characterized by deficient cortical self-regulation, e.g. attention-deficit hyperactivity disorder (ADHD). Behavorial and neurophysiological effects of an extended SCP training in ADHD children will be reported. **Methods:** 13 ADHD children, aged 7 to 13 years, participated in a SCP neurofeedback training during summer holidays. They completed 25 SCP training sessions of 50 minutes each within three weeks. Before and after training, the German ADHD rating scale was completed by parents and event-related potentials were recorded in a cued continuous performance test (CPT). For a waiting list group of 9 ADHD children, the same testing was applied also at an interval of three weeks. **Results:** ADHD symptomatology was reduced by about 25% after SCP training. Moreover, a decrease of impulsivity errors and an increase of the contingent negative variation were observed in the CPT task. **Conclusion:** Positive behavioral and specific neurophysiological effects of SCP training provide evidence that this method may become a valuable treatment module for ADHD.

S-103
Free communication II
Chairperson: Miguel Cherro-Aguerre, Montevideo, Uruguay,
macherro@mednet.org.uy

S-103-477   Topic: 25, 45
Sexual knowledge, attitude and risk behaviors amongst adolescents: A qualitative study from India with a cultural perspective
Sameer Malhotra, AIIMS, Dept. of Psychiatry, New Delhi,
India, sameersankalp@hotmail.com

Objective: In view of the HIV epidemic, increasing consumerism and vulnerability amongst adolescents, it becomes important to understand the level of sex knowledge, attitude and sexual behaviors amongst this vulnerable age group. Adolescents in India constitute about 1/5th of its population. The study was conducted to gain insights into the sexual knowledge, attitudes and behaviors amongst the adolescents in India, from a cultural perspective. **Methods:** Experiential and qualitative research. Detailed information gathered on profile, sexual knowledge, attitude and behaviors of adolescents. **Results:** Lacunae exist in the sexual knowledge amongst adolescents, particularly amongst rural girls. Masturbation is associated with a strong sense of guilt and shame. Sexual knowledge is usually acquired through mass media and friends. Parents are neither considered nor preferred as a source of such information. There are emerging trends towards recreational view of sexuality, particularly amongst male as well as female college students in metropolitan cities. Although premarital sexual experience is not as common as in the West, however, it is not as rare as perceived widely. There is a striking male preponderance amongst substance users and the sexually active. Overall, India presents a contrasting picture of sexuality notions, attitudes and behavior. The society can neither be regarded as too rigid nor too permissive with regard to sexuality, making generalizations difficult. However, growing consumerism, globalization, role of media, trends towards delay in the age of marriage, easy money, drug use etc. are seen as important contributors to sex risk behaviors in a society deep rooted in traditions. **Conclusion:** Overall, the existing literature and the study signals a need for age appropriate value based sex education in Indian schools and colleges; and focus on traditional value systems alongside globalization.

S-103-478   Topic: 42
Psychological and emotional functioning of children with congenital heart defects prior to and after surgery

Zeffie Poulakis, Royal Children's Hospital,
Community Child Health, Parkville, Australia,
zeffie.poulakis@mcri.edu.au
Sam Menahem

Objective: This study aimed to investigate the psychological and emotional functioning of children with congenital heart defects (CHD) subjected to surgey. There previously had been little attempt at examining these children with a prospective study design, and with comparison of pre-surgery and post-surgery functioning. This study reviewed these aspects, looking at the psychological and emotional functioning of these children. In addition, child and family characteristics that may confer risk or contribute resilience to adverse adaptive functioning in children who were subjected to other surgical intervention were also investigated, guided by knowledge and concepts from stress-resilience research. **Methods:** Complete data was obtained from thirty-nine families whose child underwent cardiac surgery. Information was collected from the child aged 2.5 years to 12 years and at least one parent prior to surgery, and again between eleven and fifty months post-surgery. Measures included assessment of the child's receptive vocabulary, adaptive behaviour skills, emotional and behavioural problems, temperament, and quality of life, as well as medical and surgical data. Amongst parents and families measures included parent mental health, anxiety, and locus of control, family functioning and social support. Ten children who underwent non-cardiac, non-neurological surgery comprised a control group, and underwent the same pre-surgery assessment as the CHD group. **Results:** Prior to surgery, the CHD group were comparable to normative groups on all measures, including all of the key dependent variables (receptive vocabulary, adaptive behaviour skills, and behaviour problems). CHD group parents reported higher state anxiety and a greater tendency to attribute events to luck and chance than normative groups pre-surgery. Post-surgery descriptive analyses indicated that the CHD group once again did not differ from normative data on any measures. Likewise, mothers and families of children in the CHD group were not significantly different at follow-up to norms on all of the maternal and family variables, including the Quality of Life measures, and anxiety, which had reduced to levels comparable to normative groups. Psychological and emotional functioning at follow-up was related to psychological and emotional functioning prior to surgery. In addition, significant residual defects after surgery, and the need for further surgery, were associated with poorer functioning at follow-up. **Conclusion:** Overall, the results of this study indicated that children with CHD who undergo surgery for CHD displayed psychological and emotional functioning that was not distinguishable from normative populations, and from children in a control group who were undergoing non-cardiac surgery. This finding persisted when re-assessed eleven to fifty months after surgery. Why were the children in the CHD group doing so well? It is possible that given advances in detection, these children's CHD was identified very early, and that many parents knew antenatally, or im-

mediately after birth, of their child's condition and the management required, resulting in treatment at the earliest possible stage. Advances in treatment and medical care for CHD has resulted in earlier treatment, reduced hospitalizations and better prognosis for those children born with CHD. A further theme emerging from this study was that of the pattern of variables related to the children's psychological and emotional functioning at either pre-surgery or follow-up. The strongest relationships with functioning were evident with other 'within child' variables, with few parent or family variables showing a relationship with functioning at either time point. The other general theme that emerged from this study is that mothers of children in the CHD group showed heightened levels of anxiety and psychological distress prior to their child's surgery, and a greater tendency to attribute the cause of events to luck and chance. At follow-up, months or years after their child's CHD surgery, mothers no longer reported anxiety and psychological distress at levels differing from the normal population.

S-103-479   Topic: 59, 41
Young people and their music: Experience and consumption of music by healthy and psychologically ill young people

Gottfried Maria Barth, University of Tübingen,
Child a. Adolescent Psychiatry, Tübingen, Germany,
gottfried.barth@uni-tuebingen.de
Karin Sauer; Gunther Klosinski

Objective: The meaning of media for the healthy and pathological development of young people is differently judged. It is discussed whether a connection exists between juvenile music consumption and violence or suicidal thoughts. The consumption of music by young people and its meaning was explored in German pupils. **Methods:** 243 pupils of different public schools (class 8–10) and 78 young patients of the department of child and adolescent psychiatry Tübingen were interviewed by a self constructed questionnaire about the way, importance and consequences of listening music by them. 25 in- and outpatient adolescents were additionally interviewed by a 1 hour semi standardized oral interview. **Results:** Music consumption was very similar between healthy and psychologically ill young people. Female adolescents had a greater preference for music than male. Girls were more occupied with the text of a song than boys but all prefer more the music than verbal content. Young people don't think to copy the styling of musicians. Drug abuse was mentioned only by few adolescents. Music seems to be able to elevate depressed mood and to intensify good temper. There were no signs of aggressive escalation induced by music. **Conclusion:** Listening music is of particular importance for young people. They attribute quasi therapeutic effects. There seems to be no danger of increasing aggressiveness or suicidal tendency. Recognizing patterns of music consumption and personal preferences provides diagnostic and therapeutic capabilities.

S-103-480　Topic: 83, 29

Onset on an autistic disorder after excision of a cerebellar astrocytoma – A case report

Naoufel Gaddour, CHU F Bourguiba, service de psychiatrie, Monastir, Tunisia, naoufelgaddour@historique.zzn.com
Tilouch Samia; Hannachi Rimeh; Missaoui Sonia

Objective: Autistic-like disturbances have been anecdotally reported in patients with cerebellar alterations. Recent publications based on radiological and autopsy studies demonstrated that the cerebellar vermis (especially lower lobules) is involved in the pathogenesis of infantile autism. **Results:** We report the case of a Tunisian 4 years old boy: After a normal pregnancy and delivery, and an initial normal development, he started to develop equilibrium and locomotion difficulties since age of 10 months. At age of 15 months, MRI showed a posterior fossa tumour while the patient still got normal emotional and social behaviour and his language consisted in at least 20 words. After excision of the tumour, found to be a grade 2 gemistocytic astrocytoma, the patient developed a dramatic psychological regression, with loss of acquisitions in language and social skills. Bizarre stereotypic linguistic repetitions appeared, with social and affective retire, sameness, and stereotypic movements and vocalisations. These symptoms met the DSM IV criteria for autistic disorder, CARS-T score was 35.5, corresponding to a mild to moderate autism. Further MRI yearly controls showed no recurrence of tumour. Repeated EEGs, including 24 hours recording, showed no abnormalities. **Conclusion:** This case reinforces the idea that cerebellum plays a role in the processing of complex social and emotional behaviours, and could be disturbed in autistic patients.

S-104　Topic: 82

Learning disorders

Chairperson: Gerd Schulte-Körne,
Universitätsklinik Marburg Kinder- und Jugendpsychiatrie, Marburg, Germany, schulte1@med.uni-marburg.de

S-104-482　Topic: 82

Learning disabilities in relation to social context, school organization and classroom climate

Mara Westling Allodi, Stockholm Institute Education, Dept. of Special Education, Stockholm, Sweden, mara.allodi@lhs.se

Objective: To investigate the effects on classroom climate of a heterogeneous group composition, with pupils with learning disabilities, taking account of the schools' social context. The hypothesis is that the inclusion of pupils with disabilities will favor learning environment and group climate. **Methods:** Data was collected with Questionnaire on classroom climate to 679 Swedish pupils in 38 classes in 9 municipalities. Of the pupils, 80 had special needs. Questionnaires to the teachers. Public statistic data from the recruitment areas. The data was analyzed with confirmatory factor analysis (CFA), structural equation modeling (SEM) and two-level modeling. **Results:** The results show a negative relationship between Social context and Friction, and a positive between Cohesiveness and Social context. The relations between the presence of disabled pupils, the grade of their disability and aspects of the learning environment were significant. The presence of pupils with assessed disability, as well as the degree of disability is related to less Friction and greater Cohesiveness. Segregated learning environments and higher estimations of disabilities occur more often in socially disadvantaged neighborhoods. The learning environment in disadvantaged neighborhoods is characterized by more friction and segregation: it is important to make efforts to change this situation i.e. giving space in teacher training program to issues as group processes, democratic leadership, classroom climate. **Conclusion:** A heterogeneous groups composition is associated with processes that heighten acceptance and respect for differences: a learning environment where children with varying abilities and experiences are accepted facilitate the transmission of pro-social attitudes and values. The differences between schools in the occurrence of segregation should be investigated further: does the type of support given to the pupils differs depending on social status of parents and children? Aspects of group composition – as heterogeneity in background or ability – assessment of classroom climate, and schools' strategies in managing variation in ability should be considered when studying school effectiveness or comparing pupils' performances and school outcomes.

S-104-483　Topic: 82, 23

Saccadic control as an example of sensory-motor training in Dyslexia

Monica Biscaldi, Universitätsklinikum Freiburg, Kinder- und Jugendpsychiatrie, Freiburg, Germany, biscaldi@psyallg.ukl.uni-freiburg.de
Bettina Wagner; Klaus Hennighausen; Eberhard Schulz

Objective: Many dyslexics show problems in low perceptual/motor information processing. Although perceptual/motor functions can very often be successfully trained, it is controversially discussed whether their improvement influences the reading/spelling abilities of dyslexics. This study evaluates the effects of a controlled oculomotor daily training on the reading ability of dyslexic children with poor saccadic control. **Methods:** N=22 children (8–12 y.) with significant deficits in saccadic control were randomly assigned to an experimental group I (N=11) performing 5 weeks of saccade training and 6 weeks of reading training or to a control group II (N=10) waiting 5 weeks for the 6 weeks reading training. The reading performances of all children were measured before (t1) and after (t2) the 'waiting' or 'saccade training' time and after the reading training (t3). **Results:** Nine out of 11 children of group I (with saccade training) improved saccadic control. Both groups turned out to improve significantly their reading abilities after reading training. Group I showed a tendency towards a stronger improvement, reaching statistical significance in children above 10 years. **Conclusion:** Saccade control can similarly to other sensory-motor functions be successfully trained. We found weak evidence in support of reading improvement as a consequence of better saccade control. On the other hand a systematic training of reading abilities seems to be effective. Late and lasting effects of these training programs should be further investigated.

S-104-484   Topic: 58, 41
Apathetic college students withdrawing from academic activities

Chiyoko Uchida, Ibaraki University,
University Health Center, Mito, Japan,
uchidach@mx.ibaraki.ac.jp

Objective: To evaluate the proportion of the apathetic and withdrawing students among those who leave school, take off or repeat academic years and how the situation has changed in the last 20 years, further more to find out the characteristics of high risk groups for providing them effective psychiatric support service. **Methods:** First we examined the rates of the college events as mentioned such as repeating or taking off academic years and leaving school among Japanese national college students. Our department has been in charge of collecting and analyzing data from each college for 20 years. The students were divided into 6 groups according to gender and academic major, and each rate of each group was compared statistically. Then the reasons of those events were also examined to be classified into several groups; negative reasons like "Student Apathy" positive reasons like studying abroad and so on. **Results:** Each rate of academic event such as repeating or taking off academic years and leaving school has been becoming larger in the last 20 years and a considerable number of the students showed to have been in a "Student Apathy" state, especially in men. Male science major group shows the highest rate of leaving school – mostly because of "Student Apathy". **Conclusion:** A considerable number of Japanese national college students leave school, repeating or taking off academic years because of apathetic state, especially in men. Male science major students are the highest risk group in terms of leaving school because of "Student Apathy" Intensive psychiatric support is necessary for those students.

S-104-485   Topic: 56
Quality of life among children and adolescents in a psychiatric patients outpatient sample

Thomas Jozefiak, St. Olav University Hospital,
Child & Adolescent Psychiatry, Trondheim, Norway,
jozefia@online.no

Objective: Preliminary results of a multi-informant evaluation of QoL from an ongoing longitudinal study of Quality of Life (QoL) in 300 patients aged 8–16 years will be presented. **Methods:** Participants: By October 2003, 83 patients, their parents, teachers and clinicians were consecutively recruited into the study. Instruments: The Inventory of Life Quality in Children and Adolescents (ILC) by Mattejat & Remschmidt (1998), the CBCL, YSR and TRF (Achenbach & Rescoria 2001), the CGAS (Shaffer 1983), the ICD-10, were used in addition to the KINDL (Ravens-Sieberer & Bullinger 2000) from June 2004. Assessment: Before, and 6 months after initiation, at the end of treatment, in addition to 1 year after treatment. Statistical methods: Descriptive statistics, parametric and non-parametric tests. **Results:** Children experienced their QoL as good in many life domains in general, but older patients, evaluated the school and mental health areas as more problematic. Mothers evaluated global QoL among their children on the ILC as significantly poorer ($p < 0.05$) than the children. No significant associations ($r = 0.18$) between the patient and mother ratings of QoL on the ILC were found. There were low to moderate correlations ($r = 0.08$ to 0.63)

between reports on the ILC, and the CBCL, YSR, TRF and CGAS. **Conclusion:** In a preliminary analysis of the data the patients reported a good QoL in general. Children reports represent a most important information source of OoL. Prospective measurement of QoL, as used in the present study, will provide more specific knowledge about how QoL changes over time for this outpatient group. The inclusion of QoL adds important information in addition to standard assessment of psychiatric symptoms and social aspects in children with psychiatric disorders. At the congress updated results will be available.

S-104-486   Topic: 82
Mental representation and cognitive abilities in Dyslexia and garden variety reading disabled children

Roberta Penge, University Rome,
Child Adolescent Neurol. Psych, Rome, Italy,
roberta.penge@uniroma1.it
Flavia Capozzi; Valentina Ivancich Biaggini

Objective: Reading acquisition and reading mastering request the integrity of both phonological based decoding skills and of more general meta-linguistic and cognitive abilities. Reading disabled children often present difficulties in different kind of tasks, often not directly related to reading skills, The ability to mentally represent different kind of stimuli and situations seems to be a promising way to study the wide range of linguistic and non linguistic problems commonly detected in those children. Aim of this contribution is the study of representational abilities in specific learning disabled (Dyslexic) and in the more general learning disabled (Garden Variety) children. **Methods:** 25 garden variety learning disabled children (mean age 10 yrs, 1 month; mean IQ 77.6) are compared with a group of 25 chronological age matched and with 25 mental age matched Dyslexic children in two different kind of tasks (Drawing a Bicycle and Narrative Comprehension) that request mental representation abilities. Results obtained from the three groups are also compared with age group norms for both tasks. Text Reading and meta-phonological (Anagram Test) abilities are also compared among the three groups. **Results:** Garden Variety reading disabled group shows marked difficulties in drawing a bicycle by memory and using a three-dimensional model, and show a lack in the comprehension and retelling of inferential aspects of the narrative task in comparison with both chronological and mental age matched dyslexic group. Reading ability does not differentiate Garden Variety from mental age matched group, while reading comprehension of dyslexic groups is always better than that of Garden Variety group. In the Anagram task, Garden Variety children show a greater number of incorrect answers than both Dyslexic groups. **Conclusion:** The significant difficulties sowed by Garden Variety reading disabled children can be interpreted as the result of underlining problems in the mental representation of linguistic and graphic tasks, while Dyslexic children (with some differences at different ages) seems to have a sufficient mental representation of the problems and difficulties (more marked in linguistic tasks) in detecting autonomously the correct way to solve them. These results can have clinical implication both in the comprehension of pathogenetic pathways to reading disabilities and in the formulation of diagnostic and rehabilitative guide lines.

S-104-487   Topic: 58
Learning disabilities from varying special educational perspectives

*Siv Fischbein, Stockholm Inst. of Education,
Dept. of Human Dev., Stockholm, Sweden,
siv.fischbein@lhs.se*

Objective: Based on the hypothesis that the school environment can increase or decrease learning disabilities the objective of this project was to investigate which children and what type of difficulties the special educators report as well as the intervention undertaken by the schools. **Methods:** Special educators working in schools located in the vicinity of Stockholm were contacted. They formed a network, met regularly and functioned as informers and co-workers and were necessary to get in touch with pupils in need of special support as well as their parents, teachers and headmasters. Information concerned type of problems, pupil experiences, home and school cooperation, teacher's and headmaster's views on special educational activities. Both quantitative and qualitative data were collected. Some of the pupils have been followed for nine years through compulsory and supplementary school. **Results:** The main result from this project is that the same type of difficulty can be devastating in one school situation while it is not considered a problem at all in another situation. Thus our initial hypothesis seems to be corroborated. We also found that there are good special educational strategies as well as bad. Good strategies enhanced a clear structure, expressed rules and engagement of the teacher and headmaster to prevent difficulties. It also involved adequate support at an early stage. Bad strategies were categorization and exclusion of pupils without adeqate support. Another risk was to wait and hope that the pupils 'mature'. **Conclusion:** These results underline the necessity to train teachers and headmasters to appreciate a large variation and find ways of including all children. In order to do that they must also be aware of specific disabilities in order to establish interdisciplinary cooperation.

S-105   Topic: 96
Comorbidity

*Chairperson: John Campo, Western Psychiatric Institute
Psychiatry, Pittsburgh, PA, USA, campojv@msx.upmc.edu*

S-105-488   Topic: 96, 26
Alexithymia among 15–16 year olds – an epidemiological study

*Matti Joukamaa, University of Tampere,
School of Public Health, Tampere, Finland,
matti.joukamaa@uta.fi
Anja Taanila; Juha Veijola; Juha T. Karvonen;
Minna Koskinen; Jouko Miettunen*

Objective: During the past years the occurrence of alexithymia among general population has been elucidated in a handful of studies. There are no data concerning the epidemiology of alexithymia among teen age people. We aimed to study the prevalence of alexithymia among a representative sample of 15–16 year olds. **Methods:** This study forms part of the Northern Finland birth Cohort 1985/86 Study. The original material (N=9362) consisted of all live-born children in the provinces of Lapland and Oulu in Finland with an expected delivery date between 1. 7. 1985–31. 6. 1986. In 2001 when the subjects were 15–16 years old a comprehensive follow up study was made. Of the subjects 6068 participated in the present study. The 20-item version of the Toronto Alexithymia Scale (TAS-20) was the measure of alexithymia. **Results:** Of the boys 10% and 7% of the girls were alexithymic. The social situation and educational status of the mothers were associated with the prevalence of alexithymia. Children living in broken families were more commonly alexithymic than other subjects. **Conclusion:** We conclude that the rate and gender distribution of alexithymia among this age group are similar than among adult people, and alexithymia is associated with poor social situation.

S-105-489   Topic: 95
Problematic peer relationships and psychopathology in preschoolers

*Edelmira Domenech Llaberia, U. Autonoma de Barcelona,
Psicologia Salut i Social, Barcelona, Spain,
edelmira.domenech@uab.es
Teresa Corbella Domenech; Maria Claustre Jané Ballabriga;
Josepa Canals Sanz; Griselda Esparo; Sergi Ballespi Sola*

Objective: Our goals are: a) to explore aggressive behaviours among preschoolers peers; b) to examine the relation of the problematic peer relationships to specific externalizing and internalizing symptoms in a Spanish population of 3–6 years old children. **Methods:** Parents and teachers completed the Spanish version of the Early Childhood Inventory (ECI-4) for preschool children (Sprafkin and Gadow, 1996) (n=1104). It includes 10 items of Peer Conflict Scale (PCS) which assess disruptiveness and aggressive behaviour among peers and 98 items of DSM-IV-based symptoms. **Results:** Both parents and teachers find more aggressive behaviours among boys (parents: p-value=0.029; teachers: p-value<0.001). According to parents, the younger the child the more peer aggressive behaviours (p-value<0.006); however, this result does not appear in teachers' answers. There are no rural-urban group differences. Results show: a) a positive relationship between PCS and hyperactivity (parents: p-value=0.006; teachers: p-value<0.001), as expected due to boys; b) a positive relationship between PCS and oppositional disorder (parents: p-value=0,003; teachers: p-value<0.001), which is meanly due to boys and c) a negative relationship between PCS and some school improvement variables. Emotional symptoms do not appear to be related. **Conclusion:** In conclusion, preschool Peer Conflict Scale (PCS) symptoms appear to be related to behavioural symptoms rather than to emotional ones.

S-105-490   Topic: 96, 68
Investigation of the risk factors of video games addiction of children in Changsha City of China

*Linyan Su, Mental Health Institute,
Dept. of Child Psychiatry, Changsha, China,
sulinyan@sina.com
Xuejun Liu*

Objective: To find the risk factors of video games dependence. **Methods:** 602 pupils (8–15 years of age) were assessed on questionnaires in the schools of Changsha City to determine their video games dependency. The odds ratios of different factors to video game dependence were calculated in various statistic methods. **Results:** The risk factors of video games addiction are depending on: frequency of playing video games per week, duration of video game playing, sessions, playing video games in a street video games bar, use of violence video games, male gender, the awareness of the benefit and harm of playing video games and the age of starting to play video games. **Conclusion:** Specific measurements should be taken into account according to these risk factors mentioned above in order to protect children from video games addiction.

S-105-491   Topic: 87, 52
Aggression in adolescents with Tourette syndrome

Yukiko Kano, Kitasato University, Developmental Psychiatry, Sagamihara, Japan, kano-tky@umin.ac.jp
Masataka Ohta; Yoko Nagai; Takashi Arai

Objective: Rage attacks frequently found in Tourette syndrome (TS) hinder TS patients' social adjustment. This study was conducted to clarify the psychological mechanism of aggression in TS adolescents in terms of rage attacks and to find a clue to appropriate treatment for that aggression. **Methods:** The subjects were 36 TS adolescents (29 males and 7 females; mean age: 13.4, SD: 3.4). Twenty-four individuals were diagnosed by DSM-IV with TS only; 6 with TS + attention-deficit/hyperactivity disorder (AD/HD); 5 with TS + obsessive-compulsive disorder (OCD); 1 with TS + AD/HD + learning disorders. A battery of tests included Rage Screening and Questionnaire by parents, Rating of Aggression related to rage attacks within one month by clinicians and Child Behavior Checklist (CBCL) by parents. **Results:** Nineteen subjects out of 36 (52.8%) were judged aggressive by clinicians. Parents reported 23 with rage attacks in the last six months. Sixteen subjects were considered aggressive by both clinicians and parents. Between the 19 aggressive and the 17 non-aggressive subjects, no significant differences were found in age, gender and diagnosis. Sixteen aggressive and 10 non-aggressive subjects were on medication. There were no significant differences in medication and its contents, either. When the CBCL ratings of 17 aggressive and 13 non-aggressive subjects were compared, t-scores of Thought Problems and Externalizing were found significantly higher in the former than in the latter and t-scores of Anxious/Depressed, Delinquent Behavior and Aggressive Behavior were nearly significantly higher in the former. **Conclusion:** Aggression in TS was found to be related to anxiety or depression and thought problems, and importance of mental health activities including intervention programs for elimination of these problems was suggested to decrease aggression.

S-105-492   Topic: 87, 95
A Study of comorbid behavioral problems in Tourette's syndrome in China

Yan Zhu, Central South University, Mental Health Institute, Changsha, China, zhuyan4895025@hotmail.com
Su Linyan

Objective: To examine comorbid behavioral problems in Tourette's syndrome (TS) and the relation between severity of tic disorder and comorbid behavioral problems. **Methods:** Sixty-nine children with TS and 69 healthy controls were assessed by the Child Behavior Checklist (CBCL) and the Yale Global Tic Severity Scale (YGTSS). Statistical analysis used compare, correlation and multiple linear regression. **Results:** Scores of social competence subscales and total score of CBCL in TS group were lower than that in the control group, and behavioral problems subscales and total scores were higher than in the control group P < 0.01. Children with more severe tic syndrome had higher CBCL Delinquent behavior, Thought problems, Externalizing and Total problems scores than those with less severe tic syndrome P < 0.05. The severity of tic syndrome was negative correlated with School and Total Competence P < 0.05, and significantly positive correlated with Social problems, Thought problems, Attention problems, Delinquent behavior, Aggressive behavior, Externalizing and Total problems P < 0.01. **Conclusion:** The findings indicate that children with TS had broad behavioral problems, and some behavioral problems were associated with the severity of tic syndrome.

S-105-493   Topic: 95, 75
Parental anxiety, depression, and somatization associated with pediatric recurrent abdominal pain

John Campo, Western Psychiatric Institute, Psychiatry, Pittsburgh, PA, USA, campojv@msx.upmc.edu
Jeff Bridge; Boris Birmaher; Carlo Di Lorenzo; Satish Iyengar; David Brent

Objective: High rates of comorbid anxiety, depressive, and other somatic symptoms and disorders have been reported in children and adolescents with functional recurrent abdominal pain (RAP). Our aim was to determine if RAP is associated with higher parental levels of anxiety, depressive, and somatic symptoms and disorders. **Methods:** Mothers of children and adolescents 8 to 15 years of age, inclusive, presenting with RAP (cases; N = 53) or for routine care in the absence of recurrent pain (controls; N = 65) who were identified by a screening procedure in pediatric primary care office waiting rooms completed self-report questionnaires assessing current anxiety, depressive, and somatic symptoms, as well as a standardized family history assessment by an interviewer blind to subject status. Comparisons were made using standard tests of proportions for categorical variables and the appropriate t-test or Mann Whitney U for continuous variables. **Results:** Mothers of RAP cases were significantly more likely to report anxiety, depressive, and somatic symptoms, and were significantly more likely to meet diagnostic criteria for irritable bowel syndrome (IBS), migraine, fibromyalgia, and anxiety, depressive, and somatoform disorders than mothers of pain-free controls. Mothers of children with RAP reported lower overall quality of life than control mothers, but the groups did not differ on measures of health or mental health service use in the prior 6 months. **Conclusion:** The observed higher levels of functional abdominal pain consistent with IBS and anxiety, depressive, and somatoform symptoms and disorders in mothers of children with RAP than in mothers of pain free controls provide support for the clinical phenotype of RAP and observed nonrandom associations with anxiety, depressive, and other somatic disorders such as migraine. Future studies, including longitudinal, family, and psychobiological studies are needed to illuminate the nature of observed comorbidities.

S-106   Topic: 63
Training and professional issues

Chairperson: Bernhard Blanz, Universität Jena Inst. für Psychiatrie, Jena, Germany, blanz@landgraf.med.uni-jena.de

S-106-494   Topic: 63, 20

E-learning and Child and Adolescent Psychiatry Integrating psychiatric cases into a somatically based system for Problem-Oriented-Learning (POL)

Laura Weninger, Universitätskrankenhaus Ulm, Kinder- und Jugendpsychiatrie, Ulm, Germany, laura.weninger@medizin.uni-ulm.de
Gerhard Libal; Anna Skrabal; Ferdinand Keller

Objective: Electronically based learning devices are increasingly introduced for teaching medicine at a graduate and postgraduate level. We describe the advantages and disadvantages of the integration of a child and adolescent psychiatry module in a pre-existing, somatically based e-learning system. The e-learning system was primarily developed for medical students with the objective to train them particularly in the field of Problem Oriented Learning (POL). **Methods:** First we developed an adjusted psychological and psychiatric decision-tree and integrated it into the somatically based e-learning system. As a second step we selected 4 (frequent) general medical problems, which lead to decision-making procedures, psychiatric diagnoses and treatment options at several difficulty levels. These specific case-scenarios are relevant for POL in the graduate, postgraduate and professional training. **Results:** We developed specific history-taking questions, psychometric questionnaires/scales (e.g. CBCL), diagnostic criteria and treatment options for the new module. We integrated case-scenarios of Anorexia/Bulimia, ADHD, Tic disorder-Tourette und Autism into the e-learning system. A preliminary evaluation demonstrates good acceptance of the new module among users. **Conclusion:** The integration of a child and adolescent psychiatry module in a somatically based e-learning system is a meaningful supplement to traditional lectures and courses, which facilitates teaching and Problem-Oriented-Learning of Child- and Adolescent Psychiatry in the graduate, postgraduate and professional training.

S-106-495   Topic: 63, 45

Current issues in training child, adolescent and family psychiatrists in Australia and New Zealand

Michael Bowden, NSW Institute of Psychiatry, Parramatta, Australia, michael@nswiop.nsw.edu.au
Howard Cooper

Objective: To elucidate current issues in training of Child, Adolescent and Family Psychiatry trainees in Australia and New Zealand, including the need for a re-examination of the training Curriculum. **Methods:** Recent changes in the training requirements for advanced trainees in Australia and New Zealand are described. The training curriculum is examined and compared with international trends. Issues particular to Australia and New Zealand are discussed in this context. **Results:** Changes in the practice of Psychiatry, particularly advances in assessment, treatment and service delivery, have led to increasing global interest in training issues in postgraduate Psychiatry recently. The need for competency-based training has been emphasised internationally. There are important issues in the implementation and evaluation of such programmes, though little has been published regarding training programmes in the specific area of Child, Adolescent and Family Psychiatry. New training by-laws for Psychiatry training in Australia and New Zealand commenced in 2004, which prompted a re-examination of the training curriculum for advanced training in Child, Adolescent And Family Psychiatry. Issues particular to Australia and New Zealand include the relatively low numbers of trainees, large differences in numbers of trainees in different academic centres that are geographically distant and that have different access to resources and the need for a uniform yet serviceable curriculum. Dealing with these issues is an ongoing, dynamic process that draws on the international experience and which also requires novel solutions to the particular issues of this region. **Conclusion:** There is a need for clarification of core competencies in Child, Adolescent and Family Psychiatry training. Elucidation of these competencies needs to result in a curriculum that equips trainees for the challenges of their future professional role and which allows adequate evaluation.

S-106-496   Topic: 63, 45

How to recruit and train child psychiatrists in remote and arctic areas. Recruitment and Training in Northern Norway

Inger Simonsen, Nordland Hospital, Training & Recruitment Project, Bodø, Norway, inger.simonsen@nlsh.no
Carl Bechstrøm; Mette Medby

Objective: To recriut and train 15 new MD's by 2006 to the empty positions of child and adolescent psychiatrists in Northern Norway, and to refrain both the existing consultants and new doctors. **Methods:** Seeking out suitable trainees with local connections and facilitate their training path. Establishing regular seminars for all the doctors in the region 3–4 times each year, using videoconferences for lectures 18 times a year, monthly meetings for the trainees with supervisor and one yearly meeting for the consultants. **Results:** The project is now in its fifth year – 2004 – and we have 10 consultant psychiatrists and 15 trainees. The number today has increased from 8 to 25, 2 more than the original objective. We also have a strong professional network. **Conclusion:** Some of the trainees have chosen to work in clinics that lack formal approval as places for training. In those cases facilitating the training path has been difficult and demanding for both the trainee, the clinic and the consultant. Without the network this would have been very difficult. It looks like working with relationships and the network as well as the training has been vital factors to the success for this project.

S-106-497   Topic: 63, 45

The effect of a new primary health care program on the trainees. The European Early Promotion Project as a training method for Primary Health Care Professionals

Ritva Erkolahti, Turku University Hospital, Adolescent Psychiatric Clinic, Turku, Finland, ritva.erkolahti@tyks.fi
Aino-Maija Salin; Päivi Rytölä; Pauliina Hiltunen; Irma Moilanen

Objective: Infancy is seen as an optimal time for prevention and there is considerable evidence of effectiveness of preventive programs in populations where several risk factors are present. The aim of European Early Promotion Project is to enable Primary Health Professionals (PHCPs) to assess and reinforce factors relevant to childrens' psychosocial development. In this research we wanted to find out the change of thinking of the PHCPs during the training program. **Methods:** 63 Primary Health Care persons were chosen to participate the training and this research. To measure the interpretation of the trainees about the expressed feelings we used the series of pictures developed by Emde (I FEEL pictures). Lot of background variables were gathered. Statistical test methods used: Kruskal-Wallis-test, Mann-Whitney U-test, Spearman correlation coefficient test. To measure the change of test scores between the first assessment before the training and the second assessment after the training we used the Friedman test and Wilcox-test. **Results:** The most popular affect category was interest (25.4%) and next sadness (10.5%). Only few answers were in the category shame/guilt (0.05%). The average amount of affect categories per figure was almost the same in both test situations. The affect category sadness changed from 10.5% to 12.0%. Statistically significant change between the affect categories was found in the category of fear (p = 0.025). In the second test situation the trainees used more answers expressing the fear of the child than in the first test. There were background variables connected to the change in the affect categories: Chronic disease in the family, sex of the trainees own children, years at work and the amount of children in the family. **Conclusion:** The results of the retest show that there are only few changes in the usage of the affect categories. It tells more about the retest reliability of the test method than about the change of thinking in the study group. Sadness and fear were the affect categories the study group used after training more than before. It was also seen that the more occupational education the trainees had the easier they recognized sadness.

S-107   Topic: 47, 49
Family issues

Chairperson: Gunther Klosinski, University of Tuebingen Child & Adolescent Psychiatry, Tuebingen, Germany, Gunther.Klosinski@med.uni-tuebingen.de

S-107-498   Topic: 41
Parental attitude, self-preoccupation, and various mood states associated with self-preoccupation among Japanese adolescents

Mihoko Oba, Nagoya University, Dept. of Psychology, Ogaki, Japan, mihokoº@ogaki-tv.ne.jp
Satomi Murase; Takashi Murakami; Jiro Takai; Hitoshi Kaneko; Shuji Honjo

Objective: Self-preoccupation is a tendency to focus more on the self and to maintain self-focused attention, and it is a cognitive trait predisposing to depression. To date, no study has examined whether self-preoccupation leads to any mood states other than depression. Furthermore, the relationship between parental attitude, self-perception and self-preoccupation has not been studied. **Methods:** Three-hundred and fifty-five undergraduates (104 males, 252 females, average age 19.9 yrs.) were administered 4 questionnaires: the Parental Bonding Instrument (PBI); Actual-Negative Ideal Discrepancy Score; the Self-preoccupation Scale (SPS); and Profile of Mood States (POMS). **Results:** Multiple regression analysis revealed that 'Rejection' measured by PBI predicts the tendency to perceive 'actual-self' as close to 'negative ideal-self', as well as self-preoccupation. In addition, t-tests showed that subjects who had high scores on self-preoccupation showed not only signs

of depression, but also other mood states measured by POMS, such as Tension-Anxiety, Anger-Hostility, Fatigue and Confusion. **Conclusion:** Finally, the current study showed that negative parental attitude results in the distortion of self-perception, which might lead to various mood states via self-preoccupation. It would be important to deal with cognitive traits and self-preoccupation as a treatment strategy.

S-107-499   Topic: 50, 45
An exploration of the factors facilitating intercountry adoption outcome

Katrina Rickards, Lothian Primary Care Trust, Dept. of Clinical Psychology, Edinburgh, United Kingdom, katrinarickards@hotmail.com

Objective: Contradictory findings have emerged in the field of adoption outcome research, raising questions about whether this experience is associated with healthy functioning and development. However, there have been few attempts to understand the experiential and contextual factors that facilitate outcome. **Methods:** This paper will explore the intercountry adjustment outcome and the contextual factors contributing to outcome in a sample of 39 children adopted from the Philippines by parents in Victoria, Australia. Complementary quantitative and qualitative methods were used in the study. Quantitative measures were employed to assess emotional and behavioural difficulties and self esteem, as well as the contextual factors of family and parent-child relationships, pre-adoptive experiences, and the acculturation of the parents to Filipino culture. Parents were interviewed about their experiences of adoption. **Results:** The children either did not significantly differ from the general population in terms of their emotional and behavioural difficulties and their self esteem, or were functioning at higher levels than the general population. They were found to have lower school competence than the general population. An association between emotional and behavioural difficulties and contextual factors was suggested, and significant associations were found among the quality of the parent-child relationship, the child's emotional and behavioural difficulties, and the parents' acculturation to the Philippines. Pre-adoptive experiences, such as age at arrival, health on arrival or number of placements were not significantly associated with emotional and behavioural difficulties. These results were confirmed and elaborated by the qualitative interview findings. However, many challenges in intercountry adoption were discussed, such as the assessment and allocation process, early transition difficulties, and intrusive community responses. Factors facilitating outcome included helping the child to understand adoption, support from others, contact with the Philippines and managing developmental issues appropriately. Many parents felt that adoption outcome was related to contextual factors such as development and parenting, and not to adoption per se. **Conclusion:** The results addressed in this paper provide support to the emerging body of literature that concludes that adoption outcome is determined by a range of developmental and contextual factors, of which adoption is just one.

S-107-500 Topic: 49

Separation of parents: How it is conveyed to children and what about the influence on the further parent-child relationship?

Gunther Klosinski, University of Tuebingen,
Child & Adolescent Psychiatry, Tuebingen, Germany,
Gunther.Klosinski@med.uni-tuebingen.de
Annhild Weber; Michael Karle

Objective: Does the way how parents inform their child about an occurring near separation influence the mother-child and father-child relationship? What do and what don't parents tell their children, when they are going to separate? **Methods:** On the basis of 1. a retrospective analysis of 45 custody expertises, pertaining to 95 children (44 girls and 45 boys, average age: 7 1/2 years old) and 2. a catamnestic survey carried out by questionnaires, including 62 parents, it was examined, how the parents told their child about the near separation and if the way the parents inform the child had an impact on coping with the separation. **Results:** Only 48.9% of the families talked about the separation. 35% of the children were not informed, 12.4% of the children were not told the truth. There was no clear correlation between the way the children were informed and their coping behavior. Yet it could be shown, that talking to the child had a positive effect on the relationship between the father and the child. If the mother left, we found only a good mother-child relationship in 18.5% and a good father-child relationship in 81.5%. But if the father was leaving family a good mother-child as well as a good father-child relationship was found in 78.4%. **Conclusion:** If the situation of separation is highly conflictous and the parents do not inform appropriately the child, there is evidence that this is of disadvantage for the parent-child relationship. This topic has neither been sufficiently considered in literature nor by parents planning a divorce.

S-107-501 Topic: 47

Consensus, hedonism: The characteristics of new families, consequences for children

Alain Lazartigues, CHU de Brest, Bohars, France,
alain.lazartigues@chu-brest.fr
Pascale Planche; Eric Lemonnier

The structure of the family has changed a lot through the last two centuries. Until the eighteen century, the traditional family relied upon the authority of the father and a long lasted mariage. After that, the modern family was organised with love between spouse and husband, and the authority of the father, which had been reduced gradually across the last century. Over the last three decades, the marital family model described by Durkheim at the end of the nineteenth century has undergone numerous changes, e.g. questioning about the principle allegiance to authority, women emancipation, occurrence of the 'new fathers', the growing influence of the media on the daily life of families, the less frequent and most precious child (couples have less children),... Through clinical psychoanalytical and developmental models we, here, analyse these changes together with their impact on the child. Historical and sociological approaches also allowed us to examine some of the effects induced by consensus and hedonism, the new familial parameters, on the child's life and development. The modern family being classically founded upon duty (central value) and the principle of authority to settle relationships between individuals, its main characteristics are opposed to those of the contemporary family. The latter, which started to emerge over the sixties, is characterised by both the prevalence of parent-child relationships symmetrization and the emergence of the search for immediate pleasure. This led us to assume new basic personalities (passive – dependent, perverse – narcisstic with psychopathic aspects) and to envision some psychopathological consequences.

S-107-501A Topic: 70, 6

Child and Family Focused Cognitive Behavior Therapy (CFF-CBT) in pediatric bipolar disorder

Mani Pavuluri, University of Illinois, Child Psychiatry,
Chicago, USA, mpavuluri@psych.uic.edu

Objective: To develop and test the efficacy of CFF-CBT versus treatment as usual in Pediatric Bipolar Disorder (PBD). **Methods:** CFF-CBT is a developmentally sensitive psychosocial treatment for PBD that is developed to be administered along with medication. It seeks to integrate principles of interpersonal psychotherapy with those of CBT. CFF-CBT actively engages parents along with children over 12 sessions. This study compared 34 subjects with PBD who had a mean age of 11.33 years (SD = 3.06) and were treated with CFF-CBT in a specialty clinic (experimental group) to 32 subjects with PBD who had a mean age of 11.34 years (SD = 3.25) and received treatment as usual in a general outpatient clinic (control group). Subjects were diagnosed using the WASH-U-KSADS. All subjects were assessed prospectively during treatment using the CGI-BP severity scales and other measures. **Results:** Controlling for differences in pre test severity ratings, the experimental group showed significantly lower overall post-test severity (🌑). There are significant differences with lower scores in experimental group compared to control group on all CGI subscales including CGI Mania subscale (1.02 vs 4.56; $p < 0.0001$), CGI Depression subscale (2.00 vs 3.03; $p < 0.05$) and CGI Aggression subscale (2.12 vs 4.84; $p < 0.0001$). At post-test, C-GAS scores for the experimental group (mean = 54.24, SD = 8.51) were significantly higher than those of the control group (mean = 39.17, SD = 11.11), indicating that the treatment group was functioning at a higher level upon termination of treatment compared to the control group ($t(64) = 7.45$, $p < 0.0001$). **Conclusion:** Preliminary results suggest that CFF-CBT may be superior to treatment as usual. Randomized studies will be necessary to conclude that CFF-CBT is effective.

S-107-501B Topic: 70, 30

Neurocognitive function in pediatric bipolar disorder

Mani Pavuluri, University of Illinois, Child Psychiatry,
Chicago, USA, mpavuluri@psych.uic.edu
Lindsay Schenkel; Ryan Shaw; John Sweeny

Objective: It is critical to evaluate neurocognitive functioning in individuals with pediatric bipolar disorder (PBD) given the neurodevelopmental abnormalities and educational difficulties of these children. Our hypothesis is that PBD is marked by impaired cognition, including deficits in spatial working memory, verbal learning and memory, executive control of working memory, set shifting, and sustained attention, similar to that we and others have reported in adult bipolar disorder. **Methods:** Forty age, sex, and race matched PBD and healthy subjects entered the study (mean age: 11±2.7 years). Groups were matched in word reading ability on the Wide Range Achievement Test-3. All subjects were euthymic during the testing period (Young Mania Rating Scale score 8 and Revised Child Depression Rating Scale Score 40). A computerized neurocognitive battery was administered (including tests from the Penn Battery and Cogtest), along with neuropsychological tests including the California Verbal Learning Test (CVLT-C), subtests from the Wechsler Memory Scale-III (WMS-III) and Wechsler Abbreviated Scale of Intelligence (WASI), and Trails A and B. **Results:** PBD subjects showed marked impairments on tasks of set shifting, and working memory; and when these elements are involved in complex tasks, psychomotor speed, visual spatial memory, verbal learning, and executive functioning are all affected. Conclusions: There are a wide range of neurocognitive deficits in PBD subjects, even in the euthymic phase of illness, that underscore the complexity of neuronal networks involved in PBD beyond affective brain systems. **Conclusion:** The results of this study indicate selected deficits in controlled use of attentional resources, in learning, and in executive functioning in clinically stabilized pediatric bipolar disorder patients. Moreover, impairment in verbal learning was the factor that best discriminated bipolar from control subjects. These results are similar to findings from the adult bipolar disorder literature. They suggest that efforts need to be made to account and provide psychoeducational support in the treatment of pediatric bipolar patients. The data also imply a potential role of frontal systems in the etiology and expression of bipolar disorder in pediatric patients.

S-108   Topic: 93
Suicide and self injurious behaviour
Chairperson: Eberhard Schulz, Universität Freiburg Kinder-und Jugendpsychiatrie, Freiburg, Germany, schulz@psyallg.ukl.uni-freiburg.de

S-108-502   Topic: 93, 41
Attending adolescent suicide attempters: Clinical and organizational problems
Giancarlo Rigon, Neuropsichiatria Infantile,
Dip. de Psichiatria, Bologna, Italy, girigon@libero.it
Stefano Costa; Alessandra Mancaruso; Roberta Mansi;
Daniele Giovanni Poggioli; Simona Chiodo

Objective: Adolescents who attempt suicide usually present a highly complex psychopathological and social pattern. In this paper we support this observation through the comparison among three different groups. **Methods:** A clinical group composed of 28 adolescents who were referred to our Service for suicide attempt; a second group composed of 26 adolescents who anonymously declared in a self report inquiry to have attempted suicide; a control group. Statistic: the difference among the groups has been estimated with the exact test of Fischer for small samples. **Results:** We found that the majority of the risk factors for suicide attempt are present both in the clinical and in the self report group, while they are absent in the control group. Adolescents who attempted suicide present simultaneously a great number of risk factors in comparison with the control group, and besides, they have school, family and peer problems. **Conclusion:** According to this complex situation, the therapeutic action have to be carried out

with a multiprofessional clinical group and in a strong full collaboration with all the local Services and Authorities.

S-108-503   Topic: 93
Comparison of two generations of adolescent suicide attempters
Maja Radobuljac, University of Ljubljana,
University Psychiatric Hosp., Ljubljana, Slovenia,
maja.radobuljac@mf.uni-lj.si
Urban Groleger; Nada Ovsenik; Martina Tomori

Objective: To compare the characteristics of adolescent suicide attempters admitted to the Adolescent Department, University Psychiatric Hospital in Ljubljana, Slovenia during the years 1975–1977 and 2002–2004. **Methods:** A general questionnaire had been routinely applied by the staff to every inpatient in the years 1975–1994. It included general characteristics of the patient, family circumstances, frequency of smoking, alcohol and substance abuse, number of previous suicide attempts and data on past violent behaviour. In 2001 a new questionnaire comprising of the same groups of data was constructed for the purposes of another study and used in adolescent inpatients admitted after a suicide attempt. We compared the data collected in adolescent suicide attempters in the years 1975–1977 with the data we collected in the years 2002–2004. **Results:** We found no statistically significant differences between the two groups in age, sex, family structure (parents divorce, parent loss, number of siblings), frequency of smoking, alcohol, soft drugs (marijuana, hashish) and hard drugs (heroin, cocaine, synthetical drugs) abuse. The two groups significantly differed in diagnoses, educational level, violent behaviour, number of previous suicide attempts, abuse of psychoactive medications. **Conclusion:** Observed findings from our study will be compared with data from the literature on changes in inpatient psychiatric population during last decades. The treshold to inpatient treatments has been raising all over the world in all age populations, including adolescents. Findings from our study on diagnosis, violent and suicidal behavior as well as other observed variables have confirmed the above mentioned findings from other studies. Results have important implications for future in- as well as outpatient programs for adolescents with psychiatric and developmental disorders.

S-108-504   Topic: 93
Model of the maintenance of self-injurious behaviour (SIB)
Barbara Haas, Linz, Austria, barbara.haas@liwest.at

Objective: The aim of this work is a combination of most models that explain the maintenance of self-injurious behavior (SIB). **Methods:** The definition of SIB excludes suicidal attempts, mental retardation and self-injuries that are accepted in culture. Via collection of actual models of the maintenance of SIB documented in literature they were tried to be combined and integrated into one explanatory model. **Results:** 17 models have been found. They included biological, psychological and social factors. Some of them were about SIB in mentally retarded that seemed to suit, too, in SIB defined above. The integrative model can be devided into negative and positive reinforcement. The first contains coping with stimulus satiation and combines hypotheses such as of biological factors, substitute activity, negative cognitions and dissociation. Some aspects of possible origins of SIB are included as well. Missing of stimuli as a cause of SIB is only expected to be relevant in early childhood and mental retardation. The model of positive reinforcement discusses the effects of SIB on the social system. **Conclusion:** It seems to be possible to create an integrative model of the maintenance of SIB. It shows that many partly very different factors play an important role at the same time in SIB. This model is seen as a hypotheses. The next step is a verification via studies.

S-108-505   Topic: 93, 20

www.youth-life-line.de: Suicide prevention by peers

Susanne Denoix, Arbeitskreis Leben, Tübingen, Germany,
susanne.denoix@youth-life-line.de
Franz Kimmig; Marc Weinhardt; Gottfried Maria Barth

Objective: Suicide prevention is an important issue in adolescence. Many young people don't dare the step to professional support. It was suggested that peer consulting could facilitate searching help. There were many questions about benefits and risks of peer consulting. **Methods:** www.youth-life-line.de is an online project for teens and young adults in life crises and under the risk of suicide. Trained young people help other peers under competent leadership by mail and chat. 21 adolescents got half a year training by psychological consultants. Then they started in March 21st 2003 internet-counselling for peers. Five days in the week they are 3 hours online, four times via mail, one day by direct chat. **Results:** In the first year requests of 500 clients reached the consulter. 1800 mails were sent in response. Most frequent issues were suicidal ideation, self-injury and problems with parents and other connected people. Most critiical events were two concrete suicide announcements which didn't lead to suicidal acts. **Conclusion:** The youth-life-line project was well accepted by peers both counselors and consulter. There was only few misapplication. Coaching of counselors was well. Suicide prevention by peers is a reasonable supplement to conventional offers of consulting. No considerable risks appeared until today.

S-108-506   Topic: 93

Juvenile Suicidal Behaviour

Günter Schmitz, Universität Kiel, Kinder- und
Jugendpsychiatrie, Kiel, Germany,
ch.haase@kiju-psych.uni-kiel.de
Berit Filschke; Conny Fliegauf

Objective: Suicidal acts of adolescents, male and female, show different patterns of psychiatric and psychodynamic aspects than adolescent suicidal behaviour 25 years ago. **Methods:** We analysed 79 patients (23 males, 56 females; 49 in patient in the period from 1999–2003 and compared these 30 inpatient patients in 1978–80. The mean age of both groups was about 15.5 years on average. **Results:** Cluster analyses suggest, that presend suicidal behaviour is associated with truancy, depressive symptoms, automutilation and dissocial tendencies. Intoxication, often in connection with alcohol, is the most common method. This syndrome was interpreted as a type of we use the term "juvenile refusal". An important aspect of these juveniles is refusal of therapeutic intervention and a low compliance. A second group shows signs of a borderline personality organisation. Former suicidal adolescents are either characterised by dissocial/depressive symptoms or histrio-

nic personality organisation. **Conclusion:** More than 70% of our patients come from families with considerable psychosocial problems and/or psychiatric disturbances. First symptoms present at ages 7 and 11 years. The preadolescent developmental period we should be a focus our diagnostic and therapeutic efforts including teachers who should pay attention to early depressive and dissocial symptoms. This is the only way for an effective prevention to minimize the severe forms of "juvenile refusal".

S-109   Topic: 57

Forensic child and adolescent psychiatry

Chairperson: Frank Häßler, Universität Rostock, Kinder-
und Jugendpsychiatrie, Rostock, Germany,
frank.haessler@med.uni-rostock.de

S-109-508   Topic: 57, 96

The problem of differentiating between sudden infant death syndrome, Munchhausen by proxy syndrome, and homicide

Frank Häßler, Universität Rostock,
Kinder- und Jugendpsychiatrie, Rostock, Germany,
frank.haessler@med.uni-rostock.de

Objective: Sudden infant death syndrome (SIDS) is the most common type of post-neonatal death in infants aged under 2 years. It is defined as the sudden death of an infant that is unexpected from the child's history and unexplained by a thorough post-mortem examination. The incidence of SIDS in Germany has fallen from 1.7 per 1000 live birth in 1990 to 0.62 in 2000. According to the literature 5 to 11 percent of deaths recorded as SIDS may be disguised homicides. These homicides can be caused by a Munchhausen syndrome by proxy (MSBP). This paper examines some difficulties in differentiating between SIDS, MSBP, and homicide using case reports. **Methods:** In a family with three children the youngest daughter suddenly died at an age of 17 month of suffocation. Before death the child was admitted 11 times to different hospitals for various reasons. As the mother reported her daughter was admitted for epileptic seizures, suffocation attacks, and diarrhoea. No remarkable organic signs and symptoms were found during the child's stays in a hospital. The girl was discharged without symptoms and without a clear-cut diagnosis every time. Toxicological analysis of the blood revealed the presence of caffeine. Clinically an accidental death appeared to be unlikely. In a second family with two children the youngest daughter was strangled at the age of 24 month. Before the child's death, it was known that the mother hated her daughter and had induced an illness to her daughter. It was also known that he child had suffered from physical and emotional neglect. **Conclusion:** For assessing cases of SIDS a MSBP or homicide practitioners should consider if one or more of the following cues are given: recurrent symptoms of illness, repeated hospitalization and/or consultation of physicians, multiple diagnostic procedures without a clear-cut diagnosis, a certain resistance to therapy, illness or unnatural death of siblings, and repeated poisoning or suffocation attempts. Differentiation between SIDS, MSBP, and homicide should be done extensively and carefully because legal consequences differ vastly according to facts of the matter.

S-109-509   Topic: 57, 85
Characteristics of emotion and behavior in Korean adolescent delinquency

Sung-Do David Hong, Samsung Medical Center, Child & Adolescent Psychiatry, Seoul, Republic of Korea, sdhong@smc.samsung.co.kr
Ji-Hae Kim

Objective: The Purpose of present study was to explore characteristics of behavior and emotion in Korean adolescent delinquency. **Methods:** Four-hundred-three adolescents participated to fill out the Latent Delinquency Questionnaire (LDQ), the Revised Children's Manifest Anxiety Scale (RCMAS), the Beck Depression Inventory (BDI), the Conner's Adult ADHD Rating Scales (CAARS), Aggression Scale, and Conflict Tactic Scale (CTS). **Results:** In male adolescent, delinquency was positively correlated with hyperactivity and aggression. In female, delinquency was correlated with all behavioral and emotional variables. Multiple regression analysis showed that hyperactivity and aggression in male, and familial abuse, hyperactivity, and aggression in female were significant predicting variables for adolescent delinquency. **Conclusion:** From our results it was inferred that Korean adolescent delinquency is correlated with behavioral problem, especially hyperactivity.

S-109-510   Topic: 57, 40
Forensic treatment of female pyromanic/fire setter

Oliver Bilke, Humboldt-Klinikum, Kinder- und Jugendpsychiatrie, Berlin, Germany, oliver.bilke@vivantes.de

Objective: The patient grew up with her two younger siblings and her mother. The unsteadiness of her mother brought about an early undertaking of responsibility for her siblings that led to growing tensions between family members. With her puberty the first apparent problems outside her family occurred – leading to school changes, repetition of classes and drug abuse. She became victim to several sexual abuses by adolescents. This fact and three suicide attempts in 2002/2003 resulted in outpatient treatment in adolescent psychiatry. The 18 assaults occurred between September 2002 and March 2003. **Methods:** The cognitive-behavioural and problem-solving therapy is planned specific to the disorder and pathology. When assuming a developing emotionally unstable personality disorder the main goals of treatment are the self-perception of emotions and self-regulation as well as the interpersonal behaviour – using parts of M. Linehans manuals. A further integral part of daily work and treatment of the patient is the experience of constant pedagogic and therapeutic relations. The explicit therapy of the chronic post-traumatic stress disorder is not yet the intention of the patient. Elements of trauma therapy would be possible for the future. In regard to a pharmacological support the patient feels very ambivalent, so that the current setting includes only sedative pharmacotherapy on demand. **Conclusion:** The successful treatment of this patient necessitates a long-termed planning that has to include the further clarification and settlement of offences. Currently no direct correlation of psychiatric disorders and offences are being observed, so that the previous therapy strategy is unchanged.

S-110   Topic: 52, 41
Adolescence, personality pathology and violence

Chairperson: Maya Krischer, Universität zu Köln Klinik für Kinderpsychiatrie, Köln, Germany, mayakrischer@aol.com

Adolescence, personality pathology and violence

Maya Krischer, Universität zu Köln, Klinik für Kinderpsychiatrie, Köln, Germany, mayakrischer@aol.com

The goal of this Symposium is to present different aspects of adolescent personality pathology and its effects on violent behavior. The realm of this symposium extends from longitudinal studies on juveniles with borderline personality disorder (1), an ongoing study on Psychopathy comorbid with ADHD (2), as well as the impact of trauma on violence, conducted with incarcerated adolescents (3) (the Cologne GAP-Study) to a new instrument to assess antisocial personality disorder in Switzerland (4).

S-110-511   Topic: 42, 80
Long-term outcome of juvenile in-patients with Borderline Personality Organization

Michael H. Stone, Columbia University, Dept. of Clinical Psychiatry, New York, NY, USA, mstonemd@aol.com

Objective: As part of the long-term (10 to 25 year) follow-up study of borderline and other patients who had been hospitalized between 1963 & 1976 at the New York State Psychiatric Institute, a large group of adolescents (between ages 13 and 18 when first hospitalized) was also traced. **Methods:** Sixty-five were borderline by the broader criteria of Kernberg ("Borderline Personality Organization" or "BPO"), but most of these also met DSM criteria for Borderline Personality Disorder ("BPD"): 60 of the 65. There were 20 males (2 of whom were BPO only) and 45 females (3 of whom were BPO only). **Results:** Among the males, 7 of the 20 were comorbid for antisocial personality disorder (ASPD), and of those 7, three committed murder during the follow-up period, and one committed suicide. Another died in a motorcycle accident. There were three other suicides, making 4 altogether (20%, that is, in the male adolescent group). The BPD x ASPD male who committed suicide had been arrested several times for selling drugs and for arson. In contrast, 9 of the male adolescents ultimately achieved outcome Global Assessment scores > 60 (including two of the ASPD males), meaning 45% were doing well, 10 to 25 years later. **Conclusion:** Of the 45 females, only three were comorbid for ASPD (one of whom committed suicide; one doing "fair", one doing well). None of the 65 has committed a serious crime. Altogether there were 3 suicides among the females (6.7%). 37 females achieved outcome GAS scores > 60, meaning that 82% were doing "well" at the time they were traced. Some of the borderline adolescents (of either sex) had very colorful life courses; a few examples of unusual and unexpected outcomes will be given.

S-110-512   Topic: 57, 80
The GAP-Study – a forensic psychiatric study on juvenile delinquents: Psychopathy in delinquent adolescents

Kathrin Sevecke, Universität Köln, Kinder und Jugendpsychiatrie, Köln, Germany, kathrinsevecke@aol.com

Objective: The purpose of this study was to study psychopathy in male and female delinquent adolescents as the first project on this topic in Germany. In our ongoing study we included 40 male and 40 female juvenile offenders in 2 German prisons shortly before their release. **Methods:** Adolescents were included in the age range of 14 to 19.11 years with a mean age of 17 years. All subjects were assessed with the Psychopathy Checklist Youth Version (PCL-YV, Forth, Kosson, & Hare, 2003, German version, Sevecke & Krischer), a self report on attention deficit hyperactivity disorder – ADHD- (SBB-HKS, Doepfner & Lehmkuhl, 2000), and a self report on Juvenile Temperament Factors (JTCI, Luby, 1999). Furthermore, they were given a self report on drug abuse and delinquency. **Results:** We looked into associations of the psychopathy score and violent behavior in the two groups, using t-tests. Furthermore, we focused on correlations between the PCL-score, temperament factors and ADHD, again comparing boys with girls. Our first results suggest that the PCL-scores range between 5 to 38 points, with a mean score of 20. The mean score of the PCL-YV does not vary in boys and girls, the overall score seems to be a little higher in boys than in girls. We analyzed differences of the subtypes of Attention Deficit Hyperactivity Disorder, the attention deficit, the hyperactivity and the impulsivity. First results suggest that there is a similar factor structure for the PCL-YV as for the PCL-R. We found a high association between drug abuse and the overall PCL-Scores. **Conclusion:** Our study showed that the psychopathy-checklist can also be used for adolescents in the German forensics, and can be considered an important instrument for the child and adolescent psychiatry and for prognostic issues. Final results of this study will be presented at the conference.

S-110-513   Topic: 52, 80
The Cologne Gap-Study: Personality pathology, violence and trauma in female and male delinquent juveniles
Maya Krischer, Universität zu Köln, Klinik für Kinderpsychiatrie, Köln, Germany, mayakrischer@aol.com
Manfred Doepfner

Objective: This study focused on associations between personality traits, impulsive behavior and traumatic experiences in delinquent adolescents. Gender differences in this population is often mentioned in the literature, but rarely empirically analyzed with similar sample sizes. Therefore we chose a group of male and a group of female offenders. **Methods:** As described in Dr. Sevecke's abstract, the sample consists of 40 boys and 40 girls, with a mean age of 17 years. We included the Dimensional Assessment of Personality Pathology (DAPP, Livesley 2000), the Overt Aggression Scale Modified (OAS-M, Coccaro, 1991) and the Childhood Trauma Questionnaire (CTQ, Bernstein 1998), a drug abuse instrument and demographic data on factors such as upbringing, household status etc. With t-tests and variance analyses we looked for associations comparing those two groups. **Results:** Not surprisingly and as hypothesized, more girls than boys claim to be traumatized earlier, and more delinquent girls are from broken homes than boys (meaning single parent households, many foster care housing). Our first results suggest that delinquent girls score almost as high as boys in dissocial behaviour and impulsivity, but show a tendency of higher problems in emotional dysregulation and insecure attachment. Furthermore they use more often hard drugs than boys. Interestingly our ongoing results found that girls show as high an aggression on a daily basis as boys (OAS-M, Coc-

caro, 1991). **Conclusion:** Conclusively our results show that the DAPP (Livesley & Jackson 2003) can be used as a valid instrument for the dimensional assessment of personality pathology in adolescents. Furthermore, we can prove some gender differences in the association of personality traits, violent behaviour and former traumatic childhood incidents. Final results of this study are to be presented at the conference.

S-110-514   Topic: 57, 37
The BARO.ch screening for adolescents with antisocial behavior
Daniel Gutschner, IFB-Institut für forensische, Kinder- und Jugendpsychiatrie, Bern 7, Switzerland, daniel.gutschner@ifkjb.ch

Objective: In Switzerland there are no criteria defined that help to evaluate an antisocial adolescent. **Methods:** The BARO.ch is a standardized instrument that screens an adolescent and helps in deciding whether a special treatment is necessary and what kind of intervention would be useful. With the BARO.ch all important areas of information are collected that are important to assess the antisocial development. The BARO was first developed in the Netherlands and adapted for its application in Switzerland. The BARO.ch contributes information on interventional measures, such as supportive treatment that has to be established for the adolescent, for example placing a juvenile under guardianship, or finding a place in a special educational setting. **Results:** Furthermore, this instrument gives supportive information in the process of finding adequate sanctions. **Conclusion:** In this paper, first results in using the BARO.ch with delinquent juveniles will be reported.

S-111   Topic: 84
Attention Deficit Hyperactivity Disorders V
Track: ADHD
Chairperson: Lioba Baving, University Utrecht Child & Adolescent Psychiatry, Utrecht, Netherlands, l.baving@psych.azu.nl

S-111-515   Topic: 84, 19
Summercamp treatment of ADHD
Klaus Schmeck, Universitätsklinik Ulm, Kinder- und Jugendpsychiatrie, Ulm, Germany, klaus.schmeck@medizin.uni-ulm.de
Cornelia König; Dörte Grasmann

Objective: There is no definite evidence that in ADHD patients behavioural therapy alone or in combination with psychostimulants yields better results than pharmacotherapy alone. This could be due to a dosage effect in outpatient behavioural treatment which usually offers one session per week. We present a treatment approach that is based on a highly intensive summer treatment program. **Methods:** The SummerCamp method (adapted from the Summer Treatment Program approach of Pelham and coworkers (1996)) is a 2-week program for children with disruptive behavioural disorders. Children aged 8 to 13 years attend the program from 8.00 a.m. until 4.00 p.m. on weekdays in groups of 6 children. During these two weeks, the children can experience functioning as a group, making friends and interacting with adults in an appropriate way. Treatment interventions comprise 20 units of psychoeducation, social skills training, project work, relaxation techniques and recreational group activities. Parent training consists of 10 sessions that start one week before SummerCamp and last until seven weeks after. The main goal of these interventions is to inform the parents and to facilitate the generalization of children's behavioural changes to different settings. **Results:** In a multicenter study conducted in 2002 (Döpfner et al., in prep.) we successfully used the SummerCamp approach for a two week day treatment of two groups of ADHD children (6 children per group). At the Ulm University we manualized the SummerCamp approach (König et al., 2003) and used it in a day treatment program with disruptive children in summer 2003 with good short-term effectiveness on social competence and self-esteem. **Conclusion:** The Summer-Camp method seems to be a promising approach for the treatment of ADHD children. Long-term stability of changes has to be checked in a longitudinal study.

S-111-516   Topic: 84, 23
Budgetary impact of treatments for Attention Deficit Hyperactivity Disorder (ADHD) in Germany: Increasing relevance of health economic evidence

Michael Schlander, Hochschule für Wirtschaft, Ludwigshafen, Germany, ms@michaelschlander.com

Objective: Like many third-party payers in health care, the German sick funds (statutory health insurance, SHI) suffer from financial constraints. Against this background, economic criteria are taken into account in various ways when medical interventions undergo prioritization. Objective: To estimate, from the SHI perspective, the economic relevance, i.e., the potential future budgetary impact of ADHD treatments in Germany. **Methods:** Based on a review of the literature on prevalence, resource utilization, and economic implications of ADHD, epidemiological data were combined with three scenarios extrapolating current trends to project future diagnosed prevalence, treatment prevalence, assumed acceptance (share) of novel drug treatments (methylphenidate modified-release products and atomoxetine), and unit costs in children and adolescents aged 6–18 (total population: 10.8 million). **Results:** The tabulations indicate that annual direct SHI pharmacotherapy expenditures for ADHD may rise from 23.7 m€ in 2002 up to 175 m€ in 2009 (low case: 70.7 m€; for comparison: assuming a treatment prevalence similar to that reported for the US (Safer et al. 1996) gives an annual drugs bill of 338.8 m€). This dramatic increase results from the multiplicative effects of three variables, increased awareness/rate of diagnosed cases, growing acceptance of pharmacotherapy, and higher unit costs for novel medications. – Currently, no reliable data are available in Germany on ADHD-related physician services, behavioral or psychological interventions. **Conclusion:** From the SHI perspective, the opportunity cost caused by ADHD treatments may escalate over the next decade. While medication costs are likely to represent a major cost driver, they are just a fraction of the total cost associated with ADHD. It is anticipated that, in the foreseeable future, reimbursement of therapeutic options will require evidence of an acceptable cost-effectiveness ratio. Providers of care in this area will have to meet new challenges in the fields of health economics and medical ethics.

S-111-517   Topic: 84, 23
Preliminary findings from attention-deficit/hyperactivity disorder observational research in Europe (adore) Netherlands: Attention-deficit/hyperactivity disorder is a significant burden on the patient and family

Stephen Ralston, Eli Lilly & Co Ltd., EHOR, Windlesham, United Kingdom, ralston_stephen_j@lilly.com
R. Rodrigues Pereira; W. Brussel; L. Vlasveld; H. G. Tuynman-Qua; M. J. Lorenzo

Objective: To present preliminary findings on Dutch patients from the ADORE study on the burden of illness associated with ADHD at baseline. **Methods:** ADORE, is a 2-year, prospective, observational study in attention-deficit/hyperactivity disorder (ADHD) with data collected by paediatricians and child-psychiatrists. To date, 67 patients from the Netherlands have been included in the database and reported. A full Netherlands dataset will be presented in the poster. **Results:** The dataset consisted primarily of 59 boys (89%) and the mean age for all patients was 8.7 years (SD 2.9). In most cases, patients were the eldest (26 [40%]) or the youngest sibling (23 [35%]) in the family, and 48 patients (72%) lived with both biological parents. First awareness of ADHD problems occurred at a mean age of 4.7 (SD 2.9) years. Treatment was first sought at a mean age of 7.2 (SD 3.2) years. For parents, 29 (45%) mothers and 13 (24%) fathers experienced an emotional problem due to the patients' symptoms. In school, only 31 (47%) patients were considered manageable in the classroom environment. For academic performance, 9 (24%) were classified as having a worse performance than 81–100% of children of the same age. In regard to bullying, 4 patients (7%) were the bully, 18 patients (30%) were the victim, and 6 patients (10%) were involved as both the bully and victim. In terms of social activity, 21% of the patients had no invites, while on the contrary, 37 (60%) patients were invited to 3 or more social activities. **Conclusion:** From the reported baseline information, enrolled patients are associated with a significant burden of illness in terms of school behavior, academic performance, and social activities. Notably, over one-third of patients with ADHD symptoms are the victims of bullying.

S-111-518   Topic: 84, 23
Preliminary findings from the Attention Deficit Hyperactivity Disorder (ADHD) observational research in Europe (ADORE) Austria Study Group

Stephen Ralston, Eli Lilly & Co Ltd., EHOR, Windlesham, United Kingdom, ralston_stephen_j@lilly.com
S. Tauscher-Wisniewski

Objective: To present the Austrian preliminary findings from the ADORE recruitment phase. **Methods:** This is a 2-year prospective, observational study in ADHD. Of the 61 patients analysed, 48 patients fulfilled either the diagnostic criteria of: ICD-10 (52%); DSM-IV (23%); both (3%); and 4 (7%) patients fulfilled a diagnosis of ADHD with unspecified criteria. The remaining 9 (15%) patients did not satisfy a diagnostic criteria. Comorbid disorders included oppositional defiant disorder (50%, N = 30), learning disorders (54%, N = 28), conduct disorder (48%; N = 27), anxiety disorder (27%; N = 16), and depression (24%; N = 14). We used Clinical Global Impression Severity Scale (CGI-S), ADHD rating scale, Child Global Assessment Scale (CGAS), and Child Health and Illness Profile (CHIP-CE) for assessment. The mean age was 9.4 years (SD 2.6; N=59), with 95% boys (N=57) and 5% girls (N=3). **Results:** The patients showed a mean ADHD rating score of 32.3 (SD 9.0) with a mean inattentiveness score of 16.5 (SD 4.8) and a mean hyperactivity/impulsivity score of 15.8 (SD 5.8). The mean CGI-S score was 4.4 (SD 1.1) at baseline. Parents first became aware of ADHD symptoms at a mean age of 4.5 (SD 2.1). At baseline, patients received psychotherapy (45%; N=25), pharmacotherapy and psychotherapy combined (13%, N=7), or "other" treatment (18%; N=10). Ten patients (18%) did not receive any form of treatment. **Conclusion:** Patients enrolled were predominantly boys with a moderate CGI severity score. Comorbid diagnoses are prevalent. Although not all of the patients fulfilled the diagnostic criteria of a DSM-IV or ICD-10 diagnosis of ADHD, their CGI-S score was moderate to markedly ill. Preliminary data suggest that ADHD is currently diagnosed at a mean age of 9.4 years although first awareness is at the age of 4.5 years. Furthermore, the delay in treatment in Austria needs to be examined in further studies.

S-111-519   Topic: 84, 3
Dialogue on the differences between Italy and the UK in ADHD practice

Stefano Palazzi, West Norfolk PCT, King's Lynn, United Kingdom, stefano.palazzi@westnorfolk-pct.nhs.uk
Ettore Guaia

Objective: ADHD involves cognitive, emotional and behavioural problems possibly extending into adulthood. Since first described, cultural and secular differences have been observed. Its true epidemiology and optimal treatment are debated. We report a synthesis of the combined clinical experience of two senior child mental health professionals who have recently traversed health system confines. **Methods:** Rhetorical dialogues date back to Plato (427–347 BC) and Galileo (1564–1642 AD). Modern medical journals also use this method, particularly in educational and health promotion articles. When groups meet in brainstorming sessions, individual perceptions and knowledge are organized into flowchart diagrams that may allow heuristic breakthrough to emerge from complex debates. On-line forums and professional chat-lines are another example of the added heuristic value of informed dialogues. Along these principles, a battery of Questions and Answers were agreed and discussed within the mentoring relationship developed between the Authors. A final refinement was made in view of the presentation to a professional audience. **Results:** Questions included the access to and use of medication and psychological treatments, the role of academic opinion leaders, the streaming of young people into the different care levels and cultural differences in interpreting the medical, social and corporate model of health care. Not all questions have yet received an answer. Major perceived dissimilarities were the attitude towards the administration of psychoactive medication to children (methylphenidate not available in Italy), the integration within the educational system (higher exclusion rates in the UK) and divergent demographic trends in the last 25 years. **Conclusion:** Our 'dialogue box' tried not to fall into the surreptitious-advocacy bias, which characterised some of the historical Socratic conversations. On the contrary, we aimed to share our increased awareness of the professional and cultural differences within the community of child mental health physicians.

S-111-520   Topic: 84, 95, 72
Comorbidity of CD and ODD among children with diagnosis of ADHD

Artur Kolakowski, Warsaw Medical University, of Child Psychiatry, Warszawa, Poland, akolakowski@wp.pl
Tomasz Wolanczyk; Agnieszka Pisula

Objective: The study addressed following questions: 1. What is the frequency of ADHD ODD/CD comorbidity in Polish Children 2. Is the ODD diagnosis is always prior to CD diagnosis 3. What developmental and family factors contribute to ADHD? 4. Does severity of impulsivity, hyperactivity and attentional problems interfere with ODD and CD symptoms? **Methods:** 525 children referred to ADHD Out-patient clinic with preliminary diagnosis of ADHD. The diagnosis du to ICD-10 and DSM-IV was confirmed with 395 children (75.24%). Some children were excluded because of other comorbid problems. **Results:** There were 348 children enrolled at study, they constitute three subgroups: "pure" ADHD – 30.7% Comorbid ADHD and ODD – 60.1% comorbid ADHD/CD group – 9.2%. All the patients with CD diagnosis meet criteria of ODD. All patients diagnosed with CD has the beginning in early childhood. ADHD patients with ODD/CD had a history of head injuries, and incidents of day or bedwetting. These group of children achieve worse academically than children with pure ADHD, present also more behavioral complaints from teachers. In families of comorbid ADHD and CD/ODD fathers are more frequently unemployed, had criminal history, and also some crime history in generation family. Mothers tend to present criminal history and smoking in their families of origin. ADHD children with comorbid CD/ODD are more frequently brought up in divorced families, and less frequently by both caretakers. There was no relation between attentional and ODD/CD problems, however there is strong association between CD/ADD and severity of impulsive and hyperactivity symptoms. **Conclusion:** As previous research has suggested, substantial comorbidity exists among childhood externalizing disorders, specifically attention-deficit/hyperactivity disorder (ADHD), oppositional defiant disorder (ODD), and conduct disorder (CD).

S-112   Topic: 84
Attention Deficit Hyperactivity Disorders I
Track: ADHD

Chairperson: Timothy Wilens, Massachusetts General Hospital, Boston, MA, USA, wilens@helix.mgh.harvard.edu

S-112-521   Topic: 84, 45, 37
A cross-cultural comparison of Brazilian and German children with ADHD using the Child Behavior Checklist (CBCL)

Tobias Banaschewski, Universität Göttingen, Kinder- und Jugendpsychiatrie, Göttingen, Germany, tbanasc@gwdg.de
Henrik Uebel; Björn Albrecht; Monika Robatzek; Andreas Becker; Aribert Rothenberger; Luis Augusto Rohde

Objective: The aim of this study was to investigate cross-cultural similarities and differences of Brazilian and German children and adolescents with the diagnosis of attention-deficit hyperactivity disorder (ADHD; combined type) regarding their psychopathological profile as reported by parents in the Child Behavior Checklist (CBCL). **Methods:** We compared the behavioral and emotional characteristics of a sample of children and adolescents with ADHD from a pediatric psychopharmacology outpatient clinic in Brazil (N=152; 21 girls and 131 boys; 8 to 13 years, mean age 10.18 (SD 1.73)) with those of a German sample from an outpatient clinic for child and adolescent psychiatry in Germany (N=136; 18 girls and 118 boys; 8 to 13 years, mean age 10.15 (SD 1.76)) as reflected by the subscales of the Children Behavior Checklist (CBCL). Furthermore receiver operating characteristic (ROC) analyses were carried out to evaluate and compare sensitivity, specificity and positive and negative predictive power of the CBCL at optimum cutoff scores. A multivariate analysis of variance was computed across the eight subscales of the CBCL. In case of significant differences between Brazilian and German participants additional univariate analyses of variance were calculated. **Results:** The multivariate analysis revealed significant differences between the two samples. While the profile in both samples was comparable, Brazilian parents reported significant higher levels of their children regarding the CBCL-subscales somatization, attentional problems, anxiety/depression, and aggression. Effect sizes (Cohen's d) were small. Results of ROC analyses will be reported. **Conclusion:** Despite differences in language, culture and the pattern of mental health services or diagnostic procedures and thresholds may, total differences between both samples concerning additional psychopathological characteristics were small. Possible explanations will be outlined.

S-112-522 Topic: 83, 15
Treatment of Attention Deficit Hyperactivity Disorder (ADHD): Modeling the cost-effectiveness of a modified-release preparation of Methylphenidate from the perspective of the National Health Service (NHS) in the United Kingdom
Michael Schlander, Hochschule für Wirtschaft, Ludwigshafen, Germany, ms@michaelschlander.com
Kristen Migliaccio-Walle; Jaime Caro

Objective: Methylphenidate (MPH) has been shown to be an effective and cost-effective treatment for children and adolescents with attention-deficit/hyperactivity disorder (ADHD). Given their short duration of action, MPH immediate-release (MPH-IR) formulations require multiple daily dosing. Studies have reported noncompliance rates of 20–65%. Objective: To evaluate, from the perspective of the UK NHS, the cost-effectiveness of MPH-OROS, a novel once-a-day formulation. **Methods:** A meta-analysis was performed to synthesize data on clinical efficacy from three randomized clinical trials, comparing MPH-OROS o.a.d., MPH-IR t.i.d., and placebo. Results were combined with unit cost data (BNF 2003, PSSRU 2003), resource utilization estimates (NHS perspective), and assumptions on treatment compliance (principal source: systematic review by Claxton et al. 2001). Data were used to populate a decision tree model adapting and extending the CCOHTA analysis (1998) of ADHD therapies. **Results:** MPH-OROS and MPH-IR were significantly more efficacious than placebo, in both community teacher and parent ratings of inattention/overactivity (IOWA Conners I/O scale; primary trial endpoint). For teacher ratings, standardized mean differences (SMD, random effects model) compared to placebo were 1.32 (1.09–1.55, 95% CI, for MPH-OROS) and 1.19 (1.00–1.38 for MPH-IR); effect sizes reported by parents were generally higher and better for MPH-OROS compared to MPH-IR. Assuming 79% compliance with MPH-OROS

o.a.d. and 65% with MPH-IR t.i.d. over one year, the incremental cost of MPH-OROS per SMD (teacher ratings) was £1,345 (for MPH-IR: £1,120); for parent ratings, MPH-OROS exhibited extended dominance over MPH-IR. Comprehensive sensitivity analyses were performed. For MPH-IR compliance rates below 57%, MPH-OROS dominated (in an extended sense) also in teacher ratings. **Conclusion:** These data suggest that MPH-OROS will be more effective than MPH-IR t.i.d. in daily practice. They indicate an acceptable incremental cost-effectiveness ratio of MPH-OROS, with extended dominance over MPH-IR under a broad range of assumptions. Real world data will have to confirm these estimates.

S-112-523 Topic: 84, 16
Effects of Atomoxetine and Methylphenidate on sleep in children with Attention Deficit Hyperactivity Disorder (ADHD)
Albert J. Allen, Eli Lilly and Company, Indianapolis, IN, USA, allenaj@lilly.com
R. Bart Sangal; Judith Owens; Douglas Kelsey; Virginia Sutton; Kory Schuh

Objective: Atomoxetine is a nonstimulant medication for treating ADHD [1, 2]. This study compared the effects of atomoxetine and methylphenidate on the sleep of children with ADHD as measured by actigraphy, polysomnography, and parent and child diaries. **Methods:** The study was a randomized, double-blind, crossover trial. After collecting baseline measures, patients were treated with each medication for about 7 weeks. Parents and patients completed diaries, patients wore wrist actigraphy monitors, and polysomnography data were collected. **Results:** Relative to baseline, the actigraphy data indicated that methylphenidate increased time to sleep onset significantly more than atomoxetine (30.14 versus 3.36 min, p<0.001). This was consistent with the polysomnographic data. Child diaries indicated that it was easier to get up in the morning, it took less time to fall asleep, and they slept better with atomoxetine. Parents reported that it was less difficult getting their children up and getting them ready in the morning and they were less irritable, children had less difficulty getting ready for bed, and had less difficulty falling asleep with atomoxetine. **Conclusion:** The main finding was that patients on atomoxetine reported shorter time to sleep onset and more normal sleep relative to methylphenidate as measured by actigraphy, polysomnography, child diaries, and parent diaries.

S-112-524 Topic: 84, 47
Relationship between self-esteem and familial expressed emotion in children with Attention Deficit Hyperactivity Disorder (ADHD)
Aliye Tugba Bahadir, Marmara University of Medicine, Child & Adolescent Psychiatry, Istanbul, Turkey, drtugbabhdr@yahoo.com
Zeynep Yaman; Ayse Rodopman Arman; Kemal Kuscu; Yanki Yazgan; Meral Berkem

Objective: Familial high expressed emotion is related with social-emotional problems in children. In children with Attention Deficit Hyperactivity Disorder (ADHD) low self-esteem is a remarkable finding. We intended to investigate the contributions of expressed emotion within the family to low self esteem in children with ADHD. **Methods:** 36 boys and 4 girls, aged 7–17, who were given the diagnosis of ADHD in Marmara University Child Psychiatry Clinic, completed Piers-Harris Self-Concept Scale (PHSCS) for the evaluation of their self-esteem. Mothers and fathers were given Expressed Emotion Scale (by O. Berksun) to determine the expressed emotion within the family. Mothers were given Conner's Parents Rating Scale (CPRS) for ADHD. Pearson correlation analysis was used. **Results:** Children's scores for CPRS and mothers' scores for expressed emotion were positively correlated and statistically significant (r=0.353, p=0.026). Children's increasing scores for CPRS and decreasing scores for PHSCS were negatively correlated and statistically significant (r=−0.494, p=0.001). Decrease in the sum of children's self-esteem scores and increase in the mothers' expressed emotion scores were negatively correlated, but were not statistically significant (r=−0.049, p=0.766). Correlations within the subgroups of the scales will be more informative. **Conclusion:** The increase in the ADHD symptom severity had a negative influence on children's self-esteem, and it made an increase in familial expressed emotion. Low self-esteem and increased expressed emotion, causes difficulties in the adjustment of ADHD children. Researches on the treatment for ADHD children, which can positively contribute to the feelings and thoughts about themselves, remain to be important.

S-112-525   Topic: 84, 16
Efficacy of Atomoxetine in placebo-controlled studies in children, adolescents and adults with Attention Deficit Hyperactivity Disorder (ADHD)

Albert J. Allen, Eli Lilly and Company, Indianapolis, IN, USA, allenaj@lilly.com
Peter Feldman; Milton Denai; Alexander Simpson; Christopher Kratochvil; Jeffrey Newcorn; Joseph Biederman

Objective: Atomoxetine is a highly specific inhibitor of the norepinephrine transporter that has been developed as a nonstimulant treatment of attention-deficit/hyperactivity disorder (ADHD). We review here the efficacy data from double-blind, placebo-controlled clinical studies conducted with atomoxetine to date. **Methods:** Eight large, acute, randomized, double-blind, placebo-controlled studies (4 in children, 2 in children and adolescents, and 2 in adults) have been conducted involving atomoxetine in the treatment of ADHD. Three trials in children were conducted with once-daily dosing (6–8 weeks), whilst the other 5 studies employed twice-daily dosing, all on a weight-adjusted basis (8–9 weeks). Adults were dosed twice daily over 10 weeks with dose escalation within a fixed range. Protocol-specified primary outcome measures in 5 of the pediatric studies were parent-reported assessments corresponding to DSM-IV symptom criteria, and 1 involved teacher-reported assessments. Adult studies were self-reported. **Results:** In all studies, atomoxetine was superior to placebo in reduction of mean symptom ratings for the primary outcome measure. The effect size for once-daily treatment was similar to that of twice-daily treatment. No serious safety concerns were observed and tolerability was good, as evidenced by discontinuation rates of less than 5% for adverse events in the pediatric studies. **Conclusion:** Atomoxetine appears to be safe and efficacious for the treatment of ADHD in children, adolescents, and adults.

S-112-526   Topic: 6, 16
Longer-term treatment with Atomoxetine in adolescents with ADHD

Timothy Wilens, Massachusetts General Hospital, Boston, MA, USA, wilens@helix.mgh.harvard.edu
Jeffrey Newcorn; Christopher Kratochvil; Douglas Gelowitz; Christine Thomason; Haitao Gao

Objective: There is a paucity of longer-term studies of ADHD, particularly in adolescents [1]. We now report on the effectiveness, safety, and tolerability of atomoxetine in adolescents treated openly for up to 2 years. **Methods:** Data from 12 to 18 year-old adolescents with DSM-IV-defined ADHD enrolled in similarly designed clinical trials of atomoxetine were pooled. Primary efficacy was analyzed using the ADHD Rating Scale (RS) based on parent reports [2] and safety/tolerability from measurement of vital signs, growth parameters, ECG, and laboratories conducted throughout the study. **Results:** Four hundred fourteen subjects were treated for greater than or equal to 1 year; 218 (53%) completed greater than 2 years of treatment at the time of analysis. The mean modal dose (±SD) of atomoxetine was 1.46 mg/kg/day (0.33). Mean ADHD RS total scores were significantly improved at endpoint compared to baseline (p<0.001); scores improved significantly over the first 3 months and remained improved up to 24 months. Adolescents discontinued the trial for reasons including lack of efficacy (N=31, 7.5%) and adverse events (N=11, 2.7%). There were no clinically meaningful effects seen in laboratory values, vital signs, height and weight, or ECG. **Conclusion:** Atomoxetine remained efficacious during the 2-year open trial and does not appear to be associated with the development of new or unexpected safety concerns. Research funded by Eli Lilly and Company.

S-113   Topic: 57, 80
EFCAP Symposium: Forensic assessment and psychopathy

Chairperson: Theodore Doreleijers, Free University of Amsterdam, Amsterdam, Netherlands, t.doreleijers@debascule.com

Forensic assessment and psychopathy

Theodore Doreleijers, Free University, of Amsterdam, Amsterdam, Netherlands, t.doreleijers@debascule.com

Psychopathy is a well-established construct in assessing adult criminal offenders and the focus upon this has, in turn led to an increased interest in the development of psychopathic traits in adolescence. The key to early intervention and prevention of the further development of both antisocial behaviours and psychopathy is the effective assessment of psychopathic traits and forensic diagnosis. This symposium will present data on the reliability and validity of Flemish versions of the Anti-social Process Screening Device and the Childhood Psychopathy Scale, as well as outlining the strengths and limitations. The development of two instruments, which aim to measure psychopathic traits in children and adolescents, will be discussed with data presented on their reliability and validity. The decisions made within juvenile courts have far reaching consequences for young people and society as a whole. Using utility as a model of quality can clarify aspects of forensic assessments for adolescents and this concept will be discussed from a Dutch perspective. The role of moral development in recidivism will be discussed along with the quality of psychiatric expertise in assessing sexual offenders.

S-113-527 Topic: 57, 80
Assessment of psychopathic traits in children and adolescents by means of multi-informant questionnaires
Patricia Bijttebier, University of Leuven, Leuven, Belgium, patricia.bijttebier@psy.kuleuven.ac.be
Steff Decoene

Objective: The emergence of psychopathy as a well-established construct in the assessment of adult criminal offenders has stimulated great interest in measuring psychopathic traits in adolescents and even younger children. To establish this, the Antisocial Process Screening Device (Frick & Hare, 2000) and the Childhood Psychopathy Scale (Lynam, 1998) have been developed. Both are multi-informant questionnaires, designed for parent-, teacher- and self-report, including items that, in line with the Psychopathy Checklist-Revised for adults (Hare, 1991), refer to antisocial/impulsive as well as affective/interpersonal characteristics of psychopathy. In the presented study, the psychometric properties of the Flemish version of the APSD will be investigated. Methods: Data were gathered in a community sample, consisting of 188 children (82 boys, 100 girls) aged as well as clinical groups, within a broad age range (9.42–19.17 yrs, M 13.16 SD 2.47) using parent-, teacher and self-report. Results: Confirmatory factor analyses was used to compare one-, two- and threedimensional models in the self-, parent-, teacher- and combined forms. Only the 3-factor model in the combined form (parent+teacher) showed an acceptable goodness of fit. Further data on reliability and convergent validity with commonly used measures of conduct problems as well as preliminary analyses of clinical data sets will be presented. Strenghts and limitations of psychopathy screening measures in adolescents and issues related to multi-informant assessment will be discussed.

S-113-528 Topic: 57, 80
Assessment of psychopathic traits in youths
Henrik Andershed, Orebro University, Orebro, Sweden, henrik.andershed@bsr.oru.se

Objective: Development and validation of two instruments aimed at measuring psychopathic traits in children and adolescents, the Child Problematic Traits Inventory (CPTI) and the Youth Psychopathic traits Inventory (YPI). Methods: Data on the reliability and validity among preschool children and adolescents of these two instruments are presented. Results: Findings show that the measured traits manifest in a constellation of (1) grandiose, deceitful, (2) callous, unemotional, and (3) impulsive with the need for stimulation traits, and that these traits relate in expected ways to antisocial behavior and other theoretically relevant dimensions in both children and adolescents. Conclusion: It is concluded that these traits can be measured with reliability and validity in children and adolescents and that they seem similar to the psychopathic traits manifested by adult offenders with full-blown psychopathy. Keywords: psychopathic traits, assessment, CPTI, YPI, children, adolescents.

S-113-529 Topic: 57, 80
Predictors for recidivism in delinquent youth according to the PCL-YV and the role of moral development
Pia Niklaus, IFB-Institut für forensische, Kinder- und Jugendpsychiatrie, Bern, Switzerland, pia.niklaus@ifkjb.ch

Objective: To examine the predictors for recidivism in delinquent youth according to the PCL-YV. Methods: 87 young delinquents (77 boys and 10 girls) who were referred to us by juvenile court for assessment had to run through a test-battery consisting of tests for intelligence (Hamburg-Wechsler, CFT 20), attention (FAIR), the Rey complex figure and a list of other questionnaires (Achenbach, Giessen-Test, FAF). Also structured interviews were held to gain information about socio-economic data and the psychopathology. Finally, the PCL-YV was rated for each individual. Results: Juvenile offenders can't be distinguished in gender, age, nationality and type of offence regarding the partitioning in psychopaths/non-psychopaths. Yet it could be shown that juvenile offenders which are defined as psychopaths carry significantly more often ICD-10 diagnoses than juvenile offenders without a psychopathy. Conclusion: Age, gender, nationality and type of offence do not explain the high scores in the PCL-YV. ICD-10 diagnoses lead to higher scores on the PCL-YV and therefore to a higher risk for recidivism.

S-113-530 Topic: 57, 37
Quality of diagnostic assessment for juvenile court
Nils Duits, Forensic Psychiatric Service, Juvenile department, Amsterdam, Netherlands, n.duits@fpd.dji.minjus.nl

Objective: To examine utility as a concept of quality of the diagnostic assessment for juvenile court in the perspective of the Dutch juvenile juridical context. Clarification of quality enables quality management. This is necessary due to the fact that these assessments are used for decisions of the juvenile court which can have far reaching consequences for juvenile delinquents and Dutch society. Methods: A double concept mapping consensus method has been done among (1) five groups of 'users' of diagnostic assessment for juvenile court: juvenile court, child protection board & juvenile rehabilitation service, mental health care professionals, therapists of penal treatment institutions and parents & juveniles (n=57) and (2) a group of 'makers' (n=25). Results: 7 different clusters are specified: juridical content, form (execution), advice, expertise assessor, form (content), advice, organisation. Users and makers do agree on some aspects but specify different aspects as most important. For example: contrary to therapists, judges and prosecutors classify foren-sic assessment a basis for treatment as not important. Ethical aspects and expertise are more important for assessors than for users. Conclusion: These specifications of utility make quality management and research possible for the diag-nostic assessment for juvenile court (quality instrument, auditing). Important issues as criminal responsibility, risk assessment, expertise, ethical aspects of assessment and formal aspects such as a 'feasible advice' can now be developed.

S-113-531   Topic: 57

The quality of psychiatric expertises in a representative sample of sexual offenders

Jörg M. Fegert, Universität Ulm, Kinder- und Judendpsychiatrie, Ulm, Germany,
joerg.fegert@medizin.uni-ulm.de
Frank Häßler; Cornelia König; Ulrich Auer;
Kathleen Schnoor; Detlef Schläfke

Objective: The objective was to analyse the differential quality of psychiatric expertises in adolescent (n = 99 < 18; 18–21:43) and adult (n: 617) sexual offenders. **Methods:** In a representative sample from the German Land Mecklenburg-Vorpommern (1994 to 1998) we find a total of 731 cases with 156 expertises. We use instruments, developed in our analysis of capital delinquency and fire setting but we extend the instruments to delict specific items. A qualitative analysis of the description of sexual fantasies is presented. **Results:** In contrast to the results in arsonists, we found that in juvenile sexual offences where more often subject of a psychiatric expertise than adult offenders. A "higher risk" of being confronted with a psychiatric expert was also related with the number of victims, low educational level, serial crimes and neurological or psychiatric disorders and prior psychiatric treatment. In 30% of the expertises the psychiatric experts did not discuss criminal responsibility with respect to a specific period of time where criminal acts had been carried out (there is an absolute necessity to do so according to German law). In 20% of the expertises we didn't find any sexual history of these sexual offenders. So from a technical point of view, in more than a quarter of the expertises there was no sound basis for a fair trial. Nevertheless, in more than 90% the courts followed the experts opinion. **Conclusion:** In psychiatric expertises on criminal responsibility and prognostic questions in sexual offenders it is a severe default not to explore sexual fantasies and not to take the sexual history of the perpetrators. Child psychiatrists often see sexual offences as a transitional behaviour of normal sexual development especially in mentally handicapped people. Therefore they might forget to explore for specific (masturbation) fantasies and prior sexual delinquency.

S-114   Topic: 40, 24

Normal adolescence in different cultures in the 21st Century

Chairperson: Füsun Çuhadaroğlu Çetin, Hacettepe University Child & Adolescent Psychiatry, Ankara, Turkey,
fusunc@hacettepe.edu.tr

Normal adolescence in different cultures in the 21st Century

Füsun Çuhadaroğlu Çetin, Hacettepe University,
Child & Adolescent Psychiatry, Ankara, Turkey,
fusunc@hacettepe.edu.tr

Sociocultural and economical changes effect psychosocial development in various societies. Among the groups who are effected the most are the adolescents with their rapid growth and developmental patterns. There has been some studies done investigating normal development in adolescence in the past. We would like to look at the changing characteristics of adolescent development brought up with the changes produced by globalization and other sociocultural factors in the 21st century. In this symposium we are going to present data related to the normal developmental processes of adolescents from several different countries and open a discussion about the similarities and differences in relation to various factors.

S-114-532   Topic: 40, 24

Adolescence in the United States

Gordon Harper, Harvard Medical School,
Dept. of Psychiatry, Boston, MA, USA,
gordon_harper@hms.harvard.edu

Objective: To review the changing course of adolescent development in the United States. **Methods:** Literature review (both scientific and popular) and interviews with clinicians were used to gather data on current trends in American adolescence. **Results:** American adolescents come of age amid unprecedented economic well-being, environmental changes possibly affecting maturation and learning, and an impinging "global communications village" that is producing communities and discontinuities not known in previous generations. The felt competence of families and the other natural caretaking communities is eroding, while documentation, advocacy, and validation of aspects of teenage life previously regarded as nonexistent or not worthy of notice have greatly increased the range of identities that adolescents can embrace. Health and mental health services are changing as are patterns of utilization. **Conclusion:** Rapid change, in unprecedented directions, challenges contemporary American adolescents. Implications for clinicians and educators will be presented.

S-114-533   Topic: 40, 24

The Bedouin adolescent in Israel

Alan Apter, Schneider Childrens Medical,
Dept. of Psychiatry, Petah Tikva, Israel, eapter@clalit.org.il
Sami Hamdan; Muhammed El-Haib

Objective: To describe the psychological aspects of Bedouin adolescence in Israel. The Bedouin population of Israel is about 150,000 strong and is part of the Arab Minority of the State of Israel. Children make up 65% of this population, which is growing by 5% per year-one of the highest growth rates in the world. These children and adolescents suffer from poverty and have tremendous unmet needs for health and educational services. This population has had to undergo tremendous cultural changes, which include having to relinquish their nomadic life style and to come to terms with increasingly dominant Western values. As a result identity problems compounded by the religious and national struggles going on around them have led to an increase in referrals for mental health assessment. **Methods:** Interviews with educationalists and psychologists working with this population were conducted. In addition Bedouin high school pupils from both the North and South were asked to make pictorial essays of their major concerns which were then collated on a website designed by the University of Toronto School of Public Health directed by Harvey Skinner Ph.D. **Results:** These concerns will shown pictorially and include thoughts about violence suicide, smoking and ecology. **Conclusion:** This bottom up strategy could be very useful in designing public health prevention programs for high risk behaviors among Bedouin adolescents in Israel.

S-114-534   Topic: 24
Developmental characteristics and some problems of Turkish adolescents

Saynur Canat, University of Ankara, Ankara, Turkey,
canat@med.ankara.edu.tr

Objective: To examine psychosocial development, some problems and risk factors of a Turkish adolescent group. **Methods:** A stratified sampling method was used to choose a repesentative sample for two cities (Ankara and Adana). The sample consisted of 248 male (46.3%) and 288 (53.7%) total 536 adolescents (students, workers and non-workers) 12–21 years of age (X=16.72 ss=2.57) in both cities. Demographic Data Form, The Questionnaire For Evaluating The Development of Adolescents, Brief Symptom Inventory, Rosenberg Self-Esteem Scale and Stability of Self-Concept Scale were administered to the adolescents. The data was analyzed by using the SPSS program. Descriptive statistics, chi-square, t-tests, correlation analysis and multivariate analysis of variances were used in data analysis. **Results:** Adolescents reported that 17% smoked and 17.3% drinking alcohol and these numbers increased with age. Smoking was more frequent in groups who had left school and who had health problems. Drinking alcohol most frequent in the high SES group. Adolescents who had witnessed violence in their families had negative psychological profiles and low self-esteem. Most of the adolescent group had self-esteem at medium level and reported no psychopathological symptoms. Stability of self concept came out to be high. These three qualities did not show any differences in terms of location, SES and gender. However according to the evaluation of developmental issues; adolescents who reported introversion, excessive daydreaming, irritability, restlessness, witnesing violence, exposure to violence, hopelessness about future showed negative pschological profile, low self-esteem, and low level of stability of self-esteem. On the other hand adolescents who reported to have close friends, and boyfriends or girl-friends had higher levels of self esteem. **Conclusion:** Although the results of this study showed that most of adolescents has no psychopathologic symptoms, had self-esteem at medium level and stability of self-concept at high level, some psychological features such as introversion, irritability, restlessness, excessive day dreaming and witnessing or being exposed to violence are found as risk factors for the adolescents' mental health.

S-115   Topic: 68
Adolescents and young adults substance use: Neurobiological, developmental and psychopathological particularities

Chairperson: Olivier Halfon, SUPEA Child & Adolescent Psychiatry, Lausanne, Switzerland,
olivier.halfon@inst.hospvd.ch

Adolescents and young adults substance use: Neurobiological, developmental and psychopathological particularities

Olivier Halfon, SUPEA, Child & Adolescent Psychiatry, Lausanne, Switzerland, olivier.halfon@inst.hospvd.ch

Fluctuations and diversifications in substance use, as well as early substance use, characterize adolescents and young adults. This type of problematic will be analyzed from different perspectives: first, several theories and models can explain the etio-pathogenesis of dependant behavior; the relationship between depressive symptoms and addictive disorders will be discussed referring to a psychodynamic point of view; second, recent data from addiction neurosciences show that some substances have a reinforcing effect in activating the dopaminergic mesolimbic system, and that chronic substance use determines adaptations that result in dependence mechanisms; third, from a psychosocial point of view, adolescent substance use can be considered as a transient "recreative" rather than a chronic behavior; moreover, according to a complex mode of interactions, personality, family and environmental factors play a significant role, both in the onset and substance use course; finally, in order to treat substance abuse adolescents a specific bi-focal approach should be favoured, associating a consideration of the external reality as well as intra-psychic conflicts. These different complementary approaches have implications both at the level of prevention and therapeutic strategies.

S-115-535   Topic: 68, 42
Family risk factors in adolescent drug users: A longitudinal assessment

Monique Bolognini, SUPEA, Lausanne, Switzerland,
mbologni@inst.hospvd.ch
B. Plancherel; Olivier Halfon

Objective: The research project developed in the French-speaking part of Switzerland (1999–2003) aims to get a follow-up on a four-year period of a regular drug or alcohol users cohort. Population: 102 adolescents aged 14–19 yrs, 66 boys and 36 girls, using drugs or alcohol weekly at least for three months, were recruited for the study. After 4 years, the attrition rate was 18%. **Methods:** Several instruments were included in the protocol in order to get a multidimensional approach referring to life problem areas relevant to the treatment needs of adolescent drug users. The most important instrument is the ADAD (Adolescent Drug Abuse Diagnosis, Friedman & Utada, 1989), a structured interview which provides a comprehensive evaluation of the subject and allows to measure evolution over time. **Results:** Family risk factors such as abuse, sexual abuse, drug and alcohol use by the parents, and mental health in the family are much more frequent in girls compared to boys and are associated with higher drug use severity as measured in time 1. Disturbances in family relationships (conflicts, lack of contact between family members) are also correlated with more substance use problems. The follow-up assessment after 4 years shows a covariation of family severity ratings and drug use severity ratings. However, family problems reported from time 1 to time 4 tend to decrease globally, except for subjects who increase substance use who report more family problems.

S-115-536   Topic: 68
Bi-focal therapy in cannabis use during adolescence

Olivier Phan, Institut Mutualiste Montsouris, Paris, France,
olivier.phan@imm.fr
Philippe Jeammet

The relationship between cannabis use and psychopathological disturbances is well established. The most fragile adolescents tend to develop more often problems of substance use or dependence. This phenomenon requires special treatment modalities, both a pragmatic approach focused on the external reality (substance use) and offering a space where the intra psychic conflicts can be elaborated. This is what is called bi-focal therapy.

S-115-537 Topic: 68, 3
Risk factors for addictive disorders
Maurice Corcos, Institut Mutualiste Montsouris, Psychiatry, Paris, France, maurice.corcos@imm.fr

Objective: Many common risk factors have been described in addictive disorders. Little is known about their respective contributions to the discrimination between addictive and healthy subjects. **Methods:** We compared two large samples including 513 healthy subjects and 374 addictive subjects meeting the DSM-IV criteria of eating disorders, alcohol or substance dependence. Twenty-six risk factors were assessed by interview or self-rating scales. A discriminant analysis determined the respective weight of each risk factor. **Results:** One discriminant function emerged and characterized a depressive dimension. **Conclusion:** The results suggest that the different risk factors described in addictive disorders were secondary to a depressive dimension. Using notably a psychoanalytic point of view, the relationships between these depressive dimension and the addictive disorders were discussed.

S-115-538 Topic: 68
Neurobiological mechanisms of addiction
Olivier Halfon, SUPEA, Child & Adolescent Psychiatry, Lausanne, Switzerland, olivier.halfon@inst.hospvd.ch
Jean-René Cardinaux; Pierre J. Magistretti

Drug addiction is one of the world's major health problems, with large direct health costs (psychiatric and physical) as well as massive indirect costs to society in terms of crime, loss of earnings and productivity, and social damage. Addiction can be best defined as the loss of control over drug use, or the compulsive seeking and taking of drugs despite adverse consequences. It is a chronic, relapsing psychiatric disorder that results from the prolonged effects of drugs on a vulnerable brain. This process is strongly influenced both by the genetic makeup of the person and by the psychological and social context in which drug use occurs. Once formed, an addiction can be a lifelong condition in which individuals show intense drug craving and increased risk for relapse after years and even decades of abstinence. An important challenge for neurobiological research is to understand what molecular and cellular adaptations contribute to the development of drug addiction. Chronic exposure to drugs of abuse causes long-lasting changes in several neuronal systems. While the full diversity of drug effects is mediated by multiple neurotransmitters acting in multiple brain regions, the critical shared substrate of the reinforcing effects of most addictive drugs is the mesolimbic dopamine system, extending from the ventral tegmental area to the nucleus accumbens, the major component of the ventral striatum. Blockade of dopamine neurotransmission in this region, also called brain reward system, attenuates most rewarding effects of addictive drugs. Moreover, adaptations in the cAMP pathway and in certain transcription factors (CREB, FosB,...) along with resulting changes in gene expression, have now been shown to underlie specific behavioral abnormalities associated with addiction. For example, prolonged activation of dopamine D1 receptors by cocaine can lead to increased expression of the neuropeptide dynorphin in the striatum. Dynorphin activates opioid receptors on presynaptic dopamine terminals, causing decreased dopamine release that may contribute to the dysphoria seen during withdrawal. Although the increase in striatal dynorphin is one of the longest-lasting gene upregulation induced by drugs, dynorphin levels return back to normal level within days if no further drugs are administered. Thus, the upregulation of striatal dynorphin by psychostimulants is an example of a reversible homeostatic adaptation that may contribute to withdrawal symptoms. However, while homeostatic adaptations to excessive stimulation may underlie important aspect of drug dependence and withdrawal symptoms, it is unlikely that they can account either for the compulsive nature of drug abuse or for the persistent tendency to relapse. In contrast, addictive drugs also engage a set of molecular mechanisms normally involved in synaptic plasticity, which allows for the association of drug-related stimuli with specific learned behaviors. Drug-associated cues and contexts activate a narrow repertoire of drug-taking behaviors in the fully addicted person. The persistence of drug addiction may thus reflect the persistence of specific altered patterns of synaptic connectivity, as is thought to occur for normal memory formation.

S-116 Topic: 42
Longitudinal studies/longterm course/follow up
Chairperson: Blaise Pierrehumbert, SUPEA Research Unit, Lausanne, Switzerland, blaise.pierrehumbert@ip.unil.ch

S-116-539 Topic: 42
Psychiatric morbidity in adulthood of former child psychiatric patients
Minna Koskinen, Tampere University Hospital, Dept. of Child Psychiatry, Tampere, Finland, minna.koskinen@pshp.fi
Irma Moilanen; Hanna Ebeling; Matti Joukamaa

Objective: We aimed to study the adulthood psychiatric disorders of people hospitalised as children because of mental disorders. **Methods:** This study is part of the Northern Finland Birth Cohort (N=12058), which covers 96% of all children born in the two northern-most provinces of Finland in 1966. Of these children we identified all those who had received a psychiatric or psychosomatic diagnosis during hospital treatment below 18 years of age (N=225). The data was gathered from Finnish Hospital Discharge Register. In light of the case notes the diagnoses were reclassified according to the ICD-10 and DSM-IV-diagnostic systems. The final, validated diagnoses are considered to define the mental disorders of the children. The adulthood psychiatric hospital diagnoses were classified in a similar way. **Results:** Of those children having received a psychiatric diagnosis during childhood, 20% had received a psychiatric diagnosis in adulthood, too (p<0.001). There was an association between severe mental disorder in childhood, internalising or externalising disorder in childhood and psychiatric hospital diagnosis in adulthood. **Conclusion:** There was an association between psychiatric hospital diagnoses in childhood and in adulthood, but it was positive that the majority of former child psychiatric patients were doing quite well in adulthood what becomes to psychiatric hospitalization.

S-116-540   Topic: 42
Child and adolescent psychiatric patients and later criminality

Ulf Engqvist, Karolinska Institutet, Women and Child Health, Stockholm, Sweden, ulf.engqvist@mh.se
Per-Anders Rydelius

Objective: To describe criminality development in a population of 1420 patients followed up 8–29 years after admission to child and adolescent psychiatric care. **Methods:** An examination of hospital records and linkage to the national prisons and probation administration register at The National Council for Crime Prevention. **Results:** 502 persons or 35.6% of the child and adolescent psychiatry patient group (1412), 348 male that is every second man and 154 female every fifth woman, had been known in the national prisons and probation administration register during the observation time, a significant higher rate than the population in general. **Conclusion:** The most important task for child and adolescent psychiatry to prevent later criminality is to identify risk groups among them who are admitted to psychiatric care to help patients and families to strengthen the social bonds and their social network and to find more effective and helpful treatment methods for those with conduct disorder.

S-116-541   Topic: 42, 43
Neurodevelopmental outcome and neonatal brain injury in boys and girls born preterm

Matthew Allin, Institute of Psychiatry,
Dept. Psychological Medicine, London, United Kingdom,
matthew.allin@iop.kcl.ac.uk
Marion Cuddy; Brigitte Vollmer; Katharine Riley;
John Wyatt; Larry Rifkin; Robin Murray

Objective: Being born preterm is associated with significant risk of brain lesions, including periventricular haemorrhage (PVH) and periventricular leukomalacia (PVL) which may subsequently affect neurodevelopment. Boys have been shown to be more vulnerable than girls to a variety of neurodevelopmental disorders, and preterm birth and low birth weight and their complications are more common in males. We examined gender differences in severity of PVH and PVL at birth and neurodevelopmental outcome at age 4 and 8 in a large cohort of children born very preterm (VPT; before 33 gestational weeks). **Methods:** A cohort of VPT individuals was recruited into a long-term follow-up program at University College Hospital, London neonatal intensive care unit between 1979 and 1991. Neonatal cranial ultrasound assessments were performed. These individuals were subsequently assessed at age 4 and 8 with neurodevelopmental assessments, rating their outcome on scale based on the presence of neurological impairments or disability. 1066 individuals (489 girls; 577 boys) were seen at 4 years; 978 (454 girls; 529 boys) at 8 years. Outcome was compared between boys and girls using Mann-Whitney U test, as the data were not normally distributed. **Results:** Boys showed more neurodevelopmental impairment than girls at 4 years ($Z = -3.15$; $p < 0.001$) and at 8 years ($Z = -2.19$; $p = 0.029$). There was a trend towards increased severity of PVH in boys ($Z = -1.80$; $p = 0.072$), but there was no significant difference in severity of PVL between genders ($Z = -0.42$; $p = 0.673$). **Conclusion:** Boys are more vulnerable than girls to the adverse neurodevelopmental consequences of preterm birth. This difference may be related to a propensity for VPT boys to suffer more severe neonatal brain injury than girls.

S-116-542   Topic: 42
Why we need to do longitudinal studies to understand the transition to parenthood and child adjustment in the first year of life

Sandra Lancaster, Victoria University, Psychology, Melbourne, Australia, sandra.lancaster@vu.edu.au

Objective: Many research studies have addressed the question of early predictors of later child adjustment. These studies have often focussed on areas such as temperament, early behaviour problems, attachment, psychosocial factors and parenting styles and their influence on later functioning. While these longitudinal studies have produced important results, in most cases these investigations have begun after the child's birth. There have however been some notable exceptions, where longitudinal studies have commenced before the birth of the child. This paper first reviews findings from previous longitudinal studies and discusses the conceptual issues, practical advantages and disadvantages associated with collecting data pre and post birth. A longitudinal study of the transition to parenthood and child adjustment is then described. The aim of this prospective longitudinal study was to examine the effects of prenatal characteristics such as mood, prenatal attachment, own childhood experience, marital relationship and social support on the transition to parenthood and the mother's postnatal attachment to the child. **Methods:** Women (n = 180) were recruited in pregnancy from antenatal clinics of a large public hospital. Questionnaires were completed by the participants in the 1st and 3rd trimesters, and 6 weeks, 6 months and 12 months after the birth. Measures used included the Parental Bonding Instrument, Life Events Questionnaire, Hospital Anxiety and Depression scale and the Edinburgh Postnatal Depression Scale, Dyadic Adjustment Scale and pre- and postnatal measures of mother-infant attachment. Data were analysed using multiple regressions. **Results:** Preliminary results are reported for the first stages of the research project. **Conclusion:** Results from this study underline the importance of beginning studies in pregnancy. Such designs allow for clearer identification of the contribution of parental characteristics to child adjustment as well as highlighting the important opportunities for preventative work during pregnancy.

S-116-543   Topic: 42, 38
Cognitive and behavioral outcomes of children born preterm

Blaise Pierrehumbert, SUPEA, Research Unit, Lausanne, Switzerland, blaise.pierrehumbert@ip.unil.ch
Ayala Borghini; Laure Jaugey; Margarita Forcada-Guex; Lyne Jaunin; Carole Müller-Nix; François Ansermet

Objective: Progress in perinatal medicine has made it possible to increase the survival of very or extremely prematurely born infants. Outcomes of the surviving infants however remain a concern. Many studies have been conducted, especially at the levels of cognitive and behavioral problems; meta-analysis clearly indicate that long-term outcomes are significantly affected by severe prematurity. We suggest however that several potentially confounding factors still have to be taken into account. The study presented here considers the latent mediating/moderating effects of variables such as the family's SES, or the parents' posttraumatic reactions following birth, and the importance of correcting for age.

Methods: Forty-seven families with a premature infant (25–33 gestation weeks) and a control group of 25 families with a full term infant participated. Children were examined when they were 6 months, 18 months (corrected ages) and 42 months (non corrected age). Developmental quotients (DQ) were computed at each age. Mothers were interviewed about their children's behavior problems and filled in a perinatal PTSD questionnaire. **Results:** Cognitive and behavior problems are somehow delayed: premature children's DQ don't differ from those of control subjects at 6 and 18 months, and become lower at 42 months; also, premature children present a higher rate of behavior problems at 18 and 42 months. However, when DQ is corrected for age and when SES is introduced as a co-variate, there are no differences left between groups at any age, and when the intensity of the mothers' perinatal PTSD symptoms is considered as a co-variate, there are no differences left between groups concerning behavior problems. **Conclusion:** These results advocate considering more carefully possible confounding factors in further comparative/control-group outcomes studies concerning the long-term effects of premature birth.

S-116-544   Topic: 42, 85
Anti-social behaviour and emotional problems: Are parental assessments good predictors?

Maria da Conceicao Taborda Simoes, Universidade de Coimbra, Faculdade de Psicologia, Coimbra, Portugal, mctabordas@fpce.uc.pt
Luiza Nobre Lima; Maria da Luz Vale Dias

Objective: Information given by parents is often used to identify behavioural problems in children and adolescents. The importance that is placed on this information is due to the fact that it is namely the parents who observe the children most in a number of diverse situations and during successive phases of their development. A question arises about whether the information supplied by the parents is useful in predicting future types of social inadaptability. Are parental assessments good predictors of all problems or of just some of them? In this study we aim to analyse the predictive usefulness of parental assessments with regards to emotional problems on the one hand, and with regards to anti-social behaviour on the other. **Methods:** Therefore data were used from a longitudinal study currently being undertaken in the Coimbra region, in the centre of Portugal, which involves several hundred children. The children were first assessed in primary school and then finally ten years later. **Results:** The results showed that the parents' assessments are relatively poor predictors of both subsequent emotional problems and anti-social behaviours. **Conclusion:** These results highlight the need to use more than one source of information in the diagnosis of psychopathology in children and adolescents.

S-117   Topic: 45
Transcultural child and adolescent psychiatry/ethnic issues

Chairperson: Rainer Georg Siefen, WKKJPP Marl Sinsen Haard Klinik, Marl-Sinsen, Germany, rainer_georg.siefen@wkp-lwl.org

S-117-545   Topic: 45, 52
Psychological consequences of "blood feud" (canonical vengeance) to children

Ariel Como, UHC "Mother Tereza", Tirana, Albania, Valbona Alikaj; Sonila Tomori

Objective: Context Kanun represents the medieval unwritten 'juridical system'. According to Kanun a person who offended another one is called 'being in blood' with the entire family of the offended one. 'Being in blood' that only by killing someone of the family 'in blood with' the offence is over. So on for centuries, families changing position, from being the ones who have to 'take the blood' means to kill a first or second range relative of the one who previously killed, to those who have to 'give' the blood, means staying hidden, generally isolated within armed fortified houses. Hypothesis I. The children living in the families of 'revenges' and the children living in the families 'to be revenged' are presenting psychological consequences of trauma with more similarity to Terr's Typo II trauma (e.g. more dissociation defenses) compared to children out of the chain of 'kanun'. II. Having a non traumatized maternal grandmother will offer the most mitigation against the development of PTSD in the grandchildren, after state/trait anxiety is factored out. **Methods:** According to official data there are around 150 families locked inside their fortified houses in order to escape canonical vengeance. According to the media, the number of families only in Shkodra district (north-west part of Albania) is 412. Children from families living in the Shkodra city will compose the study sample. Semi-structured interview with children of 8–11 years old from 12–15 families who are involved in the Kanun, living in isolation for a period of 4-24 months (6–8 families who are in the status of 'taking the blood' and 6–8 families 'to give the blood'). A control group not involved in Kanun will be matched through: Age, Sex, Neighborhood, Composition of family. The structured part of the interview will be composed by: – UCLA PTSD-index – Family Environment Scale – State/Trait Anxiety Scale – K-SCID – PTS Parental Traumatization Scale – Child Dissociation Index. The open part of the interview will be composed by: – Berkley Puppet – Open interview questions where issues about the traumatic experiences, the life style and ideas for the future will be included. The analyzing process will include correlation analyses, group differences, qualitative assessment of family belief system. **Conclusion:** Considering the number of the interviews we should point out that we are not trying to make sure any statistical sense on the results, as it might be considered as a pilot study, looking for the trend serving also as a preparation phase for a full study.

S-117-546   Topic: 45, 52
Violence exposure and psychiatric disorders in immigrant children: Towards an integrative approach on relation between diversity and psychiatric trauma

Flavia Capozzi, University of Rome, Child & Adolescent Psychiatry, Rome, Italy, flavia.capozzi@uniroma1.it
Angela Romano; Mara Roello; Francesca Piperno

Objective: Many recent immigrant children are victims of violence within their families, at school and in their communities. They often risk to be exposed to violence (a) in their countries of origin, (b) during the migration process, (c) in the host country. Moreover, once they settle in the new country, many of them live in poverty and in overcrowded housing. Such stressful living conditions can be associated with an increased violence exposure. More often, these children are silent witnesses of domestic violence. Many of these traumatized youths display PTSD symptoms. They also show several symptoms of other psychiatric disorders (Anxiety Disorders, Mood Disorders, Conduct Disorders). In Italy, immigrant children are generally a silent and overlooked population and therefore most of the abuses experienced by them are actually unknown or underestimated. Our goal is to adopt an integrative approach to provide a framework to understand psychiatric symptoms in immigrant youths and improve mental health in a context of cultural diversity. In this work, we try to investigate the role of cultural and social issues in the expression of psychological symptoms of abuse. We also suggest to form a multidisciplinary team of mental health specialists and other professionals who can take into account both the philosophical, contextual, experiential and pragmatic aspects of cultural diversity and immigrant children's daily needs.

S-117-547   Topic: 54, 1

Immigrant parents and their emigrant adolescents: The tension of inner and outer worlds

Mali A. Mann, Stanford University, Dept. of Psychiatry, USA, mannm@stanford.edu

Objective: This paper examines different experiences of immigrant families and their children in transit between the parents' ethnic world and American culture through three clinical cases. Methods: A study of three cases including a 16 year-old male whose mother is Persian and father East Indian, presenting with depression and lack of focus; an 18 year-old female whose mother is Nigerian and father Afro-American, reporting depressive symptoms and confusion about sexual identity; and an 18 year-old depressed male from an Assyrian-Iraqi background, whose both parents are from Northern Iraq but have lived in the United States for 20 years. Results: These adolescents in their strong fantasy framework strive to join their new peer group where parents do not belong, particularly when the immigrant parents present a variety of different social and cultural values discordant to the contemporary culture. The cases suggest that both positive and negative aspects of ethnic identification are diluted during adolescence when identification with parental mores occurs. Conclusion: Adolescents of immigrant families have much more complicated tasks during this phase of their lives in order to establish a future sense of self-identity. A well-consolidated sense of self-identity is more complicated for these types of multi-ethnic immigrant families. The adolescents must rely on parental ego functions and their coherent sense of identity to weather this state of their turbulent experience.

S-117-548   Topic: 45

Specific focus of expert opinion in cross-cultural child custody decision

Dieter Stösser, Universität Tübingen, Kinder- und Jugendpsychiatrie, Tübingen, Germany, dieter.stoesser@med.uni-tuebingen.de
Gottfried Barth; Gunther Klosinski

Objective: Cross-cultural problems have to be considered in child custody reports. If the parents stem from different cultures the decision on child custody has particularly far-reaching consequences and, compared to inner-cultural evaluation, needs to take additional aspects into consideration. Due to high immigration into Germany the appearance of cultural differences becomes more frequent and more complex. The consequences of this cultural mix on divorce cases have so far hardly been treated scientifically. Methods: From the expert reports dealing with family law of the department of child and adolescent psychiatry and psychotherapy Tübingen cases with cross-cultural problems were chosen and examined. At the same time expert reporters of our department were asked about their approach in their reports having to do with cross-cultural problems. The results were compared with results from scientific literature and specific problems and recommendations of how to solve these problems were worked out. Results: In cross-cultural report cases the estimation of the other culture of the one parent by the other parent plays an important role as to the appreciation of the ability of educating a child. In divorce cases the cultural differences, which were originally considered positively, become negative factors. The family of origin plays, as a rule, a particularly important role. More often than usually the role of close relatives in the education of children must also be taken into consideration. The recommendations of child custody with its effect on the cultural identity of the child can hardly be based on objective differences between the cultures because they must be looked at and qualified from their own perspective. The appreciation of the psychic stability and the ability to educate a child of the parents is the attempt to free oneself from a cultural evaluation, although it takes its roots in values of western civilisation. It is not always considered ideal for the welfare of the child if it stays in its original country. Conclusion: Family law related cases of cross-cultural families are on the increase. Family structures can greatly differ from traditional German conceptions, examples are a greater importance of a big family of more than one generation and of relatives. Values such as family honour play an important part. Of particular importance is onés own cultural integration and the psycho-social integration of the divorced parents. No prediction can be made as to which culture is better or worse for the development of the child. The objective evaluation can be endangered if the expert is culturally biased in his report (expert reporter artefact). An objective recommendation for child custody is in reality impossible.

S-117-549   Topic: 45

Ethnocultural child psychiatry: Implementation of specific services and information lines for migrant families and their children and adolescents

Rainer Georg Siefen, WKKJPP Marl Sinsen, Haard Klinik, Marl-Sinsen, Germany, rainer_georg.siefen@wkp-lwl.org
Alina Pimenov; Jenny Schwab; Hülya Bingöl

Objective: This study analyses the help-seeking behaviour of migrant families when children or adolescents suffer from psychological distress and problems. Especially referral pathways as well as obstacles to culturally fair diagnoses and therapy in child and adolescent psychiatric services were to be investigated. Methods: Overall 10 treatment records of Turkish and 10 treatment records of Russian/German ethnic origin indoor patients were analysed and compared to an equal number of ambulatory patients of the same ethnic background. Clinical pathways to admission and after treatment are described as well as hints of barriers to diagnosis and treatment related to language and culturally determined health behaviour. **Results:** In spite of special services for both ethnic groups including bilingual medical doctors of Russian and Turkish origin patients of both groups are underrepresented in indoor and ambulatory treatment. Negative expectations concerning the cultural competences of professionals are overcome more easily if participation of therapists with the same cultural background can be assured. **Conclusion:** Clinical interventions to support cultural opening of indoor and ambulant psychiatric services for children and adolescents, such as bilingual medical doctors, facilitate access. Cultural and cognitive thresholds must be additionally lowered by key persons and mediators within the respective ethnic communities. Information programs concerning child and adolescent psychiatric services should be developed and be specifically addressed to mothers who seem to be most responsible for health related decisions in migrant families.

S-118   Topic: 70
Mood disorders/Affective disorders I
Chairperson: Rémy Barbe, Pittsburgh, USA, remy.barbe@hcuge.ch

S-118-550   Topic: 70, 9
Grief among children and the effect of a support group therapy for parentally bereaved children
Heba Elkshishy, Faculty of Art Elmenia Univer., Dept. of Psychology, Elmenia, Egypt, abuhegazi@hotmail.com

Objective: The present study aims at investigating the following: a– The differences between bereaved and non bereaved children on self concept, anxiety and depression. b– The differences between bereaved children who lost their mother and those who lost their father on the previous variables. In addition, the present study aims at examining the effectiveness of support group therapy for parentally bereaved children on self concept, anxiety and depression. **Methods:** The sample consists of (180) pupils. They were divided into three groups: Group 1: 60 bereaved children (30 males and 30 females) who lost their mother. Group 2: 60 bereaved children (30 males and 30 females) who lost their father. Group 3: 60 non bereaved children. These pupils were approached with a brief description of the support group session and the benefit it was hoped they would produce. 30 bereaved children approved to participate. The author also administrated the psychological measurements on the matched control group (30 bereaved children who were not exposed to support group sessions) individually. The bereaved children were exposed to the support group sessions for 12 weekly sessions for 2 hours each week. The groups were lead by the author who has advanced training in group work, and with a psychiatrist. The content of the sessions was selected to represent the goals for bereaved support groups as suggested by Pennells and Smith (1995). **Results:** Results revealed that there were statistically significant differences between bereaved children who lost their father and those who lost their mother on anxiety and depression in favor of those who lost their mother. Results also indicated that there were statistically significant differences between bereaved children and non bereaved children on self concept in favor of control non bereaved children and on anxiety and depression in favor of the bereaved children. **Conclusion:** Finally results also indicates that participants in a support group therapy for

parentally bereaved children showed statistically significant changes in self concept anxiety and depression.

S-118-551   Topic: 70, 13
Lamotrigine treatment of mood disorders in adolescents
Ana Jovanovic, Belgrade, Serbia and Montenegro, dranajov@yahoo.com
Aneta Lakic; Vesna Milovanovic; Milorad Vukasinovic

Objective: Mood disorders among adolescents are frequently unrecognized. The four most common types of mood disorders are: Major Depressive Disorder, Dysthymic Disorder, Bipolar Disorder and Cyclothymic Disorder. For adolescents, the point prevalence of depression has been estimated at 2.9–4.7%, dysthymic disorder 1.6–8.0%, and bipolar disorder 1%. In this study we have analyzed the effects of lamotrigine as a therapy for mood disorders in adolescence period. **Methods:** Study included 10 patients, between the age of 13 and 18 years, from the Clinic of Neurology and Psychiatry for Children and Adolescent in Belgrade, diagnosed as mood disorder according to DSM-IV criteria. We have applied the following experimental procedures and tests: psychiatric and psychological exploration, electroencephalogram, laboratory tests, the Clinical Global Impression Scale (Severity and Improvement), the Hamilton Rating Scale for Depression and the Young Mania Rating Scale. **Results:** Results of the clinic-evaluation and test-evaluation indicated good recovery of the patients. We did not record any side effects of lamotrigine, except in one of the patients who had a headache at the beginning of the therapy. **Conclusion:** Patients receiving lamotrigine showed good response and remission. Lamotrigine is effective and safe for patients with mood disorders.

S-118-552   Topic: 70, 42
Predictors of long term outcome in a treatment study of adolescent depression
Rémy Barbe, Pittsburgh, USA, remy.barbe@hcuge.ch
Jeffrey Bridge; Boris Birmaher; David Kolko; David A. Brent

Objective: In this study we will investigate the long-term outcome of adolescent depression in a treatment study and determine the predictors of a poor long-term outcome. **Methods:** One hundred seven adolescents with major depressive disorder randomly assigned to 12 to 16 weeks of cognitive behavioral therapy, systemic behavioral family therapy, or nondirective supportive therapy were evaluated for 2 years after the psychotherapy trial to document the subsequent course and predictors of major depressive disorder. **Results:** Most participants (80%) recovered (median time, 8.2 months from baseline), and 30% had a recurrence (median time, 4.2 months from recovery). Twenty-one percent were depressed during at least 80% of the follow-up period. Severity of depression (at baseline), lifetime history of sexual abuse and presence of self-reported parent-child conflict (at baseline and during up period) predicted lack of recovery, chronicity, and recurrence. Despite the similarity to clinically referred patients at baseline, patients recruited via advertisement were less likely to experience a recurrence. **Conclusion:** While most participants in this study eventually recovered, those with severe depression, lifetime history of sexual abuse and self-perceived parent-child conflict were at greater risk for chronic depression and recurrences.

S-118-553   Topic: 70, 38
Predictors and patterns of depression and anxiety among pregnant and postpartum Australian adolescents

Kathryn Gilson, Monash University, Psychological Medicine, Melbourne, Victoria, Australia, kathryn.gilson@med.monash.edu.au
Sandra Lancaster

Objective: Research on depression and anxiety during pregnancy and postpartum has been restricted to adults with little attention given to adolescent mothers, despite additional challenges and hardships that are present for this age-group. Moreover, the occurrence, timing, and consequences of depression and anxiety among pregnant, Australian adolescents have not yet been examined. The stressful nature of early parenthood may further increase the risk for depression and anxiety in pregnant adolescents. Other factors associated with an increased risk for depression and/or anxiety include a history of sexual abuse, negative attitudes, and unplanned pregnancy. Antenatal depression and/or anxiety may impair an adolescent's capacity to make decisions regarding her own health and well-being, as well as that of her foetus (eg., diet, smoking, and substance misuse). Depression during pregnancy and postpartum also has implications regarding parenting difficulties. The aim was to investigate the patterns and predictors of depression and anxiety measured during pregnancy and six weeks and six months postpartum. **Methods:** As part of a longitudinal study 80 primiparous adolescents were recruited from The Young Mothers Antenatal clinic at Monash Medical Centre, Clayton, Victoria (Australia). At recruitment information was collected about childhood upbringing, abuse history, attitude towards pregnancy as well as depression and anxiety. At third trimester and at six weeks and six months postbirth the young women were again screened for depression and anxiety. **Results:** Preliminary findings, as part of an ongoing longitudinal study of adolescent mothers and their babies, are reported. Predictors of depression and anxiety at each time point and patterns across time are reported. **Conclusion:** The opportunities for early intervention are discussed as well as implications for the adolescent.

S-118-554   Topic: 70, 21
Preventing adolescent depression: Effectiveness of a school-based universal intervention

Roslyn Montague, NSW Institute of Psychiatry, Dept. of Mental Health, Parramatta, BC, Australia, rmontague@nswiop.nsw.edu.au
Ian Shochet

Objective: This study investigated the effectiveness of a universal school-based program, the Resourceful Adolescent Program (RAP), designed to prevent depression in 13–15 year olds. This study also examined the impact of the leaders' discipline on outcome and differential gender response to the intervention. **Methods:** 1003 students participated in a controlled trial of the Resourceful Adolescent Program. Students in Year 9, after gaining parental consent completed a battery of self-report measures including:

Child Depression Inventory, Reynolds Adolescent Depression Scale and the Beck Hopelessness Scale. Students in the intervention group completed an 11 session program in groups of 10–12 students with a trained leader. The self-report battery was re-administered at post-test and at a 6 month follow-up to the control and intervention groups. Qualitative evaluation of the program indicated the student's view about the program. **Results:** Small program effects on depressive symptoms for the intervention were found at post-intervention for boys and girls and for girls only at follow-up. However both boys' and girls' self-reports indicated positive overall benefits from the intervention. **Conclusion:** The Resourceful Adolescent Program is cost effective, developmentally appropriate intervention for preventing depression particularly in young women. Further research is required to understand the differential gender response to the intervention.

S-118-555   Topic: 70
Bipolar disorder in children. Does it really exist?

Cristina Maria Ribeiro Marques, Hospital Dona Estefania, Barcarena, Portugal, mmaiaesi@jnjpt.jnj.com
Teresa Cepeda

Objective: Bipolar disorder in children has been considered for many decades a rare diagnosis. However, in the past few years, an increased number of cases under the age of 12, which present clinical manifestations such as irritability, aggression, impulsiveness and 'mood swings' associated with psychotic features, made some clinicians reconsider this diagnosis in children. Nevertheless, strong controversy remains, especially in some European countries. The authors support the hypothesis that pre-pubertal children can suffer from bipolar disorders and that these may be considered as a spectrum of conditions. **Methods:** The authors evaluated a group of 10 children under the age of 12, presenting clinical features that can be included in the bipolar spectrum disorders. Clinical issues such as symptoms, diagnostic criteria, family history, co-morbidity, differential diagnosis, intervention and prognosis are evaluated and discussed. **Results:** Psychiatric assessment of these 10 children showed that the clinical picture of pre-pubertal patients suffering from bipolar disorders might present many distinctive characteristics (such as rapid and ultradian cycles) that surely contribute to make accurate diagnosis of bipolar disorders in children a difficult one. **Conclusion:** Although a variety of difficulties and doubts came along when evaluating these children and several implications have to be taken into account, diagnosis of bipolar disorders in pre-pubertal children should be considered. Nevertheless, further investigation is needed in this field.

S-119   Topic: 82
Auditory and visual processing in dyslexia

Chairperson: Gerd Schulte-Körne, Universitätsklinik Marburg Kinder- und Jugendpsychiatrie, Marburg, Germany, schulte1@med.uni-marburg.de
Andreas Warnke, Universitätsklinik Würzburg, Kinder- und Jugendpsychiatrie, Würzburg, Germany, warnke@kjp.uni-wuerzburg.de

Auditory and visual processing in dyslexia

Gerd Schulte-Körne, Universitätsklinik Marburg,
Kinder- und Jugendpsychiatrie, Marburg, Germany,
schulte1@med.uni-marburg.de

Dyslexia is a disorder resulting from a developmental impairment in the ability to read and spell despite adequate educational resources, a normal IQ, no obvious sensory deficits and adequate sociocultural opportunity. Research into the aetiology of dyslexia looked at visual and auditory processing functions, and moleculargenetic analysis has begun to delineate the genetic basis of dyslexia. The underlying basic processes of cognition and perception and their neurobiological correlates have been analysed. Recent findings of basic auditory and visual processing deficits in people with dyslexia have added new dimensions of phenotypic analyses. A speech perception deficit of the dyslexics has been repeatedly found which already occur on the level of sensory perception which is characterised by pre-attentive and automatic processing. A neurophysiological paradigm which is best suited to examine pre-attentive and automatic central auditory processing is the mismatch negativity (MMN). Visual processing is currently seen as comprising two separate but interactive subsystems with different spatiotemporal response characteristics. Considerable evidence has been put forward in favour of the magnocellular deficit theory in dyslexia. Contradictory findings, however, have resulted in continuing debate as to its role in the pathogenesis of dyslexia. A consensus has emerged that a deficit in phonological processing is a major cause for dyslexia. Phonological processing abilities promise to be an important area for genetic research and, in particular, many studies have demonstrated the importance of early sensitivity to the phonological structure of words. Phonological awareness, (the ability to identify and manipulate phoneme-sized elements of spoken language) is also strongly related to early reading acquisition and is a significant predictor in pre-school years of later success in reading and spelling development orthographic processing (the knowledge of the specific word structure) is a second major area of genetic research. Orthographic knowledge refers to the awareness of the probability of a particular letter following a given letter in any syllable. Some letter combinations are not even possible within a syllable (e.g., fn), while other combinations (e.g., th) occur with great frequency. Skilled readers and writers have implicit knowledge of which letter combinations are orthographically legitimate. In contrast to the phonological deficit hypothesis, there has been very limited research done on the role of orthographic knowledge on reading and spelling disability.

S-119-556   Topic: 82
Multimodal data analysis of phonological processing abilities of dyslexic and nonimpaired readers

Carolin Ligges, Universität Jena,
Kinder- und Jugendpsychiatrie, Jena, Germany,
carolin.gruenling@med.uni-jena.de
Marc Ligges; Ralph Huonker; Bernhard Blanz

Objective: Difficulties in phonological processing are discussed to be one of the major causes for developmental dyslexia. Previous neurobiological studies describe dyslexia-specific functional deficits as a reduction of an N400 (EEG) as well as reduced temporo-parietal fMRI activations as result of reduced phonological processing capacities. **Methods:** Following the hypothesis of a core deficit of phonological awareness in dyslexia behavioral data and changes in fMRI signal intensities were measured in 134 children, adolescents and adults. A subset of those subjects was also examined with EEG using the same paradigm. Subjects had to decide whether two visually presented items were identical or not: slash patterns; letter strings; high frequent German words; pseudowords and rhyming of pseudowords. **Results:** Behavioral, EEG- and fMRI-data showed dyslexia specific reading problems most evidently, when the reading tasks (reading of pseudowords, rhyming of pseudowords) explicitly required phonological skills for an adequate solution. The comparison of fMRI-activation patterns in dyslexics and nonimpaired readers revealed significant differences in the left inferior frontal gyrus, resulting from a hyperactivation in the dyslexics. Multimodal data analyses of one control and one dyslexic subject revealed maximal activations of the dyslexic subject primarily in frontal regions, whereas the maxima of the control subject were localized over temporo-parietal regions. **Conclusion:** Multimodal data analysis helps to shed further light on the phonological deficits that could underlie developmental dyslexia. A repeatedly described fMRI-finding for dyslexia is that of an over-activation in inferior frontal language areas. The reconstruction of fMRI-constrained current source densities revealed maximal activations for the dyslexic subject over inferior frontal regions lasting up until 2 seconds. Even though these results have to be validated in group analysis, our data could probably demonstrate that inferior frontal overactivations are the consequence of a phonological deficit and represent ongoing articulation processes in dyslexics in order to solve phonological challenging tasks.

S-119-557   Topic: 82
Brain responses at infancy predict emergent reading skills in children with risk familial dyslexia and at school age differ in poor readers

Paavo Leppänen, University of Jyväskylä, Dept. of
Psychology, Jyväskylä, Finland, paavo.leppanen@psyka.jyu.fi
Tomi K. Guttorm; Jarmo Hämäläinen; Minna Torppa;
Anne Puolakanaho; Anna-Maija Poikkeus;
Kenneth M. Eklund; Paula Lyytinen; Heikki Lyytinen

Objective: To examine the association of infant brain responses with early reading skills in children with risk for familial dyslexia and brain activation differences in poor readers with the same background. **Methods:** We earlier found differences between 6-month-old at-risk (25) and control infants (27) in event-related brain potentials (ERPs) for duration change in two-syllable pseudowords presented in a mismatch negativity (MMN)-paradigm. We used these ERPs to predict later early reading skills in children before school entry. At school-age for third graders, we used partly the same speech stimuli and comparable new paired non-speech complex stimuli. **Results:** The response latencies for the deviant/atta/and the amplitude of the standard/ata/response at 6 months were associated with reading and writing skills at 6.5–7 years, but only in at-risk children. The brain responses accurately identified 87% of the poor and 80 % of the good readers just before school start. At the third grade, preliminary results showed differences in MMN to change in pitch and rise time of the second tone in the pair. In normal readers, MMN was bilateral for pitch change and left lateralized for rise time change. Poor readers had no clear or reduced MMN response to both types of deviant stimuli. **Conclusion:** Our findings suggest differences in the early organization of the neural networks sub-serving speech perception with cascading effects on later reading skills in children with familial background for dyslexia. The results further indicate that ERPs could provide ways to identify children benefiting from early language training.

S-119-558   Topic: 82, 30
Phonological awareness and orthographic knowledge in German children with spelling disorders

Ellen Plume, Universität Würzburg,
Kinder- und Jugendpsychiatrie, Würzburg, Germany,
plume@kjp.uni-wuerzburg.de
Gerd Schulte-Körne; Helmut Remschmidt; Andreas Warnke

Objective: A German family genetic study assesses neurobiological, neurophysiological and psychological aspects of spelling disorders. Parts of this study examine the role of phonological awareness and orthographic knowledge in children with spelling disorders. **Methods:** 51 children with spelling disorders at the age of 9 to 14 years (experimental group) were compared with 31 of their non affected siblings (control group) according several variables. Phonological awareness was assessed by phoneme blending, segmentation of pseudowords, phoneme reversal and backwards pronunciation of pseudowords. Orthographic knowledge was assessed by a pseudohomophone test. **Results:** Children with spelling disorders were significantly inferior in phonological awareness and orthographic knowledge in comparison to their non affected siblings. Regression analyses showed that phonological awareness plays an important role in German primary school levels whereas orthographic knowledge is more substantial in secondary school levels. **Conclusion:** Children with spelling disorders have deficits in phonological awareness and orthographic knowledge.

S-119-559   Topic: 82, 36
Developmental dyslexia – recurrence risk estimates from a German bi-center study using the single proband sib pair design

Gerd Schulte-Körne, Universitätsklinik Marburg,
Kinder- und Jugendpsychiatrie, Marburg, Germany,
schulte1@med.uni-marburg.de
Inke R. König; Wolfgang Deimel; Ellen Plume;
Markus M. Nöthen; Peter Propping; André Kleensang;
Bertram Müller-Myhsok; Andreas Warnke;
Helmut Remschmidt; Andreas Ziegler

Objective: We assessed reading and spelling in a family sample ascertained through the single proband sib pair design (SPSP) design. 287 families with at least two siblings and their parents were recruited until April 2004 in which at least one child was affected with spelling disorder according to a one standard deviation (1SD) discrepancy criterion between the expected and the observed spelling score. **Results:** Mean values for probands and their siblings were different for both the spelling and the reading phenotype. For the probands, variances of the phenotype spelling were smaller than for their siblings. This effect became stronger when more extreme selection criteria were applied. Both siblings fulfilled the 1SD criterion for spelling and reading in 173 (60.3%) and 83 (28.9%) of the families, respectively, indicating a low cost efficiency of the extreme sib pair approach. A recurrence risk of 4.52 (95% confidence interval 4.07–4.93) was obtained for reading

when the 1SD criterion was applied to both siblings. **Conclusion:** The study demonstrates the suitability of the SPSP design for genetic analysis of dyslexia. The recurrence risk estimates may be used for determining sample sizes in gene mapping studies. Family, segregation and linkage studies all clearly indicate a genetic component for dyslexia. However, both segregation and linkage analyses show contradictory results pointing out the difficulties in studying a complex disease.

S-120   Topic: 84
Attention Deficit Hyperactivity Disorders III
Track: ADHD

Chairperson: Sung-Do David Hong, Samsung Medical Center Child & Adolescent Psychiatry, Seoul, Republic of Korea, sdhong@smc.samsung.co.kr

S-120-560   Topic: 84, 28
Studies of genetic model of Attention Deficit Hyperactivity Disorder (ADHD)

Xueping Gao, Central South University, Dept. of Child Psychiatry, Changsha, China, xuepinggao@hotmail.com
Linyan Su; Xuerong Li

Objective: To analyse the genetic model of attention deficit hyperactivity disorder ADHD and to explore the role of the genetic factors in the etiology of ADHD. **Methods:** The ADHD prevalence and disease types of the relatives of probands children in 54 ADHD families were measured using family based analysis. The single-gene segregation analysis was used to analysie the family data to prove the genetic mode of autosomal inheritance or X-linked inheritance of ADHD, and the polygenic multiple threshold model was used to explore the polygenic model and to estimate the heritability, the liability of ADHD and the recurrence risk of ADHD in each relatives. **Results:** (1) Prevalence of ADHD in the first-, second- and third-degree relatives of ADHD probands were 29.63%, 3.25% and 4.42%, respectively. The prevalence of ADHD in the first-degree relatives was significantly higher than that of the general population. The ADHD prevalence of the first- and the second-degree relatives were rapidly decreased with the increased magnitude of consanguineous relationships of each relatives and ADHD probands. (2) There were comorbid conditions among affected relatives in each familie. The comorbid disorders were Learning Disorders and Conduct Disorder in childhood, and the patterns of psychiatric disorders were Personality Disorders, Gambling and Alcohol Dependence in adulthood. (3) Among the first-degree relatives of probands children, the prevalence of male affected relatives was significantly higher than that of female affected relatives (p<0.01). There was no statistical significance in percentage of each subtype of ADHD (DSM-Criteria) between male and female relatives. In addition the ADHD fathers of ADHD probands were significantly more often effected than ADHD mothers. (4) The datie fit best with a polygenic model with major genes, while other models such as autosomal inheritance or X-linked inheritance could be rejected. The weighted mean value of heritability of ADHD was 82.47±9.78 %. (5) The expected prevalence of ADHD in each relative was 23.0%, 8.9% and 5.0%, respectively. The first-degree relatives of probands children have a high risk for ADHD. The prevalence of ADHD each relative rapidly decreased with the increased magnitude of consanguineous relationship. No differences were found between actual prevalence and expected prevalence of ADHD in each relative of probands children (p < 0.05), which suggested that ADHD was a familial disorder. **Conclusion:** (1) ADHD was a familial disorder. The first-degree relatives of probands have a high risk for ADHD. (2) Learning Disorders and Conduct Disorder were often associated with ADHD in childhood, and the patterns of psychiatric disorders in adulthood were Personality Disorders, Gambling and Alcohol Dependence. ADHD was probably associated with those disorders. (3) There was a gender difference in the prevalence of ADHD in first-degree relatives, the prevalence of ADHD in male relatives was higher than in female relatives. (4) The genetic model of ADHD was most likely polygenic inheritance with major genes. The weighted mean value of heritability of ADHD was (82.47 ± 9.78) %, which suggested that the genetic factor might play an important role in the liability variance of ADHD. Excepting that multiple genes were involved and each gene contributed a small additive effect, major genes may be involved.

S-120-561   Topic: 84, 15

Efficacy and safety of concerta in children with Attention Deficit Hyperactivity Disorder

Sung-Do David Hong, Samsung Medical Center,
Child & Adolescent Psychiatry, Seoul, Republic of Korea,
sdhong@smc.samsung.co.kr
Soyoung Irene Lee; Eui-Jung Kim; In-Hee Cho; Ji-Hoon Kim;
Se-Hyun Park; J-Wook Choi

Objective: The objective of this study was to evaluate the efficacy and safety of Concerta in initiating treatment for ADHD. **Methods:** This was a multi-center, open-label study. One hundred nineteen ADHD children were enrolled through 12 psychiatric treatment facilities. For clinical efficacy measurement, IOWA Conners Rating Scale (I/O and O/D) by parents and teachers, Peer Interaction Rating Scale by teacher, and Clinical Global Impression-severity by researchers were completed at Day 0 & 21. Neuropsychological measurement including Continuous Performance Test was also done pre- and post-medication trial. Adjustment of the dosage of Concerta was done weekly according to the clinical response. **Results:** Subjects showed significant improvement not only on clinical but also on neuropsychological measurements. The majority of the reported adverse events were mild. **Conclusion:** Once-daily Concerta treatment was well tolerated and improved attention and behavior in children with ADHD.

S-120-562   Topic: 84, 15

Switching from MPH immediate-release tablets to MPH extended-release tablets (Concerta®): A multi-center, open-label study in children with ADHD

Steffen Heger, Janssen-Cilag, Medical & Scientific Affairs,
Neuss, Germany, mstrobel@jacde.jnj.com
Andreas Schreiner; Klaus Rettig; Rossella Medori;
Helmut Remschmidt

Objective: To evaluate safety and efficacy of MPH extended-release tablets (Concerta®) in clinically stable children and adolescents with ADHD switched from MPH immediate-release tablets (MPH-IR). **Methods:** Prospective, multi-center, open-label, dose-adjustment study over 3 weeks. 213 patients with ADHD previously treated with MPH-IR were switched to Concerta® 18 mg, 36 mg or 54 mg. Primary efficacy criteria were the IOWA-Conners Inattention/Overactivity-Subscale and a global assessment of efficacy. Secondary efficacy criteria included the IOWA-Conners Oppositional/Defiant-Subscale, Peer Interaction Rating and investigators' global assessment. Safety assessments comprised recording of adverse events, height and weight, vital signs, sleep and appetite. Results were tested for significance using the Chi^2 – or Wilcoxon-test for dependent samples. **Results:** 86% of the 213 patients were male. Mean age was 11.4 ± 2.4 years. Median duration of pre-study treatment was 119 days. Before entering the study 64% of patients had received MPH-IR on a once or twice daily basis. 204 patients (96%) completed the study. From baseline to endpoint, mean I/O-Scores decreased by 2.2 (p < 0.001, caregiver's rating) and by 0.2 (n.s., teachers' rating). O/D-Scores decreased by 1.2 (p < 0.001, caregiver's rating) and by 0.1 (n.s., teachers' rating). Efficacy was rated as 'good' or 'excellent' by 55% of teachers, 79% of caregivers and 77% of psychiatrists, respectively. Effect of study medication on Peer Interaction as rated by teachers was equieffective to prestudy medication. Study medication was well tolerated. Most frequent adverse events were headache (8.9%) and rhinopharyngitis (7.0%). No unexpected adverse events occurred. An improvement in sleep quality (p = 0.07) and appetite was observed. **Conclusion:** Switching symptomatically stable patients from MPH-IR to MPH extended-release tablets (Concerta®) resulted in a significant improvement of ADHD-symptoms in the after-school sphere. At school, MPH extended-release proved to be at least as effective as MPH-IR. Tolerability was very good with a trend for improved sleep and appetite.

S-120-563   Topic: 84, 15

Treatment of Attention Deficit Hyperactivity Disorder with Amphetamine: Short term effects on family interaction

Peik Gustafsson, BUP Kliniken, Child & Adolescent
Psychiatry, Lund, Sweden, peik.gustafsson@bup.lu.se
Kjell Hansson; Lena Eidevall; Gunilla Thernlund

Objective: The aim of the study was to investigate the effect on the family interaction of amphetamine treatment of children with attention deficit hyperactivity disorder. **Methods:** 43 children (34 boys and 9 girls in the ages from 6 to 12) and their families participating in a Swedish multi-centre study concerning treatment with amphetamine of children with ADHD, were examined before start and after three months of treatment. The children's behaviour was assessed by parents with the Conner's abbreviated rating scale and by teachers with the Conner's teacher questionnaire. The family functioning was assessed with a parent self-report questionnaire (the Family Relations Scale) and by observers rating video taped family situations with two instruments (the Beavers Family Competence Scale and the Dyadic Family Interaction). Parental symptomatology was measured with the SCL-90 self-report questionnaire. **Results:** The self-report questionnaire as well as ratings of the video tapes by the observers showed that the families had more signs of family dysfunction compared to normal families. A factor defined from the observer ratings that we called hostility showed a linear correlation with the parent ratings of the child's behaviour. After three months of medical treatment both parents and teachers reported a significant improvement of the children's behaviour. The family interaction also improved according to both self-report by parents and observer ratings of the video tapes.

Mothers to the children with the most severe ADHD-symptoms had more depression, somatization and anxiety compared to mothers of children with less ADHD-symptoms, and their symptoms improved after three months of treatment. **Conclusion:** The results of our study seems to suggest that the child's ADHD-symptoms can influence the family functioning in a negative way. Treatment of the child with central stimulant medication for three months leads to an improvement of the family functioning, presumably because the child's ADHD-symptoms improve.

S-120-564   Topic: 84, 28
Association study of serotoninergic candidate genes and Attention Deficit Hyperactivity Disorder (ADHD) in a German sample

Philip Heiser, Universitätsklinik Marburg,
Kinder- und Jugendpsychiatrie, Marburg, Germany,
heiser@mailer.uni-marburg.de
A. Dempfle; Kerstin Konrad; Susann Friedel; Judith Smidt;
Justyna Grabarkiewicz; Frank Geller; Hans Kiefl;
Ulrich Knölker; U. Hemminger; K. Saar; Andreas Warnke;
Beate Herpertz-Dahlmann; Helmut Remschmidt;
Johannes Hebebrand

Objective: Alterations in the serotoninergic pathway have been implicated in the pathogenesis of attention-deficit/hyperactivity disorder (ADHD). The aim of this study was to investigate seven genetic variants in three genes (serotonin transporter (5-HTT), serotonin receptor 1B (5-HTR1B) and serotonin receptor 2A (5-HTR2A)), which have previously been shown to be associated with ADHD. **Methods:** We genotyped five single-nucleotide polymorphisms (SNPs), one deletion and one microsatellite in a sample of 102 families (80 quartets, 19 quintets, 3 sextets). ADHD was diagnosed according to DSM-IV criteria. Index patients and their affected sibs fulfilled criteria for the combined type in 69%, for the predominantly inattentive type in 27%, and for the predominantly hyperactive-impulsive type in 4%. The mean age was 11.6 yrs, with males accounting for 72%. The single parameters under investigation were:– 5-HTT: (markers: 5-HTTLPR (promoter polymorphism, 44bp del); VNTR in intron 3'UTR; SNP (rs3813034)). – 5-HTR1B: (marker: G861C (rs6296)). – 5-HTR2A: (markers: T102C (rs6313); His452Tyr (rs6314); 1438G/A (rs6311). Associations were tested by the pedigree transmission disequilibrium test (PDT). **Results:** The investigated SNPs as well as the deletion and the microsatellite showed no association to ADHD in our sample. **Conclusion:** We were not able to confirm the positive results described for ADHD in earlier studies. This discordance between previous findings and our results may reflect variation between patient recruitment, genetic heterogeneity or too low statistical power for confirmation. We cannot rule out the possibility that other variations in the investigated genes contribute to the etiology of ADHD.

S-121   Topic: 84, 15
Methylphenidate holiday in ADHD children
Track: ADHD
Chairperson: Luis Augusto Rohde, UFRGS-HCPA-Brazil
Dept. of Psychiatry, Porto Alegre, Brazil,
lrohde@terra.com.br

Methylphenidate holiday in ADHD children
James Swanson, UCLA at Irvine, Irvine, CA, USA,
jmswanso@uci.edu

To present an up date of the literature on drug holidays during methylphenidate (MPH) use. An overview of the current status of the literature on drug holidays is presented. In addition, recent findings supporting the theory of a situational effect (higher effect in settings of higher environment demand) during the use of stimulant medication are discussed. We also provide data supporting the notion that the amplification of dopamine signals enhances the saliency value of the stimuli. Data from three studies addressing MPH holidays are presented; one assessing the impact of weekend days out of methylphenidate in the MTA titration trial; the second evaluating weekend holidays during MPH use in a randomized, double blind, parallel group study, and the third assessing days without OROS MPH in a multi-center open-label 12 month study. In PET scan studies, MPH administered with salient stimuli induced greater changes in dopamine than MPH given with neutral stimuli. The MPH effects were situational dependent in a study designed to assess the efficacy of the medication, with greater effects in the classroom setting than in the playground setting. While no significant decrease in parents and teachers' account (rating) of the efficacy of the MPH regime with a weekend holiday was found in the one study, days without methylphenidate in both the MTA titration trial and the open-label study with OROS MPH were associated with a decrease of the efficacy in those days. Although there is some evidence supporting a situational effect for MPH and the adequacy of MPH weekend holidays for a special sub group of patients, possible reduced efficacy associated with MPH drug holidays should be discussed with families.

S-121-565   Topic: 84, 15
Methylphenidate effects on Dopamine:
The impact of the context (salient condition)
Nora D. Volkov, National Inst. of Drug Abuse, USA

Objective: To evaluate the hypothesis that methylphenidate (MPH)-induced dopamine increases is context dependent. **Methods:** Using PET scan technology, we measured the effects of MPH on extracellular dopamine when it was given either in a neutral condition or in a salient stimulation condition in two different experiments (one involving food deprivation and the second involving reinforced mathematical calculations). **Results:** In both experiments, MPH administered with salient stimuli induced greater changes in subjective experiences and extra-synaptic dopamine than MPH given with neutral stimuli. **Conclusion:** Taken together, these findings suggest that MPH effects are context dependent and the amplification of dopamine signals enhances the saliency value of the stimuli.

S-121-566   Topic: 84, 15
Efficacy of a new pattern of delivery of Methylphenidate for the treatment of ADHD: Effects on activity level in the classroom and on the playground

James Swanson, UCLA at Irvine, Irvine, CA, USA, jmswanso@uci.edu
S. Gupta; L. Williams; D. Agler; M. Wasdell; S. Wigal

Objective: To investigate the situational nature of methylphenidate (MPH) effects in laboratory classroom and playground settings. **Methods:** A randomized, double-blind cross-over design was used to compare two patterns of delivery of MPH to each other (an ascending pattern and a three times a day bolus pattern) and to placebo. Measures of efficacy were obtained from a MiniMotionlogger to quantify physical activity and the SKAMP rating scales to quantify behavior (problems of attention and deportment) in two different settings (classroom and playground). **Results:** The two MPH conditions did not differ significantly, but both differed from the placebo condition due to lower levels of activity and reduced SKAMP ratings. The MPH effects were situationally dependent and were smaller for the playground than for the classroom setting. **Conclusion:** The situational effects of MPH provide support for the theory of selective effects of stimulants, depending on the demands of the environment. These findings are discussed in the context of some recent neuroimaging studies suggesting that stimulant medications may not produce direct effects on specific brain regions, but instead may integrate and facilitate neural activity in segregated brain circuits elicited by environmental stimulation.

S-121-567   Topic: 84, 15
Weekend holidays during Methylphenidate use in ADHD childrens: A randomized clinical trial

Silvia Martins, Univ. of Rio Grande do Sul, Outpatient Clinic, Brazil, Silza Tramontina; Guilherme Polanczyk; Mariana Eizirik; James Swanson; Luis Augusto Rohde

Objective: To assess whether weekend drug holidays during methylphenidate (MPH) administration change the efficacy and tolerability to the medication in male children with Attention-Deficit/Hyperactivity Disorder (ADHD). **Methods:** In a 28-day, double-blind study, children with diagnoses of ADHD were randomized to receive BID MPH for 7 days a week (n = 21) or to receive BID MPH on weekdays and placebo on weekends (n = 19). Parents completed the Conners' Abbreviated Rating Scale (ABRS) to assess ADHD symptoms and the Barkley's Side Effect Rating Scale (SERS) to assess side effects on weekends. Teachers completed the ABRS on each Monday after weekends. **Results:** Both groups showed significant reduction on the ABRS over time as the dose increased. However, the group difference in the ABRS scores was not statistically significant either on weekend parent ratings (at the end point, p = 0.41; effect size = 0.26) or on teachers ratings (at the end point, p = 0.99; effect size = 0.002). The omission of MPH on weekends was associated with significantly less severity of insomnia (F = 3.96, d.f. = 1, p = 0.05) and a trend for less interference on appetite (F = 3.18, d.f. = 1, p = 0.08). **Conclusion:** Our findings suggest that weekend holidays during MPH administration reduce the side effects of insomnia and appetite suppression without a significant increase in symptoms either on weekends or in the first

school day after them. Possible explanations for these findings (rate-dependent response or impact of demands of the environment) are discussed.

S-121-568   Topic: 84, 15
Weekend days out of Methylphenidate: Findings from the MTA titration trial

Laurence Greenhill, New York State, Psychiatric Unit, New York, NY, USA, larrylgreenhill@cs.com
James Swanson; Benedetto Vitiello; Mark Davies; Walter Clevenger

Objective: To assess the impact of days out of methylphenidate (MPH) on the weekends during the titration trial of the NIMH Collaborative Multisite Multimodal Treatment Study (MTA) of children with Attention-Deficit/Hyperactivity Disorder (ADHD). **Methods:** Children with ADHD assigned to MTA medication treatment groups (n = 289) underwent a controlled 28 day titration protocol that administered different MPH doses (placebo, low, middle, high) on successive days. This methodology allows comparisons between weekend days with and out of MPH. **Results:** Parental scores on several objective ratings scales were significantly higher on weekend days on placebo than on those weekend days that subjects were receiving adequate doses of MPH (all comparisons: p < 0.05). **Conclusion:** The results of the MTA titration trial provide support for the efficacy of weekend MPH dosing.

S-121-569   Topic: 84, 15
Impact of drug holidays on ADHD children treated with OROS Methylphenidate

Stephen Faraone, Massachusetts General Hosp., Harvard Medical School, USA, James McGough; James McCracken

Objective: To assess adherence and predictors of non-adherence among children with Attention-Deficit/Hyperactivity Disorder (ADHD). **Methods:** Children with ADHD (6–13 years) enrolled in a multi-center, open-label, 12-month study received once a daily OROS methylphenidate (MPH). Drug holidays were measured as a proportion of days that medication was not taken. Baseline demographics and clinical variables were also assessed as predictors of non-adherence. **Results:** Adherence was excellent: on average, subjects took 86% of the doses, rising to 92% for subjects who did not take planned drug holidays. 32% of the subjects took drug holidays. Drug holidays were predicted by the following baseline characteristics: 1) older age (p = 0.02); 2) ADHD inattentive type (p < 0.01); 3) fewer hyperactivity/impulsivity symptoms (p < 0.05); 4) lower MPH starting doses (p = 0.03); 5) minority ethnic status (p < 0.01). Drug holidays during follow-up were associated to poorer efficacy at home (p < 0.01) but not at school (p = 0.94). **Conclusion:** Drug holidays were primarily observed for older, less impaired children and ethnic minorities. Drug holidays may adversely impact ADHD children, particularly older children, and caution is recommended.

S-121-570   Topic: 84, 15
Current aspects on Methylphenidate drug holidays in ADHD children

Luis Augusto Rohde, UFRGS-HCPA-Brazil,
Dept. of Psychiatry, Porto Alegre, Brazil,
lrohde@terra.com.br
James Swanson; Larry Greenhill; James McCracken

Objective: To present an update of the literature on drug holidays during methylphenidate (MPH) use. **Methods:** An overview of the current status of the literature on drug holidays is firstly presented. In addition, recent findings supporting the theory of a situational effect (higher effect in settings of higher environment demand) during the use of stimulant medication are discussed. Data from three studies addressing MPH holidays are presented; one assessing the impact of weekend days out of methylphenidate in the MTA titration trial; the second evaluating weekend holidays during MPH use in a randomized, double blind, parallel group study, and the third assessing days out of OROS MPH in a multi-center open-label 12 month study. **Results:** The MPH effects were situational dependent in a study designed to assess the efficacy of the medication in the classroom and playground settings. While no significant decrease in parents and teachers' account (rating) of the efficacy of the MPH regime with a weekend holiday was found in the second study, days out of methylphenidate in both the MTA titration trial and the open-label study with OROS MPH were associated with a decrease of the efficacy in those days. **Conclusion:** Although there are some evidences supporting a situational effect for MPH and the adequacy of MPH weekend holidays for a special subgroup of patients, possible lower outcomes associated to MPH drug holidays should be discussed with families.

S-122   Topic: 75
The clinical assessment of children with suspected somatoform disorder: An update

Chairperson: W. Boudewijn Gunning, Epilepsy Centre Kempenhaeghe Dept. of Epileptology, Heeze, Netherlands, gunningb@kempenhaeghe.nl

The clinical assessment of children with suspected somatoform disorder: an update

W. Boudewijn Gunning, Epilepsy Centre Kempenhaeghe, Dept. of Epileptology, Heeze, Netherlands, gunningb@kempenhaeghe.nl

The European Working Group for Consultation, Liaison and Psychosomatics (ESCAP) organized this symposium to focus on both the somatic and psychological aspects of the clinical assessment of children and adolescents with suspected somatoform disorder.

S-122-571   Topic: 74
Conversion Disorder in childhood: Diagnosed too late, investigated too much?

Michael Leary, Bristol Children's Hospital, Dept. of Neurology, Bristol, United Kingdom, mickleary@blueyonder.co.uk

The term "conversion disorder" (DSM IV) is applied when symptoms and deficits involving voluntary motor and sensory function suggest a neurological or other physical condition which is in fact not present. In Britain such cases are regularly encountered by paediatric neurologists and place significant demand on consulting time and diagnostic resources. The widely diverse manner in which organic neurological disorder may present creates a dilemma in the diagnosis and management of conversion disorders. While there is real need to exclude organic disease the thoroughness with which this is done may strengthen patient and parental conviction that there must be a physical explanation for the symptoms. Management may be further complicated by anxiety about litigation, parental refusal to accept an emotional cause for symptoms, patient refusal to accept intervention and a community shortage of resources for treating children and adolescents with emotional problems. In this study illustrative cases will be presented, recent relevant research findings reviewed and management strategies discussed.

S-122-572   Topic: 75
Recurrent abdominal pain

John Campo, Western Psychiatric Institute, Psychiatry, Pittsburgh, PA, USA, campojv@msx.upmc.edu

Objective: This presentation will examine the factors relevant to the assessment of pediatric recurrent abdominal pain (RAP), with special attention to the relationship between RAP and psychiatric disorder. **Methods:** Previous research regarding the assessment of RAP and the association between RAP and psychiatric disorder will be reviewed, followed by presentation of the results of studies conducted by the presenter and colleagues of: the adult physical and psychiatric outcomes of pediatric RAP; the relationship between RAP, anxiety, depression, and temperament in primary care; and, open label treatment of RAP and comorbid anxiety and depression with the selective serotonin reuptake inhibitor citalopram. **Results:** Childhood RAP predicts preoccupations with physical health, hypochondriacal fears, and anxiety symptoms and disorders in adulthood, and children with RAP are significantly more likely to be diagnosed with anxiety and depressive disorders in childhood and exhibit higher levels of anxiety and depressive symptoms, temperamental harm avoidance, and functional impairment than pain-free controls. Anxiety disorders tend to precede RAP onset in comorbid cases. Twenty-one of 25 RAP subjects treated openly with citalopram (84%) were classified as clinical responders, with ratings of abdominal pain, anxiety, depression, and impairment improving significantly compared to baseline, and citalopram being generally well tolerated. **Conclusion:** Youth presenting with RAP deserve careful assessment for anxiety and depressive disorders, and are at risk for emotional and somatic distress in adulthood. Citalopram is a promising treatment for pediatric RAP that deserves further study, as do other treatments proven to be efficacious for pediatric emotional disorders. Longitudinal, family, and psychobiological studies are needed to illuminate the nature of observed associations between RAP, anxiety, and depression.

S-122-573   Topic: 74, 37
Psychosocial assessment of children and adolescents with recurrent headaches

Bo Larsson, Child & Adolescent Psychiatry, Neuroscience, Trondheim, Norway, bo.larsson@medisin.ntnu.no

Objective: Recurrent headaches in children and adolescents are one of the most common health complaints. The presentation will address various psychosocial factors relevant to the assessment of recurrent, nonorganic headaches in children and adolescents with an emphasis on psychiatric aspects. **Methods:** Results from previous clinic and epidemiological studies will be reviewed, in addition to presentation of recent data from an epidemiological Norwegian study of adolescents with various forms of recurrent pains. Most common comorbid problems are depressive, anxiety and other somatic symptoms (than headaches), in particular among adolescent girls. The specificity of relationships between recurrent headaches and psychiatric disorders will be discussed. **Results:** Psychological and psychiatric problems should be assessed in children and adolescents suffering from frequent headaches (at least once a week) for a longer period of time. The assessment should also include various dimensions of impairment related to the experience of frequent headaches, e.g. school absence, reduced leisure time activities, in addition to problems with concentration, doing home work, eating regular meals and sleep. Such problems should also be included as outcome measures when evaluating the effects of various intervention (drug and psychological) strategies for children and adolescents suffering from recurrent headaches.

S-122-574   Topic: 74, 37
The clinical assessment of children and adolescents with suspected psychogenic pseudoseizures

W. Boudewijn Gunning, Epilepsy Centre Kempenhaeghe, Dept. of Epileptology, Heeze, Netherlands, gunningb@kempenhaeghe.nl

Objective: To develop guidelines for the clinical assessment of children and adolescents with suspected psychogenic pseudoseizures, and to apply these guidelines to a cohort of patients in our epilepsy centre to find out strengths and weaknesses of the guidelines. Based on a Medline search we used the following (expert-based) definition: psychogenic pseudoseizures are episodic disturbances of behaviour that mimic epileptic seizures, but are not associated with the paroxysmal EEG discharges that can occur during epileptic seizures (i.e., no ictal epileptiform discharge, and maintenance of alpha rhythm during clinical event) and have characteristics that plead for the psychogenic nature of the seizures. **Methods:** We applied our definition of psychogenic pseudoseizures prospectively to a cohort of 20 adolescents with suspected psychogenic pseudoseizures. **Results:** Consistent with prior research approximately 25% of our patients with psychogenic pseudoseizures had either active epilepsy or a past history of epilepsy. Due to the low frequency of seizures ictal EEG-video-recording was not possible in a considerable part of patients. In those cases, and in patients in which the EEG was not conclusive (simple partial and mesial frontal lobe seizures can be electrographically 'silent seizures') the initiation of treatment had to be based on the typical psychogenic nature and course of the seizures, and the exclusion of epileptic clinical characteristics. **Conclusion:** Keeping in mind that conclusive evidence for a diagnosis of psychogenic pseudoseizures can not always be produced, a structured investigation of patients with suspected psychogenic pseudoseizures will probably help to make a more precise diagnosis earlier in the course of the seizure disorder.

S-123
Free communication III
Chairperson: Aribert Rothenberger, Universität Göttingen, Göttingen, Germany, arothen@gwdg.de

S-123-575   Topic: 79, 19
Adjustment in the team in adolescent resident care: A model for systemic interventors

Raymond Traube, Centre Pédagogique et Thérapeutique, Neuchatel, Switzerland, r.traube@bluewin.ch
Jean-Marie Villat

Objective: We present a modality of organization in an educational and therapeutic in-patient unit for children and adolescent with behavioral disorders. The director and the child psychiatrist lead conjointly the network and family meetings. They share the mixed caring and framing identity as well they co-evaluate the benefits and risks of institutional options. In case of emergency due to violence, the cohesion of the multidisciplinary team can decrease and symetrical counter-reactions can occur. Namely the director has to make sure of the institutional coherence and respectively the psychiatrist worries about psychological implications on the child. **Conclusion:** The process develops in the team alliance and confrontation as well the possibilities of formulation of complementary positions. The device plans consequently times and places to reach an additional consens. A three phase model of the co-evaluation's process between systemic interventors in crisis situations can be designed. Two clinical vignettes illustrate exclusion and penal time-out processes. We apply clinicaly the concept of enmeshed hierarchy (Lerbet G, 1997, Pédagogie et Systémique, PUF, Paris) as well the split therapeutic double bind (Ausloos G, 1983, Adolescence, Délinquance et Famille, Vaucresson); We focus on coping with institutional crisis (Traube R, Villat JM, 2003, Complementarity and crisis between director and psychiatric consultant in resident care of children with conduct disoders, Neuropsychiatrie de l'enfance et de l'adolescence, Elsevier, 51, p. 257–264 as well on institutional violence (Traube R, Villat JM, Violence de l'adolescent – Contre Violence de l'institution, 2002, Psychothérapies, 22.3, p. 167–173, Genève)

S-123-576   Topic: 84, 19
The multiple identity of the child psychiatrist

Raymond Traube, Centre Pédagogique et Thérapeutique, Neuchatel, Switzerland, r.traube@bluewin.ch

In many situations the child psychiatrist is in the same time a family therapist, a systemic interventor, a child psychotherapist, a psycho-pharmaco-therapist. We illustrate our model with long term guidance of so-called hyperactive with attention deficit children. 1. The family consultation includes: a. a modelisation of the symptomatic countertransferential interaction, b. a psychotherapeutic process during family psychodramatic sessions c. an parental coaching on the educative rules, 2. the social and psychotherapeutic effects of medication, 3. a regular network monitoring with school and educational agents, 4. a developpemental space could be: a. sensory-motor or speech symbolic therapies. b. group story telling therapy. The identity of the child psychiatrist mixes biomedical responsibility, family psycho-therapy, behavioural guidance and social-psychiatric network.

S-123-577   Topic: 36, 84
Do periodic non-contingent cues improve sustained attention to response and goal-related electrodermal activity (EDA) in attention-deficit/hyperactivity disorder?

Redmond O'Connell, Trinity College, Psychology, Dublin 2, Ireland, oconnelr@tcd.ie
Mark A. Bellgrove; Paul Dockree; Ian H. Robertson

Objective: To apply a simple cognitive rehabilitation cueing technique to the remediation of the ADHD attention-deficit. **Methods:** The ability of children with ADHD to self-sustain attention was examined using a version of the Sustained Attention to Response Test (SART). Participants in this study included 15 children with ADHD and 20 matched controls. Participants completed four blocks of the sustained attention task with random non-contingent alerts introduced on two blocks as a cue for participants to take a more supervisory stance to the task at hand. Electrodermal activity (EDA) was recorded and waveform amplitudes in response to commission errors, correct withholds and alerts were analysed. **Results:** (1) The patient group showed a significantly increased propensity for error on the task suggesting poorer sustained attention ability relative to controls. (2) Variability of reaction times (RTs) in both groups was correlated with commission errors, with the patient group showing significantly greater variability than controls. (3) Non-contingent cues produced a significant short-term reduction in commission errors in the ADHD group but failed to bring about any overall reduction in commission errors. (4) EDA measurements indicated an attenuated skin conductance response (SCR) to commission errors in the patient group and this was associated with an increased rate of commission errors. (5) An investigation of RTs on the stimuli immediately before and after each target indicated significant post error slowing in both groups suggesting that error awareness was normal for the ADHD children. **Conclusion:** This study demonstrates that ADHD children can be cued to improve their top-down control over sustained attention for short periods and suggests that reduced post-error processing, as indicated by attenuated SCRs to errors, may be an important contributory factor.

S-123-577A   Topic: 19, 2
Network therapy

Raymond Traube, Centre Pédagogique et Thérapeutique, Neuchatel, Switzerland, r.traube@bluewin.ch
Mary Braunschweig; Jacques Chabanier; Germana De Leo; Margerita Ibanez; Olivette Mikolajaks; Ida Ropstad

We present the program of a postgraduate training in network interventions. It is organized by AESMEAF (European Association of Multidisciplinary Interventions in Child, Adolescent and Family Mental Health. It concerns the various professions in the psycho-social and educative fields. The first three years cycle is scheduled in Italy (Torino), Spain (Barcelona) and France (Nice), starting 2005, a week end every month, for a total of 800 hours. It is given by german, belgian, norwegian, swiss, italian, spanish, french and other european teachers Teaching includes lessons, seminars, workshops, supervisions, week trainings in different countries, and final dissertation. Themes are, among others: -risk and resilience factors -network along the life cycle: early childhood, schooltime, adolescence, and so for

– the specific contexts of intervention: family, nursery, school, residential unit, – the intra-institutional and inter-institutional interactions – the society problems, as parenthood, migration, and so on – the various professional tools in mental health – the psycho-social incidences of handicap, psychosis, violence, and so far – the local, national and european regulations regarding deontology in the multidisciplinary practice

S-124   Topic: 71
Anxiety and phobic disorders
Chairperson: J. Gerald Young, New York University, Dept. of Psychiatry, New York, NY, USA, jerry.young@nyu.edu

S-124-578   Topic: 71, 38
The relationship between maternal separation-individuation and separation anxiety in Australian adolescent mothers
Rachele Aiello, Monash University, Dept. Psychological Medicine, Melbourne, VC, Australia, rachele.aiello@med.monash.edu.au
Sandra Lancaster

Objective: Findings of fewer, less sensitive and less competent maternal attachment behaviours in adolescent mothers have been associated with non-integrated personality structures, suggesting that adolescent developmental tasks interfere with the budding mother-infant relationship. The adolescent mother's ongoing separation-individuation from her family of origin may be incompatible with her infant's need for closeness and thus make it more difficult to form a close mother-infant relationship. Previous research has reported that adolescent mothers had heightened maternal separation anxiety that was attributed to their ongoing personality development. The degree of early separation-individuation during adolescence is likely to influence the adolescent mother's response to separation (maternal separation anxiety) from her infant during the first year. The aim of this preliminary study was to investigate the relationship between maternal separation-individuation and separation anxiety in Australian adolescent mothers. **Methods:** Ninety primiparous adolescents were recruited in their first trimester of pregnancy from the Young Women's Antenatal Clinic (Monash Medical Centre, Victoria, Australia). Data on attachment to her own parents and degree of separation and individuation were collected during the first trimester. At 6 months postpartum, reactions to separation from their infant (Maternal Separation Anxiety Scale) were measured. **Results:** The paper presents preliminary findings of an ongoing longitudinal study examining adolescent mothers and their babies. Several theoretical frameworks are used to consider the reported relationships between these variables. **Conclusion:** The implications of these findings for adolescent mothers and their infants' development are discussed, with particular focus on areas for antenatal and postnatal intervention.

S-124-579   Topic: 71, 38
Phobias: Between phenomenological diagnosis and "Depth" diagnosis

Viviana Porcari, University Hospital Palermo,
Child & Adolescent Psychiatry, Palermo, Italy,
viviana.porcari@virgilio.it
Maria Patrizia Salatiello; Anna Lo Bue;
Valentina Dell'Oglio; Rosaria Cardella; Sabrina Chifari

Objective: The authors want to demonstrate how the latest international manuals for the psychiatric diagnosis based only on phenomenological parameters, do not allow to reach an exhaustive comprehension of the mental processes underlying children's Specific Phobias. **Methods:** Analysis of different clinical cases come to the Children's Psychiatry Institute at the University Hospital of Palermo for a clinical evaluation on Specific Phobia and identification of the many psychodynamic mechanisms that may underlie the symptom: phobia. **Results:** The use of this methodology demonstrates that the "Phobic Syndrome" category very often conceals variegated and more complex pathologies. **Conclusion:** The authors conclude that the actual international classifications (DSM IV and ICD 10) are often incomplete and, sometimes, misleading not only for a correct diagnosis but also for an effective therapy suitable to the children's problems. Therefore, the Authors believe that, to confront the data coming from the worldwide centres of mental diagnosis, new and more in-depth systems of classification are needed, based not only on phenomenological but also on dynamic criteria.

S-124-580   Topic: 70, 58
Depression and impact of school-factors among young adolescents

Anne Mari Undheim, NTNU, Child & Adolescent
Psychiatry, Trondheim, Norway,
anne.m.undheim@medisin.ntnu.no
Anne Mari Sund

Objective: The aims of the study were to examine the relationships between depressive symptoms and school factors like stress, satisfaction, grades and teacher support among young adolescents. **Methods:** The study is a part of a longitudinal study of depressive symptoms and disorders in 12–15 year old adolescents in Norway. 2465 students participated (50.8% girls). They filled in the Mood and Feeling Questionnaire (MFQ) to report depressive symptoms as specified by the DSM-III-R diagnostic system (Angold, 1989), and the EASQ (The Early Adolescence Stress Questionnaire (Sund et al. 2003), to capture stressful events and chronic stressors. The Class Wellbeing Scale (Ystgaard 1997) is tapping different aspects of emotional and social environment at school. Teacher support is measured by a composite variable made for this study. **Results:** Correlations between depressive symptom levels and the different school factors are all moderate, however significant $p < 0.01$. In the multivariate linear regression analyses the highest contribution to the variance was school stress ($t = 14.14$), followed by being a girl ($t = 12.31$), classroom wellbeing ($t = 11.99$), teacher support ($t = 3.78$) and low grades ($t = 2.65$), all $p < 0.001$. When teacher support was entered, the strengths of the associations between school stress, classroom wellbeing, grades and depression symptom level were slightly reduced: School stress beta 2.22, $t = 15.33$, to beta 2.12, $t = 14.47$, classroom wellbeing beta 0.802, $t = 0$ 13.23 to beta 0.73, $t = 11.70$, and grades beta 0.278, $t = 04.57$ to beta 0.242, $t = 3.951$, all $p < 0.001$. **Conclusion:** The results show how depressive symptomatology might reflect the school climate although the direction of the effects is uncertain. Teacher support reduced the effect of school stress, low classroom wellbeing and low grades on depressive symptom level. Teacher support may counteract the impact of these negative factors, which is important information for the schools.

S-124-581   Topic: 71, 42
A two year follow-up study of anxiety disorders in a Chinese Elementary School Pupils aged 8–10

Linyan Su, Mental Health Institute,
Dept. of Child Psychiatry, Changsha, China,
sulinyan@sina.com
Kai Wang; Xuerong Luo

Objective: To understand the stability of anxiety disorders in Chinese children over two years. **Methods:** Two hundreds and six pupils (105 boys and 101 girls) from an elementary school in Changsha city with the mean age 8.72 ± 0.92 completed the 41-item version of SCARED. Their parents completed Achenbach Child Behavior Checklist (CBCL). **Results:** Fifty-five pupils were with a total score higher than cut-off point of SCARED in the first survey, the positive rate was 26.7%, and 48 pupils (23.3%) during the follow-up. Symptoms of anxiety of 19 pupils (9.22%) persisted for two years. The Anx group exhibited higher levels of attention problems, delinquent behavior, aggressive behavior subscale, externalizing and total problems of CBCL than that in Non-Anx group (pupils with a total score were lower than cut-off point of SCARED) in the first survey. Significant differences were found that withdrawn, somatic complaints, anxious/depressed, attention problems subscale, internalizing and total problems were higher than Non-Anx group two years later. **Conclusion:** The anxiety symptoms were found frequently in elementary school children in China. 9.22% of children with anxiety disorders persisted in two years follow-up. Young children with anxiety symptoms have more externalizing problems, children with anxiety symptoms have more internalizing problems during development.

S-125   Topic: 84
Attention Deficit Hyperactivity Disorders II
Track: ADHD

Chairperson: John Fayyad, St. George Hospital Psychiatry
and Psychology, Beirut, Lebanon, jfayyad@inco.com.lb
Ralf Dittmann, Lilly Deutschland GmbH Medical
Department, Bad Homburg, Germany, dittmann@lilly.com

S-125-582   Topic: 84, 10
The effect of modifying maternal expressed emotion on outcome of preschool hyperactivity

Joanne Barton, North Staffs Comb. Healthcare,
Child & Adoles. Mental Health, Stoke-on-Trent,
United Kingdom, joanne.barton@nsch-tr.wmids.nhs.uk

Objective: The theoretical basis of this study draws upon empirical evidence for the role of mother-child interaction in the development of child self-regulatory capacity. The aim of the study was to examine the effect of an intervention designed to modify maternal negative expressed emotion (EE) on outcome of hyperactive preschool children.

Methods: A pragmatic controlled intervention design was employed. Forty-seven subjects and 13 wait list controls aged three to five years and their mothers were recruited from a specialist treatment centre. The primary outcome measures were child behavioural adjustment measured by the Parental Account of Childhood Symptoms (PACS), maternal EE and mother-child interaction. Intervention comprised a ten week combined parent training and child behavioural programme (Preschool Overactivity Programme, POP). Subjects were reviewed at one, six and 12 months post intervention; controls were assessed at baseline and ten weeks later. The nature of the data required the use of nonparametric statistics. Time series analyses (Friedman Tests) were used to examine change in primary outcome measures across time. Kendall's Tau B statistic was used to examine associations between outcome measures. **Results:** The sample was aged between 36 and 69 months (mean 47.37, SD 7.04), predominantly male (6:1) and of lower socioeconomic status. High levels of hyperactivity (HA) and conduct problems (CP) associated with high levels of maternal criticism and low maternal warmth were present at baseline. Intervention was associated with statistically significant reduction in criticism ($p < 0.0001$) and increase in warmth ($p < 0.0001$) together with significant reductions in HA ($p < 0.0001$) and CP ($p < 0.0001$) which were maintained at follow-up. **Conclusion:** Although methodologically limited this study demonstrates an association between a purpose designed intervention and reduction in maternal EE and child disruptive behaviour. Maternal EE is important in mediating child disruptive behaviour in the preschool period and is amenable to intervention.

S-125-584   Topic: 84, 30
Impact of emotional valence on episodic memory in ADHD patients

Lioba Baving, University Utrecht, Child & Adolescent Psychiatry, Utrecht, Netherlands, l.baving@psych.azu.nl
Kerstin Krauel; Stephanie Santel; Thomas Rellum; Emrah Duezel; Hermann Hinrichs

Objective: The current study investigated the influence of the emotional valence of visual stimuli on episodic memory processes in ADHD patients. **Methods:** Male ADHD patients (n = 18, age 11–16) and matched control subjects performed a levels-of-processing paradigm involving negative, neutral, and positive visual stimuli. The depth of processing during encoding was manipulated by the instruction to either attend to perceptual aspects ('shallow processing') or semantic aspects ('deep processing') of the pictures. Perceptual processing of highly emotional, salient stimuli puts high demands on cognitive control processes. Episodic memory performance was assessed by recognition of the previous presented pictures mixed with new distractor pictures immediately after the encoding phase. **Results:** About 50% of the ADHD boys showed considerably reduced recognition rates compared to healthy controls whereas the other half performed as well as the control subjects. Controls showed superior memory performance for pictures from the semantic task compared to the perceptual task (levels-of-processing effect), for negative, neutral, and positive pictures. In ADHD patients, however, regardless of their overall recognition performance, the levels-of-processing effect was present only for neutral and positive pictures whereas negative pictures from the perceptual and the semantic condition were remembered equally well. These findings were reflected in

differential ERP and fMRI activation patterns. **Conclusion:** ADHD patients showed deep processing of negative stimuli even if they were instructed to perceptual processing, possibly due to deviant cognitive control processes.

S-125-585   Topic: 84, 16
Attention Deficit Hyperactivity Disorder (ADHD) in children: German open-label data from an international atomoxetine relapse prevention study

Ralf Dittmann, Lilly Deutschland GmbH, Medical Department, Bad Homburg, Germany, dittmann@lilly.com
Christoph Bartel; Katja Becker; Iris Linde; E. Friederichs; Martin Schmidt

Objective: To present a German subsample of data from an international study of atomoxetine in the treatment of children with attention-deficit/hyperactivity disorder (ADHD). **Methods:** This is a 10-week, open-label, lead-in period to a large multicenter relapse prevention trial of atomoxetine (1.2–1.8 mg/kg/day) in children (6–15 years) with DSM-IV diagnosis of ADHD and an ADHD Rating Scale severity score of at least 1.5 SD. We used the ADHD Rating Scale (ADHDRS-IV-Parent: Investigator administered, response criterion: ≥40% reduction in ADHD Rating Scale), the Clinical Global Impression-ADHD-Severity Scale (CGI-ADHD-S), the Conners' Parent Rating Scale-Revised:Short Form (CPRS-R:S), the Children's Depression Inventory (CDI), the Children's Depression Rating Scale (CDRS), and the Multidimensional Anxiety Scale (MASC) to assess the efficacy of atomoxetine. Safety was assessed based on spontaneous adverse events (AE), weight, and vital signs. **Results:** 34 of 604 patients from the entire sample were treated in Germany. 85.3% of the patients were between 6 and 12 years old. Response rate at Week 10 was 67.6% (N = 23/34). Mean final dose was 1.39 mg/kg/day. The mean ADHD-RS-hyperactivity/impulsivity score decreased from baseline to Week 10 by 12.3 ± 8.4 points ($p < 0.001$), and the ADHD-RS-inattention score by 13.9 ± 8.1 points ($p < 0.001$). There were significant improvements in CGI-ADHD-S, CPRS-R:S, CDI, and CDRS scores (all $p < 0.01$). An improvement was observed in the MASC total score ($p = 0.08$). Most common spontaneously reported treatment-emergent AE were headache (N = 12, 35.3%), abdominal pain (N = 11, 32.4%), and decreased appetite (N = 8, 23.5%). Mean weight loss was −0.3 ± 1.2 kg. There were significant increases in diastolic blood pressure and pulse. There were no discontinuations due to AE in this acute treatment period. Nine (26.5%) patients discontinued their treatment due to lack of efficacy. **Conclusion:** Based on this open-label German subsample data, atomoxetine appears to be efficacious and safe in the treatment of ADHD in children. Adverse event rates and vital sign changes were as clinically expected.

S-125-587   Topic: 84, 16
Update: Long-term safety of Atomoxetine in children and adolescents with Attention Deficit Hyperactivity Disorder (ADHD)

Mark Bangs, Eli Lilly and Company, Lilly Research Laboratories, Indianapolis, IN, USA, bangsme@lilly.com
David Michelson; Haitao Gao; Peter Feldman

Objective: Atomoxetine is a nonstimulant noradrenergic reuptake inhibitor that has been approved in the United States for treatment of attention-deficit/hyperactivity disorder.

This analysis examined the tolerability and safety of atomoxetine during treatment lasting up to at least 2 years. **Methods:** The long-term safety of atomoxetine was assessed using data from all clinical trials to date: 15 in children and adolescents, and 3 in adults. **Results:** A total of 3262 children and adolescents and 471 adults have been exposed to atomoxetine in these studies, with over 1200 patients treated for at least 1 year and over 400 for at least 2 years. Discontinuations due to adverse events were uncommon (4.1%). Events more commonly associated with atomoxetine (gastrointestinal events, decreased appetite, somnolence) were predictable from pharmacology, occurred more frequently during initial treatment, and tended to resolve during ongoing treatment. Controlling for age-appropriate increases, blood pressure during long-term atomoxetine treatment (greater than or equal to 2 years) was stable (from baseline [end of acute treatment], systolic: +2.9 mmHg; diastolic: +0.2 mmHg). Atomoxetine did not significantly affect QT interval. The initiation of treatment was associated with a modest decrease in growth velocity that normalized over time. **Conclusion:** Atomoxetine was well tolerated during long-term use, with no evidence of unexpected risks or serious safety concerns. Research funded by Eli Lilly and Company, Indianapolis, Indiana, USA.

S-126 Topic: 57
EFCAP Symposium: Forensic practice

Chairperson: Theodore Doreleijers, Free University of Amsterdam, Amsterdam, Netherlands, t.doreleijers@debascule.com

Forensic practice

Helmut Remschmidt, Universität Marburg, Kinder- und Jugendpsychiatrie, Marburg, Germany, remschm@med.uni-marburg.de

The aim of this symposium is to outline the issues currently facing psychiatry in the European forensic systems. The screening of young people in contact with the justice system has established a high level of mental health need and psychopathology among them, begging the question of how we can work to address their needs. Within the symposium a proposed structure aiming to address the psychiatric needs of young people who have been detained will be outlined, as well as the quality of psychiatric expertise in the context of criminal trials. The role of a community-based multidisciplinary forensic child and adolescent mental health team will also be presented.

S-126-588 Topic: 57
Community based forensic child and adolescent mental health services in the UK

Kenny Ross, BSTMHT, FACTS, Manchester, United Kingdom, kenny.ross@tesco.net

Objective: To describe a community based multidisciplinary forensic child and adolescent mental health team that provides a range of services for young people aged between 11 and 18 who display high-risk forensic behaviours in the context of mental health difficulties. **Methods:** A UK based community based multidisciplinary forensic child and adolescent mental health team with national referrals was systematically evaluated in terms of the types of referrals and how these are addressed. **Results:** The majority of referrals undergo a multidisciplinary (psychiatrists, nurses, psychol-

ogist, art therapist, social worker) semi-structured assessment that includes the utilisation of research-validated evidence-based needs assessment (SNASA) and risk (SAVRY) and recommendations from the assessment become part of the multi-agency care-plan formulated by health, youth justice, education, social services, etc. in the young person's local area. Many of the young people seen by our service are in secure accommodation and we provide input into a Local Authority Secure Unit. **Conclusion:** There are advantages for young people families and professionals of a multi-partnership care approach and the advantages of a clinical team being involved in research and training.

S-126-589 Topic: 57
New developments in the youth forensic field in The Netherlands

Theodore Doreleijers, Free University, of Amsterdam, Amsterdam, Netherlands, t.doreleijers@debascule.com Robert Vermeiren

Objective: Since offenses committed by juveniles are becoming more violent and research has elicited that a very high percentage of these minors suffer from co-occurring psychiatric disorders, measures have been designed for more adequate professional assistance. A masterplan of the Ministry of Justice directs several projects. This paper reviews the current developments in the youth forensic field in The Netherlands, from the practical as well as from research point of view. **Methods:** Care for juvenile offenders is provided by the child welfare council, youth welfare and mental health care institutions, and ambulatory and residential justice facilities. Where in the seventies and eighties these instances provided care on an institution centered base, we nowadays try to collaborate in a way that continuity of (juvenile centered) care is warranted. An overview will be given of the results of the recent research projects which have provided more insight in this matter so that a more rational policy can tailor future programmes and provisions. **Results:** Prevalence studies have been carried out in groups of pretrial juvenile delinquents as well as in samples of convicted youths. The high percentages of psychic disorders in these kids made the child welfare council decide to implement a device and a protocol to detect disorders in an early stage of the procedures after a police arrest. At several moments in the 'justice chain' protocolised assessments are provided, for instance at the entrance of a remand institution for juveniles. After a period of forced treatment risk assessment is carried out by means of (evidence based) instruments. Large scale follow up studies are provided. **Conclusion:** The Netherlands have been forced to sum up and integrate all efforts made by many different agencies to tackle the troubles caused by an increasing amount of offending minors. A lot of work has been done, much more work has to be done yet in the future. Child and adolescent psychiatrist, psychologists and social workers should play an important role in planning these provisions and carrying out the care.

S-126-590 Topic: 57, 80
Psychopathology and delinquency: Where do we go from here?

Hans Steiner, Stanford University, School of Psychiatry, Stanford, CA, USA, steiner@stanford.edu

Objective: Recent representative state of the art screening studies in several countries on several continents have established the high prevalence rates of psychopathology among delinquents. This can now be regarded as a well established fact. The objective of this presentation is to discuss the next steps addressing this problem. **Methods:** This discussion will be based on the findings of a report on the state of the Mental health System of the California Youth Authority, commissioned by Governor Gray Davis. Site visits, staff and inmate interviews and satisfaction surveys served as the modes of assessment. The background was provided by a large scale screening study of 850 youths who were studied by structured interviews. **Results:** We found a considerable mismatch between levels of psychopathology encountered and resources available to treat these problems. In addition, there was a lack of matching what resources were available appropriately to the extant problems. Tese findings extended from entry to exit and affected all mental health interventions. **Conclusion:** We will discuss a proposed structure which has greater promise in addressing the psychiatric needs of incarcerated youths. This investment is justified as juvenile crime turned chronic is an extremely costly adverse health outcome.

S-126-591   Topic: 57
The quality of psychiatric expertises in adolescent and adult arsonists and murderers
Jörg M. Fegert, Universität Ulm,
Kinder- und Jugendpsychiatrie, Ulm, Germany,
joerg.fegert@medizin.uni-ulm.de
Frank Häßler; Kathleen Schnoor; Elisabeth Rebernig;
Cornelia König; Ulrich Auer; Detlef Schläfke

Objective: In a representative sample from the German Land Mecklenburg-Vorpommern in the north-east of Germany, we examined the quality of psychiatric expertises in the context of a criminal trial. In addition we carried out interviews with lawyers and psychiatric experts with regard to their multidisciplinary cooperation. **Methods:** We conducted a complete analysis of all cases of murder, manslaughter and fire setting between 1994 and 1998 in Mecklenburg-Vorpommern. In 208 files we found 109 written expertises, interview data stem from 89 lawyers and 11 psychiatric experts. We carried out descriptive statistics and described significant differences between adolescents and adults. **Results:** The sample is characterised by unemployed men of low educational status in most of the cases the consumption of alcohol played a certain roll. The ratio of cases with expertises was higher in capital offences than in fire setting. Juvenile arsonist were significantly less examined with regard to their criminal responsibility in comparison to adult arsonists. In the expertises we detected quality problems: lack of forensic history or lack of transparency (e.g. if there was no diagnostic according to ICD-10 or DSM-4. **Conclusion:** Also we found numerous problems in the expertises we analysed. The courts didn't question these results. Even in the interviews the lawyers and the psychiatric experts had the impression that they worked together very well. There are some doubts whether there is really a communication between psychiatric experts and lawyers or whether the expertise is just a necessary piece in the puzzle of the trial and finally for the decision making the psychiatric quality of the expertise doesn't play a major role.

S-126-592   Topic: 1
Attachment styles and parental cares in adolescents at psychosocial risk in Italian professional schools: A comparative study
Giovanni Battista Camerini, Psychiatry and Mental Health, Modena, Italy, giovanni.camerini@libero.it

Objective: In populations of adolescents with high psychosocial risk, family conditions of abuse and neglect with pathological attachments strategies can frequently be observed. Those situations assume an important role in terms of risk factors able to determine antisocial behaviours and a bad social and adaptive functioning in adolescence and in adulthood. A comparative study was realized to investigate the presence of those risk factors in two adolescent populations. The first group is formed by unaccompanied minors (any parent present in Italy) living in minor communities; this group can be defined at high psycho-social risk. The second group is formed by minors having at least one or both biological or foster parents living with them. **Methods:** In both groups a test battery was applied: SAT Separation Anxiety Test by Bowlby and Klagsbourn; Parent Child Conflict Tactic Scale by Straus; CBCL Teacher Report Form and Young Self Report by Achenbach. **Results:** The comparison between the two groups allows the possibility to recognize the presence and meaning of different psychosocial and psychopathological risk factors. **Conclusion:** These elements can be an important contribution to clinical and forensic assessment and to future research related to minors with legal problems.

S-127   Topic: 72
Obsessive-compulsive disorder
Chairperson: Aribert Rothenberger, Universität Göttingen, Göttingen, Germany, arothen@gwdg.de

S-127-593   Topic: 72, 45
Early onset obsessive compulsive disorders and family accommodation to symptoms in a Spanish child sample
Soraya Otero, Centro Hospitalario Padre Menn,
Salud Mental Infanto Juvenil, Santander, Spain,
samijsa@mennisant.com
Ana Rivas; Guadalupe Pombo

Objective: Obsessive compulsive disorder (OCD) is a frequent illness in children and adolescents but somehow hidden. Family involvement in symptoms is clinically relevant in this type of disorders. This is a preliminary report of a follow-up study of early onset OCD that aims to identify prognostic factors such as phenomenology, co-morbidity, period between symptoms onset and treatment seeking, and to measure the influence of the family accommodation on symptoms and its evolution. **Methods:** 15 children with early onset OCD (before age 14) from an Outpatient Children and Adolescent Mental Health Clinic. Instruments: Yale-Brown obsessive compulsive disorders, Family accommodation scale (FAS), and K SADS PL version. The FAS (Calvocoressi et al. 1995, 1999) was translated and adapted to be used with a Spanish child and adolescent sample by the authors. Descriptive statistics and non-parametric test (Spearman's correlation; M-W test) were carried out in order to test the hypothesis. **Results:** The average time between symptoms onset and treatment seeking is 7.5 months. The average onset of symptoms onset is 9 years, and that of clinically relevant symptoms is 11 years. 11 cases have got family history of OCD and in 5 cases the mother and/or the father are on a OCD treatment. 8 cases present a history of Separation Anxiety Disorder previous to OCD onset. There is a significant correlation between symptoms severity (YB-OCD) and the degree of Family Accommodation to OCD symptoms (FAS), mainly with the obsessions' scale. **Conclusion:** The FAS has shown to be a good measure of Family involvement in OCD symptoms. This sample of kids with Early Onset OCD has a high prevalence of both family OCD history and personal history of Separation Anxiety Disorders. The average time between OCD onset and treatment seeking is not so high as other studies suggested.

S-127-594   Topic: 72, 13
Combined psychopharmacotherapy of refractory Obsessive-Compulsive Disorder (OCD) with Fluvoxamine and Nefazodone in adolescents

Maruke Yeghiyan, ACPP – Psychiatry and Medical Psychology, Yerevan, Armenia, acpp@netsys.am
Gasparyan Kachatur; Arman Danileyan

Objective: SSRIs are the first-line treatment for OCD in adults with well-established efficacy and greater tolerability compared to clomipramine. However, approximately 40–60% of patients with OCD, treated with SSRIs, do not respond adequately to the therapy. Augmentation of SSRI therapy with a specific (triple action) antidepressant may be effective due to blockade of post-synaptic 5HT2A receptors which may be involved in OCD pathogenesis. To investigate the efficacy of combined use of Fluvoxamine (Luvox) and Nefazodone (Serzon) in adolescents with refractory OCD. **Methods:** We conducted an open study of 14 adolescents (13–16 year old) with refractory OCD. Nefazodone was added after 12 weeks of treatment with Fluvoxamine (50–150 mg/day) because of the low response rate. Doses of Nefazodone ranged between 50–100 mg/day. The response rate after augmentation with Nefazodone was assessed by CY-BOCS and Zung Depression Self Rating Scale. **Results:** More than third of patients receiving both agents reported greater improvement of symptoms than when treated with Fluvoxamine alone. We found significant improvement in both OCD symptomatology in 11 out of 14 patients (Total score – CY-BOCS decrease, 42%, P = 0.003, as well as in overlapping depressive syndromes (average SDS index of Zung score, before was 65, after treatment: 54). Efficacy of Fluvoxamine and Nefazodone combined therapy in case of refractory OCD may be explained by ability of Nefazodone to blockade the post-synaptic 5HT2A receptors. **Conclusion:** Polypharmacotherapy of OCD in adolescents with treatment-resistant symptomatology may be a good strategy. In this open study we reported the effectiveness of Fluvoxamine in combination with Nefazodone in cases of refractory to treatment OCD in adolescents. Due to the small number of patients and the open design, the results of our study have only a preliminary character. Controlled studies with larger samples are necessary.

S-127-595   Topic: 72
Symptom patterns in children and adolescents with Obsessive-Compulsive Disorder (OCD)

Tord Ivarsson, OCD-Anxiety Program, Child & Adolescent Psychiatry, Göteborg, Sweden, tord.ivarsson@vgregion.se
Robert Valderhaug

Objective: Obsessive-Compulsive Disorder is unitary on the level of diagnostic criteria but encompassing children and adolescents with widely divergent symptoms, ranging from stereotypic touching to obsessions and compulsions that are cognitively complex. Moreover, adult studies have shown that the symptoms tend to have specific patterns. The study aims to describe symptom pattens in pediatric OCD. **Methods:** Two samples of patients with primary OCD evaluated at the OCD clinic in Göteborg (n = 182) and enrolled in a treatment study in Trondheim (n = 29) were included. The patients and primary caretakers responses on the Children's Yale-Brown Obsessive Compulsive Scale (CYBOCS) were used to generate a severity rating for symptoms (0 = not present, 1 = present, 2 = present and severe, and 3 = present and worst) for 75 OCD symptoms which were analysed using cluster analysis (Ward method crossvalidated with K-means analysis based on Ward cluster centers – generating a Kappa of 0.90). The clusters were studied in respect of symptom profiles using non parametric statistics. **Results:** A five clusters solution was judged clinically and theoretically most relevant and were named: (1) Low obsession touching & mental rituals (n = 62); (2) Contamination & Cleaning (n = 69); (3) Disaster Prevention & Superstitious (n = 25); (4) Multiple Mixed (n = 33) and (5) Hypochondric (n = 24). The groups differed not only in regard to symptom patterns, where groups 2, 3 and 5 were especially unitary, but also in regard to severity (group 1 lowest), number of symptoms (group 4 highest), avoidance (group 1 lowest), exaggerated sense of responsibility (Multiple Mixed group highest) and age (group 1 lowest). However, therer were no gender differences. **Conclusion:** OCD might, in spite of unitary defining criteria, not be a unitary phenomenon and the sub groups we found might respond differentially to treatment as well as have different etiological pathways. Further studies need to replicate our findings and extend the studies of correlates (e.g. co-morbidity, temperament and treatment response) Our findings differ in important respects with previously published adult studies, indicating that pediatric OCD might have developmentally specific traits.

S-127-596   Topic: 72, 28
Transmission disequilibrium studies pertaining to children and adolescents with obsessive-compulsive disorder and candidate genes of the serotonergic system

Susanne Walitza, Universitätsklinik Würzburg, Kinder- und Jugendpsychiatrie, Würzburg, Germany, walitza@kjp.uni-wuerzburg.de
Christoph Wewetzer; Andreas Warnke; Manfred Gerlach; Frank Geller; Nikolaus Barth; F. Hahn; Beate Herpertz-Dahlmann; Christian Fleischhaker; Eberhard Schulz; Helmut Remschmidt; Anke Hinney

Objective: The serotonergic system was shown to be involved in the etiology of obsessive compulsive disorder (OCD). Here, we analysed transmission disequilibrium of alleles of single nucleotide polymorphisms (SNPs) in three candidate genes of the serotonergic pathway. SNPs within the tryptophan hydroxylase 1 (rs1800532), the serotonin transporter (SNP in the promoter region; 5-HTTLPR) and the serotonin 1 B receptor (rs6296) were studied. **Methods:** We genotyped 64 trios comprising patients with early onset OCD and both of their parents for SNPs in the 3 genes of the serotonergic pathway by PCR based detection methods (PCR-RFLP and ARMS-PCR). All patients fulfilled the diagnostic DSM-IV criteria for OCD. To confirm the criteria all patients were interviewed with the Y-BOCS and DIPS. For statistical analyses the transmission disequilibrium test (TDT, Spielman et al., 1993) was applied. **Results:** We found no evidence for transmission disequilibrium for any of the alleles of the analysed SNPs. **Conclusion:** There is strong evidence for an involvement of the serotonergic system in the development of OCD. In a previous study, we demonstrated association of the A-allele of a promoter polymorphism (1438G/A) of the 5-HT2A receptor with OCD in children and adolescents (Walitza et al., 2002). Here, we did not detect transmission disequilibrium of the investigated polymorphisms in OCD. Hence, these polymorphisms do not appear to play a major role in the genetic predisposition to early onset OCD (Walitza et al., 2004 in press).

S-127-597   Topic: 72, 6

Group cognitive-behavioral therapy versus Sertraline for the treatment of children and adolescents with obsessive-compulsive disorder

Fernando Asbahr, Univ. of São Paulo Med. School, Dept. of Psychiatry, São Paulo, Brazil, frasbahr@usp.br Ana Regina Castillo; Ligia Ito; Maria do Rosário Latorre; Michelle Moreira; Francisco Lotufo-Neto

Objective: To compare the effectiveness of group cognitive-behavioral therapy (GCBT) and of sertraline in treatment-naive children and adolescents with obsessive-compulsive disorder (OCD). **Methods:** Forty children and adolescents aged between 9 and 17 years were randomized to GCBT (n=20) or to sertraline (n=20) condition. The GCBT consisted of a manualized 12-week cognitive-behavioral protocol adapted for groups, and the sertraline treatment involved medication intake along 12 weeks. Patients were assessed before, during and after the acute treatments and at 1, 3, 6, and 9 months following their conclusion utilizing diagnostic and symptom severity interviews, and self-report measures. **Results:** Significant improvement on OCD and secondary measures were observed along the 12-week treatments and follow-up period in both treatment conditions, with no significant differences on OCD symptom severity between groups (Table). Treatment gains were maintained up to 9 months of follow-up, with a significant lower rate of symptom relapse in the GCBT group than in the sertraline condition. **Conclusion:** The treatment with GCBT is effective in decreasing obsessive-compulsive symptoms in childhood OCD, and should be considered as an alternative to individual cognitive-behavioral therapy or a medication, such as sertraline. Results support the efficacy and the maintenance of gains of GCBT in treating youngsters with OCD.

Table 1: Comparison of Scores of Patients at in the Group Cognitive-Behavorial and in the Sertraline Conditions before (Baseline) and after (Week 12) the Acute Treatment: Means, Standard Deviations, and Statistical Results

	Evaluation	GCBT[a] (n=20) Mean (sd)	Sertraline (n=19) Mean (sd)	Test Value[b] Group Time Group×Time	p-Value
CY-BOCS Total[c]	Baseline	26.30 (4.90)	27.26 (6.73)	F=0.7671	0.387
	Week 12	10.85 (7.96)	13.37 (8.58)	F=163.3272	<0.001
				F=0.4588	0.502
CY-BOCS Obs[d]	Baseline	12.95 (3.02)	13.53 (3.19)	F=0.7240	0.400
	Week 12	5.30 (4.59)	6.42 (4.22)	F=109.2660	<0.001
				F=0.1489	0.702
CY-BOCS Comp[e]	Baseline	13.35 (3.13)	13.74 (3.91)	F=0.6369	0.429
	Week 12	5.55 (3.97)	6.95 (4.62)	F=156.4901	<0.001
				F=0.7508	0.392
CGI[f]	Baseline	5.35 (0.88)	5.32 (0.75)	F=1.1061	0.299
	Week 12	2.50 (1.67)	3.26 (1.48)	F=140.9038	<0.001
				F=3.7272	0.061
NIMH-GOCS[g]	Baseline	10.10 (1.89)	9.79 (1.84)	F=0.2298	0.634
	Week 12	5.40 (2.37)	6.32 (3.02)	F=107.0769	<0.001
				F=2.4103	0.129
MASC[h]	Baseline	67.15 (22.38)	57.68 (24.48)	F=3.0607	0.088
	Week 12	49.60 (26.56)	35.16 (20.58)	F=37.7714	<0.001
				F=0.5823	0.4502

[a] Group Cognitive-Behavioral Therapy; [b] ANOVA two-way; [c] Children's Yale-Brown Obsessive-Competitive Scale total score; [d] CY-BOCS Obsessions subtotal score; [e] CY-BOCS Compesult total score; [f] Clinical Global Impression-Severity Scale; [g] National Institute of Mental Health Global IOCD Scale; [h] Mean dimensional Anxie Scale for Children.

S-127-597A   Topic: 72, 40

Hallucinations in non psychotic children

Sophie Symann, Clinique Universitaire St. Luc, Dept. de Pédopsychiatrie, Bruxelles, Belgium, sophiesymann@hotmail.com Jean-Yves Hayez; Dominique Charlier

Objective: To illustrate that hallucinations in childhood are not necessarily an indication of psychosis and can be associated with other mental health problems. **Methods:** We will describe the case of an eleven-year-old boy presenting auditory and visual hallucinations accompanied by compulsive-type behaviours and anxiety. **Results:** We will discuss the therapeutic choices we made after diagnosis and the course of the therapy. **Conclusion:** Hallucinations may occur as a feature of common psychiatric disorders without the unfavourable prognosis of childhood psychosis. Children with such presentations run the risk of being misdiagnosed as having early onset schizophrenia and being subjected to the inherent risks of treatment with antipsychotic.

S-128   Topic: 74, 75

Dissociative and somatoform disorder in adolescents

Chairperson: Franz Resch, Universität Heidelberg Kinder- und Jugendpsychiatrie, Heidelberg, Germany, franz_resch@med.uni-heidelberg.de

Dissociative and somatoform disorder in adolescents

Franz Resch, Universität Heidelberg,
Kinder- und Jugendpsychiatrie, Heidelberg, Germany,
franz_resch@med.uni-heidelberg.de

This symposium aims to present various studies concerning stress-related and somatoform disorders in childhood and adolescence. The basic concept of the development of dissociative symptomatology in adolescence will be outlined and major empirical findings based on a literature review will be presented (Presenter 1). Exposure to violence and its relationship to posttraumatic symptoms and the mediating role of dissociative reactions for antisocial behavior in youth has been investigated in non-clinical adolescent samples in comparison to a clinical sample of adolescent psychiatric patients (Presenter 2). Findings from an experimental study regarding the biological stress reactivity of adolescents with dissociative symptomatology are presented (Presenter 3). Furthermore, the results of a randomized, placebo-controlled treatment study with regard to children migraine will be presented (Presenter 4).

S-128-598   Topic: 74

Disassociation: An important concept in child and adolescent psychiatry

Belinda Plattner, Universitätsklinik Wien,
Abt. Neuropsychiatrie, Wien, Austria, bplattner@gmx.at
Astrid Elisabeth Schallauer

Objective: The objective was to give an overview of dissociation, in a way that respects the diversity of the topic and yet outlines the basic concepts. **Methods:** Literature-search with PubMed from summer 2003 to summer 2004. About 100 classic and recent articles are incorporated in the overview. **Results:** It is argued that dissociation plays an important role in child and adolescent psychiatry, because (1) the prevalence of Dissociative Disorders is higher than generally expected, (2) dissociative scores are correlated with other psychopathology (depression, PTSD, anxiety, etc.) and problematic behaviors (aggression etc.), (3) dissociation might be an underlying mechanism of various trauma-related disorders. In order to minimize the confusion about the concept dissociation three different but related concepts are offered: (1) dissociation as an underlying, hypothesized mechanism (e.g. memories are disassociated in the unconscious), (2) dissociation as observable phenomenons, that range from normal, everyday-experiences (e.g. daydreaming) to pathological symptoms (e.g. depersonalization), and (3) Dissociative Disorders, a special pattern of dissociative symptoms as defined by the ICD 10 and DSM IV (e.g. Dissociative Identity Disorder). Diagnostic tools are discussed (SCID-D, DES, Attachment Story completion Task). Furthermore we present empirical data about the etiology (trauma, attachment, inherent characteristics) and the pathomechanism of dissociation (defense mechanism, failure in information processing). An overview of therapy will be covered. **Conclusion:** Dissociation seems to be a crucial concept when trying to make predictions about the outcome of and choosing the right therapy for trauma-related psychopathology. Therefore clinicians should get familiar with the concept of dissociation.

S-128-599   Topic: 74

Exposure to violence, antisocial behavior and dissociation in adolescence

Beat Mohler, Uster, Switzerland, beat.mohler@kjpdzh.ch
P. Staub

Objective: Correlations between trauma experience and dissociation are well described in literature. This paper is presenting results on how much the relationship between exposure to trauma and anti-social behavior correlates with dissociative experience in adolescence. **Methods:** The study population includes 208 youth from a randomized general population sample, 30 delinquent youth, and 45 adolescent psychiatric patients, aged between 11 and 19 years. Exposure to violence and posttraumatic symptoms were assessed using the adapted version of a structured interview developed in the U.S. ("My ETV"). Dissociative experience was assessed with the german version of the "Adolescent Dissociative Experience Scale" (SDEJ). The "Self Report of Offending (SRO)", an adapted version of an instrument developed by Huizinga (1991), included questions about 32 forms of delinquent and antisocial behavior. **Results:** The study results support a relationship between exposure to trauma, dissociative experience and antisocial behavior. Most delinquent youth reported exposure to violent events, psychiatric symptoms similar to adolescent psychiatric patients, and more dissociative experience compared to youth from normal population. **Conclusion:** The paper discusses the importance of the combination of trauma history and high levels of dissociative experience as a risk indicator for antisocial behavior in youth.

S-128-600   Topic: 74

Physiological stress reactivity in adolescent psychiatric patients with dissociative symptomatology

Romuald Brunner, Universität Heidelberg,
Kinder- und Jugendpsychiatrie, Heidelberg, Germany,
romuald.brunner@med.uni-heidelberg.de
Carsten Müller; Peter Parzer; Franz Resch

Objective: The aim of the study was to investigate reactivity of the autonomous nervous system to a nonspecific laboratory stressor in a clinical group of adolescents with dissociative symptomatology. **Methods:** The effects of an attentional task on heart rate and skin resistance level administered with and without noise, and level of subjective distress were studied in adolescent psychiatric patients with a high (N=19) and low (N=20) degree of self-reported dissociative symptoms as measured by the A-DES (Adolescent Dissociative Experiences Scale). **Results:** Subjects with a high degree of dissociative symptoms demonstrated significantly higher changes in heart rate during the task, while the noise had no effect on heart rate. **Conclusion:** Additional noise led to an increase in skin resistance levels and subjective distress in both groups. The results of the present study suggest that the intensity of the stress response partly represents a sensitivity to stress which could correlate with the exacerbation and fluctuation of dissociative symptomatology.

S-128-601   Topic: 74
Prospective evaluation of different therapeutic approaches in childhood migraine: Which therapy is really helpful?

Rieke Oelkers-Ax, Universitätsklinik Heidelberg, Kinder- und Jugendpsychiatrie, Heidelberg, Germany, rieke°elkers@med.uni-heidelberg.de
Peter Parzer; Jochen Fischer; Uta Hermanns; Anne Nickel; Hans Volker Bolay; Franz Resch

Objective: Prophylactic therapy in childhood migraine is often inappropriate, and prospective, placebo-controlled investigations in childrens are rare. The drugs which are recommended for prophylaxis in children (beta-blockers, calcium antagonists) have a lot of side-effects. Evaluation of psychotherapeutic concepts mostly does not match the criteria of evidence-based medicine. This study evaluates a psychotherapeutic concept (music therapy) and a phytotherapeutic agent (Petadolex) in a randomized, placebo-controlled and (for Petadolex and placebo) double-blind three-arm parallel-group design. **Methods:** The patients (n=60) were aged 8–12 years and suffered from migraine with or without aura for at least one year with an actual headache frequency of two attacks or more per month. Patients were randomized and treated with placebo, Petadolex or music therapy for 12 weeks. Headache was monitored continuously using a headache diary from 8 weeks before (baseline, T0) until 8 weeks after treatment (postline, T1), and again 6 months later for 8 weeks (follow-up, T2). All patients were included in a setting with monthly consultations during baseline, treatment and postline concerning headache management and attack medication. Emotional problems were investigated using the Child Behavior Check List (CBCL). The time-course of the frequency of headache attacks was compared between treatment groups using a random effect regression, treatment effects were evaluated using variance analysis for repeated measurements. **Results:** Headache frequency was significantly reduced in all treatment groups versus baseline (Placebo T1 33.5%, 95% CI [15.6; 50.7], T2 29.7%, 95% CI [12.3; 47.4]; Petadolex T1 34.8, 95% CI [17.7; 51.9], T2 58.6%, 95% CI [36.8; 74.8], music therapy T1 64.2%, 95% CI [44.7; 81.8], T2 64.8%, 95% CI [46.0; 85.4]). At T2, music therapy (p<0.01) and Petadolex (p<0.05) were both superior to placebo. The main reduction of attack frequency, however, occurred during the baseline period. Petadolex and placebo were well tolerated in all patients. **Conclusion:** The applied design allows to separate an unspecific effect of medical consultations, headache diary and expectations concerning effective treatment (setting effect) and the placebo effect in a narrow sense. Petadolex and music therapy are both superior to placebo and may therefore be useful for prophylactic treatment of childhood migraine without serious side effects. A substantial reduction of headache attacks, however, is achieved by a semi-structured setting including the headache diary. Implications for primary care of pediatric migraine are discussed.

S-129   Topic: 70
Mood disorders/Affective disorders II

Chairperson: Miguel Cherro-Aguerre, Montevideo, Uruguay, macherro@mednet.org.uy

S-129-602   Topic: 70, 95
Symptoms and co-morbidity in a clinical sample of depressed children – age and gender differences

Merete Juul Sørensen, Child Psychiatric Hospital, Research Dept., Risskov, Denmark, mjs@buh.aaa.dk
Judith Becker Nissen; Ole Mors; Per Hove Thomsen

Objective: The objective of the present study was to determine the incidence of depressive disorders in child psychiatric patients, and to analyze effects of age and gender on depressive symptoms and psychiatric co-morbidity in child psychiatric patients with major depressive disorder (MDD). **Methods:** One hundred ninety-nine consecutive child psychiatric patients were interviewed using a semi-structured diagnostic interview (K-SADS-PL). Co-morbidity and symptoms were compared across age and gender using Chi-square analysis. **Results:** Current or partly remitted MDD was found in 42 children (21%). Thirty-eight (90%) had co-morbid psychiatric disorder(s). Generalized anxiety disorder, separation anxiety disorder and anorexia nervosa were significantly associated with MDD. Onset of the co-morbid disorder was prior to onset of depression in 37 (74%) of 50 cases with lifetime MDD. No significant gender-differences were found, but anhedonia, hypersomnia and decreased ability to concentrate were more frequent in the older age group. In contrast feelings of worthlessness and symptoms of oppositional defiant disorder were more frequent in the younger age group. The number of melancholic symptoms was significantly associated with age. **Conclusion:** MDD is frequent in child psychiatric patients age 8–13. Age – but not gender – had significant effects on melancholy-score and the prevalence of specific symptoms. Results emphasize the need for systematic assessment of depressive symptoms in children referred to child psychiatric care, and the importance of specialist treatment of children with multiple disorders.

S-129-603   Topic: 70, 26
Prevalence and characteristics of depressive disorders among adolescents in the general population

Anne Mari Sund, Faculty of Medicine, Dept. of Neuroscience, Trondheim, Norway, anne.m.sund@medisin.ntnu.no
Bo Larsson; May Britt Drugli; Lars Wichstrøm

Objective: To estimate prevalence and characteristics of depressive disorders among 13–16 year old adolescents in the middle of Norway. **Methods:** In the "Youth and Mental Health" study a representative sample of 2433 adolescents (Mean age=14.9 years; 87% response rate) were screened with the Mood and Feelings Questionnaire (MFQ). Three hundred and forty four (MFQ=>25: N=220, MFQ= 7–24: N=74 and MFQ<7: N=50) adolescents were interviewed with the Kiddie–SADS (PL). 95% of the adolescents and 79% of the parents who were invited participated in the interview. **Results:** Thirty-six adolescents received a Major Depression (MD) diagnosis (86% girls), 22 dysthymia (82% girls) and 33 (82% girls) depression NOS, defined as having less symptoms during a minimum of 14 days. Estimated 2 month prevalence rate for MD was 2.3%, for dysthymia 1.0% and for depression NOS 4.9%. The mean length of the MD episodes was 15.5 months (SD 22.4, range 0.6–99.6), of the dysthymic episodes 3.8 years (SD 2.2, range 1.48–10.8) and of the NOS episodes 13.2 months (SD 1.6, range 0.5–67.9). The mean C-GAS (Children Global Assessment Scale) score was 59 (SD 6.0) in the MD group, 63 (SD 9.6), in the dysthymic group and 68 (SD 8.4) in the depression NOS group. Suicidal thoughts were most prevalent in the dysthymic group (41%). Only adolescents with MD or dysthymia showed suicidal (13.9% and 13.6%, respectively) or self-harm (13.9% and 18.2%) behavior. Concomitant manic and psychotic symptoms were rare. 13% of those having a depressive diagnosis had currently contact with specialty mental health services. Only one adolescent received antidepressant medication. **Conclusion:** The prevalence rates were fairly low as compared to studies in other countries. Overall, the episodes lasted longer than previously reported. Few adolescents received help from the specialty mental health services.

S-129–604   Topic: 70, 93
Depression and self harming in homeless young people: An investigation into mediators and underlying psychological mechanisms

Matthias Schwannauer, University of Edinburgh,
Dept. of Clinical Psychology, Edinburgh, United Kingdom,
m.schwannauer@ed.ac.uk
Emily Taylor; Rob Wrate

Objective: Design, Implementation and evaluation of a drop-in clinical service was designed for single young homeless in Edinburgh who were suffering from significant emotional distress and/or engaged in self-harming behaviours **Methods:** 120 single young homeless people we interviewed and assessed to determine to determine the prevalence and severity of significant emotional distress in this group, and further to investigate the psychological and social factors most closely associated with the level of distress and to design a tailored psychological intervention for this high risk population. 65 young people were subsequently seen in an open drop in service attending for psyciatric and psychological intervention. A number of standardised psychometric tests as well as qualitative interviews were utilised to determine levels of need. **Results:** Utilising structural equation modelling techniques a model of complex interaction emerged between significant negative life experiences and how the individual is affected by those and the quality of their social network and the way in which individuals process and conceptualise their experiences. Twenty-eight people (24%) did not identify any mental health problems, the majority of reported problems related to affective disorders: depression, anxiety and stress, but there was also a degree of psychotic illness. Results from the Beck Depression Inventory suggested that only 13% of people did not suffer significant depressive symptoms, 27% suffered mild depressive symptoms, and 60% suffered clinically significant moderate to severe depression and emotional distress. **Conclusion:** A better understanding of these interactions and factors will facilitate the development of better ways of preventing and alleviating the extraordinarily high levels of clinically significant emotional distress and maladaptive coping strategies in this highly vulnerable group of young people. 29% of the young people interviewed reported at least one hospital admission for mental health difficulties in the past 5 years, 66% of whom had been admitted to hospital more than once. It has been demonstrated that the amount of contact with clinical services is disproportionately low when compared with the prevalence of mental health problems in the sample.

S-130   Topic: 69
Psychotic disorders in children and adolescents
Track: Psychotic disorders
Chairperson: Helmut Remschmidt, Universität Marburg,
Kinder- und Jugendpsychiatrie, Marburg, Germany,
remschm@med.uni-marburg.de

Psychotic disorders in children
Helmut Remschmidt, Universität Marburg,
Kinder- und Jugendpsychiatrie, Marburg, Germany,
remschm@med.uni-marburg.de

The aim of this symposium is the analysis of psychotic disorders in children and adolescents and their relation to schizophrenia. This will be done by applying the current diagnostic criteria according to ICD-10 and DSM to the different disorders. The introduction will describe four groups of psychotic disorders from which some have a direct relationship to schizophrenia and others do not. In the first paper, H. Remschmidt (Germany) will address neurobiological aspects of early-onset schizophrenia and will delineate very early-onset schizophrenia as a progressive-deteriorating developmental disorder. The second paper (A. Apter, Israel) will focus on depression in child and adolescent schizophrenia. Especially at onset of schizophrenic disorders in this age-group, depression is a highly frequent co-morbid disorder or also a precursor symptom of schizophrenia. But also during the course of schizophrenic disorders, depression is a very frequently occurring complication. Also the differential diagnosis between bipolar disorders and schizophrenic disorders de-serves special attention. The third paper (J. Buitelaar, Netherlands) is devoted to differential diagnostic problems in relationship with child and adolescent-onset schizophrenia. In this context, not only autism, desintegrative disorder, Asperger's disorder, drug-induced psychoses and organic brain disorders have to be discussed, but also multiplex complex developmental disorders (MCDD) resp. multiple development impairment (MDI). The last paper (E. Schulz and C. Fleischhaker, Germany) will describe the results of several follow-up studies in child and adolescent-onset schizophrenia. It will also specifically address the problem of stability and change of diagnoses during the long-term course of schizophrenia and other related psychotic disorders.

S-130-607   Topic: 69, 29
Neurobiological and clinical aspects of early-onset schizophrenia
Helmut Remschmidt, Universität Marburg,
Kinder- und Jugendpsychiatrie, Marburg, Germany,
remschm@med.uni-marburg.de

Objective: To evaluate neuropsychological factors, symptoms, course and long-term outcome in patients with early-onset schizophrenia. **Methods:** (1) Review of the literature with regard to clinical features, neurobiological and neuropsychological findings in childhood and adolescent schizophrenia. (2) Review of the results of two studies of the authors on precursors, clinical symptoms, course and long-term follow-up in two independent samples of patients with early-onset schizophrenia. Methods used were a standardized symptom list, the Instrument for the Retrospective Assessment of the Onset of Schizophrenia (IRAOS) and the Scales for the Assessment of Positive and

Negative Symptoms (SAPS and SANS) as well as the Brief Psychiatric Rating Scale (BPRS). **Results:** (1) Developmental events and precursors of schizophrenia cover a wide range of dysfunctions and disturbances, including elevated rates of soft neurological signs, birth complications, slow habituation and high-baseline autonomic activity, a high rate of developmental disorders and overall and specific cognitive deficits. (2) Positive and negative symptoms can be retrospectively identified months or even years before the first clinical manifestation of the schizophrenic disorder. During the course of the disorder, there is a shift from positive to negative symptoms, and the long-term outcome of children with very early-onset schizophrenia is poor as compared with the outcome of schizophrenia with manifestation during adolescence or adulthood. **Conclusion:** As in very early-onset schizophrenia (manifestation before the age of 13), cognitive and morphological changes are progressive, this disorder can be understood as a progressive-deteriorating developmental disorder.

S-130-608   Topic: 69
Insight and suicidal behavior in adolescent schizophrenia
Alan Apter, Schneider Childrens Medical, Dept. of Psychiatry, Petah Tikva, Israel, eapter@clalit.org.il

Objective: To evaluate the prevalence, nature and correlations of suicidal behaviors in adolescent inpatients diagnosed with schizophrenia. More specifically we examined the relationship of suicidal behavior to phase of illness, presence of and type of depression and degree of insight into illness. In addition the influence of post psychotic depression and negative signs were assessed. **Methods:** In three related studies we examined 200 first-admissions to an adolescent psychiatric inpatient unit. Patients with schizophrenia were compared to adolescents with major depressive disorder, other psychiatric diagnoses and normal controls. Depression defined as a score of >6 on the Calgary Depression Scale for Schizophrenia (CDSS). The following assessments were used: the Childhood version of the schedule for schizophrenia and affective disorders (K-SADS), the Blatt, depressive equivalent scale (DES), the childhood suicide potential scale (CSPS), the suicide risk scale (SRS), the Beck depression inventory (BDI), hopelessness scale (HS), the cognitive checklist (CCL), the positive and negative symptom scale (PANSS) the CDSS and the scale of awareness and understanding of mental disorder (SAUMD) as well as a semi-constructed interview aiming to gather demographic details and data about the outburst of the disease. **Results:** Thirty five percent of the schizophrenic patients met provisional DSMIV criteria for "post-psychotic depression". There were differences in quality and content of depression from those found in the depressed patients In addition we found that it is possible to separate between negative symptoms and depression. Furthermore, we found that post-psychotic depression and suicidal behavior phenomenon is directly correlated with the extent of the awareness and insight into the psychosis. There were differences in the quality of depression and reaction to life stress between schizophrenic subjects and those with major depression. **Conclusion:** Depression and suicidal behavior are common in adolescent schizophrenia. These behaviors have specific features that are important to consider when developing preventative measures.

S-130-609   Topic: 69
Differential diagnosis of psychotic phenomena in children and adolescents
Jan Buitelaar, University Medical Center, Psychiatry & Adolescent, Nijmegen, Netherlands, jb@psy.umcn.nl

Objective: To discuss the differential diagnosis of these phenomena. **Methods:** This presentation is based on a selective review of textbooks and research papers. **Results:** Psychotic phenomena in children and adolescents may be subdivided into signs of formal thought disorder and disturbances in the content of thought, i.e. delusions and hallucinations. Examples of formal thought disorder include illogical thinking, incoherence and loose associations. Signs of formal thought disorder may be apparent from spontaneous speech but may also be elicited and scored by specific procedures as the Kiddie Formal Thought Disorder Story Game (Caplan et al., 1989). Formal thought disorder has been observed in the context of psychotic disorders (early-onset schizophrenia, affective psychoses, and organic psychoses) but also in autistic spectrum disorders, multiple complex developmental disorder, developmental language disorders, personality disorders in adolescence, and ADHD. Hallucinations may be difficult to distinguish from illusions, dissociative states and vivid imagings, and may be occurring in normally developing children on falling asleep (hypnagogic hallucinations). Recent surveys indicate that hallucinations (hearing of voices) may be found in normally developing children in the general population, but may also reflect severe reactions to stress, bereavement, dissociations, and more severe psychopathology as early-onset schizophrenia and depression. More systematic delusions with persecutory or paranoid character often accompany hallucinations and index severe psychopathology as schizophrenia or other psychotic conditions. Background: The diagnostic status of socalled psychotic phenomena and particularly of "hearing voices" in children and adolescents is unclear.

S-130-610   Topic: 69
Results of two follow-up studies in child and adolescent onset schizophrenia
Eberhard Schulz, Universität Freiburg, Kinder- und Jugendpsychiatrie, Freiburg, Germany, schulz@psyallg.ukl.uni-freiburg.de Christian Fleischhaker; Matthias Martin; Klaus Hennighausen; Helmut Remschmidt

Objective: The aims of our two studies were to investigate treatment, course and outcome in early-onset- and very-early-onset schizophrenia. **Methods:** In the Study-VEOS, all inpatients with DSM-III-R diagnosis of very-early-onset schizophrenia (n=76) consecutively admitted between 1920 and 1960 to the Department of Child and Adolescent Psychiatry, Philipps-University Marburg, were included. In the Study-EOS, all inpatients admitted between 1983 and 1988 with DSM-III-R diagnosis of early-onset schizophrenia (n=101) were investigated at follow up. To assess premorbid adaptation, precursor symptoms of schizophrenia, treatment and outcome we administered the Instrument for the Retrospective Assessment of the Onset of Schizophrenia (IRAOS). This instrument was modified by our group for investigating children and adolescents. SANS, SAPS and BPRS were used to measure symptomatology. Additionally, the Global Assessment of Functioning (GAF) was performed. **Results:** After a mean duration of early-onset schizophrenia of 9.5 yrs (sample EOS), out of the study group, 81 patients (80.2%) could be investigated. Assessment of the highest level of adaptive functioning revealed outcome as following: very good and good (19.8%), fair and poor (38.3%) and very poor and grossly impaired (42%). In the VEOS sample (age at onset: 5–14 yrs; follow-up of 42 yrs) the overall outcome revealed that only 16% of patients had a fairly good outcome, whereas a poor and moderate outcome was observed in 60% and 24% of this sample, respectively. Premorbid adaptation and the presence or absence of premorbid developmental delays are of special relevance for long-term course of EOS and VEOS. **Conclusion:** Our data clearly demonstrate, that VEOS and EOS have a worse outcome than in adults, though this appears to be more in the degree of disability and a chronic course of the disorder than in the rate of recovery.

S-131 Topic: 84
Attention Deficit Hyperactivity Disorders IV
Track: ADHD

Chairperson: Peter Jensen, Columbia University Ctr
for Advancement Child MH, New York, USA,
pj131@columbia.edu

S-131-611 Topic: 84, 28
Genetic and environmental contributions to stability and change of ADHD symptoms

Jan-Olov Larsson, Karolinska Institutet, Dept. of Child
Psychiatry, Stockholm, Sweden, jan-olov.larsson@kbh.ki.se
Henrik Larsson; Paul Lichtenstein

Objective: The aim was to study the genetic and environmental contributions to stability and change of ADHD-symptoms between 8–9 and 13–14 years of age. **Methods:** The sample included all 1,480 twin pairs born in Sweden between May 1985 and December 1986. At baseline in 1994, when twins were 8–9 years old, 1,106 (75%) of the parents responded to a mailed questionnaire, and at 1999 when the twins were 13–14 years old 1,063 (73%) responded. At baseline and at follow-up checklists based on the DSM-III-R symptoms for ADHD (Attention Deficit Hyperactivity Disorder) were completed by the parents. Structural equation modeling was used to analyze the data. **Results:** There were relatively high heritability estimates for ADHD-symptoms at 13–14 years of age: for boys 74% and girls 61%. The longitudinal data from 8–9 to 13–14 years of age showed a strong continuity that was mainly genetically mediated. Change in ADHD-symptoms was explained by genetic factors and to some extent by non-shared environmental effects. **Conclusion:** The genetic stability highlights the importance of continuous search for genes and quantitative risk factors, or endophenotypes, which are correlated with ADHD.

S-131-612 Topic: 84, 35
ADHD in adolescence and young adulthood: Pathophysiological changes in the dopaminergic system and the influence of psychostimulants.
A [18 F]-L-DOPA-PET study

Andrea G. Ludolph, Universität Ulm,
Kinder- und Jugendpsychiatrie, Ulm, Germany,
andrea.ludolph@medizin.uni-ulm.de
Felix Mottaghy; Susanne Kraemer; Dieter Claus;
Bernhard Krause; Jörg M. Fegert; Klaus Schmeck

Objective: Some SPECT and PET studies indicate the involvement of the dopaminergic system in the pathogenesis of ADHD, especially an increased density of the presynaptic dopamine transporter (DAT) is assumed. Methylphenidate binds at the DAT with high affinity thus enhancing the dopamine concentration in the synaptic cleft. Therefore we examine young male adults recently diagnosed with ADHD by [18 F]-L-DOPA-PET in comparison to healthy controls to investigate pathophysiological changes in the presynaptic dopaminergic system. **Methods:** We enrolled 7 male patients with ADHD (mean age 21.4 y, SD 3.3, range 18–25) and 6 healthy male controls (23.5 y, SD 0.8, range 22–24). Six of the patients had never received any psychostimulant treatment, one was actually treated with methylphenidate. ADHD was diagnosed according to ICD-10 diagnostic criteria. To measure the efficacy of the presynaptic dopaminergic system we performed [18F]-L-DOPA-PET scans in patients and controls. One hour prior to scanning and 5 min before i.v. application of [18F]-DOPA (mean 190 MBq) 100 mg and 50 mg respectively of carbidopa were orally administered to prevent peripheral decarboxylation of DOPA. A dynamic acquisition protocol was used (i.e. 25 frames for a total of 94 min) and data were submitted offline to a model independent graphical analysis the Gjedde-Patlak plot. The achieved influx constants (Ki) of [18F]-DOPA into the striatum (subdivided into caudate nucleus and putamen) were compared. **Results:** Comparisons in the unmedicated ADHD group to controls revealed a trend to an overall increased uptake of [18F]-DOPA in medication naive ADHD patients. The ADHD patient receiving methylphenidate was not different from the group of healthy volunteers. **Conclusion:** Clearly there was an upregulation on the presynaptic side of the dopaminergic system in ADHD. The one treated ADHD patient did not differ from the controls. If there is a long term effect of psychostimulant treatment besides an actual downregulation remains to be further investigated.

S-131-613 Topic: 84, 95
ADHD, co-morbidity and family environment

Irma Moilanen, University of Oulu, Dept. of Child
Psychiatry, Oulu, Finland, irma.moilanen@oulu.fi
Anja Taanila; Tuula Hurtig; Hanna Ebeling

Objective: To clarify the role of social and psychological factors in manifestation and co-morbidity of ADHD in The Northern Finland 1985/86 Birth Cohort (N=9432). **Methods:** At 8 years' age, questionnaires were filled in by the parents and teachers, including data on family type and behavioural questionnaires according to Rutter. At 15 years' age, questionnaires were filled in by the parents and by the adolescents themselves, including data on family type, ADHD-symptoms (SWAN) and mental well-being (YRS, Achenbach). Clinical examination, including Kiddie-

SADS and neuro-psychological test protocol, was performed at 15-17 years' age to 272 'cases', defined as upper 5%ile in SWAN and to 199 'controls' from the lower 90%ile. **Results:** At 8 years' age, family structure correlated with the hyperactivity scores given by teachers, intact family protecting against hyperactivity. At 15 years' age, family structure correlated with hyperactivity, inattention and total ADHD-scores of SWAN, especially among boys. According to Kiddie-SADS, ADHD in boys was often co-morbid with externalising disorder (conduct disorder, oppositional disorder, substance abuse) and in girls with internalising disorder (depression, anxiety) if the adolescent was living in any other family type than an intact one. **Conclusion:** The correlations between family environment and adolescents' behaviour can explained by the common genetic origin. However, also psychological and environmental causes can be suggested to explain some of the results.

S-131-614   Topic: 84, 79
Hyperkinetic conduct disorder at younger schoolboys with a residual-organic psychosyndrome
Anna Malakhova, Ekathrinsburg, Russia,
malakhova@front.ru

Objective: The purpose of the present research consists in studying a typology of hyperkinetic conduct disorders at younger schoolboys and its influence on processes of social adaptation. **Methods:** The present work generalizes and systematizes results from a 4-year-long study. The basic methods of research involved clinical and experimental-psychologic procedures, neuropsychological and electroencephalographic recording measures. In addition the medical documentation, and pedagogical characteristics on children were studied. The somatic, neurologic and mental status of all children with hyperkinetic distresses of behaviour were investigated. In the present work descriptive statistics were used. Children with hyperkinetic conduct disorders (n=71; ICD-10) were divided into 2 groups: (1) children for whom hyperkinetic conduct disorder was accompanied by attentional impairments; (2) children for whom a clinical attributes of attention deficiency were not marked. **Results:** The most significant biological factors influencing hyperkinetic conduct disorders, arose from the residual-organic cerebral failure caused by influence on the brain of pre- and perinatal pathogenic factors. The origin and development of hyperkinetic conduct disorders occurs against a background of maturational interactions with psycho-organic distress. At an early age symptoms of neuropathy prevail. Across the preschool age a hyperdynamic set of symptoms predominate. In group-1 socialised and unsocialised forms of behavioural stress prevailed, in group-2 – in opposition – provocation stresses were marked. Organic dysfunction in the brain was confirmed by neurologic, electrophysiological and neuropsychological data. **Conclusion:** The level of a social disadaptation is higher in children with hyperkinetic conduct disorders and impaired attention. The high prevalence of a given pathology, conservation of signs in teenagers and adults, and the high probability of development of maladaptive social behaviour require early diagnosis and the development of effective methods of treatment of the sources of distress.

S-131-615   Topic: 84, 10
Preschoolers with ADHD in the community: Do their parents perceive ADHD symptoms as abnormal behaviours?
Katerina Maniadaki, Psychological Center, Athens, Greece,
katerina@arsi.gr
Efthymios Kakouros

Objective: The onset of Attention Deficit/Hyperactivity Disorder (AD/HD) usually occurs during the preschool years but the diagnosis of the disorder is rarely made before the child enters the primary school (APA, 1994). Even in the DSM-IV, the validity of the diagnosis for this age is not adequately established, as the presentation of preschool children in the DSM-IV field trials was relatively low. However, early diagnosis and intervention may increase the likelihood of successful outcomes. Thus, it is crucial to investigate how parents, who are the main referring agents, perceive the nature and severity of AD/HD symptoms at preschool years. **Methods:** Parents (both fathers and mothers) of 295 preschoolers, aged 4–6, enrolled in kindergartens in Athens completed: a) the Strengths and Difficulties Questionnaire (SDQ; Goodman, 1997) regarding their own child, for the screening of AD/HD and b) a questionnaire composed by a vignette displaying a five-year old child presenting AD/HD symptoms, and three rating scales assessing perceptions of the nature and the impact of these symptoms. **Results:** Results showed that parents whose child presents AD/HD at preschool age perceive AD/HD symptoms as less severe, untypical and with less negative impact on the child's life than parents whose child doesn't display such behaviours. **Conclusion:** The primary symptoms of AD/HD at preschool years are often perceived by parents as normal developmental characteristics of the child's behaviour at this age. Such false beliefs may delay the early diagnosis of the disorder, which would lead to the implementation of an intervention program and to the prevention of secondary difficulties, like learning and behaviour problems that often develop when these children enter primary school. The potential contribution of the nursery teachers to the early identification of AD/HD and to the referral of the child is discussed.

S-131-616   Topic: 84
Cost-effectiveness of Attention Deficit Hyperactivity Disorder (ADHD) treatments: Estimates based upon the MTA study
Peter Jensen, Columbia University, Ctr for Advancement Child MH, New York, USA, pj131@columbia.edu
Joe Albert Garcia; Sherry Glied; Maura Crowe;
Michael Schlander; E. Michael Foster

Objective: ADHD is associated with a significant economic burden, both from the societal as well as from a health care payer's perspective. To date, few economic analyses have addressed the cost-effectiveness of ADHD treatments. Objective: to provide first estimates of the cost-effectiveness of the major proven forms of ADHD treatments based on the MTA Study. **Methods:** 579 children with ADHD, combined type, were assigned to 14 months of medication management (MM), intensive behavioral treatment (BEH), the two combined (COMB), or routine community care (CC). Treatment success was evaluated according to the primary study endpoint, normalization rates being defined by a rating of less than 1 on the SNAP scale (Swanson et al., 2001): CC, 25%; MM, 56%, BEH, 34%; COMB 68%. Direct costs were determined as follows: resource utilization data came from the MTA protocol excluding the research component of the study, and unit costs were calculated from the U.S. societal perspective, adjusted to year 2000 dollars using the consumer price index (CPI). **Results:** Our preliminary calculations indicate, compared to CC as the reference case, an incremental cost-effectiveness ratio (ICER, US-$ per patient normalized) of 610 US-$ for MED (vs. CC) and 46,964 US-$ for COMB (vs. MED), with BEH being dominated by MED. An extrapolation from these data using similar utility estimates as Lord and Paisley (2000) yields an incremental cost per quality-adjusted life year (QALY) of 5,211 US-$ for MED (vs. CC) and >>100,000 US-$ per QALY for COMB (vs. MED). **Conclusion:** By currently accepted thresholds for ICERs, MED appears to be cost-effective compared to CC for routine treatment of children with ADHD, dominating the BEH strategy. Further analyses, including patient subgroups with co-morbidities and clinical endpoints other than SNAP normalization rates, are underway to better understand the cost-effectiveness of COMB and BEH treatment strategies, in particular.

S-132　Topic: 84, 7
ADHD –
Perspectives from the psychodynamic viewpoint

Track: ADHD

Chairperson: Annette Streeck-Fischer, NLKH Tiefenbrunn Psychotherapie von Kindern, Rosdorf, Germany, annette.streeck@t-online.de

ADHD –
Perspectives from the psychodynamic viewpoint

Annette Streeck-Fischer, NLKH Tiefenbrunn, Psychotherapie von Kindern, Rosdorf, Germany, annette.streeck@t-online.de

Up to the present there has only been limited mention of the attention-deficit disorder (ADHD) in the psychodynamic literature. First it is discussed why this diagnosis did not gain acceptance in the psychodynamic diagnostics. Diagnostic classifications and consequences of single-track treatment in ADHD, including existing comorbidities, are dealt with critically and compared with psychodynamic approaches. Treatment procedures and steps of psychodynamic psychotherapy are presented by means of evaluated case reports.

S-132-617　Topic: 84
The argument about "ADHD" – An attempt to portray the opposed positions systematically

Peter Riedesser, UKE Hamburg-Eppendorf, Abt. Psychiatrie, Hamburg, Germany, riedesser@uke.uni-hamburg.de

Objective: The diagnostic construct "ADHD" is the focus of discussions, which are lead with keenness and an emotional verve, which are rather rare in our discipline. The evolving polarization of professionals finds its succession in the public debate. **Methods:** The aim of the paper is to add to the objectification of the matter: The most important reasons for and against the validity of the construct, the diagnostic instruments employed, and the increasingly often used term comorbidity are described systematically.

Then, the opposed hypotheses on the etiology are depicted and – based on this – mechanisms of current interventions are considered. **Conclusion:** Pathways to research strategies with an orientation towards developmental psychopathology are proposed, which could contribute to bridge the controversial positions.

S-132-618　Topic: 84
Dangers of a monofocal view of ADHD

Dieter Bürgin, Universitätsklinik Basel, Kinder- u. Jugendpsychiatrie, Basel, Switzerland, dieter.buergin@unibas.ch

Objective: ADHD is a multifaceted syndrome and not a disease. A lot of patients with neurotic and/or personality disorders show troubles in attention as a main symptom, some also difficulties in motor functions, including hyperactivity. **Methods:** A first step in making a diagnosis is therefore not only to elaborate in detail the intrapsychic functions and structures of the patient, but also the environmental situation, including the mode of relationships inside of the family and the performance and situation in the peer group at school. Then only, a differentiated plan of therapy can be worked out and attempts can be made to get to a shared view with the parents about the situation and the treatment. Whatever the proposed and to be realised therapeutical measures will be, the patient too needs for an optimal collaboration – to get necessary information. **Conclusion:** Under this aspect, a booklet for children edited by a pharmaceutical firm seems to be rather onesided. It demonstrates in a simplicistic way how this information rather exemplifies a restricted approach of the authors than helps to inform young patients in an adequate manner.

S-132-619　Topic: 84, 24
ADHD and psychopathology

Bernard Golse, Hôpital Necker, Dept. of Pédopsychiatrie, Paris, France, bernard.golse@wanadoo.fr

Objective: ADHD is actually emblematic for the different approaches in the field of child psychiatry. There is undoubtedly an emphasis accorded to this diagnosis about which it is difficult no to take into account different sociologic and cultural influences. **Methods:** About ADHD, but not only about it, we can observe a change of splitting from a former one between organogenesis and psychogenesis, to a later one between a semiology of the moment and a semiology of the individual history. **Conclusion:** Anyway, ADHD can be understood in different psychopathological perspectives, and these perspectives help us to choose the suitable therapeutic interventions. There is not only amphetamine-like treatments able to be selected. Various other possibilities have to be kept in mind, alone or jointed to the drug treatment, and this is a crucial point in order to be really helpful for the children and also to value the psychopathological point of view of our actions.

S-132-620   Topic: 84

Psychodynamic perspectives of children with ADHD in psychodynamic treatment

Annette Streeck-Fischer, NLKH Tiefenbrunn,
Psychotherapie von Kindern, Rosdorf, Germany,
annette.streeck@t-online.de

Based on the assumption that children with the diagnosis of ADHD are primarily treated with medications such as methylphenidate as well as with behavioral therapy, and that these are the best approaches available, applications for analytic psychotherapy were reviewed. 100 applications were evaluated using the Bados of the DGKJP, BKJPP and BAGG and the SDQ for parents. Of 100 cases 19 with the diagnosis of ADHD (child psychiatrist, pediatrician) were found. The results correspond in some important aspects (Axis V: abnormal psychosocial circumstances) to the findings in the literature. Some children were treated with Ritalin during psychotherapy or already had taken the drug for several years before. The 19 applications evaluated along with a further 30 were analyzed for their ACE (adverse childhood experiences), psychodynamic diagnoses, multimodal approaches and treatment success (10 follow-up applications). Specific treatment steps which lead to overcoming the symptoms are described. Some conclusions are made from the results on the diagnostic construct ADHD.

Workshops

WS-001   Topic: 1, 2
Child and adolescent mental health ATLAS: A project of the WHO in collaboration with the IACAPAP and other organizations

Track: Therapy and intervention

Chairperson: Myron Belfer, Harvard Medical School Dept. of Social Medicine, Boston, MA, USA, myron-belfer@hms.harvard.edu

Child and adolescent mental health ATLAS: A project of the WHO in collaboration with the IACAPAP and other organizations

Myron Belfer, Harvard Medical School, Dept. of Social Medicine, Boston, MA, USA, myron-belfer@hms.harvard.edu

The World Health Organization's Project ATLAS is an initiative designed to document the resources available for mental health care within countries. The data will provide crucial information for program development and can serve as a baseline for monitoring changes over time. Project ATLAS is not an epidemiological survey, but rather is a systematic means of collecting basic information on mental health resources from all countries to construct global and regional databases, maps and country profiles. The goal is to help in the prioritzation of needs and to facilitate program planning. The adult focused ATLAS is completed; the information has been published in the form of two books and an interactive website is established (http://www.cvdinfobase.ca/mh-atlas/). This workshop (symposium) will focus on the child and adolescent mental health ATLAS data gathering techniques and findings. The ATLAS survey is unique in its global scope, and comprehensiveness. The available data will be presented and the likely use of these data in advocacy, programme planning, and regional comparision will be highlighted. Examples from two countries will be given to illustrate this process. It is hoped that the ATLAS will serve as a stimulus for countries to assess their needs and resources in a more systematic fashion and to develop policy to enhance services capacity in line with the findings of the ATLAS survey. ATLAS data instruments are dynamic and designed so that data can be updated, corrected, and tailored to meet specific country needs.

WS-002   Topic: 84, 42
Attention Deficit Hyperactivity Disorder (ADHD) in Life-Span

Track: ADHD

Chairperson: Sam Tyano, Geha Mental Health Center, Petah Tiqva, Israel, styano@post.tau.ac.il
I. Mano

Attention Deficit Hyperactivity Disorder (ADHD) in Life-Span

Sam Tyano, Geha Mental Health Center, Petah Tiqva, Israel, styano@post.tau.ac.il
I. Manor

ADHD is a well-known, common disorder of childhood and adolescence, but in the past ten years began to be known as an important disorder of adulthood. It is getting a lot of attention from several fields of research, and the amount of new data as well as changed information is quite overwhelming. Hence, we would like to present a workshop on ADHD in the light of some intriguing and renewing aspects: 1. The clinical characteristics of ADHD in the ends of the age spectrum, e.g. preschoolers and adults; 2. The diagnosis of ADHD as an integrative procedure; 3. The treatment of ADHD: new drugs, old therapies. The workshop will last 3 hours and the discussion leaders will be Prof. Tyano and Dr Manor from Israel.

WS-003   Topic: 28
Everything you wanted to know about basic molecular biology

Chairperson: Paul Lombroso, Yale University Child Study Center, New Haven, CT, USA, paul.lombroso@yale.edu

Everything you wanted to know about basic molecular biology

Paul Lombroso, Yale University, Child Study Center, New Haven, CT, USA, paul.lombroso@yale.edu
Matthew State

Objective: The participant in this work-shop will learn basic concepts in molecular biology as they relate to Child and Adolescent Psychiatry. **Methods:** The lectures will give an overview of genetics and of recent advances in molecular biology. Specific topics to be discussed are the organization of genes, how mutations in various genes lead to specific disorders, and some of the new technologies that are being used such as how and why to make knock-out mice. **Results:** Major advances have occurred over the last decade in molecular biology with the discovery of imprinting and triplet repeat expansions. We will discuss specific disorders affected by these types of mutations, including Prader Willi Syndrome, Angelman Syndrome, and Fragile X Syndrome. **Conclusion:** It is important for clinicians in Child and Adolescent Psychiatry to have a working knowledge of the tremendous recent advances that have occurred in biology. The advances in this field will have an ever-increasing impact on our work. this work-shop is geared for the clinician who "knows nothing" and went into psychiatry because they didn't particularly like biology.

WS-004   Topic: 65, 57
Ethical issues in child and adolescent psychiatry

Chairperson: Jocelyn Hattab Yosse, Jerusalem Mental Health Center Child & Adolescent Psychiatry, Jerusalem, Israel, jocelyn@vms.huji.ac.il

WS-004-001   Topic: 65, 45
Ethical issues considering Multicultural Societies

Jocelyn Hattab Yosse, Jerusalem Mental Health Center, Child & Adolescent Psychiatry, Jerusalem, Israel, jocelyn@vms.huji.ac.il

Objective: Most diagnostic procedures and treatment protocols have been developed in western countries and tested on American/European populations although most of the world population lives in China, India and other eastern countries and Africa. **Methods:** Along centuries they developed their own models of coping with psychic dysfunctions with probably no les success than ours. **Results:** The large and continuous movement of migration of the last century brought a mix of people into several American and European countries. Before imposing upon them and their children our views and understanding concerning mental health and mental disorders we do have to learn their own models and respect their ways of coping so far there is no obvious harm to these children. In a continuous process of integration and culturation they will adapt themselves to their new countries and their specificity including models of mental health. It is well admitted that the efficacy of treatments largely depends on the acceptation and identification of the patient with it, and probably also through the affective collaboration between the patient and his/her therapist. Imposed treatments can be detrimental and have to be avoided even if the therapist does believe in its efficacy. **Conclusion:** As mental health professional we support these populations either in their own countries or in ours in full respect of their identity and specific values and with humility concerning ours and our model. This symposium will bring together experts from all over the world who will share their views and experiences working in various countries and cultures.

WS-004-002   Topic: 65, 83
Ethics and autism

Jocelyn Hattab, Jerusalem Mental Health Center,
Child & Adolescent Psychiatry, Jerusalem, Israel,
jocelyn@vms.huji.ac.il

Objective: Ethical issues dealing with autism. **Methods:** Autism is specific enough to raise specific ethical considerations I will elaborate on what makes autism so attractive to research, treatment, public interest, almost magic. Research: Autism is defined by WHO as a rare disease and as such it is recommended to increase its research. It is more moral to help minorities. Informed Consent. We follow Klin and Cohen who 'believe that research involving individuals with Autism and similar disorders must pass the highest standards of ethical review. Our experience with parents of autistic children shows us some peculiarities relevant to this discussion. Their Consent is never an acceptation but the result of a harsh and positive discussion. **Results:** Once establish a clear presumption of autism, we have to act therapeutically with patient, parents and other professionals in the most known efficient way through continuous observation and assessment with readiness to modify it. Truth telling: The disclosure of the disorder will change totally these parent's lives. They will have to organize themselves, their career, their other children's schooling and social life around this autistic child. There is an absolute value answer: telling truth because it is the truth and this knowledge belongs to the patient and, as a minor, to his family without any other justification. There is a practical answer that includes the value of truth telling. Genetic counseling: Our role is certainly not to increase fears nor strengthen denial, in any case not to impose our own views and beliefs on birth rate per family etc. We only can help them face the dilemma overtly, to examine all known aspects and ensure them of our caring assistance in any case, and hope with them that statistics will be on their side. **Conclusion:** There is no curative treatment for autism but autistic persons have to be treated. However, along the years efficient therapeutic procedures emerged from researches of different types and are used worldwide. We adopt without any condition Klin and Cohen's order; 'No unproven or nonstandard behavioral or biological treatments should be used'. We elucidate

some of the dilemmas we are confronted with and proposed possible answers.

WS-004-003   Topic: 65, 93
Ethics of preventing youth suicide

Cynthia Pfeffer, Cornell University, Weill Med. College,
Psychiatry, White Plains, NY, USA, cpfeffer@med.cornell.edu

Objective: This presentation will highlight complex ethical issues relevant to preventing suicide among children and adolescents. **Methods:** This presentation will integrate empirical data from studies of youth suicide with clinical experience to discuss ethical issues in preventing youth suicide. **Results:** This presentation will discuss how suicide prevention methods must consider multiple issues that are integral to an ethical approach of intervention. These ethical issues include: patient's rights of autonomy and privacy, an equal opportunity to evaluation and treatment, establishment of rules for confidentiality, minimization of stigmatization, respect for individual differences, respect for cultural practices, minimization of stigmatization, practices of informed consent, and equal opportunities for participation in research. It is also imperative to identify specific developmental factors that affect ethical considerations for suicide prevention. These include understanding of cognitive, social, and emotional states of children and adolescents and adoption of prevention methods that may differ from those used for adults. Although not a main focus of this presentation, the ethics of children's rights to assisted suicide will be briefly discussed. **Conclusion:** This presentation will emphasize that holding ethical issues as a major priority in instituting suicide prevention efforts for youth, more effective methods can be developed. Such methods will thereby be more effectively disseminated and utilized in different countries.

WS-004-004   Topic: 65, 28
Ethics of genetics in child psychiatry

Jocelyn Hattab, Jerusalem Mental Health Center,
Child & Adolescent Psychiatry, Jerusalem, Israel,
jocelyn@vms.huji.ac.il

Objective: Ethics is based on the assumption of human free will arguing that people are responsible for their choice to behave badly or according to morality. Genetics contains a presumption of pre-birth determinism. One fifth of our genes are supposed to command our psychic life, behaviour, affects, fantasies, dreams. **Methods:** Without entering a deep philosophical dissertation, we will first clarify these arguments. Claiming for genetic origin of psychological traits and diseases leads to defectuous attitude both in child development and in treatment. We will elaborate on the genetical and environmental origin of various child mental diseases, A.D.H.D., Autism, Schizophrenia and others, and demonstrate the intrication of many factors in shapping genotype into phenotype. **Results:** The ethical attitude is one of optimism and belief in potential to change, mainly for children whose brain plasticity and openness for external influences are crucial in their development either normal or modified by illness or diseases. Research in genetics in general and in child mental health specifically, either through epidemiology or molecular genetics, involve children. What is the relevance of informed consent of children or their parents in these researches, what are the long term consequences of having samples of DNA of children, could they refuse or destroy these samples at any time. To what extent the reading of these samples will determine their future in schools, in society, in their professional activities. **Conclusion:** Finally we acknowledge the importance and benefices children can draw from genetics research and findings in their search for a better life and society. Our 3 steps model of ethical attitude will help us weighing the values involved in our discussion on Ethics and Genetics of Child Mental Health and modeling an acceptable attitude.

WS-004-005   Topic: 65, 57
Informed Consent: Its relevance in child mental health
Jocelyn Hattab, Jerusalem Mental Health Center, Child & Adolescent Psychiatry, Jerusalem, Israel, jocelyn@vms.huji.ac.il

The history, theories, philosophy, legacy, of informed consent is an expression of ambivalence between two values: the value of a person's autonomy, self-determination, free will, which means providing complete and comprehensive information to the patient, and, the value of offering aid the patient receives regarding his sickness, which means, giving the patient the best known treatment while avoiding her opposition to this treatment if he will know "too much" about it. People are ambivalent concerning their will and right for information concerning diseases and treatment. Child Mental Health is the field where this ambivalence comes to its most extreme level. According to the Code of Nuremberg: "Ethical practice requires the investigator to inform the participant of all features of the research. . . . Openness and honesty are essential characteristics of the relationship between investigator and research participant . . . Ethical research practice requires the investigator to respect the individual's freedom to decline to participate . . . or discontinue. . ." . . . The participation of the child in decisions which concern him should be encouraged and developed for ethical and for legal reasons. Studies of the child's consent must therefore be placed in a far more general current of thought, which reconsiders the status of the child within the family. Recognition that the interests of parents and children are not always coextensive (this is obvious in cases of abuse or neglect) must lead to greater attention being paid to the child's opinions. Even in its politically correct formulation, there is a flavor of coercion, persuasion, if not manipulation in informed consent as stated by Faden and Beauchamp. People are forced to sign a form that is more useful for the physician than for the patient and certainly the young mentally ill kid. This lecture, that was first presented at the memorial conference for Professor Donald Cohen at Yale Child Study Center, will develop history, philosophy and practice of informed consent in medicine and child mental health and its pitfalls. Recommendations for a better and more honest practice will be proposed.

WS-004-006   Topic: 65
Ethical issues regarding children's rights in Japanese psychiatry
Ken Takaoka, Gifu, Japan, takaoka@cc.gifu-u.ac.jp

Objective: To review children's rights issues in Japanese psychiatry. **Methods:** Selective review of discussions in the Human Rights Committee of the JSCAP. **Results:** The following four points are presented and discussed: (i) The human rights of the children of emigrants or illegal workers in Japan have so far not been of particular concern due to the government's strict immigration management policy restricting import of labor. However, it is surmised that some children from Asian or South American countries are alienated due to differences between their respective ethnic communities and Japanese society and insufficient education system measures for integrating such children into the society; (ii) The human rights of children from minority religious background have generally not been significantly violated, thanks to Japanese society's relative tolerance of religious diversity. However, children whose parents believe in certain cults or minor religions are sometimes discriminated against; (iii) More importantly, group-oriented education adversely affects children's mental health in most schools. In particular, bullying, which is prevalent in group-orients education, erodes children's self-esteem, in the worst cases even causing them to commit suicide; (iv) In addition, the human rights of children admitted involuntarily to psychiatric wards or reformatories are insufficiently protected. This is partly due to the shortage of child and adolescent psychiatrists to provide appropriate treatment for detained children. **Conclusion:** Global standards encapsulated in the Convention on the Rights of the Child should be considered and observed to protect children living in Japan.

WS-005   Topic: 3
Collaborative care models for extending access to high quality mental health care for children and adolescents in rural regions: New models for psychiatric and pediatric practitioner collaboration
Track: Therapy and intervention
Chairperson: Craig Donnelly, DHPA – Dartmouth Medical Center, Dept. of Psychiatry, Lebanon, NH, USA, craig.l.donnelly@dartmouth.edu

Collaborative care models for extending access to high quality mental health care for children and adolescents in rural regions:
New models for psychiatric and pediatric practitioner collaboration
Craig Donnelly, DHPA – Dartmouth Medical, Center, Dept. of Psychiatry, Lebanon, NH, USA, craig.l.donnelly@dartmouth.edu

Objective: This symposium will teach the fundamentals of collaborative care models of psychiatric service delivery to children and adolescents, especially in regard to rural regions of the world in which access to expert psychiatric services are limited. Specific goals include teaching: 1. Greater understanding of and sensitivity to psychosocial and developmental issues and problems that present themselves to pediatricians in practice; 2. Enhanced skill in discriminating between transient disturbances and more serious psychiatric disorders, such as childhood depression, autism, schizophrenia, attention disorders, anxiety disorders, conduct disorders, eating disorders, and somatizing disorders; 3. Enhanced skill in managing developmental crises such as separation, discipline, school achievement, sexuality, body image, adolescent autonomy, divorce, and family dysfunction; 4. Greater understanding of psychosocial issues in chronic illness and disability: family dynamics, developmental effects, behavior problems, school issues, limits of available services; 5. Greater understanding of family dynamics, including abuse, through a family system approach to evaluation and management; 6. Enhanced skill in interviewing and counseling techniques; 7. Increased ability to recognize serious psychopathology and to better understand the scope of the pediatrician's competency in matters requiring intervention; 8. Increased awareness of the impact of such factors as personal bias and values on the pediatrician's relationship with children and families; 9. Specifically, how to develop productive collegial relationships between pediatrics and psychiatry; including consultation with vs referrals to child psychiatrists; 10. Increased awareness of, utilization of, and collaboration with community mental health resources for children on a local, regional, and state-supported level; 11. Facilitation of a more comprehensive approach to children's health supervision 12. Understanding of the utility of the DSM-IV/ICD 10 codes for practicing pediatricians. 13. Development of collaborative 'spinoff' projects which impact screening, access, delivery and outcomes for pediatric mental health services in the community. **Methods:** We will outline the approach that we have utilized for the past 12 years in establishing a collaborative group of pediatricians and child psychiatrists to extend care to rural regions in the northeastern area of the United States. We will outline the optimal group membership, leadership of the group, timetable for meetings and details of using a collaborative model for evaluation and treatment of children and adolescents, using psychiatrists to extend services to pediatricians in rural settings. Utilizing twice monthly meetings with a case discussion format will serve as the primary educational format of the collaborative group. Child Psychiatrists will learn the utility of a monthly collaboration meeting where they will travel to meet with pediatricians in isolated regions. We will discuss the specifics of the collaborative process: Led by the psychiatrist, the pediatrician moderator, and the child psychiatry moderator, the group then discusses the case from multiple perspectives, including data gathering, assessment instruments, DSM-IV/ICD-10 diagnosis, individual psychodynamics, family and cultural factors, and possible interventions by the pediatrician or consultant. Options to be considered and discussed include pediatric counseling; school-based interventions; referral to community agencies or mental health providers; and psychopharmacology. The group also considers topics such as the role of the pediatrician, the relationship between pediatrics and mental health providers, communication issues. **Results:** We will discuss evaluation of the collaborative model and adaptation to specific practice settings, how to monitor the sessions for content and objectives. Year-end self-assessments and qualitative feedback to moderators will be used to assess the utility of the group process in meeting these objectives. As part of our proposal to create more collegial relationships with our local mental health professionals (MHP) and to establish ongoing conferences of Pediatric Primary Care Providers with MHPs, we will demonstrate a pre- and post-conference survey of conference participants used to determine the several outcomes measures.

WS-006   Topic: 11
Fixing Treatment Planning
Track: Therapy and intervention

Chairperson: Gordon Harper, Harvard Medical School Dept. of Psychiatry, Boston, MA, USA,
gordon_harper@hms.harvard.edu
Füsun Çuhadaroğlu Çetin, Hacettepe University Child & Adolescent Psychiatry, Ankara, Turkey,
fusunc@hacettepe.edu.tr

Fixing Treatment Planning
Gordon Harper, Harvard Medical School,
Dept. of Psychiatry, Boston, MA, USA,
gordon_harper@hms.harvard.edu

Treatment planning based on categorical diagnoses, though increasingly prevalent around the world, is ill-suited to children's needs. Conventional treatment planning works against collaboration, fails to emphasize strengths and a developmental perspective, fails to express the voice of the child, and promotes monomodal interventions. In this workshop, participants will learn an alternate approach, drawing on experience in the US and Turkey, that uses categorical diagnoses but that also fosters interdisciplinary collaboration, promotes strengths and a future perspective, and captures the individual child's point of view. The workshop will consist of a presentation of this method followed by practice sessions in which participants will apply this method to cases from their own practice.

WS-007   Topic: 7, 45
Psychodynamic therapies in the developing world
Track: Therapy and intervention

Chairperson: Myron Belfer, Harvard Medical School Dept. of Social Medicine, Boston, MA, USA,
myron-belfer@hms.harvard.edu

Psychodynamic therapies in the developing world
Myron Belfer, Harvard Medical School, Dept. of Social Medicine, Boston, MA, USA, myron-belfer@hms.harvard.edu

Objective: To describe the current role and potential of psychodynamic therapy in the spectrum of care in developing countries. **Methods:** It is little appreciated that psychodynamic therapy has flourished in many countries for decades and to this day influences the overall orientation of care provided. These therapies now coexist or compete with the more biologically oriented therapies being introduced. The current interplay and understanding of the development of comprehensive systems of care perhaps incorporating pluralistic models need to be explored. Of even more unique interest is the upsurge in interest in psychodynamic therapy in countries where there was no prior organized training and where it did not appear to be a significant orientation in an otherwise biologically oriented system. Special attention will be given to the emerging interest in China of psychodynamic therapy and psychoanalysis. A focus on a broader understanding of mental disorder has led to an active interest in dynamic therapy. Data from pilot studies will describe 'the need to understand' from both the patient and therapist perspective. **Conclusion:** The workshop will provide an opportunity to hear about an overview of psychodynamic therapy in developing countries and discuss the place of psychodynamic therapy in systems of care.

WS-007-007   Topic: 7
Psychoanalysis in China
Wenhong Cheng, Shanghai Mental Health Center, Shanghai, China, chengwhb@online.sh.cn

In the past two decades China's mental health professionals have engaged in an expanded dialogue with their counterparts in other countries. Psychotherapy, and psychology in general, are of great interest. Particular interest is shown in ways that facilitate the expression of emotion and pain which was long ignored. Psychoanalytically oriented psychotherapy in large cities in China is of increasing popularity. Therapists themselves are also seeking through the dynamic approaches a better understanding of their own experiences. Psychoanalytic training has been made available in China. The presentation will provide the evidence on the development of psychoanalysis in China and present data from patients about the usefulness of this approach.

WS-007-008   Topic: 7, 2
Psychoanalysis in Bulgaria
Nadia Polnareva, Medical University, Sofia, Bulgaria, polnarev@medun.acad.bg

In Bulgaria there has been a longstanding, though less acknowledged interest in psychoanalysis and psychodynamic therapy. These therapeutic approaches have been utilized in settings that are quite varied. Training now exists for work with families, couples and individuals, not only in the large cities but in outlying areas. The approaches follow a classic French psychoanalytic paradigm. The experience in Bulgaria will be compared to that in other former Eastern bloc nations. In addition, the ways and reasons for the support of psychoanalytic based treatments will be described.

WS-007-009   Topic: 7
Psychoanalysis in Brazil
Salvador Celia, Instituto Leo Kanner Ltoa, Child Psychiatry, Porto Alegre, Brazil, sahc@terra.com.br

In Brazil psychodynamic theory and practice have been well established, particularly in the South. Teaching about psychoanalysis and psychodynamic therapy begins in the first year of medical school. This experience includes mother child observation and home visiting. They learn about transference and counter-transference. Pediatricians are also interested and exposed to training in psychoanalysis and psychodynamic therapy. The presentation will describe the nature of the training experience and the use of classic references from Winnicott, Lebovici, Cramer, Fraiberg, Stern and others. The nature of interventions will be described.

WS-008   Topic: 63
Medical Student/Residency Workshop
Chairperson: Eli Breger, AACAP Internat. Relations Committee, Hilton Head Island, SC, USA, bregerhhi@hargray.com

Medical Student/Residency Workshop – Student Tutorial Program
Eli Breger, AACAP, Internat. Relations Committee, Hilton Head Island, SC, USA, bregerhhi@hargray.com

To provide special recognition, sense of inclusion and global congress experience for young colleagues in child and adolescent psychiatry and allied professions. A 2-hour workshop of scientific presentations of doctoral and masters theses or other pertinent research. Four presentations – in English – will be selected and discussed with the participants. It will also be possible to present a project in form of a poster.

WS-009
Forensic psychiatric inpatient treatment: A documentary by the Flemish television
Chairperson: Robert Vermeiren, University of Antwerp Child & Adolescent Psychiatry, Antwerp, Belgium, robert@vermeiren.name

Forensic psychiatric inpatient treatment: A documentary by the Flemish television.
Robert Vermeiren, University of Antwerp, Child & Adolescent Psychiatry, Antwerp, Belgium, robert@vermeiren.name
Dirk Leestmans

Objective: To present and discuss a documentary on a forensic residential adolescent unit in Antwerp, Belgium. **Methods:** In 2002, a documentary was made on the adolescent forensic psychiatric unit Het Spoor in Belgium, Antwerp. Het Spoor is a 8-bed unit for delinquent adolescents with a psychiatric disorder. The documentary was made in order to give the public an impression of the population in this unit and of the life of the youths who live there. This 40-minute documentary consists of short interviews of some of the youths by the journalist (DL). In between the interviews, different aspects of the day program are presented briefly. For reasons of anonymity, the youths are filmed in a way that recognition is impossible. **Results:** The reports by the youths demonstrate that these youths bear severe problems both as offenders and as victims. When considering their problems, it is obvious that intervention and treatment is complex. The documentary does not go into detail on the specific treatment modules that are offered, since the goal was to show this documentary on public television. This documentary has been successful, however, in giving a convincing and interesting view on the overall day life within the unit. **Conclusion:** This documentary has succeeded in giving a very interesting impression of the population and the life in the forensic psychiatric unit Het Spoor. The documentary will be shown as starting point of a discussion on the development of forensic psychiatric treatment programs.

WS-010   Topic: 7
Child analytic workshop under the auspices of the American Association of Child Psychoanalysts (Part I)
Track: Therapy and intervention
Chairperson: Veronica Mächtlinger, Karl-Abraham Psychoanalytisches Inst., Berlin, Germany, maechtlinger@t-online.de

Child analytic workshop under the auspices of the American Association of Child Psychoanalysts
Veronica Mächtlinger, Karl-Abraham, Psychoanalytisches Inst., Berlin, Germany, maechtlinger@t-online.de

Representing the American Association of Child Psychoanalysis the workshop offers two detailed clinical reports given by two members of the International Psychoanalytical Association and recognised Child Psychoanalysts. The papers describe their intensive, in-depth psychoanalytic work with two severely disturbed patients – a 9 year old child and an adolescent. The adolescent patient, presented by Dr. Erika Hartmann (Berlin), was referred for treatment because of the relatively unusual symptom of "Stalking" and the paper describes the slow and painstaking, but fascinating development of a relationship to the analyst, in which words could gradually be found to express the feelings and inner conflicts which had led to the symptom. In the paper by Dr. Renate Kelleter (Darmstadt) which describes the psychoanalytic treatment of a latency child suffering from Traumatic Epilepsy, in whom the epileptic attacks persisted in spite of medication, the analytic work shows how the attacks were precipitated by recapitulations of earlier traumatic experiences and how these could be understood in an intensive psychoanalytic therapy.

WS-010-010   Topic: 96
Stalking as a symptom in a 13 year old girl
The gradual development of a language for expressing feelings during an intensive psychoanalytic treatment
Erika Hartmann, Berlin, Germany,
dr.e.hartmann@t-online.de

This single-case-study uses the psychoanalytic narrative method to describe the symptom of stalking in a 13-year old girl in the overall context of a broader psychopathology with its underlying psychodynamic conflicts and the interplay between family-background and other environmental factors, which together led to a severe developmental disturbance in puberty. The 13 year old patient was brought to treatment by her parents, because for 2 years she had been stalking two older girls to an unbearable degree. The symptom was accompanied by severe disturbances of social relationships e.g. inhibitions in initiating verbal and visual contact. School-performance and other interests were gravely interfered with by constant pre-occupation with thoughts about the girls, who felt increasingly persecuted. The patient appeared to have little access to her own feelings and apparently no idea that her behaviour, for which she could offer no explanation, might be disturbing for the girls. The patient's development in the course of an intensive psychoanalytic treatment, which started with a severe suicidal crisis, will be described with a focus on the development of a language for expressing feelings. Parallel to this development in the psychoanalytic relationship she was gradually better able to understand her conflicts, centred around hate of her own body. Her social capacities as well as her relationships to class-mates, teachers and to her mother as a primary object all improved. In the ongoing treatment, the stalking impulse still occasionally occurs, however the constant pre-occupation with thoughts and memories of the girls has ceased and her school-performance has improved, so that she will be promoted into the next class, something that seemed quite impossible when treatment began.

WS-011   Topic: 79
Deaf children: Communication and mental health
Track: Therapy and intervention
Chairperson: Johannes Fellinger, Krankenhaus St. John Abt. für Schwerhörige, Linz, Austria,
johannes.fellinger@bblinz.at

Deaf children: Communication and mental health
Johannes Fellinger, Krankenhaus St. John,
Abt. für Schwerhörige, Linz, Austria,
johannes.fellinger@bblinz.at

The aim of this workshop is to provide an overview of the issues surrounding the assessment and treatment of deaf children and adolescents regarding their communication development and Mental Health problems. The challenging field of deaf children with special needs, like deaf children with Autism will also be covered. It is our believe that this interactive workshop would help to promote Mental health and Well being in deaf children.

WS-012   Topic: 91, 95
Psychiatric disorders and epilepsy:
Clinical aspects, comorbidity, therapeutics
Chairperson: Roberto Canitano, General Hospital of Siena Dept. of Child Neuropsychiatry, Siena, Italy,
r.canitano@ao-siena.toscana.it
Mario Speranza, General Hospital of Versailles, Versailles, France, mariosperanza@wanadoo.fr

Psychiatric disorders and epilepsy:
Clinical aspects, comorbidity, therapeutics
Roberto Canitano, General Hospital of Siena, Dept. of Child Neuropsychiatry, Siena, Italy, r.canitano@ao-siena.toscana.it

It's well recognised that epilepsy is a strong risk factor for emotional and behavioural disorders in children and this has been demonstrated by different epidemiological studies. The relationships between psychiatric disorders and childhood epilepsy are complex and controversial. The aim of this workshop is to provide an overview of this topic according to recent findings, and to treat specific issues based on the clinical and research experience of the speakers. The program of the workshop will be as follows: introduction will be an up to date overview on psychiatric disorders in epilepsy; two interventions will deal with specific topics: one regarding epilepsy and pervasive developmental disorders, epidemiology, clinical and neurophysiologic data and risk factors implicated. The association of epilepsy and language impairment will be considered in early childhood and pre-school children with autism spectrum disorders. Another intervention will cover the topic of epilepsy and psychosis, the relationships between early onset schizophrenia and temporal lobe and other types of epilepsy will be presented. Theoretical implications, consequences for treatment choices will be discussed. Emotional disorders in childhood epilepsy is the last topic of the workshop, it will be considered in terms of a comprehensive clinical approach and within the context of liaison consultation, thus it will be divided in two parts with contribution by two speakers. Several difficulties in managing children and adolescents with epilepsy are discussed in view of the various therapeutic options. We will address the link between epilepsy and cognitive impairment (difficulties in learning capabilities and implication for school success) as well as between medications for epilepsy and their side effects and compliance. The issue of stigma will be addressed, in addition problems of conduct, family factors and other relevant emotional factors will be dealt with.

WS-012-012   Topic: 91, 83
Epilepsy in pervasive developmental disorders

Roberto Canitano, General Hospital of Siena, Dept. of Child Neuropsychiatry, Siena, Italy, r.canitano@ao-siena.toscana.it

Objective: Approximately 20–30% of individuals with autistic spectrum disorders suffer from seizures, moreover paroxysmal discharges on EEG without seizures have been reported more often in autism than in any other psychiatric disorders in childhood. There is a significant variability of prevalence among studies depending on differences of samples examined, there are two peaks of seizures onset, in infancy up to 5 years and in adolescence. The cognitive level and the type of language disorder are the other two factors influencing the appearance of epilepsy in autism. All seizure types have been described including partial, generalized, absence seizures and infantile spasms. Autistic regression is reported in one third of patients, epileptiform abnormalities may be detected in a proportion of them, and it is debated if they may be implicated in the clinical course. **Methods:** We present the data of the study on epilepsy in autism conducted in our department to determine the prevalence rates of seizures and epileptiform abnormalities, their characteristics and the relationships with regression. **Results:** Seizures and paroxysmal abnormalities were observed in a significant percentage of the children with autism examined. Regression rate was independent to the presence of epilepsy and paroxysmal abnormalities. **Conclusion:** Epilepsy in autism is frequent but it still unclear its effect on the core symptoms of the disorder. Treatment of seizures do not differ from that of other children with epilepsy and usually is not particularly difficult. On the contrary many questions are unanswered regarding the treatment of subclinical epilepsy with or without regression, i.e. how and when it should be started, whether it should be administered only when regression is occurring and whether it affects the general clinical outcome. As well the treatment choice when comorbid disorders are present is not still defined and is mainly empirical.

WS-012-013   Topic: 91, 69
Epilepsy and psychosis – early onset schizophrenia

Mario Speranza, General Hospital of Versailles, Versailles, France, mariosperanza@wanadoo.fr

Objective: Psychotic disorders are described in association with temporal lobe as well as with frontal lobe epilepsy. Symptoms may appear during ictal, interictal and post-ictal phase of the seizure disorder; when hallucinations and delusions are occurring as expression of a seizure usually impairment of consciousness, fear and anxiety are concomitant. Interictal symptoms are predominantly delusions, hallucinations and disorganised behaviour, while negative symptoms frequently observed in childhood schizophrenia are rare in epileptic psychoses. Children with complex partial seizures have been demonstrated to present formal thought disorders with increasing severity related to incomplete seizure control and age of onset. The increased risk of a schizophrenic outcome of temporal lobe epilepsy were observed more often in females with left temporal lesions and childhood epilepsy. With respect to the chronological sequence psychotic disorders usually follow the epileptic syndrome unfolding. **Methods:** Clinical cases from a study on early-onset schizophrenia carried out in our department are presented and discussed. **Conclusion:** Epilep-

tic disorders involving temporal and frontal lobe structures are likely to interfere with the developing brain and may be implicated in the co-occurrence of psychosis probably sharing a common neurobiological substrate. An overview of the current concepts dealing with the association of psychosis and epilepsy will be presented in order to provide an in depth update of the topic.

WS-012-014   Topic: 91, 86
Emotional disorders in childhood epilepsy

Milica Pejovic-Milovancevic, Institute of Mental Health, Dept. Children & Adolescents, Belgrade, Serbia and Montenegro, mpejovic@eunet.yu
Olivera Aleksic

Objective: Children and adolescent with epilepsy could have different problems such as progressive structural changes in neural system, disturbances of frontal processes and mental confusion resulting in attention difficulties, lessens of memory capacity and consequently in learning difficulties. The weakness of motor function of dominant arm, and other abnormalities of motor functioning are also recognized. Mild to severe depression could be one form of learning helplessness, and close relatives could seen them as inattention and keen to social withdrawal. As a result of brain disabilities school performances could be detect in a form of lower school achievement, more absences from school. **Methods:** We would present the data from five years longitudinal study who examines the relation between depressive symptoms, averse life experiences, hopelessness life style and explanatory system. **Results:** The result shows that in early childhood and negative life events produce depressive symptoms. Isolation, stigma, parental overprotection, development of separation anxiety, and fear of convulsion are some other aspects of emotional disturbances. All together those problems could be seen as adjustment problems of children and adolescents with epilepsy either on intrapsychic or interpsycic functioning. **Conclusion:** Factors that could be seen as important in treating those incapability are: variables connected directly to children (sex, age, individual psychological characteristics), family, demographical; and psychosocial factors (the diagnosis of stigma and coping reactions) and environmental factors (stressors, capacity and adaptation).

WS-012-015   Topic: 91, 22
Psychiatric consultation – liaison for epilepsy

Emmanouel Tsalamanios, University of Athens, Dept. of Child Psychiatry, Athens, Greece, emtsalamanios@hotmail.com
V. Hatzara; L. Zacharaki; I. Andriotis; A. Covanis; John Tsiantis

Objective: This study has been conducted in Greece in "St Sophia" Children Hospital of Athens from 2001–2004. We examined all children who were referred to Child psychiatric clinic from the Neurology Clinic of "St. Sophia" Children Hospital of Athens. **Methods:** Participants were 45 boys and 40 girls, 6 to 14 years old from the Neurology Clinic. We examined the demand, the comorbidity, the presence of "pseudo" seizures, the socioeconomic status of the family, the way of treatment and the difficulties of continuity of care. Two case studies will be presented. **Results:** Results showed that children with epilepsy presented: a) emotional and conduct disorders, and b) special learning difficulties. **Conclusion:** Children with epilepsy is at risk for developing mental health difficulties. The complexity of needs require the combined skills of the neuro paediatrics and child psychiatry team.

WS-013   Topic: 65, 63
Partnering with the pharmaceutical industry
Chairperson: Barry Herman, Pfizer, Inc. Medical Dept., Radnor, PA, USA, barry.herman@pfizer.com

Partnering with the pharmaceutical industry
Barry Herman, Pfizer, Inc., Medical Dept., Radnor, PA, USA, barry.herman@pfizer.com

Objective: Most psychiatrists do not understand the role of pharmaceutical industry physicians and of the types of alliances that can be developed with them. The current relationship between pharmaceutical industry physicians and psychiatrists ranges from total unfamiliarity of the role of industry physicians to a collaboration and partnership between the parties. Building relationships has been difficult in some instances due to perceptions of troublesome conflicts of interest by the pharmaceutical industry. **Methods:** This program will explore ways in which psychiatrists can develop effective alliances with their physician counterparts in industry. Three types of relationships in particular will be examined – the psychiatrist as researcher, consultant, and speaker on behalf of industry. **Results:** The discussion will be facilitated by two pharmaceutical industry physician "insiders" (former psychiatrist practitioners) who have enjoyed positive working relationships with practicing psychiatrists, and by a psychiatrist researcher who will offer a perspective on partnership relationships with the pharmaceutical industry. The focus will be on strategies to optimize pharmaceutical alliances rather than interactions intended to affect the prescribing and professional behavior of practicing psychiatrists. **Conclusion:** It is important to understand the role of physicians working at pharmaceutical companies. This information can be used to begin building long-term, effective relationships with the pharmaceutical industry and may result in improved clinical trials, educational initiatives, value-added programs, and other benefits.

WS-013-016   Topic: 65, 63
Life in the "inside": The diverse roles of physicians in the pharmaceutical industry
Barry Herman, Pfizer, Inc., Medical Dept., Radnor, PA, USA, barry.herman@pfizer.com
Objective: Most psychiatrists are not familiar with the various roles of physicians who are employed by the pharmaceutical industry, and of the various resources that are available to physicians. **Methods:** This program will discuss "life on the inside": the diverse roles of physicians working in industry. The pharmaceutical industry "toolkit," an array of valuable resources and programs that are available to physicians will be described. **Conclusion:** It is important to understand the role of physicians working at pharmaceutical companies. This information may be used to begin building valuable relationships with the pharmaceutical industry.

WS-013-017   Topic: 18, 65
Partnership building: Creating alliance to promote research; consulting with and speaking on behalf of the pharmaceutical industry
Barry Herman, Pfizer, Inc., Medical Dept., Radnor, PA, USA, barry.herman@pfizer.com

WS-013-018   Topic: 34, 65
A researcher's perspective on pharmaceutical industry partnerships
Jörg M. Fegert, Universität Ulm, Kinder- und Jugendpsychiatrie, Ulm, Germany, joerg.fegert@medizin.uni-ulm.de

Objective: Advances in child and adolescent psychopharmacology are impossible without a steady partnership between industry and academia. Nevertheless there might be conflicts of interest and there might be divergent primary goals. The presentation tries to classify potential projects in projects likely to be done by industry in cooperation with academia and other projects where academia or governmental organisations have to give impulses to industry. **Methods:** Improving psychopharmacological research for the benefit of children and adolescents. **Results:** Usually new therapeutic agents are introduced in adults. An aim of child and adolescent psychiatric research is to study the specific efficacy and the safety profile of a drug in children. The GCP-guideline forced the different parliaments in Europe to introduce the notion of "class benefit" to the national legislations finally allowing placebo controlled trials in children and adolescents if there is an expected benefit to the group. The SSRI crisis demonstrates that from an ethical point of view class benefit can be only accepted if the results of research in the given class are published so that the class and their caregivers can profit from the results of research. Defining the status of the pharmaceutical sponsor the GCP-guideline and the corresponding national laws will make investigator initiated studies in these fields nearly impossible, the state will have more importance in stimulating studies of treatment combinations and in rare diseases. **Conclusion:** There are possible ethical and legal pitfalls in the cooperation with industry but without this cooperation advancement in child and adolescent psychopharmcotherapy would nearly be impossible. Doctors should strictly disclose all their contacts with industry and should try to make all research contracts transparent for example in their faculty. In research with children and adolescents doctors should not sign any contract reserving the publication of results to the decision of a pharmaceutical company.

WS-014   Topic: 40, 51
Assessment of risk of violence in youth: Practice issues
Chairperson: Sue Bailey, BSTMHT/UCLAN Gardener Unit, Manchester, United Kingdom, ntattersall@gardener.bstmht.nhs.uk

Assessment of risk of violence in youth: Practice issues
Sue Bailey, BSTMHT/UCLAN, Gardener Unit, Manchester, United Kingdom, ntattersall@gardener.bstmht.nhs.uk

The objectives of this workshop will be to increase skills in assessing needs and risks of violence in adolescents through the use of systematic assessment processes, which will enhance the ability to plan effective interventions. Through working with the Structured Assessment of Violent Risk in Youth (SAVRY) the aims of this workshop will be achieved via knowledge sharing and practical application using case scenarios. Based on professional judgement, the SAVRY is designed to assist in making decisions regarding a young person's risk of violent behaviour and can be applied to mental health services, social services, schools and criminal justice services.

WS-014A   Topic: 54
Refugee children and their families

Chairperson: Gudrun Fischer-von der Marwitz, KJP Bremerhaven, Bremen, Germany,
g.fischer@kjp-bremerhaven.de

Refugee children and their families

Gudrun Fischer-von der Marwitz, KJP Bremerhaven, Bremen, Germany, g.fischer@kjp-bremerhaven.de
Andrea Schneider

Experiences during war, oppression, persecution, torture or flight exercise a special grade of traumatization on people. This workshop will be focusing on living conditions and special problems of traumatized refugee children and their families. Case stories will provide details about symptoms and signs of post-traumatic stress disorder with special regard to children and adolescents. Diverse therapeutic interventions for children as well as day-by-day support for the parents will be demonstrated. The topic will be rounded by suggestions on how to deal with or manage traumatized refugee families in a psychiatric office for children and adolescents.

WS-015   Topic: 7
Child analytic workshop under the auspices of the American Association of Child Psychoanalysts (Part II)

Track: Therapy and intervention
Chairperson: Veronica Mächtlinger, Karl-Abraham Psychoanalytisches Inst., Berlin, Germany, maechtlinger@t-online.de

Child analytic workshop under the auspices of the American Association of Child Psychoanalysts

Veronica Mächtlinger, Karl-Abraham, Psychoanalytisches Inst., Berlin, Germany, maechtlinger@t-online.de

The workshop will be continued by a discussion about the presented cases and general aspects of psychoanalytic treatment in children and adolescents.

WS-015-019   Topic: 7
The analysis of a 9 year old boy with traumatic epilepsy following a newborn stroke

Renate Kelleter, Frankfurter PA Institut, Darmstadt, Germany

The 9 year old patient, born prematurely, was tube fed for a month as he was unable to suck. Investigations revealed a peri-ventricular brain haemorrhage with resulting cerebral seizures, which medication could not control. He has an IQ of 85 and multiple psychological and psycho-physiological symptoms. The epileptic seizures – which occurred by full consciousness and lasted about 30 minutes – were accompanied by unilateral motor paralysis and loss of speech. The attacks, usually observed by the parents during the morning waking phase, occurred at 4 to 6 weekly intervals. The parents are very cooperative. The mother tends to deny the mental consequences of the physical trauma but the father is increasingly anxious about these. In the first year of this ongoing, intensive psychoanalytical treatment the patient has communicated his inner world to the analyst in the form of obsessive drawings and paintings, through which he was able to convey his anxieties and experience during his seizures. This communication has become increasingly verbal. Within the protected analytic setting and in the transference relationship a developmental process has begun in which the patient's severe anxieties and his bodily confusion can be named and talked about in an increasingly differentiated verbal manner. He has been able to use his creative potential in the originality of his paintings and drawings, whose formal characteristics are well in advance of his age. He has become the best in his class in a school for retarded children and has had no seizures since September 2003 – although his medication has not been changed.

WS-016   Topic: 20
The PRINCE: A computerized clinical chart for infant mental health units

Track: Therapy and intervention
Chairperson: Mirelle Keren, Geha Mental Health Center Infant Mental Health Unit, Petah-Tiqva, Israel, ofkeren@internet-zahav.net

The PRINCE: A computerized clinical chart for infant mental health units

Mirelle Keren, Geha Mental Health Center, Infant Mental Health Unit, Petah-Tiqva, Israel, ofkeren@internet-zahav.net

The need for comparing and evaluating clinical data, both in terms of diagnostic and treatment issues, is more and more imperious while infant mental health units become more common in different places in the world (as it is reflected in the increasing number of Affiliates of WAIMH), and cross-cultural epidemiological studies depend on sound data base collection. In parallel, there is an increasing need to show the content and the rationale of our daily work to professionals, mental health ones as well as others. We are also expected to be able to determine the efficacy of our clinical work, not as part of a funded and time-limited research protocol...but as part of our routine. These various motives brought us to develop a clinical standardized and computerized chart, potentially usable in various infant mental health units from different countries, for data base collection, comparison and eventually joint research projects. We suggest here a workshop where both the "container", saying the computer software, and the "content" of this chart will be presented. The rationale the software was to create a tool that is friendly, easy to use and flexible enough to allow units from different places to work in a standardized manner but at the same time to keep a potential space for adding "free text" and for introducing changes. The rationale of its content (evaluation, on-going treatment sessions and summary of treatment) was that it needs to reflect a multidisciplinary approach, a conceptualization of infant mental health in psychodynamic as well as in nosological terms.

After the presentation of the tool, we will share with the audience its advantages and its limitations as we are experiencing while using it.

WS-017   Topic: 4, 6
WPA Global program on child and mental health: Application of evidence-based interventions across different counties and cultures:
A multi-site feasibility study
Track: Therapy and intervention

Chairperson: Peter Jensen, Columbia University Ctr. for Advancement Child MH, New York, USA, pj131@columbia.edu

WPA Global program on child and mental health: Application of evidence-based interventions across different counties and cultures:
A multi-site feasibility study
Peter Jensen, Columbia University, Ctr. for Advancement Child MH, New York, USA, pj131@columbia.edu

Mental disorders among children and youth, coupled with lack of effective services to address them, exert a great toll across the world. To close the gaps between countries' needs for children's mental health services and actual implementation of effective policies and practices, the World Psychiatric Association, in collaboration with the WHO and IACAPAP initiated a Presidential WPA Program on Global Child Mental Health. This symposium describes one of the 3 components of the WPA initiative, the activities of the Task Force on Mental Health Intervention Services and Policy. **Methods:** State-of-art evidence-based assessment, treatment, and organizational practices applicable across countries with relatively few mental health resources have been distilled into 3 manuals: 1) an intervention manual for disruptive behavior disorders (using behavioral therapy methods), 2) an intervention manual for internalizing problems (using cognitive behavioral procedures, targeting anxiety and depression), and 3) an implementation manual and protocol linking all procedures, along with appropriate assessments, clinician supervision, clinic staff training, and fidelity and outcome measures. **Results:** The 2 intervention manuals are derived from established, evidence-based treatment manuals, but adapted to make them briefer (6–8 sessions), more user-friendly, and portable across different cultural and service system contexts. The implementation manual emphasizes the application and local adaptation of healthcare and service organization principles from system of care and chronic illness care models. **Discussion:** Challenges encountered in developing and implementing this project are summarized, manuals' contents are reviewed, and the program's portability to other countries' service contexts is discussed.

WS-018   Topic: 92
Psychological aspects of cleft lip & palate and craniofacial anomalies
Chairperson: Paul Wharton, University of Florida Dept. of Pediatrics, Jacksonville, FL, USA, paul.wharton@jax.ufl.edu

Psychological aspects of cleft lip & palate and craniofacial anomalies
Paul Wharton, University of Florida, Dept. of Pediatrics, Jacksonville, FL, USA, paul.wharton@jax.ufl.edu

The authors will present a review of the current psychological literature on cleft lip and palate and other craniofacial anomalies. Parental issues of acceptance/rejection, peer relationships, cognitive function, emotional development and self concept will be discussed. Additionally, commentary will be offered from the presenter's personal perspective regarding specific psychosocial issues.#

Courses

C-001   Brain imaging in child and adolescent psychiatry
C-002   Eating disorders
C-003   Recognition and treatment of depression in children
C-004   Approaches to managing ADHD
C-005   Psychopharmacology I: Stimulants and medications in PDD
C-006   Psychopharmacology II: Antidepressants, mood stabilizers, antipsychotics
C-007   Autism and related disorders
C-008   Elimination disorders (enuresis and encopresis)
C-009   Tourette's syndrome: The self under seige
C-010   Dyslexia

C-001   Topic: 35
Brain imaging in child and adolescent psychiatry
Course leader: Alexander C. McFarlane, University of Adelaide Queen Elizabeth Hospital, Woodville, Australia, alexander.mcfarlane@adelaide.edu.au

Brain imaging in child and adolescent psychiatry
Alexander C. McFarlane, University of Adelaide, Queen Elizabeth Hospital, Woodville, Australia, alexander.mcfarlane@adelaide.edu.au

The decade of the brain has brought together the confluence of a series of technologies that have enabled far more sophisticated methods of measuring and conceptualizing brain function. It is now possible to demonstrate the patterns of cognition in real time, as well as defining the critical brain networks with precise anatomical locations and underpin many different cognitive and emotional processes. This course will focus on a description of the different forms of neuroimaging and their particular strengths and associated limitations. The functional methods of imaging which provide excellent spatial resolution during particular tasks have impacted broadly on mental health professionals. However, positron emission tomography and fMRI are limited in their capacity for temporal resolution. In general, it is difficult to gain an activation that lasts for less than two seconds of duration because of the very small shifts in metabolic activity measurable using these approaches. Event related potentials on the other hand, provide excellent temporal resolution, but have poor spatial resolution. Many of the technical issues to do with the collection of EEG data and its modeling, have recently been overcome. The challenge for the clinician is to understand both the strengths and weaknesses of the various methods of neuroimaging, so that the significance of the published studies can be appropriately interpreted. One of the challenges is that different provocation paradigms are used by many different researchers leading to apparently contradictory results. The bewildering array of findings can sometimes be a major challenge to individuals who are primary clinicians to make sense of the emerging findings. In this course the neuroimaging studies arising from the impact of trauma will be focused on to highlight these issues. The value of an integrated neuroscience approach, which limits the range of paradigms used and establishes large normative data bases, will be highlighted as a potential solution to some of these methodological challenges. In particular, the interaction between the neural circuitry involved in the management of cognitive functioning and affective modulation will be highlighted. The notion of working memory is a useful construct in understanding how individuals negotiate their world through the complex maze of perceptual inputs that require constant organisation and deconstruction. The participants in the course will be equipped to better analyse and critique the emerging neuroscience literature as a consequence of their participation in this workshop.

C-002   Topic: 78
Eating disorders
Track: Eating disorders
Course leader: Beate Herpertz-Dahlmann, RWTH Aachen Kinder- und Jugendpsychiatrie, Aachen, Germany, bherpertz-dahlmann@ukaachen.de
Johannes Hebebrand, Universitätsklinik Marburg Kinder- und Jugendpsychiatrie, Marburg, Germany, johannes.hebebrand@uni-duisburg-essen.de

Eating disorders
Beate Herpertz-Dahlmann, RWTH Aachen, Kinder- und Jugendpsychiatrie, Aachen, Germany, bherpertz-dahlmann@ukaachen.de

1) Diagnosis of eating disorders: We will discuss the different weight criteria used for a diagnosis of anorexia nervosa. We propose using the 10th BMI centile throughout all age ranges. Finally, the prognostic significance of body weight during the acute stage of the disorder will be discussed. 2) We will discuss alternative diagnostic criteria for anorexia nervosa. The need to do so stems from the fact that some of the phrasings used in the current DSM-IV criteria are not empirically based. 3) We will also refer to bulimia nervosa and binge and night eating disorder in childhood and adolescence. 4) Epidemiology: Some recent epidemiologic data in eating disorders especially on the prevalence of childhood binge eating will be presented. 5) Symptomatology: Because symptoms in anorexia nervosa are closely intertwined with those of semi-starvation, a precise knowledge of somatic and psychopathological symptoms. 6) Hypoleptinemia, which sets in during the early stages of anorexia nervosa, presumably represents the major trigger for the development of amenorrhea. Preliminary evidence in patients suggests that hypoleptinemia also contributes to the hyperactivity in patients with anorexia nervosa. 7) Comorbidity: Eating disorders are associated with many comorbid disorders, especially depression, anxiety disorders, obsessive-compulsive disorders and substance abuse. On one side the influence of starvation will be discussed, on the other hand important diagnostic and therapeutical implications are demonstrated. 8) Treatment: A multimodal inpatient and outpatient treatment model based on several components will be introduced: – nutritional rehabilitation and treatment of physical complications – nutritional counselling – individual therapy – family counselling and/or therapy – treatment of concomitant psychopathology 9) Recent results of pharmacological treatment studies and own research results will be discussed. 10) Last not least findings of inpatient outcome studies may be described.

C-003   Topic: 1, 3
Recognition and Treatment of depression in children
Course leader: Alan Apter, Schneider Childrens Medical Dept. of Psychiatry, Petah Tikva, Israel, eapter@clalit.org.il

Recognition and Treatment of depression in children
Alan Apter, Schneider Childrens Medical, Dept. of Psychiatry, Petah Tikva, Israel, eapter@clalit.org.il

The course will cover the following topics and will attempt to be as practical and as interactive as possible Epidemiology Course Risk for Prolonged Episode Risk for Recurrence Risk Factors: Family History Genetic and Biological risk Factors

Medical Treatments and Conditions associated with childhood depression Adverse Outcomes Depression and Suicidal Behavior Suicidal Behavior: Risk Factors Bipolar Disorder Assessment Treatment-overview and phases Treatment Approaches: Psychoeducation Efficacious Treatments for Child and Adolescent Depression Cognitive Theory of Depression CBT Therapeutic Structure Adaptation Of CBT to Younger Populations: Role of Family Typical Elements in CBT Treatment of Depression Prevention of Depression Results of CBT trials inn depressed children Poor Response to CBT Effects of Maternal depression on childhood depression Effects of abuse on response to treatment Autobiographical memory and depression in adolescents Mindful based therapy for childhood depression Dialectical behavior therapy Interpersonal therapy Psychoanalytic theories Efficacy of SSRI in depression SSRI Side Effects SSRIs and Suicidality Rates of Suicidality in Antidepressants ical Efficacy Trials SSRI-Drug Interactions Approach to therapy with SSRI Importance of Adequate Duration and Dosage of SSRI Pharmacokinetics Poor Response to SSRI Approach to the Treatment Resistant Depressed Adolescent: Enhance Compliance Relapse/Recurrence Rate Follow-Up Impact of CBT Booster CBT Prevention of Relapse Mindfulness based therapies (MBCT) and prevention of relapse What is not Known Pharmacogenetic predictors

C-004　Topic: 84
Approaches to managing ADHD
Track: ADHD
Course leader: Eric Taylor, Institut of Psychiatry
Child & Adolescent Psychiatry, London, United Kingdom,
d.kingsmill@iop.kcl.ac.uk
Henrikje Klasen, Child and Family Service, Chichester,
United Kingdom, h.klasen@iop.kcl.ac.uk

Approaches to managing ADHD
Eric Taylor, Institut of Psychiatry,
Child & Adolescent Psychiatry, London, United Kingdom,
d.kingsmill@iop.kcl.ac.uk

Approaches to Managing ADHD 1. Education and Advice (ET) Terminology; DSM-IV and ICD-10; non-ADHD The new biology of genes, environment and neuroimaging Limitation of knowledge; descriptive vs explanatory concepts Discussion: What kind of patients do you see? How do you advise families and children? How do you advise schools? (Handouts: schools information, assessment measures, lists, manuals) 2. Initial Treatment (ET & HK) Protocols and guidelines Drugs vs behavioural approaches as initial therapy (Handouts: algorithm, auditable protocol) 3. Developing Clinical Services (HK) 4. What To Do When Stimulants Fail (ET) Current dilemmas Non-stimulant drugs (Handouts: algorithm) 5. Future Expectations Genomics; Early Intervention & Prevention; Educational Changes Further reading: Hill & Taylor Euro Guidelines Consensus paper

C-005　Topic: 15
Psychopharmacology I:
Stimulants and medications in PDD
Track: Therapy and intervention
Course leader: Jan Buitelaar, University Medical Center Psychiatry & Adolescent, Nijmegen, Netherlands, jb@psy.umcn.nl

Psychopharmacology I:
Stimulants and medications in PDD
Jan Buitelaar, University Medical Center, Psychiatry & Adolescent, Nijmegen, Netherlands, jb@psy.umcn.nl

The aim of this course is to review the possibilities and the limitations of using medication in treating target symptoms in subjects with PDD. Medications to be reviewed include conventional and new antipsychotics, psychostimulants, presynaptic noradrenergic blocking agents (clonidine and guanfacine), selective serotonin reuptake inhibitors, and mood stabilizers. The participants will be requested to prepare questions on medication in PDD from their own clinical practice and to bring one of more case descriptions to be used in the discussion. More scientific issues will be discussed as well, such as the question: why have the effects of medication in autism been disappointing in improving the core deficits? The explanation for the medication-refractory status of social and communicative deficits should be sought in at least two related factors: (1) the as yet unidentified neurochemical basis of autism, and (2) the obvious uninvolvement of the main neurotransmitter systems (dopamine, noradrenaline, and serotonin) in the pathophysiology of social and communicative behaviour.

C-006　Topic: 14, 12
Psychopharmacology II: Antidepressants,
mood stabilizers, antipsychotics
Track: Therapy and intervention
Course leader: Stanley P. Kutcher, Dalhousie University, Halifax, Nova Scotia, Canada, stan.kutcher@dal.ca

Psychopharmacology II: Antidepressants,
mood stabilizers, antipsychotics
Stanley P. Kutcher, Dalhousie University, Halifax, Nova Scotia, Canada, stan.kutcher@dal.ca

This course will consist of a review of the advances in the psychopharmacologic treatment of youth with psychotic (schizophrenia and schizoaffective disorder) and mood (depression and bipolar) disorders. It will review the recent (over the last two years) treatment literature on these topics and address in detail seminal studies in these areas. In addition, it will provide practical approaches to the treatment of these disorders using the recent literature as a foundation for treatment. If time permits, case based discussion will be included.

C-007　Topic: 83
Autism and related disorders
Track: Pervasive developmental disorders (PDD)
Course leader: Joaquin Fuentes, Policlinica Gipuzkoa Child & Adolescent Psychiatry, San Sebastian, Spain, jfuentes@servitel.es

Autism and related disorders
Joaquin Fuentes, Policlinica Gipuzkoa, Child & Adolescent Psychiatry, San Sebastian, Spain, jfuentes@servitel.es

Objective: To provide a state of the science review of the area of autism spectrum disorders (ASD), including clinical and research aspects, that could be applied by participants in their daily professional practice. **Methods:** The course will cover the following sections: diagnostic concepts in ASD; early detection and assessment procedures; current understanding of the psychological and the neurofunctional basis for the symptoms; educational, pharmacological and psychosocial treatments. The review will end by proposing likely roads for research advancement, and systems for services delivery to persons with autism and their families. To accommodate this agenda to the available timing, the course will be basically structured as a formal verbal presentation by the speaker, but a brief time for discussion will be made available after each of the sections, in order to clarify questions while fostering participation of the group. A short mid-course break will be made available. Participants will receive a paper printed copy of the supporting slides, as well as bibliographic references of the topics covered. An attendance certificate will be delivered. **Results:** Participants will be asked to fill a form by the end of the course, that will permit the assessment of their degree of satisfaction, and gather their suggestions for further initiatives in this area that should be undertaken by IACAPAP. **Conclusion:** The course may be a rewarding experience for those professionals, not specifically specialised in this area, who share an interest in supporting children and adolescents with autism spectrum disorders and want to update their knowledge about these conditions.

C-008   Topic: 88
Elimination disorders (enuresis and encopresis)
Course leader: Alexander von Gontard, Uniklinik des Saarlandes, Homburg, Germany, alexander.von.gontard@uniklinik-saarland.de

Elimination disorders in children and adolescents
Alexander von Gontard, Uniklinik des Saarlandes, Homburg, Germany, alexander.von.gontard@uniklinik-saarland.de

Elimination disorders are among the most common disorders of childhood. Of seven year olds, 10% wet at night, 2–3% during daytime and 1–2% soil. Often these disorders coexist. Despite a high remission rate, still 1–2% of all adolescents are affected by nocturnal enuresis, and <1% by either daytime wetting or soiling. The vast majority of elimination disorders are functional, i.e. not due to neurological, structural or medical causes. According to standard classification schemes such as the ICD-10, enuresis is defined as wetting from the age of 5 years onwards (encopresis: 4 years) – after organic causes have been ruled out. In the past two decades, several distinct subtypes of elimination disorders have been identified which differ regarding aetiology, clinical symptoms and treatment. While some disorders (such as nocturnal enuresis) are primarily genetically determined, in others (such as voiding postponement) environmental factors predominate. Also, the rate of comorbid behavioural disturbances differs greatly from one syndrome to another: in some (such as encopresis) the rate of concomitant behavioural disorders is high, while in others (such as primary monosymptomatic nocturnal enuresis) no more children are disturbed as controls. Because of this variety and heterogeneity, each elimination disorder requires specific approaches in assessment and treatment. The aim of this course is to provide an evidence-based, state-of-the-art overview on the different elimination disorders. It will provide practical de-

tails regarding the paediatric and child psychiatric assessment and treatment of enuresis, functional urinary incontinence and encopresis. Guidelines will be discussed and short case vignettes will be presented.

C-009   Topic: 87, 3
Tourette's syndrome: The self under seige
Course leader: James Leckman, Yale University Child Study Center, New Haven, USA, james.leckman@yale.edu

Tourette's syndrome: The self under seige
James Leckman, Yale University, Child Study Center, New Haven, USA, james.leckman@yale.edu

As our knowledge of Tourette's syndrome (TS) increases, so does our appreciation for the pathogenic complexity of this disorder and the challenges associated with its treatment. Advances in the neurosciences have led to new models of pathogenesis, while clinical studies have reinvigorated earlier hypotheses. The interdependent roles of genes and environment in disease formation have yet to be fully elucidated. Recent epidemiological studies have prompted a debate on how best to characterize and diagnose this disorder. The absence of ideal anti-tic medications combined with the knowledge that uncomplicated cases of childhood TS often have a favorable outcome has led to marked changes in the care and treatment of patients with TS. This workshop focuses on these changing views and offers a new perspective on our understanding of the pathogenesis of TS and on principles for therapeutic management of patients with this disorder.

C-010   Topic: 82
Dyslexia
*Course leader: Gerd Schulte-Körne, Universitätsklinik Marburg, Kinder- und Jugendpsychiatrie, Marburg, Germany, schulte1@med.uni-marburg.de
Andreas Warnke, Universitätsklinik Würzburg, Kinder- und Jugendpsychiatrie, Würzburg, Germany, warnke@kjp.uni-wuerzburg.de*

Dyslexia
Gerd Schulte-Körne, Universitätsklinik Marburg, Kinder- und Jugendpsychiatrie, Marburg, Germany, schulte1@med.uni-marburg.de

Participants of this course will get a clinically oriented introduction to the main topics of dyslexia like diagnostics, etiology and remediation. Dyslexia is one of the most frequently diagnosed developmental learning disorders which clearly affects the psychosocial development of the affected children. Diagnostics and classification are based on the ICD-10 criteria but also DSM IV criteria were considered. Based on case reports and longitudinal studies the development of dyslexic children will be demonstrated. One major topic of this course are the different etiological models of dyslexia. Results of recent genetic, neurophysiological, brain imaging and neuropsychological studies were presented. The theoretical and empirical link between the results of these basic research and therapeutic concepts will be discussed. The last major topic will be actual results of treatment evaluation. Effective remediation will be shown for programmes at school, at home and in the outpatient department.

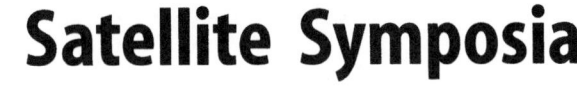

Satellite Symposia

IS-001   Topic: 84
Objective measurement in ADHD
(sponsored by Janssen-Cilag and QbTech)
Track: ADHD

Chairperson: Helmut Remschmidt, Universität Marburg Kinder- und Jugendpsychiatrie, Marburg, Germany, remschm@med.uni-marburg.de

Objective measurement in ADHD

Helmut Remschmidt, Universität Marburg, Kinder- und Jugendpsychiatrie, Marburg, Germany, remschm@med.uni-marburg.de

ADHD is a behavioural defined disorder based on the symptom triad attention deficit, hyperactivity and impulsiveness. There are some differences in the definition of the syndrome according to the currently used classification systems ICD 10 and DSM IV which lead to a more frequent diagnosis, when the DSM system is used. There are numerous symptom check-lists, scales and interviews aiming at the diagnosis of the behavioural pattern of ADHD. Nearly all of them are based on the judgement of observers (parents, teachers, doctors, psychologist) or on self-ratings. In contrast to this approach, objective measurements try to register the behaviour pattern and the possible basic processes underlying the disorder by neurobiological and neuropsychological parameters. The papers presented in this Symposium will be focused on the simultaneous measurement of the symptom triad of ADHD, the measurement of motor activity using the Doppler-Radar-Technique, molecular-genetic findings, results of neuro-imaging techniques and neuro-psychological measurements.

IS-001-001   Topic: 84, 30
Simultaneous objective measurement of attention, hyperactivity and impulsiveness

Philip Heiser, Universitätsklinik Marburg, Kinder- und Jugendpsychiatrie, Marburg, Germany, heiser@mailer.uni-marburg.de
Joachim Frey; Helmut Remschmidt

Objective: The purpose of this study was to investigate whether the parameters of the OPTAx test differentiate between unmedicated and medicated status of children with hyperkinetic disorder (HD) treated with methylphenidate (MPH). **Methods:** The OPTAx test is an infrared motion analysis to record the movement pattern during a continuous performance test. We tested 25 children between 6 and 12 years with HD (ICD-10: F90.0 or F90.1) before and after treatment with MPH. The parameters under investigation were activity (microevents and spatial scaling), impulsiveness (errors of commission), and attention (accuracy and variability). For statistical analysis a one-tailed matched pairs test (adj. p=0.01) was conducted to discriminate differences found from those occurred at random. A post hoc partial correlation of absolute differences in the respective parameters and the daily dose of MPH (adj. for BMI) was performed if p<0.01. **Results:** Statistically significant results were found for microevents, spatial scaling, errors of commission, accuracy, and variability. The partial correlation showed significant results for microevents and variability. **Conclusion:** The mean prepost changes found in all parameters investigated consistently correspond with benefits desired from medication with MPH in children with HD. Absolute differences in microevents and variability

seem to depend on the daily dose of MPH after adjustment for BMI.

IS-001-002   Topic: 84
Studying attentional deficits with functional magnet resonance imaging (fMRI) in children with ADHD

Kerstin Konrad, RWTH Aachen, Kinder- und Jugendpsychiatrie, Aachen, Germany, kkonrad@ukaachen.de
Susanne Neufang; Gereon R. Fink;
Beate Herpertz-Dahlmann

Objective: Functional imaging provides an intriguing tool for studying the neural basis of cognitive processes in normal children and children with neuropsychiatric disorders. **Methods:** We therefore used event-related functional imaging (fMRI) to investigate the neural correlates of attentional deficits in healthy children and treatment-naïve children with Attention Deficit/Hyperactivity Disorder (ADHD), aged 8 to 12 years. **Results:** Behaviorally, children with ADHD showed a normal alerting effect, a tendentially impaired reorienting effect (p=0.06) and a significantly larger interference effect (p=0.001) compared to healthy controls. FMRI data suggested deviant brain activation patterns with regard to all attentional processes investigated: Healthy children activated significantly more the right medial frontal gyrus during the alerting condition and the fronto-striatal circuitry during the conflict condition. However, ADHD children activated frontal areas and the putamen more during the reorienting condition. **Conclusion:** Thus, our data suggest that children with ADHD tend to rely on different attentional strategies leading to unspecific brain activation patterns which are not necessarily evident in behavioural data.

IS-001-003
Electrophysiological measurements in ADHD

Andreas J. Fallgatter, Universität Würzburg, Psychiatrie und Psychotherapie, Würzburg, Germany, fallgatterª@klinik.uni-wuerzburg.de
Ann-Christine Ehlis; Christina Baehne; Jürgen Seifert; Peter Scheuerpflug; Martin J. Herrmann; Andreas Warnke

Objective: Deficits in response inhibition, working memory, time processing and delay aversion are considered as candidate endophenotypes of altered brain function in Attention Deficit Hyperactivity Disorder (ADHD). Based on their superior time resolution, electrophysiological methods like Event-Related Potentials (ERPs) are adequate for the measurement of abnormalities in brain functions underlying those deficits. **Methods:** We employed a multi-channel EEG during performance of a Go-NoGo task to assess the electrophysiological basis of response inhibition in healthy subjects as well as in patients with ADHD. The ERP-measure derived from this protocol was termed NoGo-Anteriorisation (NGA) and is characterized by a high interindividual stability, high short- and long-term test-retest reliability and, moreover, is independent from age- and gender. **Results:** In 24 adult patients with personality disorders and additional hints for an ADHD during childhood the NGA was diminished as compared to age- and sexmatched healthy controls. Furthermore, a three-dimensional source location analysis with LORETA indicated an electrical dysfunction of the ACC in this patient group. A corresponding alteration of prefrontal brain function was also found in boys with ADHD in comparison to healthy boys in the same age range. **Conclusion:**

These results exemplify the measurement of disease related disturbances in brain function in ADHD. Future studies will show whether such electrophysiological endophenotypes may contribute to the diagnosis of subgroups of ADHD and to the measurement of treatment effects on ACC-function.

IS-001-004   Topic: 84, 28
Molecular genetic findings in Attention Deficit Hyperactivity Disorder (ADHD)

Johannes Hebebrand, Universitätsklinik Marburg, Kinder-und Jugendpsychiatrie, Marburg, Germany, johannes.hebebrand@uni-duisburg-essen.de

Several formal genetic studies have addressed the contribution of both genetic and environmental factors to the development of ADHD using both categorical and dimensional definitions. Twin studies have come up with concordance rates between about 50 and 80% for monozygotic (MZ) versus 30 to 40% for dizygotic (DZ) twins. MZ and DZ correlations for quantitative traits of ADHD of between 0.48 and 0.92 and 0.16 and 0.57, respectively, also indicate substantial heritability, which has been estimated at approximately 0.8. These results warrant large scaled efforts to identify the molecular basis of ADHD; molecular genetic studies of ADHD have been ongoing for approximately 10 years. Currently, two genome scans have been published, one of which was extended to include an additional sample of families. Whereas single peaks with lod scores >3 have been identified the genes underlying these linkage findings have not yet been delineated. Some linkage regions for ADHD overlap with those obtained in autism and learning disorders thus suggesting joint underlying genetic mechanisms. We will compare recent data of a German genome scan performed with 100 families with two or more affecteds with published linkage findings. Association studies (case-control study, haplotype relative risk method, transmission disequilibrium test) of specific candidate genes have formed the major focus of molecular genetic studies in ADHD. Within the context of the symposium we will dwell on the question which of the respective findings can be considered "objective". Single findings pertaining to mostly candidate genes of the dopaminergic system have repeatedly been confirmed; however the findings are not consistent. Meta-analyses suggest a role of the dopamine D4 receptor gene and the dopamine transporter gene.

IS-001-005   Topic: 34, 38
Objective measures of ADHD – Simulating the clinical eye: A new approach to assess motor activity using frequency shifts in Doppler-radar

Michael Huss, Charite Berlin, Kinder- und Jugendpsychiatrie, Berlin, Germany, michael.huss@charite.de
Ekkehart Jenetzky

Objective: With regard to the core symptoms of ADHD (hyperactivity, impulsivity, inattention) hyperactivity is the most 'physical' one. Therefore, it should be the easiest to assess objectively. However, most devices to measure motor activity (actometers) did not prove to be valid enough in order to be used clinically. A systematic analysis of former instruments revealed a series of limitations (i.e. assessment of single muscle groups, behavior-device interaction), which may have been the reason for shortcomings

of validity. In order to improve objective measure of hyperactivity, we developed a new device based on Doppler-radar (international patent pending), which overcomes the former limitations. **Methods:** Each movement of the body causes a frequency shift of reflected radar waves. This shift is registered with a receiver and transformed by an electronic circuit into a rectangle signal indicating the movement. Global activity scores are calculated by recording all movements from the body irrespectively from which muscle they stem (analogue the clinical eye). Data are evaluated with diagnoses using the semi-structured interview K-SADS. **Results:** The index of global motor activity shows promising screening properties (for cut-off 8.4% motor activity: specificity=98%; sensitivity=50%) in boys. Furthermore, the device proved to be highly sensitive for medication effects. Effects of age, gender and intelligence have to be taken into account as covariates. **Conclusion:** Doppler radar is a cheap, easy, and useful method to assess global motor activity without behavioral interference. Screening properties and drug sensitivity are promising. In combination with other objective measures it may contribute substantially to improve the diagnostic process.

IS-001-006   Topic: 84, 30
The role of neuropsychological tests in diagnosing ADHD and evaluation of treatment responses

Geir Øgrim, Halden, Norway, gei-oe@online.no

In this 30 min lecture the role of neuropsychological tests will be examined. Testing is not required to put forward a diagnosis of ADHD, but can convey important information especially concerning differential diagnosis and comorbidity. As a rule of thumb tests rule in, but do not necessarily rule out a diagnosis of ADHD. The existing "gold standard" of diagnosing ADHD relies almost exclusively on parent and teacher information, which is considered a weakness. When diagnosing also include evaluation in a broader sense, neuropsychological tests have a still more important role in describing individual strengths and weaknesses, and should be used in treatment planning and evaluation. Examples of tests will be demonstrated, and main findings from the research literature will be presented. Some studies compare ADHD with normal controls, others with other diagnostic categories. Specificity is lower in these last mentioned studies. Clinical cases will illustrate tests as part of the diagnostic process, and their usefulness in the evaluation of treatment effects will also be described. Based on 20 randomly selected cases data will be presented that correlate test results with the diagnosis of ADHD: What tests or cluster of tests seem to be the best predictors? Data that show what tests are most sensitive to the effect of methylphenidate will also be shown.

IS-002   Topic: 84
Current trends in ADHD treatment research (sponsored by Medice)

Track: ADHD

Chairperson: Manfred Döpfner, Universität zu Köln Psychiatrie und Psychotherapie, Köln, Germany, manfred.doepfner@t-online.de
Gerd Lehmkuhl, Universität Köln Kinder- und Jugendpsychiatrie, Köln, Germany, gerd.lehmkuhl@medizin.uni-koeln.de

IS-002-007 Topic: 84, 3

Long-term effects stimulant medication on ADHD symptoms and physical growth revealed by the MTA follow-up

James Swanson, UCLA at Irvine, Irvine, CA, USA,
jmswanso@uci.edu

The Multimodal Treatment study of ADHD (MTA) is one of the largest randomized clinical trials yet conducted to evaluate the long-term effects of the two primary treatments for Attention Deficit Hyperactivity Disorder (ADHD), defined by state-of-the-art pharmacological intervention with stimulant medication (MedMgt) and psychosocial intervention with behavior modification (Beh) when this study started in the mid-1990s. 579 children with ADHD were assigned to one of 4 treatment conditions, MedMgt, Beh, the Combination (Comb) or to a Community Comparison (CC) condition, and after a 14 month treatment phase are being assessed regularly using a naturalistic follow-up design. Outcomes measures of efficacy (symptoms of ADHD) and growth (height and weight) obtained at the first two follow-up assessments (24-month and 36-month after entry into the study) will be presented. Intent-to-treat analyses of the 4 randomly assigned groups as well as analyses of naturalistic subgroups (defined by actual treatment patterns over time that differ from assigned treatment) will be discussed.

IS-002-008 Topic: 84, 3

The Cologne adaptive treatment study (CAMT) – Long term outcome of multimodal treatment

Tanja Wolff Metternich, Universität zu Köln, Köln, Germany

Objective: To evaluate the long-term outcome of ADHD children treated with an adaptive and individually tailored multimodal intervention. **Methods:** The original sample consisted of 75 school-children aged 6–10 years with a diagnosis of ADHD/HKD. After an initial psychoeducation these children were assigned to either behaviour therapy or medical management with methylphenidate plus psychoeducation. Depending on the effectiveness, the treatment was either terminated (if totally effective) with long term aftercare and continuation of medication if needed, or (if partially effective) the other treatment component was added (combined treatment), or (if ineffective) the treatment components were replaced. Thus a treatment rationale was applied which resulted in an adaptive and individually tailored therapy – similar to a strategy that may be useful in clinical practice. 60 of these 75 children could be reassessed 7 years after the termination of the intensive treatment. **Results:** A small percentage of children still use medication. ADHD symptoms and ODD/CD symptoms decreased during treatment and remained stable in the follow-up. Most of the adolescents had an adequate global social and academic functioning. **Conclusion:** Most of the ADHD children had a quite good prognosis after multimodal treatment with an individually tailored aftercare.

IS-002-009 Topic: 84, 3

The German multicentre summer camp study on the effects of long acting stimulants

Manfred Döpfner, Universität zu Köln,
Psychiatrie und Psychotherapie, Köln, Germany,
manfred.doepfner@t-online.de

Objective: This investigation was conducted to assess the efficacy and the duration of action of a new extended-release formulation of methylphenidate (Medikinet retard) as a once-daily treatment for children with attention-deficit/hyperactivity disorder (ADHD). **Methods:** This was a randomized, double-blind, crossover multicentre study with three treatment conditions: once-daily extended release methylphenidate, twice-daily immediate release methylphenidate and placebo given to 79 children (8–14 years old) with ADHD. Daily assessments in an analogue classroom setting included blind ratings of attention and deportment and a performance measure (math test) obtained 5 times over an 8-hour period. Secondary measures included an ADHD rating scale, based on DSM-IV/ICD-10 separately rated for the morning and the afternoon. **Results:** Both active treatment conditions displayed significant time course effects and were superior to placebo in improving all efficacy measures. Once a day extended release methylphenidate was not different from the same dose of twice daily immediate release methylphenidate. **Conclusion:** These data provide support for the benefit of this novel, once-daily methylphenidate preparation in the treatment of ADHD. The longer duration of action of Medikinet retard has the potential to simplify psychostimulant treatment, thus reducing dose diversion and eliminating the need for in-school administration.

IS-002-010 Topic: 84, 3

Recent studies comparing stimulant medication, behavior modification and their combination in ADHD

William B. Pellham, State University of New York, and Buffalo, New York, USA

Behavioral and pharmacological treatments both have an evidence base for the treatment of children with ADHD. However, the combination of the two treatments has been relatively understudied. In particular, multimodal studies with long acting stimulant preparations have not been conducted. In this investigation, placebo and three doses of methylphenidate were crossed with three levels of behavioral modification (BMOD) in the context of a summer treatment program (STP). Participants were 27 children aged 612 and diagnosed with ADHD. Children received four medication conditions in random order with conditions changing daily. BMOD conditions were implemented for 3-week blocks, with order randomized across groups. Both treatments produced large and significant effects on children's behavior and performance in the STP. Combined treatment was superior to either treatment alone, and a low dose of methylphenidate (average of 5 mg MPH t.i.d.) combined with BMOD produced equivalent effects as those of a high dose (average of 15 mg MPH t.i.d.) alone.

IS-003   Topic: 84
Children with ADHD: Tailoring care
for optimal outcomes (sponsored by Celltech)
Track: ADHD
Chairperson: Jörg M. Fegert, Universität Ulm
Kinder- und Judenpsychiatrie, Ulm, Germany,
joerg.fegert@medizin.uni-ulm.de
Laurence Greenhill, New York State Psychiatric Unit,
New York, NY, USA, larrylgreenhill@cs.com

IS-003-011   Topic: 58
Preschool diagnosis and management
Laurence Greenhill, New York State, Psychiatric Unit,
New York, NY, USA, larrylgreenhill@cs.com

IS-003-012   Topic: 24
Maximising learning potential
Christopher Gillberg, University of Göteborg, Göteborg,
Sweden, christopher.gillberg@pediat.gu.se

IS-003-013   Topic: 15
New options with methylphenidates
James Swanson, UCLA at Irvine, Irvine, CA, USA,
jmswanso@uci.edu

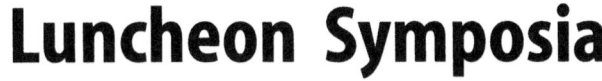

Luncheon Symposia

LS-001   Topic: 84
EINAQ – A European CME/CPD programme on ADHD for practitioners (sponsored by Thomson Advanced Therapeutics Communications)
Track: ADHD
Chairperson: Aribert Rothenberger, Universität Göttingen, Göttingen, Germany, arothen@gwdg.de

LS-001-001   Topic: 84, 63
The need for CME/CPD: Background, development, European implementation and the future of EINAQ
Aribert Rothenberger, Universität Göttingen, Göttingen, Germany, arothen@gwdg.de

LS-001-002   Topic: 84, 30
Neuropsychological models of ADHD: Relevance for daily clinical practice
Joseph Sergeant, Netherlands

LS-001-003   Topic: 84, 37
The role of assessment in identifying the needs for intervention in ADHD
Hans-Christoph Steinhausen, ZKJP Universität Zürich, Kinder- und Jugendpsychiatrie, Zürich, Switzerland, steinh@kjpd.unizh.ch

LS-001-004   Topic: 84, 3
Multimodal treatment of ADHD: A European perspective
Manfred Döpfner, Universität zu Köln, Psychiatrie und Psychotherapie, Köln, Germany, manfred.doepfner@t-online.de

LS-002   Topic: 19
Enhancing patient benefits through novel treatment paradigms: A new era in the treatment of behavioural symptoms in the pediatric patient population (sponsored by Janssen-Cilag)
Track: Therapy and intervention
Chairperson: Lawrence Scahill, Yale Child Study Center, New Haven, CT, USA, lawrence.scahill@yale.edu

LS-002-005   Topic: 19, 83
Understanding epidemiology and symptoms of Disruptive Behaviour Disorders (DBDs) and Pervasive Developmental Disorders (PDDs)
James McCracken, UCLA, Division of Child Psychiatry, USA, jmccracken@mednet.ucla.edu

LS-002-006   Topic: 19, 85
Expanding the evidence-base: Short-term and long-term trials in Disruptive Behaviour Disorders (DBDs)
Robert Findling, University Hospitals of Cleveland, Cleveland, OH, USA, robert.findling@uhhs.com

LS-002-007   Topic: 19, 83
Optimizing clinical outcomes in children with autism and behavioural problems: Results from two multi-centre trials
Lawrence Scahill, Yale Child Study Center, New Haven, CT, USA, lawrence.scahill@yale.edu

LS-002-008   Topic: 19, 23
Key considerations in a patient-centered approach: Treatment guidelines for optimal management of behavioural disturbances in children and adolescents
Jan Buitelaar, University Medical Center, Psychiatry & Adolescent, Nijmegen, Netherlands, jb@psy.umcn.nl

LS-003   Topic: 84
ADHD management, still a major concern in paediatric psychiatry (sponsored by Janssen Cilag)
Track: ADHD
Chairperson: Helmut Remschmidt, Universität Marburg Kinder- und Jugendpsychiatrie, Marburg, Germany, remschm@med.uni-marburg.de

ADHD management, still a major concern in paediatric psychiatry
Helmut Remschmidt, Universität Marburg, Kinder- und Jugendpsychiatrie, Marburg, Germany, remschm@med.uni-marburg.de

Attention-deficit/hyperactivity disorder (ADHD) is one of the most prevalent childhood disorders, affecting 3–5% of school-aged children. The condition, which is characterized by developmentally inappropriate levels of inattention, hyperactivity and impulsiveness, can have a profound impact on patients and their family. The multimodal treatment of ADHD (MTA) study demonstrated that pharmacotherapy, as the cornerstone of a multimodal treatment approach, is the most effective way of treating ADHD in children. The study concluded that methylphenidate should be given tid and titrated to the dose that delivers maximum therapeutic efficacy and should be offered in the long term for effective treatment of this chronic condition. This program will review the current feeling in Europe around this approach and the challenges of finding the optimal dose of MPH. Newer long acting agents have significantly advanced the pharmacological treatment of ADHD. Although stimulants are the gold standard for the treatment of ADHD, recently a non-stimulant has been approved. The differences and similarities will be discussed. The long term safety and tolerability of medications used to treat chronic conditions are always key considerations. We will review these important aspects of the latest treatments. Educational Objectives: Explain why pharmacologic treatment is the foundation for a multimodal approach towards the treatment of ADHD. List the challenges faced by patients and their families in terms of its impact on behavior and function. Discuss the benefits of titrating to an optimal dose. Explain why long-acting stimulants are the mainstay of treatment. Explain positioning of stimulants and non-stimulants in the treatment paradigm. Establish the safety and tolerability of stimulant medication.

LS-003-009 Topic: 84, 19
European position to the multimodal treatment approach in ADHD
Jan Buitelaar, University Medical Center, Psychiatry & Adolescent, Nijmegen, Netherlands, jb@psy.umcn.nl

LS-003-010 Topic: 84, 15
Dosing schedules:
How to get most out of the current medication
*Michael Huss, Charite Berlin,
Kinder- und Jugendpsychiatrie, Berlin, Germany,
michael.huss@charite.de*

LS-003-011 Topic: 84, 15
Optimising ADHD management:
Stimulants versus non-stimulants
Ken Steinhoff, USA

LS-003-012 Topic: 84, 15
Long term safety and tolerability of OROS methylphenidate
Timothy Wilens, Massachusetts General Hospital, Boston, MA, USA, wilens@helix.mgh.harvard.edu

LS-004 Topic: 84
ADHD: Sorting out the differences among patients and treatments (sponsored by Eli Lilly)
Track: ADHD
Chairperson: Albert J. Allen, Eli Lilly and Company, Indianapolis, IN, USA, allenaj@lilly.com

ADHD pharmacotherapeutic options:
Beyond acute efficacy
Albert J. Allen, Eli Lilly and Company, Indianapolis, IN, USA, allenaj@lilly.com

At present, agents such as methylphenidate or amphetamine salts represent the only products approved for the treatment of attention-deficit/hyperactivity disorder (ADHD) in most of Europe. Atomoxetine, approved for the treatment of ADHD in the United States in November 2002, is expected to receive first European approval shortly, representing the first new chemical entity for the treatment of ADHD in decades. We will review the modern drug development process in the United States and Europe, focusing on practical issues as well as FDA and CPMP regulations and guidance for developing a drug with a primarily pediatric indication. In addition, we will review available data for stimulants and atomoxetine, examining the benefits of continuing treatment beyond acute response. Finally, we will present data from completed clinical trials that may provide insight into selecting treatments based on patient characteristics. This is an accepted Lilly industry-sponsored symposium.

LS-004-013 Topic: 84
How long should you use pharmacotherapy in a child with ADHD?
Jan Buitelaar, University Medical Center, Psychiatry & Adolescent, Nijmegen, Netherlands, jb@psy.umcn.nl

Objective: Attention-deficit/hyperactivity disorder (ADHD) is a chronic disorder and patients with ADHD are typically treated for extended periods. The efficacy of pharmacotherapy, however, has mainly been demonstrated in acute settings. **Results:** The most systematic long-term study is the recent landmark Multimodal Treatment Assessment study (MTA Cooperative Group, 1999), which assessed the value of different interventions and provided data over 14 months of treatment. That study, however, did not include placebo control, and did not re-randomize acute treatment responders to assess the value of maintenance treatment in relapse prevention. One long-term, placebo-controlled relapse prevention study has been reported, a single-site study of amphetamine (Gillberg et al., 1997). An additional large, international relapse prevention study has recently been completed, which provides evidence of the efficacy of atomoxetine in maintaining treatment responses for up to 1 year following an initial 3-month treatment period. This study also included a second randomization of patients who satisfactorily completed 12 months of atomoxetine treatment. Atomoxetine was superior to placebo in preventing relapse; however, for both treatment groups, relapse rates were low, and among patients randomly assigned to discontinuation, mean magnitude symptom return was to a level of severity markedly less than that observed at study entry. **Conclusion:** These findings support the usual clinical practice of maintaining treatment for extended periods in patients whose symptoms respond after an initial treatment trial.

LS-004-014 Topic: 17, 40
Differentiating among treatment options –
Considerations for selecting the best pharmacotherapy for each child
Jeffrey Newcorn, Mount Sinai School of Medicine, USA

Objective: At present, psychostimulants are the only medications approved for the treatment of ADHD in Europe. Atomoxetine, recently approved for the treatment of ADHD in the United States, is expected to receive its first European approval soon. Atomoxetine and stimulants work via different mechanisms. Stimulants bind to dopamine (DA) transporters in the striatum, thereby enhancing synaptic DA. However, stimulants also increase norepinephrine (NE) in the prefrontal cortex (PFC) by binding to the NE transporter. Atomoxetine is a highly selective blocker of the NE transporter, which increases both DA and NE in the PFC, secondary to the dependence of DA on NE transporters in this region. However, in contrast with stimulants, atomoxetine has no effect on DA in the striatum, nucleus accumbens, or other regions (Bymaster et al., 2002). These differences in mechanism of action suggest that there is likely differential response and tolerability, with some individuals tolerating or responding preferentially to one treatment over the other. **Methods:** We will review data that provide insight into selecting treatments based on patient characteristics. Results will be discussed in the context of emerging biological findings regarding response to atomoxetine and stimulants.

LS-004-015   Topic: 31
An overview of the drug development process for a product with a primary pediatric indication

Albert J. Allen, Eli Lilly and Company, Indianapolis, IN, USA, allenaj@lilly.com

This presentation will review the drug development process in the United States and Europe, focusing on practical issues as well as FDA and CPMP regulations and guidance for developing a drug with a primarily pediatric indication. Atomoxetine, a novel treatment for attention-deficit/hyperactivity disorder (ADHD) approved in the United States in November 2002 and expecting first European approval in 2004, will be used to illustrate how the modern drug development process works. It will also highlight changes in the development of ADHD treatments since the introduction of stimulants over 50 years ago. In addition to dealing with unique regulatory requirements and guidance, developing a drug for use in a pediatric population poses special challenges in diverse areas including biomedical ethics, developmental pharmacology, and clinical trial design and implementation.

Poster

P-001 Care, treatment and prevention I
Track: Therapy and intervention

P-001-001   Topic: 13, 34
Indication for use of Sertraline in child and adolescent psychiatry

Olivera Aleksic, Institute for Mental Health, Belgrade, Serbia and Montenegro, imz@imh.org.yu
Milica Pejovic-Milovancevic; Smiljka Popovic-Deusic; Biljana Pirgic; Ivana Sojic

Objective: One of the most powerful medications that have very broad aspects of clinical application are the selective serotonin reuptake inhibitors (SSRI). We use SSRI as a first choice agents in treatment of depression, obsessive-compulsive disorders and some anxiety disordes. Objective: To analyze the outcome of treatment of adolescent depresion with SSRI's, considering the age group, disorder categories, response to treatment and side effects. **Methods:** A retrospective epidemiological investigation was conducted by means of medical records for all adolescent treated with sertraline during six months period at the Department of Child and Adolescent Psychiatry in Belgrade. The clinical response to treatment was rated by Beck Depression Inventory and Hamilton Depression Rating Scale. **Results:** 5 boys and 10 girls (mean age 15.7) were treated with sertraline during the first episode of depression; administred doses were 50–75 mg per day. 86% of patients improved, 10% droped out because of economic reasons, and 4% experienced side affects (nausea, vomiting, headache). **Conclusion:** Sertraline is potent, safe and effective in the treatment of young people with first episode of depression.

P-001-002   Topic: 12, 41
Changes in body composition and serum lipids in children and adolescents treated with second-generation antipsychotics

Christoph Correll, The Zucker Hillside Hospital, Dept. of Psychiatry Research, Glen Oaks, NY, USA, ccorrell@lij.edu
Umesh Parikh; Vladimir Olshanskiy; Bhrigu Chopra; John M. Kane; Anil K. Malhotra

Objective: Although second-generation antipsychotics (SGAs) are widely utilized in youth, limited comparative data exist on their effects on body composition and lipid metabolism. This study aimed to prospectively evaluate the effects of the three most widely prescribed second-generation antipsychotics on body composition and lipid metabolism in this particularly vulnerable population. **Methods:** 12-week, prospective, open-label study in subjects 5–18 years old with a DSM-IV diagnosis of psychotic, mood and/or disruptive behavior disorders necessitating initiation of SGA-treatment. At baeline and monthly, height, weight, body mass index (BMI), fat mass and percentage (bioimpedantiometry), waist circumference, as well as lipid profile, leptin and SGA levels (ensuring compliance) were measured. **Results:** In 174 youngsters (mean age: 13.8 ± 3.4 years, 60.6% male, 45.7% Caucasian) who completed 8-13 (mean: 11.8 ± 1.6) weeks of SGA-treatment, weight, BMI, fat and percentage, and waist circumference increased significantly ($p < 0.0001$, respectively). All measures increased with olanzapine the most (7.6 ± 4.3 kg=2.6 ± 1.5 BMI-points, n=57), followed by risperidone (4.7 ± 3.9 kg= 1.6 ± 1.4 BMI-points, n=47) and quetiapine (2.7 ± 5.0 kg=

0.7 ± 1.9 BMI-points, n=70) ($p < 0.0001$, respectively). Extreme weight gain (7%) occurred in 80.7%, 57.1% and 42.6% of patients, respectively ($p < 0.001$). Further, total cholesterol ($p = 0.04$), LDL-cholesterol ($p = 0.004$) and triglycerides ($p = 0.03$) significantly increased compared to baseline for all three drugs combined. In post-hoc analyses in pre-treated and antipychotic-naïve youth, only changes in the olanzapine group remained significant. Nevertheless, 19.9% of youth experienced new-onset dyslipidemia (i.e., cholesterol > 200 mg/dL and/or triglycerides > 150 mg/dl), with similar rates for all three SGAs ($p = 0.91$). Correlates of weight gain at endpoint ($R2 = 0.73$, $p < 0.0001$) were weight increase at 4 weeks ($p < 0.0001$), baseline-to-endpoint increases in leptin ($p < 0.0001$), antipsychotic-naïveté ($p = 0.007$), olanzapine treatment ($p = 0.007$), and divalproex co-treatment ($p = 0.04$). New-onset dyslipidemia was associated with weight gain only ($p < 0.0006$). **Conclusion:** In youngsters, SGAs adversely affect all components of body composition and lead to dyslipidemia, which further increases the cardiovascular risk profile. High-risk individuals are antipsychotic-naïve, leptin-resistant youngsters treated with olanzapine and co-treated with divalproex who experience significant early weight gain. Careful use of SGAs, regular monitoring of these side effects, and pretreatment dietary/lifestyle counseling are warranted.

P-001-003   Topic: 12, 27
Malignant neuroleptic syndrome in children and adolescents: Problems in diagnosis and differential diagnosis

Sonja Sieslack, Universität Tübingen, Kinder- und Jugendpsychiatrie, Tübingen, Germany, sonja.sieslack@med.uni-tuebingen.de
Gottfried Maria Barth; Gunther Klosinski

Objective: Malignant neuroleptic syndrom (MNS) is a rare complication in antipsychotic therapy of children and adolescents which induces specific problems regarding diagnosis and especially differential diagnosis. **Methods:** A review of the present standard of knowlegde about MNS in Childhood and adolescence and about etiology of MNS is given. Two case reports of MNS in childhood and in adolescence demonstrate the problems in differential diagnosis of MNS, especially the discrimination between MNS, catatonia and encephalitis. Consequences for pathogenetic concepts are drawn. **Results:** In individual cases it can be very difficult to distinguish between MNS, malignant catatonia and encephalitis. In pathogenesis of MNS the underlying etiological processes are not well understood until today. Each individual case requires accurate examination of psychic and somatic causes additional to neuroleptic medication (e.g. autoantibodies against CNS). MNS probably results from the interaction of different factors. **Conclusion:** Antipsychotic treatment of children and adolescents should be sensible for a possible appearance of MNS. Careful and extensive diagnostics are necessary. Early symptoms should be recognized because of the better course and prognosis of early intervention.

P-001-004 Topic: 13

Efficacy, tolerability and pharmacogenetic profile of Citalopram for the acute treatment of anxiety disorders and depression in children and adolescents

Shella Sadigorsky, Schneider Children's, Medical Center, Tel Aviv, Israel, shella@012.net.il
Sefi Kronenberg; Amos Frisch

Objective: To assess the efficacy and tolerability of citalopram for the acute treatment of children and adolescents suffering from anxiety disorders and depression. Furthermore, to determine the pharmacogenetic profile of citalopram regarding treatment response and adverse effects. **Methods:** One hundred subjects, aged 7 to 18 years, who showed significant functional impairment and were diagnosed with a DSM-IV-TR anxiety or depressive disorder, were recruited from a psychiatric outpatient clinic. Subjects were treated in an open trial with citalopram for 8 weeks. Dosage was adjusted during the first 4 weeks of the trial according to a fixed protocol (max. dose 40 mg/day). Outcome measures included the Screen for Child Anxiety Related Emotional Disorders (SCARED), the Children's Yale Brown Obsessive Compulsive Scale (CY-BOCS), the Children's Depression Rating Scale Revised (CDRS-R), the Child Depression Inventory (CDI) or Beck Depression Inventory (BDI), respectively, and the Clinical Global Impression Scale (CGI). Side effects were assessed weekly using a rating scale based on common adverse effects of SSRIs. Blood samples were taken from all participants and genetic material was extracted using PCR (Polymerase Chain Reaction). Genetic polymorphisms for TPH, 5-HTT, 5-HTR1A and 5-HTR2A, were determined with RFLPs (Restriction Fragment Length Polymorphisms) and VNTRs (Variable Number of Tandem Repeats). Statistical methods included one-way ANOVA with repeated measures and paired-sample t tests. **Results:** Sixty-nine subjects completed the study (mean age in years 14.04 ± 2.67). Citalopram produced clinically and statistically significant improvement (CGI$\leq$2) in 46 out of 69 subjects (67%). 23 subjects (33%) showed little or no improvement (CGI$\geq$3). No major adverse reactions were associated with citalopram use. Results of the genetic investigations are pending and will be presented at the congress. **Conclusion:** Citalopram is useful and well tolerated for the acute treatment of anxious and depressed children and adolescents. The pharmacogenetic profile of citalopram for treatment response and adverse effects will be delineated in the process.

P-001-005 Topic: 17, 6

A comparison of cognitive-behavioural therapy and pharmacotherapy for adolescent depression:
The time for a future project

Nicola Williams, Monash University, Developmental Psychology, Melbourne, Australia,
nicola.williams@med.monash.edu.au
Bruce Tonge; Neville King; Glenn Melvin; Amanda Dudley; Michael Gordon; Ester Klimkeit

Objective: The present study compared the efficacy of cognitive-behavioural therapy (CBT) with a selective serotonin reuptake inhibitor [sertraline] (MED) and a combination of both treatments in a clinical sample of adolescents with major depressive disorder, dysthymic disorder or depressive disorder not otherwise specified. It was hypothesised that (1) all three treatments would result in significant gains following treatment and that (2) COMB would lead to superior outcomes compared to CBT or MED alone. **Methods:** 73 depressed adolescents aged 12-18 years were randomly allocated to a treatment group. A multi-method, multi-informant assessment package was completed pre-treatment, post-acute treatment and at a six-month follow-up to assess treatment outcome and maintenance of gains. CBT consisted of 12×50 minute individual sessions for both young person and parents, followed by 3 booster sessions at one-month intervals. Sertraline was administered for 12 to 24 weeks and was monitored weekly to fortnightly for side-effects and response. Data was analysed using an intent-to-treat strategy with the last observation carried forward method. **Results:** The first hypothesis was supported. At post-treatment and follow-up assessment significant gains were evident on the outcome measures for all treatment groups. The second hypothesis was not supported. COMB did not result in outcomes that were significantly different to either CBT or MED. Rather, CBT showed a superior response to treatment compared with MED at post treatment assessment for those with major depressive disorder, however no difference was evident at follow-up. Sertraline was generally well tolerated. Side effects were responsible for treatment discontinuation for three adolescents. **Conclusion:** Both CBT and MED were effective in the treatment of adolescent depression. Explanations for the lack of superiority of COMB and clinical implications are presented.

P-001-006 Topic: 15, 84

The COMACS study: Effect of ADHD subtype on the treatment effects

Simon Hatch, Celltech Americas, Inc., Clinical Development, Rochester, NY, USA, simon.hatch@celltechgroup.com
John Breddy; Heleen DeCory; Sara Cameron; Mary Solanto

Objective: he COMACS study compared the effects of Metadate(r) CD (methylphenidate HCl, USP) Extended-Release Capsules (expected to be marketed as Equasym(r) XL in Europe, MCD) and Concerta(r) (methylphenidate hydrochloride) Extended-Release Tablets (CON) in 184 children aged 6 to 12 years with ADHD. Overall, the preparation with the highest predicted methylphenidate plasma concentration showed the greatest treatment effect at any given assessment time. The objective of this *post-hoc* analysis was to investigate the effect of ADHD subtype on these observations. **Methods:** The COMACS study was a multi-center, double-blind, double-dummy, randomized, placebo-controlled, three-way crossover study. Children were stratified, based on their pre-study methylphenidate dosage, to comparable daily doses of MCD and CON or to placebo. On the 7th day of each treatment week, children attended an analog school for assessments (Swanson, Kotkin, Agler, M/Flynn, Pelham [SKAMP] scale and academic performance) at 1.5-hour intervals. For the *post-hoc* analysis, SKAMP Deportment and Attention scores at each session (all dose levels combined) were analysed using a random-effects repeated measures general linear model with between-subject fixed effects of site and ADHD subtype and within-subject fixed effects of treatment and session. All two-way interactions of between-subject effects and within-subject effects were included in the model. The interaction of ADHD subtype, treatment and session was also fitted. **Results:** The effect of ADHD subtype was statistically significant on Deportment scores [$F(2,145) = 3.61$;

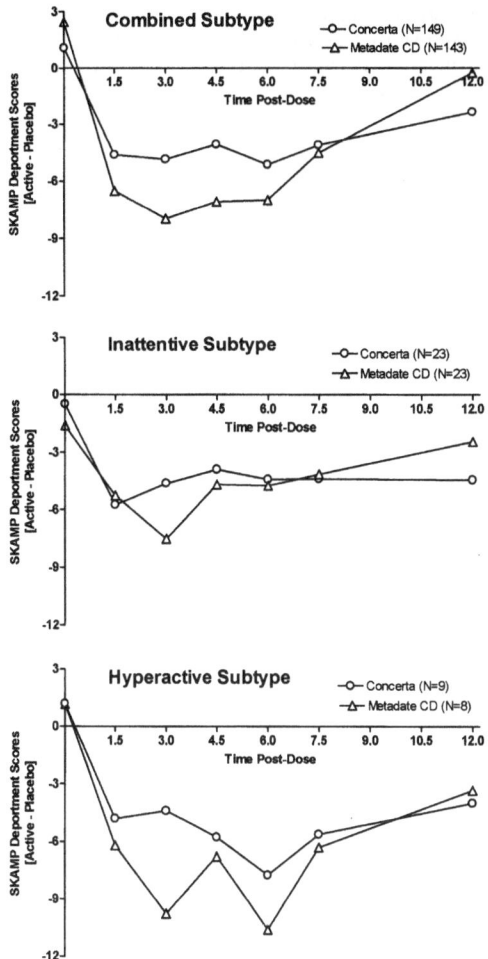

p=0.0294] but not on Attention scores [F(2,144)=1.73; p=0.1814]. The interactions of ADHD subtype and treatment and ADHD subtype, treatment and session were not statistically significant for Deportment scores [F(4,290)= 0.42; p=0.7932; and F(24,1740)=1.08; p=0.3562, respectively] or Attention scores [F(4,288)=0.85; p=0.4918; and F(24,1728)=0.91; p=0.5829, respectively]. **Conclusion:** While there was an overall difference between subtypes in overall mean change in Deportment scores, there were no significant differences between subtypes in the time-course of treatment effects for either Attention or Deportment scores.

P-001-007   Topic: 15
The efficacy of methylphenidate for ODD comorbid with ADHD

Maria Serra-Pinheiro, Rio de Janeiro, Brazil, totasp@hotmail.com
Isabella Sousa; Paulo Mattos; Fernanda Gomes; Giuseppe Pastura

Objective: To assess the efficacy of methylphenidate in causing a remission of ODD comorbid with ADHD. **Methods:** Patients with ADHD and ODD defined by DSM-IV criteria were assessed and treated with incremental doses of methylphenidate until they achieved remission of

ADHD, defined by less than 5 symptoms graded as 3 on the DuPaul rating scale. At least four months after remission of ADHD, they were reassessed for ODD. **Results:** Nine of the 10 patients achieved remission, no longer fulfilling diagnostic criteria for ODD. **Conclusion:** Methylphenidate is an efficient therapy for ODD comorbid with ADHD

P-001-008   Topic: 12, 69
Risperidone in treatment of children and adolescents with refractory psychotic disorders

Smiljka Popovic-Deusic, Institute for Mental Health, Belgrade, Serbia and Montenegro, imz@imh.org.yu
Olivera Aleksic; Milica Pejovic-Milovancevic; Vesna Milinkovic

Objective: Efficacy and safety of Risperidone is the main reason to be used as first or second choice in treatment of children and adolescents with psychosis, especially those sensitive to classical antypsychotics. It is also used in treatment of mood disorders, early child psychosis, conduct disorders etc. To investigate the efficasy of Risperidone in tretament of children and adolescents with schizophrenia and refractory psychotic disorders. **Methods:** We treated 25 children and adolescents with schizophrenia and refractory psychotic disorders with Risperidone (dose range 3–6 mg/day). Monthly evaluation with PANSS (Positive and negative syndrome scale for schizophrenia) and CGI (Clinical global impression) were used to measure treatment efficacy. Side effects were carefuly monitored. **Results:** 70% of patients decreased in total PANSS score. Positive and negative symptoms persisted with social impairment: CGI severity from 0,75 to 2,00 (index of effectivity). **Conclusion:** Risperidone was effective in 70% of cases with a wide range of psychotic disorders. It proved to be useful and safe for patients sensitive to classical neuroleptics. The advantage of Risperidone was presence of its solution enabling easier administration of medication to young psychotic children.

P-001-009   Topic: 12, 69
Toxic megacolon and other severe gastrointestinal side effects of clozapine – case report and review of the literature

Oliver Bilke, Humboldt-Klinikum, Kinder- und Jugendpsychiatrie, Berlin, Germany, oliver.bilke@vivantes.de
Sibille Kühnel; Bernhard Winterfeld

Objective: To evaluate the relevance of gastrointestinal side effects of clozapine in adolescent schizophrenic disorders that can be easily misdiagnosed as body-hallucinations or gynecological problems. A single case study with very severe symptoms illustrates the topic. **Methods:** Literature research: We screened the regular data bases, thoroughly asked the pharmaceutical firm producing clozapine in Switzerland and searched the internet. Case study: A 16 year old girl with schizo-affective disorder and anorexia (BMI=15) who did not respond on olanzapine and other new atypic neuroleptics was treated successfully with clozapine with a dosage of 300 mg/day. When fluoxetine was added due to depression, she suddenly developed a severe toxic megacolon (Ogilvie-syndrome)that had to be treated as an emergency in the internal department. **Results:** Gastrointestinal side effects such as constipation are a well known problem in clozapine treatment. The cumulative incidence of ileus or other possibly life-threatening side effects on the other hand is indicated as 0.02–0.05% of all reported cases. Clozapine being combined with SSRIs in the treatment of postschizophrenic depression possibly increases the incidence of gastrointestinal side-effects, as several publications indicate. Although clozapine is a well known drug, severe gastrointestinal side effects being rare but dangerous should be focused in adolescent patients. **Conclusion:** Constipation and undecisive abdominal pain in clozapine patients have to be taken very seriously, as they may be signs of a beginning ileus or other obstructive process which can be fatal when not detected and sufficiently treated.

P-001-010   Topic: 13, 75

An open trial of Citalopram for pediatric recurrent abdominal pain

John Campo, Western Psychiatric Institute, Psychiatry, Pittsburgh, PA, USA, campojv@msx.upmc.edu
James Perel; David Axelson; Jeff Bridge; Boris Birmaher; Neal Ryan; David Brent

Objective: To assess the potential efficacy, acceptability, and safety of citalopram as a treatment for functional recurrent abdominal pain (RAP) and comorbid anxiety and depression in children and adolescents. **Methods:** Twenty-five clinically referred children and adolescents with RAP aged 7 to 18 years, inclusive, participated in a 12-week, flexible dose, open-label trial of citalopram. Primary outcome measure was the Clinical Global Impression Scale-Improvement (CGI-I), with responders defined by ratings of 1 (very much improved) or 2 (much improved). Secondary measures included self and parent reports of abdominal pain, anxiety, depression, other somatic symptoms, and functional impairment. Side effects were assessed using a standardized checklist. Data were analyzed using an intent-to-treat format and the last measurement carried forward procedure. **Results:** Twenty-one subjects (84%) were classified as responders. Abdominal pain, anxiety, depression, other somatic symptoms, and functional status all improved significantly over the course of the study compared to baseline. Citalopram was generally well tolerated. Four subjects withdrew prematurely, one due to reported visual side effects. Suicidal thinking decreased progressively from baseline, and all subjects denied suicidal ideation at study completion. **Conclusion:** Citalopram is a promising treatment for functional pediatric RAP and deserves additional study via a randomized, placebo controlled clinical trial.

P-001-011   Topic: 15, 34

An efficacy comparison of Equasym XL capsules and Concerta tablets: A re-analysis of the COMACS study

Simon Hatch, Celltech Americas, Inc., Clinical Development, Rochester, NY, USA, simon.hatch@celltechgroup.com
Edmund J.S. Sonuga-Barke; Dorothea Y. Sanchez

Objective: The COMACS study compared the clinical effects of nearly equal daily doses of two once-daily extended-release formulations of methylphenidate HCl in 184 children with ADHD; (Equasym® XL [also marketed as Metadate® CD] and Concerta®). In clinical practice total daily doses of Concerta (CON) are generally higher than total daily doses of Equasym XL (EQSXL); the objective of this post-hoc analysis was to compare the efficacy of non-equivalent dose strengths of EQSXL and CON. **Methods:** The COMACS study was a multi-center, double-blind, randomized, placebo-controlled, three-way crossover study. EQSXL, CON, and placebo were each given for one full week. On day 7 of each week, children attended an analog school for assessment of attention and behaviour (SKAMP scale). For this post-hoc analysis, total SKAMP scores at each session were analysed across doses using Analysis of Covariance. **Results:** The comparison of EQSXL-20 mg and CON-36 mg revealed that EQSXL was superior to CON at 1.5 hours and that the 2 treatments did not differ from 3 through 7.5 hours after dose administration ($p < 0.05$). However, CON was superior to EQSXL at 12 hours. The comparison of EQSXL-40 mg and CON-54 mg revealed no difference from 1.5 through 6 hours. CON was superior to EQSXL at 7.5 hours and at 12 hours. While comparison of EQSXL-40 mg and CON-18 mg revealed that EQSXL was superior at all early time points, there was no difference between formulations at 7.5 and 12 hours (similarly for EQSXL-60 mg versus CON-36 mg). **Conclusion:** These results suggest that the delivery profiles of EQSXL and CON can be exploited to limit total daily exposure to MPH while targeting a specific period of the day for maximum efficacy. Further studies with random assignment to doses are necessary to confirm these findings.

P-001-012   Topic: 17

Open label prospective trial of Risperidone in combination with Lithium or Divalproex Sodium in pediatric mania

Mani Pavuluri, University of Illinois, Child Psychiatry, Chicago, USA, mpavuluri@psych.uic.edu
David B. Henry; Julie A. Carbray; Gwendolyn Sampson; Michael W. Naylor; Philip G. Janicak

Objective: This prospective 6-month open trial examined the safety and efficacy of two combination therapies for manic or mixed episodes of pediatric bipolar disorder: 1) divalproex sodium plus risperidone (DVPX + isp), or 2) lithium plus risperidone (Li + Risp). **Methods:** Thirty-seven (37) subjects aged 5 and 18 (age = 12.1 ± 3.5 years) with DSM IV current mixed or manic episode and Young Mania Rating Scale (YMRS) score >20 were sequentially assigned to either DVPX + Risp or Li + Risp in a 6-month, prospective open-label trial. Outcome measures included the YMRS, Clinical Global Impression Scale for Bipolar Disorder (CGI-BP), Child Depression Rating Scale-Revised (CDRS-R) as well as measures of safety and tolerability. **Results:** Effect sizes (Cohen's d) based on change of YMRS scores from baseline were 4.36 for DVPX+Risp and 2.82 for Li+Risp. Response rates (50% change from baseline YMRS score at the end of study) were 80% for DVPX+Risp and 82.4% for Li+Risp. Both combination treatments were well tolerated. Significant improvements ($p < 0.001$) from baseline were seen for mean scores on all efficacy measures, i.e., YMRS, CGI-BP and CDRS-R. There were no significant group differences in safety or tolerability, and no serious adverse events during the 6-month trial. **Conclusion:** Both DVPX+Risp and Li+Risp show strong effects coupled with safety and tolerability in treating children and adolescents with manic or mixed episodes associated with type I bipolar disorder.

P-001-013   Topic: 12, 28
Clozapine-induced weight gain:
A study in MZ twins and same-sexed sib pairs
Stefan Gebhardt, Universität Marburg, Klinik für Psychiatrie, Marburg, Germany, stefan.gebhardt@med. uni-marburg.de
Frank Theisen; Michael Haberhausen; Monika Heinzel-Gutenbrunner; Peter Wehmeier; Jürgen-Christian Krieg; Wolfgang Kühnau; Jörg Schmidtke; Helmut Remschmidt; Johannes Hebebrand

Objective: To assess the relative contribution of genetic factors in antipsychotic-induced weight gain, we explored the similarity in BMI (kg/m^2) change under clozapine of 5 monozygotic (MZ) twins in comparison with 7 same-sexed sibs. **Methods:** Twin and sib pairs were identified by a telephone screening of 786 practicing psychiatrists. Measured data on weight and other clinical variables were obtained cross-sectionally and retospectively from medical records. Clozapine ΔBMI (treatment period with clozapine) and total ΔBMI (pretreatment with other antipsychotics plus treatment with clozapine) were investigated. **Results:** We found greater similarity in total ΔBMI in MZ twins (intrapair difference 2.78 ± 3.41 kg/m^2) than in same-sexed sibs (5.55 ± 4.35 kg/m^2), resulting in heritability estimates of $h2=0.8$ and $A=0.45$ (ACE twin model). However, intrapair differences in clozapine ΔBMI were similar between twins and sibs. **Conclusion:** We hypothesize that the weight plateau achieved under clozapine is influenced by genetic factors. The weight gain achieved during pretreatment with other antipsychotics seemingly limits clozapine-induced weight gain, thus presumably explaining why heritability is greater for total ΔBMI than for clozapine ΔBMI.

P-001-013A   Topic: 13
Serum levels of SSRI in adolescents
with psychiatric disorders
Hans-Willi Clement, Uni-Krankenhaus Freiburg, Kinder- und Jugendpsychiatrie, Freiburg, Germany, clement@psyallg.ukl.uni-freiburg.de
Christian Fleischhaker; Klaus Hennighausen; Eberhard Schulz

Objective: Selective-serotonin-reuptake-inhibitors (SSRI) are found to be effective in the treatment of depression, obsessive compulsive disorder, and anxiety. In this study the serum levels of SSRI were correlated to the therapeutic window suggested by the tiaft (The International Association of Forensic Toxicologists) for adults. **Methods:** Serum levels of the SSRI's fluvoxamine, citalopram, paroxetine, sertraline, and its metabolite norsertraline, have been studied using HPLC with UV-detection. **Results:** At doses of citalopram between 10 and 40 mg/day serum levels between 8 and 144 ng/ml serum have been found. Most often used is fluvoxamine, with serum levels between 14 and 275 ng/ml serum with doses between 25 and 250 mg/day. Especially in the case of fluvoxamine, but also for citalopram, strong interindividual variations of the serum levels, up to tenfold, could be observed, indicating that monitoring of the serum levels is helpful in dose adjustment. **Conclusion:** In adolescents the serum levels of sertraline and norsertraline are found to be significantly lower as compared to adults. For Paroxetine serum levels seem to be no good indicator for therapeutic response. In summary it seems to be useful to establish therapeutic windows for SSRís for adolescents.

P-002
Care, treatment and prevention II
Track: Therapy and intervention

P-002-014   Topic: 4, 23
Which physicians cooperate with child and adolescent psychiatry?
Reiner Frank, Med. Universität München, Kinder- und Jugendpsychiatrie, München, Germany, reiner.frank@med.uni-muenchen.de
Belda Karamete

Objective: The aim of the present study is to describe pathways of cooperation between an outpatient department of child and adolescent psychiatry and physicians and to describe, how these physicians perceive the cooperation with our department. We present preliminary results. **Methods:** From 121 patients and their parents, who had been in our outpatient department during the years 1999 and 2000, satisfaction with treatment was elicited. From a chart review, all physicians known to be in contact with these patients were identified. A questionnaire was developed analogous to the questionnaire for the evaluation of patient satisfaction with treatment (Mattejat and Remschmidt 1998). A postal survey was done with up to three mailings. **Results:** For 121 patients we identified 186 physicians, about 1,5 physician per patient. There were six groups of physicians: general practitioners, paediatricians, physicians working at hospitals for child and adolescent psychiatry, physicians at hospitals in different somatic fields – such as paediatrics, surgery or neurology –, child and adolescent psychiatrists in private practice and 'others'. The first two groups are engaged in primary care (n=93, paediatricians=63, general practitioners=30). They send patients to our institution. We pass some patients for inpatient treatment to the department for child and adolescent psychiatry outside the Umiversity. Within the clinicum of the University patients from different specialties are sent for evaluation and support and go back for conjoint care. **Conclusion:** The outpatient department of child and adolescent psychiatry is a point of intersection between outpatient primary and specialized care and inpatient hospital care. In a next step the degree of satisfaction concerning the cooperation with our institute will be analyzed.

P-002-015   Topic: 2
The Maja-project: A new working method
to handle increasing numbers of patients
Gunnel Löndahl, Malmö University Hospital, Child & Adolescent Psychiatry, Malmö, Sweden, gunnel.londahl@skane.se
Peik Gustafsson; Anneli Parnegård

Objective: Viewing increasing numbers of new patients to child and adolescent psychiatry in Sweden during the 1990s, without the equivalent increase in resources, the department in Malmö started a 3-year project in autumn 2001 in order to develop methods for diversified care and treatment in groups for patients and their parents. The objectives are to integrate new ways of evidence based treatment in ordinary routine work and to offer qualitatively good care for more patients. **Methods:** COPE – A parent education program; Cool Kids – group program for children with anxiety disorders; group programs for adolescents with depressive and eating disorders. Meetings for information to parents. BCFPI (Brief Child and Family Phone interview) - a databased screening interview. **Results:** The total project will be evaluated after the summer of 2004. We have however noticed very content patients and parents so far, noticing better quality in care and better structured treatment. Some 85% of the staff working with outpatients are involved and are content with the way of working. **Conclusion:** We have found a way of dealing with overwhelming large numbers of patients. The methods will be developed further and more patients will be included in group therapy.

P-002-016 Topic: 4
Day care treatment in psychiatry of developmental age: Analysis of therapeutic factors

Giancarlo Rigon, Neuropsichiatria Infantile,
Dip. de Psichiatria, Bologna, Italy, girigon@libero.it
Simona Chiodo; Alessandra Mancaruso;
Daniele Giovanni Poggioli; Stefano Costa

Objective: In this paper the authors analize diagnosis, the entry reasons, the level of functioning (with CGAS scale) of 178 patients, followed in the day hospital of the Child and Adolescent Psychiatry and Psychotherapy Department, during the year 2002. **Methods:** Different therapeutical factors of the intensive treatment have been analized: individual psychotherapy, parents support, psychopharmacology, educational intervention. **Results:** The authors have underlined the specific and aspecific therapeutical factors and their respective influence on the result of the treatment. A statistical analysis has been done.

P-002-017 Topic: 4, 2
Connection model for primary health care: Child and Adolescent Psychiatry Unit Hospital Garcia de Orta, Portugal

Pedro Pires, Hospital Garcia de Orta, Unidade de
Pedopsiquiatria, Almada, Portugal, marymary@clix.pt
Isabel Brito; Isabel Carvalho; Sara Almeida; Paula Zaragoza

Objective: A Child and Adolescent Psychiatry Unit, recently constituted, located in a Primary Health Care Centre with connection to the area Hospital, established as main target the empowerment of its Primary Health Care professionals. The authors present a connection model between the child and adolescent psychiatry and the primary health care. **Methods:** A Primary Health Care Centre was chosen as a pilot for the implementation of the connection model. It was designed an articulation protocol in which were defined the creation of a mental health care team in this institution. It was established that there would be a monthly joint meeting between the health care technicians and the child and adolescent psychiatry unit, in which a theoretical theme on mental care issue, previously defined, would be discussed along with some clinical cases. Afterwards, there would be a more restricted reunion between the mental health care centre team and the child and psychiatry unit. A previous technical knowledge evaluation was performed by the primary health care professionals, with a multiple answer questionnaire. This evaluation will be repeated at the end of one year. **Results:** Six months after the implementation of this project, it has been taking place an active participation from the technicians, resulting in: – Better data gathering for child and adolescent psychiatry cases; – Psychiatric interventions with greater efficiency; – Maximization of human and com-

munity resources; – Discussion of clinical cases evolving different health care areas; – Anguish contention of the health care technicians. **Conclusion:** Preliminary results reinforce the importance of establishing well defined criteria in the articulation between the child and adolescent psychiatric unit and primary health care. This relationship should be privileged inside this kind of psychiatric units.

P-002-018 Topic: 9, 11
Training of emotional competency

Yury Shevchenko, Ass. of Child Psychiatrists, and
Psychologists, Moscow, Russia, acpp@online.ru
Vasilisa Korneeva

The proposed technique is conceptually based on the thesis that verbal and emotional processes are interrelated. The training is carried out in groups and using video equipment. The goal is to improve the participants' capability to acquire and distinguish non-verbal signs of emotions, identify and reproduce them arbitrary and thus adequately comprehend and assess personal needs-related context of the communicative situation. The training includes three levels (stages). The first level. Development of emotional impressiveness-expressiveness. 1. One of the participants within a group has to produce non-verbal reaction to a phrase conveying the idea of accusation or hindrance addressed to him. All other participants within the group translate it into the words of natural language thus trying to guess the meaning of response. 2. The protagonist chooses the best "translation" of his non-verbal response repeating its wording. The group assesses the congruency of the meaning of the phrase to the intonation with which it had been pronounced. The second level. Extending emotional-behavioral "repertory". Frustrating stimulus as well as unexpected provocations of positive emotions are introduced. 1. Within a minute the probationer has to give three alternative congruent replies. 2. The reply then is deciphered and its emotional quality is found out. Then the identified emotion is brought into correlation with cognitive meaning of the situation stimulating emotion. 3. Within one minute each of the participants should give three alternative responses to the situation stimulating emotion, verbalize its attendant emotion as well as his own cognitive appraisal of the situation and suggests course of its development. The third level. Cognitive-behavioral training. 1. Getting familiarized with the basic theses of the Theory of Emotions by P.V. Simonov and Conception of Frustration Tolerance by C. Rosenzvage. 2. Classifying frustration reactions being demonstrated according to their type and orientation in standard situations, individual conflicts and spontaneous conflicts during the group trainings. 3. Training of constructive behavior and finding balance between adaptation to emotionally significant situation and mastering it.

P-002-019 Topic: 6, 78
Behavioural therapy of Anorexia Nervosa (AN) in a 13-year old girl: Short-term aims in inducing weight gain and combinations of behavioural procedures

Miodrag Stankovic, Clinic for Mental Health,
Dept. of Child Neuropsychiatry, Belgrade,
Serbia and Montenegro, s-misa@eunet.yu
Aneta Lakic; Vesna Milovanovic; Sandra Stankovic

Objective: There are widely divergent views of the nature of anorexia nervosa. There is, therefore, no comprehensive approach to treatment of anorexia nervosa based on a sound empirical research. Objective of our research was to examine the behavioral therapy of anorexia nervosa in reducing fattening phobia and inducing weight gain in one inpatient girl. **Methods:** A 13-year old girl was accepted to the Child and Adolescent Neuropsychiatry Clinic with a 2-year history of disturbed eating behavior and a 6-month starvation with recent rapid weight loss up to 29 kg (BMI = 11). The patient met the ICD-10 and DSM-IV criteria for a restrictive type of anorexia nervosa according Structured Interwiev on Anorexic and Bulimic Disorders (SIAB-EX). We also carried out standardized psychopathological examinations as well as family functioning. After 3 weeks of baseline period of hospitalisation, during the next 7 weeks we combined behavioural therapy procedures: operant conditioning, flooding, relaxation in reduction of fattening phobia and planning a short term aims of weight gain with patient. **Results:** During the first 3 weeks of an inpatient treatment, patient ate three regular meals and two snacks. Her eating was monitored, but she gained no weight because she started vomiting and doing exercise. During the next 7 weeks weight gain was significantly induced by planning a short term aims of weight gain and combining of behavioural therapy procedures. Assertive training was beneficially influenced in social/family communications skills. After 10 week of inpatient treatment, discharge was followed by 9 kg weight gain and eating behavior was normalized. During 12 weeks of outpatient period her weight was maintained. **Conclusion:** Induction of behavior therapy procedures was characterized by great benefit in this case after 3 weeks of baseline period of hospitalisation with no weight gain. Planning a short term of weight gain together with patient has been showed as especially useful procedure.

P-002-020   Topic: 9, 11
Technique of self-regulation of emotional states
Vasilisa Korneeva, Ass. of Child Psychiatrists and Psychologists, Moscow, Russia, acpp@online.ru
Yury Shevchenko

Developing self-regulation, e.g. ability to voluntary control one's emotions as well as their outer expression constitutes one of the essential stages in the process of forming emotional and volitional sphere. The proposed technique is purposed to be used with adolescents and adults. The goal of psychotherapeutic measures is to learn how to master negative emotions evolved irrespectively to the situation present. 1. The client makes a list of negative emotions and marks out those which are the most frequent with him and which he most suffers. 2. The individual is proposed to create symbolic images of these states. Accomplishment of this task is facilitated by the algorithm according to which the qualities are determined on the basis of principle pair of comparison. After this work had been done the client is to make out or to draw a picture (make a photo) of 'still life' of the items associated with these qualities. 3. Then the qualities of positive emotions are analyzed. For each negative state there should be selected the corresponding one from the whole spectrum of positive emotions, the one with the most similar qualities and the least different. Then the 'still life' representing the negative emotion is altered so that 'minus-signed' mood is turned into the 'plus signed' one. The proposed technique is based on the principle rather similar to that of the well-knows techniques developed to facilitate fears fighting (metaphoric materialization, operations with the displacing object, desactualization). The basic

difference between them is that the first one implies materialization not of an object stimulating the emotion but the emotion itself, e.g. deals with generalization and abstraction on the higher level. Second, this technique is based on combining abstract conceptual thinking with sensual-concrete, creative and spatial one and thus stimulates interhemispheric activity. Third, working on the 'still life' task the patient 'turns' into an artist creating a small 'work of art' which not only helps harmonization of emotional sphere of a person but also contributes to one's individual development because that, in some indirect way, effects one's ideology.

P-002-021   Topic: 9
Ontogenesis-oriented technique of emotional development
Vasilisa Korneeva, Ass. of Child Psychiatrists, and Psychologists, Moscow, Russia, acpp@online.ru
Yury Shevchenko

As related to its ontogenesis development of emotions includes not only differentiation in their qualities and complication of objects causing the emotional response but also development of capability of controlling emotions as well as their appearance. According to neuropsychological researches verbal and emotional processes are interrelated. Within the frameworks of an integrated program aimed at harmonization of emotional and volition sphere of an individual we have developed the certain correction and teaching technique which helps not only to fight alexithymia but also to improve intellectual sphere because it employs various mental operations such as properties distinguishing, comparison, analyses, synthesis, etc. This technique has been tested with a sampling group of children from 5 to 15 years old having neurotic, behavioral and psychosomatic disorders developed on the background of residual-organic cerebral insufficiency and proved to have considerable correctional effect. The technique is intended for the group work which includes the following impressive and expressive tasks: 1) Problem comprehension tasks: the discussions the point of which is to help children understand that all emotions of an individual can be divided into positive and negative ones. 2) Tasks aimed at differentiation of negative and positive emotions. For each emotion its particular features are found out by pair comparison and consequently each of these emotions gets correlated with certain sensory characteristics. 3) Tasks aimed at defining material correlations to the emotions referred to. Selecting visual (imagined) or physical equivalents of the emotional state (metaphoric images of emotions). 4) Tasks aimed at expression of emotions. Expressing emotions by of nonverbal means of expression using allegories in traditional and non-traditional combinations. 5) Tasks aimed at integration of the acquired skills. Creating "mise en scene" as well as game expression of respective emotional states using musical and sound supplement series.

P-002-022   Topic: 4
Daily purposes and therapeutic goals during inpatient treatment
Bernard Hobrücker, Universität zu Kiel, Kinder- und Jugendpsychiatrie, Kiel, Germany, hobruecker@t-online.de

Objective: The study refers to whether there is a relation between the extent to which daily purposes are realized, and other variables, especially the way in which children evaluate their treatment goals. It is hypothesized that the consistency of the evaluations as well as the relationship between importance and availability of goals may indicate a child's motivation to cooperate in therapy. **Methods:** The sample consists of 40 children aged 7 to 12, who had got an inpatient treatment for at least 6 weeks. Evaluation of goals is measured both by direct rankings and the method of paired comparisons. Realization of daily purposes is recorded in a simple ratio of "complete","partial" and "no success" to the number of days in treatment. **Results:** Results show that, beside clinical classification, it is especially the correlation between the ratings for importance and availability of treatment goals that may predict a child's realization of daily purposes: children who rate certain goals both as highly important and easily available tend to be weak "realizers" of daily purposes. Vice versa children with a zero or negative correlation between importance and availability of goals more often have succeeded in realizing their purposes. **Conclusion:** Evaluation of therapeutic goals as well as the application of daily purposes are useful means to enable children to take part in the therapeutic community of an inpatient treatment. In addition, they are apt to indicate children's motivation in therapy. Further research should concentrate upon the relation between these variables and direct measurement of children's motivation to cooperate.

P-002-023   Topic: 9

Possibilities of solution-focused group therapy with young sexual offenders

Filip Caby, Marienkrankenhaus,
Kinder- und Jugendpsychiatrie, Aschendorf, Germany, filip.
caby@t-online.de

Objective: We will present our experience with a solution-focused group therapy approach with young sexual offenders. **Methods:** The speech will discuss the results of a 3-year-experience working in an outpatient setting with sexual offenders, between 15 and 22 years of age. All participants have been accused officially, or have been sentenced to undergo psychotherapy. The presentation will show how to handle this very touchy matter in a solution-focused way, without neglecting the severeness of the crime. The systemic approach will already be outlined by the subjects involved: victim, legal system, family and working or studying environment of the offender. **Results:** Among other aspects, we will try to answer the following questions: How can it be achieved to integrate all subjects involved into the therapeutic process? Will a therapy contract be necessary? For how long should therapy be offered? Which criteria can we define for discharge? **Conclusion:** Working with young sexual offenders in a solution-focused setting is another helpful approach in order to deal with this sensitive pyschiatric matter.

P-002-024   Topic: 4

Emergency concept in child and adolescent psychiatry

Jean Chambry, Fondation Vallee, Gentilly, France,
jean.chambry@wanadoo.fr
Stéphane Laudrin; Catherine Graindorge

Objective: The emergency concept in child psychiatry is difficult, especially like the model of the medical urgencies. It is also applicate for dibtem suffering from psychotics episodes. However, this type of pathology does not seem to constitute the majority of the requests for hospitalisation. The mean objective is to show that emergency in child psychiatry exists in old pathologies, which results in crises. The secondary objective is to show the specificity of this work and the significance of psychoanalytical approach. **Methods:** 107 patients hospitalised between 1/01/03 and 12/12/03 in the emergency unit of child and adolescent psychiatry Fondation Valleé Kremlin Bicêtre France. Descriptive statistical analysis: For the qualitative variables we determined the distribution frequencies of each variable and for the quantitative variables we calculated a measurement of central tendency (mean) and a measurement of dispersal (standard deviation). Three cases report will be approached to illustrate the conclusions of this study. **Results:** 107 patients, age between 10 and 18 years, sex ratio: 1, 55% already consulted, duration of hospitalisation 21 days (range: 1 à 107 days) 75% return to parent's residence. A patient is brought to emergency hospital, generally for disorders, which have a behavioural expression: suicide, conduct disorders. The request is generally carried by the parents, which wish a solution with the problem arising from this abnormal behaviour. Solution, which extends from the consultation that will make it possible to the young person to evacuate all his psychic difficulties. Requests where it is necessary to transform the urgency to act in urgency of listening. The urgency is generally side of external reality and not side of internal reality. We have to look how to investigate the model of the therapeutic consultation described by Winicott. We constitute an intermediate surface between the child, his external family and referents. We open the subject with the value of psychic operation. The teenager keeps in him this time of experiment to develop it elsewhere. **Conclusion:** This type of unit takes value of transitional space for the adolescent who can develop its subjectivity what affirms the value of the therapeutic process in the tradition of the institutional cure. It offers also a third space to the referents teams that find their therapeutic dimension thus. With the interface of external reality and internal reality, this unit conceived starting from a model of care heir to the psychoanalysis, takes all its value then: a true care in the care, a true care of the care.

P-002-025   Topic: 7, 11

Psychotherapeutic intervention to maltreated children and adolescents in residential care

Arata Oiji, Japan Women's University, Dept. of Psychology,
Kawasaki City, Japan, aoiji@fc.jwu.ac.jp
Yukiko Morioka; Ami Murata; Madoka Sato;
Yume Hashizume

Objective: Most of maltreated children and adolescents separated from their parents are cared in "child nursing homes" in Japan. The authors tried to extract common therapeutic factors and problems in psychotherapeutic intervention to maltreated children and adolescents in residential care. **Methods:** The authors examined case records of children and adolescents (n = 32) who have been maltreated by their parents and received individual psychotherapy in a child nursing home. Two of the authors have been conducting individual psychotherapy for them. The first author has been supervising their psychotherapy and psychiatric consultant for the home. **Results:** The authors extracted ten therapeutic factors as follows: (1) reenactment of traumatic experiences, (2) testing therapists and staff, (3) recollection of traumatic experiences, (4) regression, (5) "sibling rivalry", (6) question about meaning of the birth and life, (7) acquiring ability of expressing their emotions and pains verbally, (8) acquiring self control and self esteem, (9) questing for sexual and gender identity, (10) perspective for the future. The authors found four therapeutic problems as follows: (1) regressive behaviors, (2) sexual acting out, (3) violent acting out, (4) confidentiality. **Conclusion:** In the psychotherapeutic intervention to maltreated children and adolescents, we should have knowledge about psychological effects of traumatic and/or neglectful environment to children, group dynamics, child and adolescent psychiatry and developmental psychology. We should pay close attention to psychotherapeutic process of each child or adolescent and share information about the process with care taking staff.

P-002-026 Topic: 5, 3
The organization of the rehabilitation process in the residential home for children and adolescents "Leppermühle"

Katarina Müller, Buseck, Germany,
katarina.mueller@lepper.med.uni-giessen.de
Willigis Werner; Matthias Martin; Eva Mattejat

Objective: The residential home for children and adolescents "Leppermühle" in Buseck near Giessen, Germany is an institution which focuses mainly on the rehabilitation of psychiatrically ill children and adolescents. The long-term goal is the intergration of the handicapped and those threatened by handicap into occupational and social life. The main emphasis is on the rehabilitation and long-term treatment of adolescents with chronic schizophrenia spectrum disorders, who require special care after the acute hospitalisation phase. **Methods:** Treatment comprises medication (psychopharmacological therapy, especially treatment with atypical antipsychotics), psychotherapy including behaviour modification methods, general care and physical therapy, educational guidance with training of social skills, school attendance and occupational rehabilitation. The poster gives an overview of the main components of the rehabilitation programme. **Results:** Two conditions turned out to be a major basis for a successful rehabilitation process: 1) The cooperation of different professions in a "multi-professional team" including medical specialists in child and adolescent psychiatry, psychotherapists, educators, teachers and (e.g. sport) instructors; 2) the organization of a sequence of decisions about interventions as "decision-making processes" in interaction between patients, their parents, the youth welfare department and the rehabilitation team.

P-002-027 Topic: 9
Psychotherapeutic group intervention in adolescents with eating disorders

Myriam Olivieri, A.O. Umberto Primo, Dipt. Clinica
Psichiatrica, Torrette-Ancona, Italy,
myriamolivieri@yahoo.com
Annalisa Simoncini; Sonia Marchegiani;
Marco Lazzorotto Muratori; Gabriele Borsetti

Objective: Eating disorders involve and throw into confusion the connection between mind, body and relation; their outbreak coincides often with the time of adolescence, that is that phase of growth which sees the body as receptacle of emotional discordances and individual and relational problems. In adolescence, experiences of separation, non-command, confusion between oneself and the Other flare up again; in this emotional chaos the group

culture holds a primary role, the tendency to gather is particularly felt and the conviviality with people of the same age encourages the process of separation from the parental figures. **Methods:** Convinced that the group setting could be the privileged place to receive and contain the suffering, and also a place where an individual can take again her history, we have formed a group, psychodynamically-oriented, addressed to adolescents suffering from eating disorders, who come to our clinic at the Psychiatric Department in Ancona. The participants, at present-day, are 7, all females, from 16 to 21 years old, coming from middle-class families and good schools; they distinguish for their conditions and for the duration of their disease. The group, guided by two therapists, is open, with 80 minutes weekly sessions, which take place in an institutional environment. **Results:** The psychotherapeutic work intends to develop the cohesion of the group to encourage its members to feel safe and to experience their diversities, and to create a work group which could face each time the emerging problems. The process of subjectivation of the adolescent affects and complicates the function of the group, which, besides letting express different moments of identification, facilitates the access to the dimension of the inner cluster and to its potentialities. The group device stimulates the production of reveries, helps to create images, metaphors, dreams, offers opportunities to symbolize, facing the frequent condition, in adolescence, of the loss of the symbolic thought and the limit between inside and outside.

P-002-028 Topic: 3, 84
Behavioural intervention versus Multimodal Treatment Approach (MTA) for Egyptian children with ADHD

Shewikar Farrag, University of Sheffield, Mental Health &
Learning Dis., Sheffield, United Kingdom,
shewikar_farrag@hotmail.com

Objective: To compare the effect of behaviour intervention on its own with the medication treatment combined with behaviour intervention applied by parents and teachers of children with ADHD. **Methods:** One hundred and twelve Egyptian children were selected from two settings (schools and clinic) in Alexandria & Mansoura, Egypt. Both research groups (Medication group and non-medication group)were placed on educational training program received by their parents and teachers in five weeks period. Behaviour assessment was done before and after the program using the Abbreviated Conner's parent teacher rating scales (10-items). Parents were interviewed before the induction of training program to know more information about child's history, condition, parenting styles utilised, and parents' perception of child's behaviours. Research has assessed parents' mental health condition during the interview using the Arabic version of GHQ-12. **Results:** Children with ADHD showed a marked behaviour improvement in both groups although the combined treatment (MTA) group showed better results as evidenced by their parents' and teachers' reports on the ACPTRS (10-items). **Conclusion:** The research findings support the idea that MTA approach is the best model of treatment to manage problems of children with ADHD.

P-002-029 Topic: 10

Supporting parenthood: The adversities and achievements of a group of parents of individuals suffering from eating disorders

*Myriam Olivieri, A.O. Umberto Primo,
Dipt. Clinica Psichiatrica, Torrette-Ancona, Italy,
myriamolivieri@yahoo.com
Riccardo Coltrinari; Gabriele Borsetti*

Objective: We'd like to propose a reflection on the utility of a work of collaboration/support to the families in this type of psychopathology. **Methods:** In our outpatient' department we had a triennal experience in dealing with a group of 14 parents of teenagers suffering from eating disorders. At the moment, we're working with a new psycho-analytical-group (10 parents), half-opened, carried out by a therapist and a silent-participant. In a first instance, we receive and contain confusional and catastrophical anxieties and we direct our work towards the building of an alliance with the parents, aiming to sustain those parental skills that have been jeopardised by the emotional troubles within the family relations. **Conclusion:** The opportunity of sharing one's own suffering with other members within the group, creates strong bonds and an atmosphere of mutual trust that allows the gradual storage within the group matrix, of conjugal and trans-familiar conflicts as far as including the trans-generational dimensions of the familiar conflict, radicated in the family history. This reference to family's history does not aim to an archeological research but to understand the presence of a process of recurrence of the past, a past that recurs as an ineluctable fate. This reference allows to recognise and separate the known but not thought experiences of the parents' childhood, from their daughter's different needs, character and existential reality, previously mistaken for their own children's and adoloscent sides that have not been elaborated and therefore, separated and projected. In these teenager's families we witness a conflictuality embodied in eating problems referring to a confused and problematic parents' Oedipus condition, which results, so often, in an eating disorder or in a depression in the mother's versant. Therefore, the confusion derived from the parents' projections have soaked up all those energies that should have been available to the formation and growth of their daughter.

P-002-030 Topic: 6

Impact of cognitive behaviour therapy of children with depressive symptoms

*Doa Habib, Child Mental Health, Association Alexandria,
Alexandria, Egypt, doa11@yahoo.com*

Objective: To evaluate the effectiveness of cognitive behaviour therapy for children with depressive symptoms, and gender response to the program. The WHO report 2001, mentioned that depression is among the most common and more disabling disorder globally. Childhood depression ranged 2–6% of school age population, and indicated that it has a serios significance on the child development and should not be reported as a transient phase of normal experience where it may have serious percusion in adult life. **Methods:** A randomised controlled sample conducted during the academic year 2003/2004, for students at their first year in middle-one in two schools from a poor district in Alexandria. One for boys (n = 198) the other for girls (n = 130). Child Depression Inventory (CDI) and Child

Self-Esteem (Cooper Smith Inventory) were used as tools to measure depression and self-esteem among the studied samples, in addition to a questionnaire developed including (recent life events & stressors, socio-demographic data and scholastic performance). Those showed high scores are subjected to 8-sessions for cognitive behaviour therapy (CBT), and assessed three months after intervention using the same tools of assessment. **Results:** Suggest the short-term effectiveness of cognitive behavioural approaches for managing depressive symptoms among school children, and it can be delivered on school campuses for preventig depression.

P-002-031 Topic: 2, 41

A five-year review of adolescent mental health usage in Singapore

*Daniel Fung, Institute of Mental Health, Child Guidance
Clinic, Singapore, Singapore, daniel_fung@imh.com.sg
Nelson Lee*

Objective: To provide a review of adolescent mental health service utilisation in a child and adolescent mental health outpatient clinic in Singapore. **Methods:** Data from all new adolescent cases seen over a five-year period in the Child Guidance Clinic were analysed. A review of services provided is also included. **Results:** Adolescent mental health usage has been on an increase with a rise in the number of cases diagnosed to have depression. There has also been an increase in the number of forensic cases seen in the department. **Conclusion:** There is a growing demand for adolescent mental health services. As the demands and stresses on today's youth increase, there is likely to be a continued increase in the demand for such services. The challenge in the future is to provide adolescent mental health services in cost effective packages that will meet the needs as well as stay financially viable.

P-002-032 Topic: 6

LINK-VIS: A computer program for visualizing the psychotherapeutical process of cognitive behavioral therapy (CBT)

*Susanne Ohmann, Medizin. Universität Wien,
Inst. für Neuropsychiatrie, Wien, Austria,
susanne.ohmann@meduniwien.ac.at
C. Popow; M. Lanzenberger; H. Herzog; S. Schuch;
S. Miksch*

Objective: Analysis of the psychotherapeutical process is a laborious task involving a large number of complexly related parameters and variables. Classical descriptive and test statistics can only insufficiently describe the multifacorial and multilayered transcations. Our project aims to visualize process variables of single and group therapies in order to make the course of psychotherapy intra- and interindividually comparable. **Methods:** We develped LINK-VIS, a computer program that visulaizes up to 13 variables within one glyph using Chernoff faces and related parallel coordinates and scatter plots. The data are derived from psychodiagnostic tools that are deployed before, during and after therapy. The program consists of various modules that allow for data input, interactive data selection, mapping and display. **Results:** We used the data collected in CBT group therapy of girls with AN for exploring the functionality and power of LINK-VIS and present examples of predictor and process analysis. **Conclusion:** LINK-

VIS is a powerful tool for analyzing tpsychotherapeutic processes. It facilitates cognition and allow for a more intuitive and deeper level of understanding.

P-002-033   Topic: 2, 41
A study of educational needs in adolescents in Mazandran state 2003
Fatemeh Abdollahy, Mazandaran University of Medical Sciences, Sari, Islamic Republic of Iran,
abdollahy@yahoo.com
S. Khani; B. Shabankhani

Objective: Hence planning for adolescent's preparing to pact with puberty must anticipate on careful in formation of their behaviour and educational needs and then proved educational information. This study done to determine KAP girls Secondary students about puberty health in Mazandaran State 2003. **Methods:** This research is an analytic study on 1708 Mazandaran adolescents (KAP) to education planning. Sampling was done by sequential method. Data was based on questionnaire, demographic data, awareness, attitude and peractic about puberty health. Based on results determined educational needs, data were analyzed with the SPSS, statistical analyse was done with variance analyses and regression based methods. **Results:** Mean age and mean age of menarche was 13/33 and 12/2 year respectively. Educational states of most parents were low (35%), 5.8% of girls knew a little about puberty and puberty health awareness was low (33.4%). Knowledge about bath and nutrition during menses was quit low (p < 0.0001). Instead of positive attitude to menstruation (73.3%) emotional attitude about that was weak (67.8%). Mothers were the first source of information in 62% of girls, resembling the suspected source of adolescent information for mestruation (p < 0.0001). A significant relationship was found between awareness and health practice (p < 0.0001). **Conclusion:** Despite of the wish of most girls to know more about puberty, their health information and practice about puberty was quite low. Mother were often the primary resource of health care information. The other important point is that informations were not limited to knowledge of puberty and menses mechanism, but rather are helped to a deeper understanding of physical and psychological changes and theirs connection with sex, fertility, marriage and health.

P-002-034   Topic: 2, 5
Inpatient care in a child and adolescent psychiatric unit: A 5 years revision
Joao Guerra, Porto, Portugal, joao.guerra@netc.pt
Claudia Fontes; Vania Martins; Ana Teles;
Corina Rodrigues; Zulmira Correia

Objective: The authors intend to review the admission causes and present the results of 3 years work in their inpatient unit. **Methods:** Revision of the literature concerning hospitalization in child and adolescent psychiatry and revision of the clinical files using astandardized form created for this purpose. **Results:** The majority of the sample was of the female sex and came mainly from the emergency unit in our hospital. The most prevalent admission cause was suicide attempt by drug ingestion. **Conclusion:** In our unit we adopted a comprehensive evaluation and treatment mode. This kind of unit is better adapted for this age group and pathology than a pediatric or an adult

psychiatry unit. The authors believe that this poster may be useful to improve our work and compare it with other units.

P-002-035   Topic: 7, 48
"Touch me not!": A gesture of detachment in Picasso's "La vie" suggesting a narcissistic defence mechanism in a conflict between mother and son
Peter Wehmeier, Marburg, Germany,
wehmeier_peter@lilly.com
Gereon Becht-Jördens

Objective: To analyse Picasso's painting "La Vie" from 1903 from an iconographic and psychoanalytic perspective. This painting is considered by many art historians to be the most important painting from the Blue Period and one of the most important works ever created by the artist. **Methods:** The approach is based on the combination of an iconographic analysis and an interpretation of the results by means of psychoanalytic concepts. **Results:** We have made an iconographic discovery which allows an entirely new approach to the interpretation of this painting. The gesture at the centre of the painting, never previously interpreted correctly, refers to the "noli me tangere" gesture often seen in European paintings from earlier periods. The gesture must be interpreted as a gesture of detachment, separating the young man (and the young woman) on the left from the mother figure on the right hand side of the painting. **Conclusion:** a) All art, including modern art, can be analyzed in terms of meaning. b) Hermeneutic approaches can lead out of the dilemma of entirely subjective and therefore arbitrary interpretation. c) Biographical factors play an important role in Picasso's work. d) Picasso reverts to the iconographic tradition both to make his personal statement and treat the topic of human suffering in an indirect way. d) The gesture at the centre of the painting must be seen in the iconographic tradition of the gesture "noli me tangere" (touch me not!) and therefore suggests detachment. e) The painting deals with the dissociation of a dyadic relationship between mother and son. f) The painting also deals with the problem of loss and the resulting narcissistic reaction as a defence mechanism.

P-002-036   Topic: 6, 92
An evaluation of a model of group cognitive therapy for children and adolescents with Insulin Dependent Diabetes
Catherine McElearney, National Children's Hospital, Child & Adolescent Psychiatry, Dublin 24, Ireland,
cjmulligan@eircom.net
Michael Fitzgerald Henry Marsh

Objective: The aim of the programme was to evaluate a group cognitive therapy programme. Research indicated that metabolic control is problematic in late childhood. The impact of altering individual's negative attitudes and beliefs about their diabetic management on their diabetic control has been reported in the literature. A four session programme was devised and delivered in a group setting. The group met weekly. Sessions ran for 90 minutes. The study aim was to evaluate if participation in the group would produce. A positive change in the children's self-efficacy as measured by the self-efficacy for diabetes scale. Blood glucose control as measured by the HBAic. Self-esteem as measured by the Cooper Smith Scale **Methods:**

This was a prospective study. The efficacy of the treatment group was compared to the control group. Ethical approval was granted by The Children's Hospital incorporating The Adelaide and Meath Hospital, Dublin. 15 participants were randomised to treatment (n=8) or control (n=7) Participants completed questionnaires and metabolic measures were obtained at the pre-treatment, posttreatment and four week follow-up. All participants attended the outpatient department and had a pattern of poor blood glucose control. The data was analysed using SPSS. (2*2 ANOVA being the appropriate test). **Results:** Analysis of the results indicated a trend towards an improvement in the blood glucose level in the treatment group compared to the control group. An improvement in selfefficacy was noted post therapy in the treatment group, however this was not maintained at follow-up. **Conclusion:** The burden of regular hospital appointments and the impact on the day to day lives of children and families attending the diabetic centre heightened the attractiveness of delivering a programme over a four week period. The outcome of this study identified a definite trend towards an improvement in the HBAic result.

P-002-037   Topic: 6, 41

A specialized behavior-oriented treatment unit for adolescents with elements of the Glen Mills Schools Program

Alexander Naumann, NLKH Lüneburg, Kinder- und Jugendpsychiatrie, Lüneburg, Germany, alexander.naumann@nlkh-lueneburg.niedersachsen.de Dirk Holst; Annette Engbarth

At the clinic for child and adolescent psychiatry and psychotherapy at the Landeskrankenhaus Lüneburg in Germany, a specialized unit for patients between ages of 16 and 20 with behavioral disorders and comorbid psychiatric disorders was conceptualized in 1996. Based on a behavioristic understanding, a peer-group oriented concept integrated experiences of the US-American Glen Mills Schools, teaching adolescents to develop positive social behavior and to possibly rise in status in the group hierarchy. This is supported by a 24-hour-behavioristic contingency program. Differences to the Glen Mills Schools consisted mainly in the process of admission and the possibility for the patients to reach the status of staff member which would be the highest level in the hirarchy. For years, up to ten adolescents at one time with principal diagnoses that require inpatient treatment for example emotional disturbances, expansive behavioral disorders, psychoses, suicidality and self-harming behaviors have been treated successfully (3 to 6 month of treatment). There are still many patients with behavioral disorders as secondary diagnosis, but compared to the time when the unit was first opened, they are less frequent. Treatment goals are: 1. to become able to stay in and learn from the group process, 2. to be successful in school or at a job trial, 3. to master every day life tasks and especially the problems connected with the specific disorder. The intense learning program and the therapeutic interventions are as far as the outpatient follow-up of the treated adolescents shows, a successful and well accepted characteristic of the unit. In this presentation, elements of the every day life of this unit, especially the so called "stamp-program and the levels of hierarchy are discussed.

P-002-038   Topic: 2

Care systems in mental health and the GP

Tiberiu Mircea, University of Medicine, Dept. of Child Psychiatry, Timisoara, Romania, roxana@mail.dnttm.ro

Objective: 20% of GP's patients have a psychiatric component of their disturbance, and 50% from the psychiatric patients contact at first time the GP. The GP is the very first counseler and applies the first intervention steps in mental health. Three years after conceiving and spreading a "Mental Health Guide for GP" by psychiatric practitioners in adult psychiatry and child and adolescent psychiatry in Timis county (Romania), we intended to evaluare it's efficiency for GPs. **Methods:** Three years after the Guide's spreading, at 50 GPs we evaluated with a questionnaire how they involve themselves in prevention, care and treatment and how they collaborate with the psychiatric practitioner. The evaluation was during one year and we calculated also the specialised consultations done after GP's recommendation, what kind of psychopathology was mostly detected and imposed hospital care. **Results:** we see the GP has an important role in prevention. He recognises better ADHD and anxiety disorders in children. Care involvement is especially based on the specialist's recommendations, and the treatment is the one prescribed by the specialist. **Conclusion:** A periodic information of the GP abous various forms of developmental psychopathology is necessary. The relationship is more efficient through medical letter and direct information.

P-003

Care, treatment and prevention III

Track: Therapy and intervention

P-003-039   Topic: 11

Play observation in psychiatric evaluation of children in an Indian set up

Ashima Nehra, India, savitam@sancharnet.in Savita Malhotra; Subho Chakrabarti

Objective: Use of play in diagnostic assessment has a contributory role. Child psychiatric clinics in India are less in number with inadequate facilities. Play rooms are not available everywhere and there is shortage of trained personnel. To find if the play room observation makes a significant contribution towards mental status examination of particularly young children and if it contributes to a better description and characterization of child's current mental functioning. **Methods:** This is a retrospective study on 140 children seen in the Child and Adolescent Psychiatric Clinic of the psychiatry department, PGIMER, Chandigarh, India. All patients underwent play room observation. Children were observed/evaluated on measures like types of play material used i.e. projective techniques, family-related and nurturance toys, expressive and constructive toys, aggressive and educational toys, other multi-use toys etc. They were also assessed on the parameters like level of activity, behaviour and interaction in play room, relationship capacity, speech and content of talk etc. **Results:** Thirty three children were sent for help in diagnostic clarification (out of 140). Out of these; 72.73% cases, the play room observation corroborated the clinical diagnosis. In many children the findings helped in better psychological understanding of the cases leading to formulation of a more focused and specific psychotherapy plan. **Conclusion:** In a few children the findings formed the basis for choosing play therapy as the main mode of treatment and it also helped in deciding the nature of play therapy to be used. Role of play observation in psychiatric evaluation of children is discussed.

P-003-040   Topic: 11, 41
Long-term psychotherapy in disturbed adolescents and role of compliance in therapy

Shashi Kiran, NIMHANS, Psychiatry, Bangalore, India, skiran@nimhans.kar.nic.in
Srinath Shoba

Objective: A naturalistic study of the developmental trajectories of two adolescents with emotional and behavioral disturbances in long-term psychotherapy. **Methods:** Two male patients who presented in their early adolescence with features of emotional, interpersonal and academic disturbances. Both had criteria of mixed emotional-conduct disorder but not adequate for a clinical diagnosis. However they fulfilled criteria for a diagnosis of adjustment disorder, which resolved rapidly subsequently. Both boys had anomalous family situations with clear insight into their problems. Both the boys were taken up for therapy, which was essentially eclectic with components of supportive, cognitive-behavioral therapies and family counseling. Both boys have been in contact with therapist over the past five years. One of the patients was compliant and involved in therapy, and tried to involve his family in the therapeutic process. The other patient developed a good rapport with the therapist but was irregular and often unilaterally called off therapy sessions. Neither he nor his family show interest in participation in therapy unless there was a crisis. **Results:** The first patient has shown a significant improvement in all his symptoms and his academic performance despite persisting family related problems. He continues to be in contact with the therapist. The other boy has continued to have interpersonal, academic and emotional and behavioral problems with inadequate family engagement. He was last seen in a clinical setting about 6 months ago. There was no psychopharmacological intervention in both the boys. **Conclusion:** The commitment and consequent compliance or non-compliance to therapy seemed to have had a major influence in their developmental trajectories, as there was no attempt to change their environment by therapist

P-003-041   Topic: 23, 84
Treatment with stimulants in a county department of child and adolescent psychiatry

Allan Hvolby, Dept. of Child Psychiatry, Esbjerg N, Denmark, ahv@ribeamt.dk
Jan Ib Jorgensen

Objective: Children and adolescent with ADHD are more often treated with stimulants. This presentation will describe the results from an examination of literature and the subsequent clinically rehearsal. The purpose was to optimise the medical treatment. **Methods:** After examination of the literature we established some clinically lines of directions for the treatment with stimulants. In this project we included 38 patients where medical treatment already was established and 24 patients which commence treatment during the project. Age of the probands was between 5 and 18 years. We registered among other items, time between control and efficacy

of treatment. **Results:** We found that we, could improve our treatment. We found that a more systematically follow up on this treatment results in a better outcome of the medical treatment. **Conclusion:** By examining the literature we found that a profoundly performed treatment with stimulants was more effective than behavioural therapy and almost as effective as the combination of the two. We did also find that we, by following the clinical lines of direction, could offer a more effective and regular treatment. Finally we found that with the more systematically offer of treatment our patients achieved a better symptom reduction.

P-003-042   Topic: 23, 42
First year outcome of children in a Partial Time Care Unit

Marco Medeiros, Dona Estefânia's Hospital, Child & Adolescent Psychiatry, Lisboa, Portugal, arleteamaro@hotmail.com
Arlete Correia; Maria Gabilondo; Pedro Caldeira da Silva; Augusto Carreira

Objective: Partial Time Care Units (PCTU), associated to the maintenance of the regular school setting, are an increasingly used treatment modality for psychiatric disturbed children. Created in October of 2000, the *Área de Dia* is a PTCU for children with disruptive behaviour disorders. It provides a multimodal intervention for the child-family-school triad (Figure 1). Of the 3 year-old experience, team general appreciation is that the children and their families benefit from the treatment. The purpose of our study is to evaluate more precisely the evolution of the children who attend this unit. We aim to test the following hypothesis: children who attend the *Área de Dia* have a favourable evolution. **Methods:** Our study is a prospective study that evaluates, at admission and at the end of the first year of treatment, twenty children who are in their first year of the program. The following assessment instruments are used: the Strengths and Difficulties Questionnaire (SDQ), a signs and symptoms checklist, the Functioning Global Assessment Scale (FGA), and a content analysis of the teacher's academic report. Parental satisfaction and parental cooperation are also evaluated. Statistical Package for the Social Sciences (SPSS) is used for statistical analysis. **Results:** First year of program ends in June 2004. Results will address measurable changes in children's clinical status and general and academic functioning, as well as parents' satisfaction and cooperation with the therapeutic intervention. **Conclusion:** Objective improvement in the main focuses of the treatment, will allow us to confirm our hypothesis.

Children	Family	School
Psychomotor intervention ⇆ *snack* ⇆ **expressive activity** **(plastic arts, dramatic expression, occupational therapy)**	Parents' group	Periodic meetings with teachers

P-003-043   Topic: 22

Child psychiatric consultation in a General Hospital

Jae-Won Yang, Samsung Medical Center,
Dept. of Psychiatry, Seoul, Republic of Korea,
psyche731@medimail.co.kr
Yeoung-Rang Kim; Sung-Do David Hong; Sang-Sin Lee;
Seong-Hu Lim; Jeoung-Hwan Park

Objective: This study was to investigate the clinical characteristics of psychiatric consultation for children and adolescents in a general hospital. **Methods:** Hospital records of 302 children and adolescents who were referred for psychiatric consultation in a general hospital over 5 years were reviewed and analyzed. **Results:** The mean referral rate for psychiatric consultation for school age children and adolescents was 2.06%. While more girls were referred in middle and high school age group, more boys were referred, in pre-school age group. Fifty percent of the consultation was requested from department of internal medicine and pediatrics. Main reason for requesting psychiatric consultation was for the assessment of the patients from psychiatric point of view (31.1%), followed by the management of depression (11.6%) and anxiety (11.3%). Most frequently rendered psychiatric services for the treatment was psychosocial intervention and supportive therapy (21.2%). **Conclusion:** There are differences in clinical nature of psychiatric consultation and referral patterns between adult patients and child and adolescent patients. Future research is needed to strengthen the services for child and adolescent psychiatric consultation.

P-003-044   Topic: 11

Children with script of aggression, maltreatment and trauma

Vera Trbic, Institute of Mental Health,
Dept. Sustance Abuse, Belgrade, Serbia and Montenegro,
danicica@eunet.yu
Danica Boskovic

Objective: Considering scripts of aggression, maltreatment and trauma, autors have in mind family, nation and cultural frame of reference, which deefly influence cognition and emotional development of children. They also find it an ethical issue to work on this kond of "inheritance" and to try to deconstructe it, and to deloborate enormeus energy, which was entrapped in those rigid patterns. **Methods:** The part of therapeutic session with Kosovo refugee family is videotyped and avaluible to be presented. **Results:** Taking stance of curiosity and multipositionong, therapists took adventure to co-construct a new scripts more resilient and less opti creative, during narrative and storytelling.

P-003-045   Topic: 23

Effectiveness evaluation of an adolescent psychiatric treatment (Marburger-Routine-Project)

Jan Pauschardt, Universitätsklinik Marburg,
Kinder- und Jugendpsychiatrie, Marburg, Germany,
pauschar@med.uni-marburg.de
Fritz Mattejat; Kurt Quaschner; Helmut Remschmidt

Objective: The current study will examine data from a 5-year longitudinal outcome study regarding the effectiveness of psychiatric treatment for children and adolescents at the Clinic for Psychiatry and Psychotherapy of the Philipps-University Marburg. All inpatient and day patients undergoing clinical treatment took part in comprehensive follow-up evaluations as part of their treatment. Treatment outcome will be assessed from different perspectives, namely those of the children, adolescents, care givers and therapists. **Methods:** Data was collected at the onset and termination of treatment from a referral population (N=2637). Follow-up data was collected from patients and caregivers by telephone at 4 weeks and 2 years after termination. Multiple questionnaires and rating scales were used, including an inventory to assess life quality (Inventar zur Lebensqualität bei Kindern und Jugendlichen), a rating list regarding psychopathological symptoms in the last six months (Marburger Symptom Liste), a questionnaire to assess treatment quality (Fragebogen zur Beurteilung der Behandlung), the Child Behavior Checklist (CBCL) and the Youth Self Report (YSR). **Results:** Positive outcomes were found for all primary measures regarding the effectiveness of child psychiatric treatment, as well as from all measured perspectives. Results demonstrated medium to high effect sizes, suggesting improved quality of life and decreased number of symptoms. These results were maintained at the two year follow-up. **Conclusion:** Results from this study demonstrate support for the positive effects of treatment for a referred psychiatric child and adolescent population.

P-003-046   Topic: 11

Hospital, Volkswagen, Community:
Integrative experiental therapy in child and adolescent psychiatry – children need objectives

Erika Lischka, Fachkrankenhaus Uchtspringe,
Kinder- und Jugendpsychiatrie, Uchtspringe, Germany,
dr.e.lischka@uchtspringe.de
Mechthild Bauer; Franka Petzke

Objective: Two thirds of the 400 patients who are treated in the child and adolescent psychiatry Uchtspringe per year are adolescents. They are in a phase of their lives, in which it is very important for them to find out about their own interests and abilities. This is very important for their

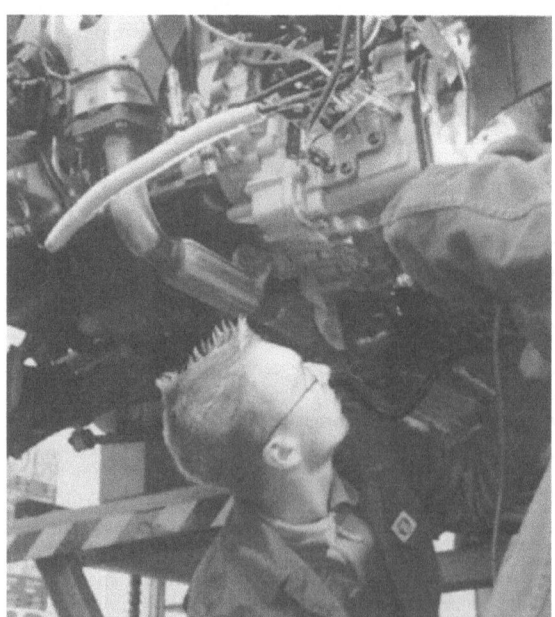

relationships, leisure behavior and professional orientation. Because of their mental illness most of the patients are not self-confident and motivated enough to test new behavior. That's why activating therapies are part of the concept of our clinic. A multiprofessional therapeutic team enables the patients to integrate new experiences in their personality concept under conditions very close to real life. The poster demonstrates different successful projects which have been realized through an integrative therapeutic approach. **Methods:** The therapeutic and experiential project AUTO Uchtspringe or TERRA-U. started in 2001. Young patients can try themselves under conditions very close to reality. They discover their interests and technical abilities under professional supervision. For this purpose, we have a Volkswagen Lupo, which can be disassembled, reassembled and tested several times. The project was sponsored by the Volkswagen car dealer Rosier in Stendal, a coaching partner, who assists the project staff in case of problems. Other partners are the training team of Volkswagen-Coaching Gesellschaft mbH Wolfsburg, the Employment Exchange Stendal and the Ministry of Labor of Sachsen-Anhalt. Another project is the integrative play and leisure center Uchtspringe. It doesn't matter whether one is a patient in Uchtspringe or one is living just around the corner in the village. The adolescents planned and realized the project mainly by themselves. The project was sponsored by the Federal Republic of Germany and approved by the Ministry of Health and Social Welfare of Sachsen-Anhalt. **Results:** We have no empirical data yet, since we are still in the process of preparing an outcome study. But we find it worthwhile to present this unusual project to a broader professional public. **Conclusion:** We believe that this kind of practical activity is very stimulating for the motivation of rather reluctant adolescents. That's why we are planning to enrich the offers.

P-003-047   Topic: 11, 96

Psychiatry and psychotherapy with deaf children and adolescents

Erika Lischka, Fachkrankenhaus Uchtspringe, Kinder- und Jugendpsychiatrie, Uchtspringe, Germany, dr.e.lischka@uchtspringe.de
Britta Wehrmann

Objective: Since March 1993, we have treated 154 girls and boys in the "German Center for Psychiatry and Psychotherapy for deaf children and adolescents" at the Uchtspringe Psychiatric Hospital. We are the only institution in Germany, which meets that challenge. The disorders are quite differently, but at time of admission aggressive behavior is prevailing. **Methods:** Essential information results from medical, psychological and pedagogical diagnostics, behavior observation and behavior analysis, which are necessary for a successful treatment. All members of the therapeutic team use bearing language. Fellow patients also learn that language, so that communication is possible and fears of the hearing adolescents can be discussed and reduced. Many questions are still unclear, for example the diagnostics of "central auditive perception disturbances". To find out more about this problem, we established a study group in Sachsen-Anhalt, which coordinates the efforts of the ear-clinic at the St. Salvator hospital Halberstadt, the "Landesbildungszentrum für Hörgeschädigte" Halberstadt and our child and adolescent psychiatry. The poster presents the results regarding the disorders, specific diagnostics and therapy of deaf patients treated until now

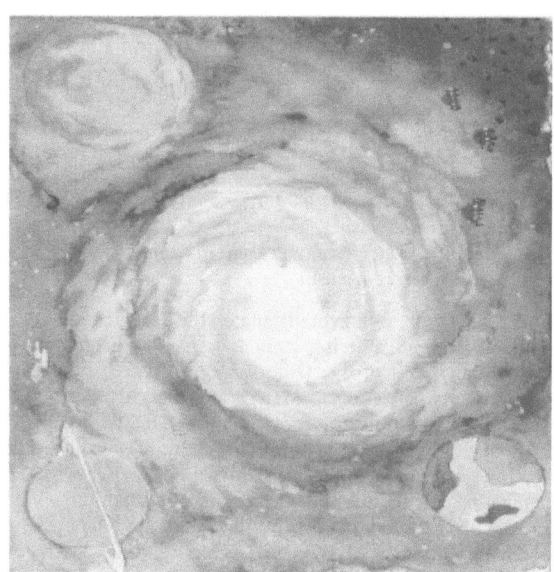

and offers some ideas for further studies. **Results:** The poster presents a description of the patients pool of the last ten years. **Conclusion:** Since our clinical experience is very encouraging, we plan a broader empirical evaluation study.

P-003-048   Topic: 23, 4

Analysis of the therapeutic aspects in child psychiatric in-patient unit in Lithuania

Sigita Lesinskiene, Vilnius University, Dept. of Clinic of Psychiatry, Vilnius, Lithuania, sigita.lesinskiene@vrc.vu.lt
Laura Paskauskaite

Objective: The aim of the study was to assess aspects of the therapeutic quality, short and long term effect of the in-patient treatment in Child Developmental Center in Vilnius. **Methods:** 22 children and 24 parents were interviewed using CBCL/4-18, YSR/11-18 together with the semistuctured interview at the beginning of in-patient treatment (first day), at the end of treatment (last day) and 6 weeks after the discharge. Children were interviewed and filled the questionnaires separately from the parents. Parents were also interviewed using second questionnaire developed by the authors that focused on the family changes during the period when child was getting in-patient treatment. Third questionnaire was developed for the team workers of the unit to analyse their view to family changes during the hospitalisation of the child. Data from medical records were also used. **Results:** Significant positive change was found comparing CBCL/4-18 data of the fist and second stages while data after 6 weeks showed significant change almost to the previous level of the first stage. Significant positive change comparing YSR/11-18 data of the fist and second stages were also found but this positive change remained at the third phase. Analysis of the data from the family changes questionnaire and team workers of the unit will be also presented. **Conclusion:** Children tended to rate effect of the treatment more positively than parents, especially 6 weeks after the in-patient treatment. There is a need to evaluate the long term effects of the tratment after the half year and one year. Changes in family system had impact on the dynamics of the child symptoms There was a need for systematic outpatient work with families and children after the in-patient treatment.

P-003-049   Topic: 11, 83
Aquatic environment and autism

Luisa Garcia-Giralda Bueno, Torremolinos, Spain, mlggbueno@wanadoo.es
Juana Montiel Gonzales; Javier Gallego Cumbres; Francisco Gutierrez Asensio

The Aquatic Environment facilitates the essential development of persons suffering from Autism. The professionals in the Daily Unit of the 'Quinta Alegre Centre', belong to the Autism Association of Malaga, are carrying out a programme of Hydrotherapy for people suffering from autism. It was started in the year 2000. Originally belonging to the 'Socrates Project', the programme is now carried on independently due to the positive results of its activities. Dr. Luisa García-Giralda from The Physiotherapy Department of Health Sciences at Málaga University collaborates on educating trainers as well as on supervising the programme. We emphasize the role of the aquatic environment as a favourable resource for the essential development of the patients who are participating in the Hydrotherapy programme demonstrate. It is divided into the following stages: Psychic Adaptation, Flotation, Rotations, Balance Reactions, Swimming and Diving. The result of the investigation demonstrate that the participants have improved in several aspects relative to: personal autonomy, self-control of corporal scheme, movements coordination, social and communicational skills, expression of positive feelings, and boosting to improve their quality of life.

P-003-050   Topic: 20, 3
Emotional stress of peer counselors in www.youth-life-line.de-project

Gottfried Maria Barth, University of Tübingen, Child a. Adolescent Psychiatry, Tübingen, Germany, gottfried.barth@uni-tuebingen.de
Susanne Denoix; Franz Kimmig; Marc Weinhardt

Objective: In the peer-counseling-project www.youth-life-line.de trained adolescents give online support for suicidal young people. Question arises whether these young counselors will be overstrained. **Methods:** 21 adolescent counselors were tested by questionnaires regarding depression, anxiety and psychic state in the weeks before first online consulting and during consulting. They had the possibility to call a psychiatrist if they would have psychic problems. **Results:** The young counselors demonstrated no extreme emotions in the questionnaires. There was no sign for emotional excessive demands. One of the 21 participants called the psychiatrist. His problems didn't arise from counseling in contrast counseling was able to stabilize preceding problems and opened the way to an own therapy. **Conclusion:** Results show no excessive demand for young counselors. Therefore there ist no reason to prevent them from own counseling. In contrast training and counseling seems to be supportive for their own psychic maturing.

P-003-051   Topic: 23, 25
Outpatient treatment settings in Berlin: A cooperation initiative

Peter Greven, Gemeinschaftspraxis, Kinder- u. Jugendpsychiatrie, Berlin, Germany, dr.greven@web.de
Stefan Buchmann; Nurgül Atas; Ute Jonkanski; Bodo Pisarsky; Silvia Treuter

Objective: The presentation introduces a cooperation network of child and adolescent psychiatrists focusing on aspects of quality management, interdisciplinary exchange, continued education and in consequence an improvement of mental health care in the community. The profile and structure of the initiative are demonstrated. **Methods:** In the German mental health system, outpatient treatment of children & adolescents in the community is a main field of child psychiatric specialists set up in their own practice, in single or group practice, or in accordance with the "social psychiatry agreement" with additional qualified staff like psychologists, child guidance workers, social workers, occupational therapists and many more. **Results:** The initiative was started in 2003 as a primarily informal activity of interested specialists aiming for internal quality assurance in the first place. Almost inevitably, matters of cooperation with clinical departments, paediatricians and general practitioners, school, health and family care services or practical therapists as substantial fundamentals of outpatient work have become important topics. Interdisciplinary activities concerning continued education are organized regularly now. **Conclusion:** The common presentation as a professional group shows to be beneficial for mediating professional contexts and objectives in community health care. Meanwhile, with quite a large number of patients treated by the involved practices and with the support of a renowned scientific board from several universities, certain research questions are in continuing process. Possible research partners will be welcome with their contributions.

P-003-052   Topic: 21, 41
Child and adolescent psychiatry of trench

Josep Cornellà, Girona, Spain, cornella@comg.es
Alex Llusent

Objective: To direct the attention of doctors of the "Outpatient Department" to the State Secondary Schools (SSS), in order to overcome the psychological and bureaucratic barriers that prevent the access of the young people to the "Outpatient Department". **Methods:** The activity in the SSS has been developed in two different facets. One of them, with an eminently preventive activity, constitutes different types of workshops, whose theme has been Self-esteem and Project of Life, Drugs, Sexuality and Abandonment of the Tobacco Smoke Habit. The second facet has been the establishment of an Open Doctor's Office in each one of the SSS, with confidential and gratuitous character. **Results:** This project has been developed during three years consecutively in five SSS of the city of Girona. During this period of time, 1080 consultations from the part of the students have taken place. The main reasons for consultation have been: substance abuse, preoccupation with weight and self-image, problems of attention and concentration, difficulties in the family interaction, difficulties in the personal relations, sexuality, and bulimic behaviour. **Conclusion:** From a welfare point of view, 90% of the consultations were successful "in situ", and 10% needed successive visits in the Hospital Unit. From our point of view, this work of prevention and early detection, is one of the best forms to approach the services of health for young people. The program is highly estimated by the SSS and is now part pf their equipment.

P-003-053   Topic: 22
Is child psychiatry necessary?: Pediatricians' perceptions towards child psychiatry consultation services
Lara Condesso, Lisboa, Portugal, lara@keyboard-pro.com
Pedro Caldeira da Silva; António Trigueiros

Objective: Dona Estefânia Pediatric Hospital was founded in Lisbon 125 years ago, and its Child and Adolescent Psychiatry Liason Unit (LU) began functioning in 1988. This study attempts to evaluate qualitative and quantitative aspects of child psychiatric liaison work, including pediatricians' perceptions and expectations of child psychiatry consultants within our hospital. Our main goal was to obtain direct feedback that could help us enhance the quality of consultation services at our facility. **Methods:** A self-report questionnaire was delivered to members of the pediatric teams of the hospital (pediatricians, residents in pediatrics and pediatric nurses). It included sections allowing the respondent to comment on the efficacy and usefulness of several consultation activities, positive and negative consequences of the LU intervention, problems making psychiatric referrals, etc. **Results:** 164 people returned the questionnaire. Overall, LU was found useful in all the clinical situations presented, especially when patients present with behavior problems and when families are of difficult approach. LU was considered effective in almost all clinical situations presented. Most of the respondents feel that consultation services provide a deeper understanding of the patient, and ensure a more comprehensive therapeutic plan after discharge. In this sample, 7% of the respondents is not aware of the presence of the psychiatric yard, and 15% is not aware of the existence of permanent emergency psychiatric assistance. **Conclusion:** In spite of insufficient and suboptimal communication between the two disciplines, well reflected by the findings concerning awareness of specific psychiatry units inside the hospital, the results suggest that pediatricians consider psychiatric consultation activities an important contribution to patient care. The present study supports the need for improvement in the relationship between pediatricians and child psychiatrists.

P-003-054   Topic: 23, 42
Treatment outcome and treatment satisfaction in different diagnostic groups: current results of the Marburger treatment evaluation project
Klaus Schütz, Universitätsklinik Marburg, Kinder- und Jugendpsychiatrie, Marburg, Germany
Fritz Mattejat; Kurt Quaschner; Helmut Remschmidt

Objective: Since 1999 the Clinic for Psychiatry and Psychotherapy of the Philipps-University Marburg accomplishes a catamnestic study ("Routine-evaluation-project") including all inpatient and day patients regarding the effectivness of psychiatric and psychotherapeutic treatment. The current study examine the differences in measures of treatment outcome and treatment contentment in different psychiatric disorders of childhood and adolescence. First results were presented in the german congresses in Berlin 2002 and Wien 2003. **Methods:** Psychometric data were collected at three different times (begin of treatment, end of treatment respectively 4 weeks after, 2 years catamnesis) from therapists, patients and their parents. Multiple questionnaires and rating scales were used, including an inventory to assess life quality (Inventar zur Lebensqualität bei Kindern und Jugendlichen; ILK), a rating list regarding psychopathological symptoms in the last six months (Marburger Symptom Liste; MSL), a questionnaire to assess treatment quality (Fragebogen zur Beurteilung der Behandlung; FBB), the Child Behavior Checklist (CBCL) and the Youth Self Report (YSR). **Results:** Different psychiatric disorders were compared regarding treatment outcome and treatment contentment. Previous results were confirmed and related to newer findings.

P-003-055   Topic: 19
The mental health of children in long-term foster and kinship care: The children in care study
Michael Tarren-Sweeney, University of Newcastle,
Medical Practice, Callaghan, Australia,
michael.tarrensweeney@newcastle.edu.au
Philip Hazell

Objective: Describes the findings of the baseline survey of a prospective, epidemiological study of the mental health of children in long-term foster and kinship care. The baseline component sought to examine relationships between the mental health of children in care, and retrospective and cross-sectional estimates of their exposure to multiple risk and protective variables. The study addresses several limitations of prior research, including a need to control for the effects of multiple adverse events (such as maltreatment, emotional deprivation and loss). **Methods:** Carers of children in long-term care were recruited to a state-wide mail-out survey in NSW, Australia. Children's mental health was estimated from two carer-report checklists: the Child Behavior Checklist (CBCL); and the Assessment Checklist for Children (ACC). The ACC was designed to measure problems specific to this population (namely self-injury, sexual behaviour, dissociation, trauma-related anxiety, attachment problems, suicidal behaviour, and abnormal food behaviour). Over 150 study factors were measured from a survey questionnaire and from the state's child welfare database. **Results:** 347 index children were recruited to the baseline survey (56% response rate), and the characteristics of non-respondent index children were characterised. Boys and girls were reported to manifest exceptionally high externalising and internalising problem behaviour. These estimates were at the upper limit of those reported previously for children in care. ACC scores suggested high rates of attachment disturbance, self-injury, dissociative behaviour and age-inappropriate sexual behaviour. CBCL and ACC scale scores correlated highly. Retrospective predictors of mental health included 'age at entry into care', 'number of maltreatment notifications', and 'history of sexual abuse'. **Conclusion:** Children in long-term care manifest significant and complex psychopathology, following early exposure to multiple adverse experiences. Children who enter care as infants fare remarkably better than later-placed children. The phenomenology of psychiatric disturbance among children in care is re-considered in light of these findings.

P-004
Scientific disciplines/approaches I

P-004-056   Topic: 28, 83

Brachidactyly-mental retardation syndrome and autism: Evolutionary course in 2 unrelated patients

Luigi Mazzone, University of Catania, Paediatrics, Catania, Italy, mazzone@unict.it
Diego Mugno; Liliana Ruta; Valentina Genitori D'Arrigo; Perrotta Concetta Simona; Teresa Mattina; Domenico Mazzone

Objective: Brachidactyly-Mental Retardation Syndrome (OMIM 600430) is associated with deletion at chromosome 2q37 and characterised by phenotypic overlapping with Albright Hereditary Osteodystrophy (OMIM 103580). **Methods:** We describe two cases of autism in unrelated children with BDMR syndrome, showing progressive reduction of autistic symptoms. **Results:** Patient 1: Chromosomal analysis showed 46, XY, de novo del(2)(2q37-qter). Cognitive evaluation demonstrated moderate mental retardation. At first assessment (4 years of age) he met the DSM IV criteria for Autistic Disorder (F84.0); CARS global score was 46 (severe autism). At 5 years he met criteria for Autistic Disorder; CARS global score was 33.5 (mild-moderate autism). At 6 years he met criteria for Pervasive Developmental Disorder NAS (F84.9); CARS global score was 30.5 (mild-moderate autism). Patient 2: Chromosomal analysis revealed 46, XX, de novo del(2)(2q37-qter). Cognitive evaluation demonstrated moderate mental retardation. At the age of 3 years 4 months (first assessment) she met the DSM IV criteria for Autistic Disorder; CARS global score was 49.5 (severe autism). At follow up (4 years of age) she met criteria for Autistic Disorder; CARS global score was 43 (severe autism). **Conclusion:** There are limited detailed reports in the literature of an association between deletion of 2q37 to the telomere and autism. Both children showed physical, cognitive, behavioural, and evolutionary homologies. Long term follow up and further studies are necessary to better describe the BDMR syndrome related phenotype and genotype-phenotype correlation. Genes in the 2q37 region may contribute to the aetiology of autism.

P-004-057   Topic: 36, 38

Event-related potentials in children with Dyslexia compared to an age and sex matched control group

Ralf Nordbeck, Groß Kussewitz, Germany, ralf.nordbeck@med.uni-rostock.de
Wolfgang Gierow; Frank Haessler; Johannes Buchmann

Objective: Children with dyslexia show a strong discrepancy between their performance of reading and writing in contrast to their performance in the other subjects. It's not yet clear, which part of the cerebral information processing is disturbed in Dyslexia. With the recording of visual and acoustic event-related potentials could be analysed on one hand the focused and sustained attention and on the other hand the cerebral information processing. **Methods:** 30 children aged from 8.0 to 14.1 years (mean/sd: 11.7 years +/– 20 month) were enrolled in this study. 15 children with dyslexia were compared with an age- and sex-matched control group. Children in both groups had a normal intelligence and no neurological, other psychiatric or AD(H)D diseases. Subject of the study was a visual and acoustic stimulus-reaction-task (go/nogo). 500 randomized stimuli were offered with an constant interval of 1.65 sec.: 115 attention-stimuli (yellow light or deep tone of 600 Hz), 75 go-stimuli (red light or high tone of 2400 Hz after attention-stimulus), 40 nogo-stimuli (no red light or high tone of 2400 Hz after attention-stimulus) and 270 random-stimuli (green light or middlehigh tone of 1200 Hz). The children should press a button as quickly as possible after the combination attention-go. The EEG was recorded in the Ten-Twenty-System using an Electro-Cap. Data were analysed by "Brain-Vision"-software. **Results:** Visual task: The dyslexia-group shows after the attention-stimulus a significantly stronger negativation in Fz and Cz ($p = 0.01$). Acoustic task: The control-group shows after the attention-stimulus a significantly stronger negativation in Fpz ($p = 0.001$). After the nogo- and go-stimulus we found in the control-group a stronger negativation in Fpz, Fz und Cz ($p = 0.01$). The dyslexia-group shows after the nogo- and go-stimulus also a fewer strong negativation in the 300 ms-area in the frontal and central electrodes ($p = 0,01$). **Conclusion:** Dyslexic children seems to need more effort for sustained attention in visual tasks – we conclude this from the stronger frontal and central negativation after the attention-stimuli at comparable amount of errors (false and omissions, Poster Horn, D et al.). Based on our findings (P300-amplitude not significantly different in Cz/Pz) we discuss a normal cerebral processing in visual tasks. In contrast, in dyslexic children attention is not affected in acoustic tasks, but in relation to reduced P-300-amplitudes we discuss a impaired cerebral processing of acoustic task dependend stimuli in these children.

P-004-058   Topic: 31, 83

Carbohydrate-Deficient Transferrin (CDT) in serum: Preliminary results for children and adolescents

Lucia Bliznakova, Zentralinstitut für, Seelische Gesundheit, Mannheim, Germany, bliznak@zi-mannheim.de
Yvonne Grimmer; H.J. Roth; Christine Jennen-Steinmetz; Martin H. Schmidt; Katja Becker

Objective: By examining Carbohydrate-Deficient Transferrin (CDT) in serum, adults engaged in heavy alcohol consumption can be identified and abstinence can be monitored. For children and adolescents, CDT normative data are not available yet. The main goal of this study was to obtain CDT values in 10 to 18-year-old children and adolescents in a first step. **Methods:** In a present prospective study the CDT-values of 10 to 18-year-old children and adolescents were examined. % CDT concentration were obtained by means of the AXIS Shield % CDT TIA. As an instrument for screening alcohol abuse, the section related to alcohol abuse in the KIDDIE-SADS-PL was used. Additionally the AUDIT was used to assess alcohol consumption. **Results:** CDT-data of 63 inpatients (39 boys, 24 girls) were analysed. 61 (38 boys, 23 girls), did not show alcohol consumption. The non-drinking girls (mean age 15 years; range 11.0 to 17.1 years) demonstrated CDT-values lower than 2,5% CDT (mean 2.1%). The non drinking boys (mean age 13.5 years; range 10.0 to 18.2 years) showed CDT-values lower than 2.5% CDT (mean 1.9%). **Conclusion:** Preliminary data of CDT values in a group of 10 to 18-year-old psychiatric inpatients without excessive alcohol consumption in the last six weeks showed comparative results to adults with moderate alcohol consumption (CDT < 3.2%). Prospective analysis of a healthy control group to get normative data will be performed as well as further analysis of cut-off levels in children and adolescents.

P-004-059   Topic: 34
Effects of Methylphenidate, Methylenedioxymethamphetamine (MDMA) and Fluoxetine in cultured mesencephalic neurons

Andrea G. Ludolph, Universität Ulm, Kinder- und Jugendpsychiatrie, Ulm, Germany, andrea.ludolph@medizin.uni-ulm.de
Alexander Storch; Tobias Boeckers; Joachim Kirsch; Jörg M. Fegert

Objective: The psychostimulant methylphenidate (MPH) is used for the long-term treatment of ADHD. Probably MPH binds with high affinity to the presynaptic dopamine transporter (DAT) of dopaminergic neurons, thereby blocking dopamine reuptake and thus increasing the availability of dopamine in the synaptic cleft. Similarly, the drugs 3,4 Methylenedioxymethamphetamine (MDMA, "Ecstasy") and fluoxetine have been implicated in interfering with serotonin reuptake by inhibition of the serotonin transporter (SERT). Therefore, we investigated the short- and long-term effects of MPH, MDMA or fluoxetine treatment in mixed cultures of dopaminergic and serotonergic neurons. **Methods:** We cultured rat embryonal (E14) mesencephalic neurons for up to 25 days in vitro and investigated whether MPH, MDMA or fluoxetine affected the survival of mesencephalic neurons by visual inspection and cell counting. Immunocytochemistry was used to characterize the transmitter phenotypes of mesencephalic neurons and for monitoring the subcellular localization of DAT in the presence or absence of the drugs. **Results:** We confirmed the presence of tyrosine hydroxylase (TH) positive neurons and demonstrated synaptogenesis within one week in culture. Neither short-term nor long-term MPH treatment in doses up to 1000 μM had any detectable effect on cell viability. MDMA elicited massive cell death within 24 h at doses ranging from 10 μM to 1000 μM. Similarly fluoxetine leads to the loss of TH positive neurons in concentrations between 10 μM and 1000 μM. Moreover, DAT immunoreactivity was first detected in TH positive neurons at day 4 in vitro. Most intensive labelling was observed in intracellular vesicles. An accumulation at nerve terminals was not observed at the developmental stages investigated. The same DAT distribution was observed in neurons treated with increasing concentrations of MPH, however the intensity of the intracellular immunoreactivity was increased depending on the MPH concentration and the time for which the drug was applied. **Conclusion:** In contrast to MDMA and fluoxetine, which both induced neuronal cell death in our cultures, MPH treatment of mesencephalic neurons elicited no obvious neurotoxic effects over the time period of our experiments. It is likely that MPH affects the targeting and/or turnover of DAT in TH positive neurons. Moreover, MPH could influence DAT expression at transcriptional or translational level.

P-004-060   Topic: 28
Psychic desadaptation and phenotype

Oksana Drevitska, Kyiv, Ukraine, opppa@ukr.net

Objective: 600 children, aged 10-12, from schools and hospitals were studied. Investigation included: a chat with the child; characteristics of the teacher and parents; study of

health condition, including mental status; study of the condition of central and vegetative nervous systems, verbal and non-verbal psychological tests; measurement and fixing of the some of phenotypic signs. **Methods:** Among the socially unsuccessful and less adapted pupils we found an accumulation of the quantity of recessive phenotypic signs. There was a statistically significant accumulation of the following exterior singularities: asthenical type of constitution, left handedness, chronic tonsillitis at the stage of decompensation; recessive phenotypic signs of child face features according to the McKusick enumeration, empirically established peculiarities of the palm. **Results:** As a rule, the parents of less satisfied children also had problems of psychological adaptation, they had biological singularities of psychological reactions, for example, increased stimulation or rigidity. Psychological and social help to the pupils with hampered adaptation will be more effective with allowance of scientific data about their singularities of mental reactions. **Conclusion:** Scientific data show a role of genetic factors in many psychiatric disorders, but the mechanism of influences of genetic factors have not been identified yet. We cannot see severe isolation of different psychic disorders, but gradual transition. The basic psychiatric disorders have a more or less stable frequency in populations. Predisposition to psychiatric disorders can be associated with accumulations of homozygous recessive genes. We try to go from phenotype, from clinic, from empirical material to the genotype. The different combinations of these phenotypic signs lead to a mosaic of clinical manifestations and developmental disorders and is a problem for genetic analysis.

P-004-061   Topic: 30, 37
Card Sorting Tests for executive functions: Classic and new proposed scoring parameters

Carlo Cianchetti, University of Cagliari, Dept. of Child Neuropsychiatry, Cagliari, Italy, cianchet@unica.it
Simona Corona; Maria Foscoliano; Daniela Contu; Giuseppina Sannio Fancello

Objective: The Wisconsin Card Sorting Test (WCST) and its simplified the version Modified Card Sorting Test (MCST) according to Nelson (Cortex 12:313-324,1976) are instruments largely used in the study of executive functions. In particular, they explore the subject's perseverations and capability to categorize. The capability to categorize is evaluated by the number of categories achieved and the number of errors made. However, in subjects reaching the top number of categories (10 in WCST and 6 in MCST) no differentiation is made regarding the number of cards used for reaching the goal. This is relevant in the MCST, since 1/3 of children being 10 years old reach the top of 6 categories; however also with WCST a consistent percentage of adolescent reaches the top of 10 categories. **Methods:** We integrated the scoring criteria with two new ones, named "categorizing efficiency" and "categorizing efficiency plus". "Categorizing efficiency" is used when the subject reaches the top of 6 categories in MCST: for each not-used card a supplementary point is added to 36, which corresponds to the number of correct responses in 6 categories. "Categorizing efficiency plus" integrates the score of categories adding a small score inversely related to the number of errors made, applied both when the 6 categories are reached and not. We studied the effects of calculating these new parameters in a population of 1126 children aged 4 to 13 years and in 23 adults evaluated with the

MCST. **Results:** All classic and new parameters show strong correlation (or inverse correlation) with age; however, categorizing efficiency and categorizing efficiency plus are shown to be the most sensitive to age variation especially for older children. Moreover, especially for ages 10 to 13, the distribution of the scores in categories completed is strikingly asymmetrical, as well as that of non-perseverative errors, while that of categorizing efficiency and of categorizing efficiency plus is approaching to a normal distribution. **Conclusion:** Our data suggest that "categorizing efficiency" and "categorizing efficiency plus" may give more information on performance on MCST, respect to similar parameters like the number of categories completed, number of correct responses and of non-perseverative errors. This may help to a better evaluation of the subject's executive function capability to categorize.

P-004-062   Topic: 30

A neuropsychological and neurolinguistic follow-up of a sample of children affected by Benign Myoclonic Epilepsy of infancy

Anna Costa, Univesity of Rome, Child Adolesc. Neur. Psych., Rome, Italy, costanna1@virgilio.it
Mara Roello; Angela Romano; Anna Fabrizi; Andrea Pelliccia; Maria Matricardi

Objective: The aim of this study is to investigate the presence and the features of language disorder in a sample of children with Benign Myoclonic Epilepsy of Infancy. **Methods:** We report clinical an neuropsychological follow-up of a sample of 10 children, aged between 12 months and six years, who have been diagnosed with benign myoclonic epilepsy of infancy according to Dravet's criteria. No one had evidence of clinical or radiological evidence of brain lesion. **Results:** The first fit occurred before 18 months and was a febrile seizure in half of the patients. After the age of 30 months non-febrile myoclonic seizures occurred. In all the cases the ictal EEG showed atypical spike-wave paroxysms. This type of epilepsy had a favourable evolution in all cases under treatment (VPA, LTG, VPA + LTG). The children underwent age-related psycho-diagnostic assessment: cognitive tests, neuropsychological and neurolinguistic tests. **Conclusion:** All the patients had a normal cognitive development. The evolution is characterized by the absence of fits and the appearance of a developmental language disorders.

P-004-063   Topic: 36, 75

Measurement of parasympathetic activity by heart rate variability and its impact on understanding psychic disturbance

Gottfried Maria Barth, University of Tübingen, Child a. Adolescent Psychiatry, Tübingen, Germany, gottfried.barth@uni-tuebingen.de
Nickola Matthias; Gunther Klosinski; Timo Lesnick; Matthias Gass

Objective: Parasympathetic nervous system generally is disregarded in psychiatric investigation. Regardless there is no doubt about the close junction between affects and autonomic nervous system. Testing parasympathetic activity could provide insight in unconscious affective states. **Methods:** After describing the way of recording parasympathetic activity by heart rate variability (HRV) today standard of knowledge and own results are demonstrated. Measurement of HRV was performed in psychiatric young patients. HRV of

patients with vegetative dystonia was compared with controlled and HRV in double blind methylphenidate application was detected. **Results:** Diagnosis of ADHD was connected with elevated parasympathetic activity, psychosis with depressed parasympathetic activity. Correlation between anxiety or depression and parasympathetic activity was detected. And the parasympathetic part of psychosomatic symptoms of vegetative dystonia was analysed. **Conclusion:** Measurement of parasympathetic activity by analysing heart rate variability discloses a link between body and mind. Parasympathetic nervous system constitutes an indicator and at the same time an influencing factor of the affective state and symptomatic occurrence of psychic disturbance. It provides a way to the unconscious part of affectivity.

P-004-064   Topic: 36, 82

The diagnostic significance of P300 evoked potentials for brain cognitive dysfunction in children with learning disorder

Linyan Su, Mental Health Institute, Dept. of Child Psychiatry, Changsha, China, sulinyan@sina.com
Jishui Zhang; Daxing Wu; Xuerong Luo

Objective: To study the diagnostic significance of P300 evoked potentials for brain cognitive dysfunction in children with learning disorders. **Methods:** The diagnosis of learning disorder (LD) was made according to the DSM-IV criteria. The LD group comprised of 30 children, 25 male, 5 female, 7~15 (10.69 ± 2.34) years old. The control group included 30 healthy children, 24 male, 6 female 7~15 (10.47 ± 2.16) years old. All the children were evaluated with the Wechsler Intelligence Scale for Children, Chinese Revised (WISC-CR). With the 32-channel Neuroscan 4.1, all the subjects underwent P300 evoked potentials at Fz, Cz, C3, C4 and Pz, respectively. Then we compared the latency, amplitude, waveform and topography of P300 in LD children with that in healthy control subjects. **Results:** The latencies of P300 at Fz, Cz, C3, C4 and Pz in LD children were significantly longer than those of healthy control subjects ($1.87 \le t \le 2.43$, $P < 0.05$). The amplitudes of P300 at Fz, Cz, C3, C4 and Pz in LD children were significantly lower than those in healthy control subjects ($2.76 \le t \le 3.69$, $P < 0.01$). The incidences of abnormal waveform ($X2 = 22.50$, $P < 0.001$) and topography ($X2 = 26.79$, $P < 0.001$) of the P300 evoked potentials in LD children were significantly higher than those in healthy control subjects. **Conclusion:** Our results showed that LD children suffered from cognitive dysfunction indicated with P300.

P-004-065   Topic: 30, 69

Memory deficit in early onset schizophrenic spectrum

Ignazio Ardizzone, Rome, Italy, ignazio.ardizzone@fastwebnet.it
Paola D'Oto; Francesca Priskich; Elvira Rigillo; Nadia Tomassetti; Francesca Vagnoni

Objective: To identify the presence and the features of memory deficit in eoss using a battery of neuropsychological measures as the principal method of evaluation. **Methods:** Fifteen treated symptomatically stable, schizophrenic (dsm iv) adolescent inpatiens, fifteen age-matched ocd and fifteen healthy subiects, were administered: wisc-r, wcst, tower of london, tema. The battery included the measuring of working memory, declarative memory and procedural memory. **Results:** (Statistical data are not available at the moment) Preliminary results: compared with control and ocd sample patients seem to show global impairment in all neuropsychological tasks. In the schizophrenic patients, as a group, it's possible to define differents features in declarative, procedural and working memory functyioning. **Conclusion:** According to recent international literature, eoss is chareterized by paculiar memory deficits. On the basis of the quantitative and qualitative analysis of different deficits in declarative, procedural and working memory our findings support the differentiation of subsyndromes in eoss and suggest that memory impairment in schizophrenia may reflect the involvement of different memory systems. To understanding better these findings for tha sake of prevention, we need to explain these result to shed light upon the links between the neuropsychological features of premorbid, prodromic development and bio-psychosocial features of adolescent development.

P-004-066   Topic: 36, 68
Visual and acoustic evoked event-related potentials in young-adult drug users

Ralf Nordbeck, Groß Kussewitz, Germany,
ralf.nordbeck@med.uni-rostock.de
Wolfgang Gierow; Frank Haessler; Johannes Buchmann

Objective: Young and adolescents drug users often report about a better attention and performance under the influence of psychotropic substances like Cannabis or "Ecstasy". With the recording of visual and acoustic event-related potentials could be analysed on one hand the focused and sustained attention and on the other hand the cerebral information processing. **Methods:** We investigated 8 male adolescents (mean/sd: 17.9 years ± 20.1 month) with a continuous drug-consumption and compared with an age-matched control group. All were of normal intelligence and had no neurological, psychotic or AD(H)D diseases. All drug-users were positiv tested in a 24-houres-intervall on actually drug consumption befor the investigation. Subject of the study was a visual and acoustic stimulus-reaction-task (go/nogo). 500 randomized stimuli were offered with an constant interval of 1.65 sec.: 115 attention-stimuli (yellow light or deep tone of 600 Hz), 75 go-stimuli (red light or high tone of 2400 Hz after attention-stimulus), 40 nogo-stimuli (no red light or high tone of 2400 Hz after attention-stimulus) and 270 random-stimuli (green light or middlehigh tone of 1200 Hz). The children should press a button as quickly as possible after the combination attention-go. The EEG was recorded in the Ten-Twenty-System using an Electro-Cap. Data were analysed by "Brain-Vision"-software. **Results:** Visual task: The P300-amplitude after the attention-stimulus in Fz, Cz and Pz was strongly higher in the control-group. The "nogo"-P300-amplitude was higher in Cz and Pz in the drug-user group. There were no significant differences between drug-users and control-group after the go-stimulus. Acoustic task: The "attention-P300-amplitude in Fz, Cz and Pz was strongly higher in the control-group again. Also the P300-amplitude after the go-stimulus was in Fpz and Cz higher in the control-group. **Conclusion:** Based on our findings we suppose that the sustained attention is impaired in drug-users especially in acoustic tasks. We conclude this in relation to the reduced P300-amplitude after the attention-stimuli. We discuss the nearly equal configuration of ERP after the go-stimulus in the visual task in this way, that psychotropic substances seems not to affect the information processing of task related visual stimuli.

P-004-067   Topic: 36, 82
Language comprehension in dyslexic children as revealed by event-related brain potentials (ERPs)

Beate Sabisch, Max-Planck-Institut, Human Cogn. and
Brain Sciences, Leipzig, Germany, sabisch@cns.mpg.de
Anja Hahne; Lisa Glass; Angela D. Friederici;
Waldemar von Suchodoletz

Objective: Reading and writing are complex activities that require the involvement of similar subprocesses. A current neurobiological model of language comprehension (Friederici, 2002) distinguishes three functionally different processing phases that are reflected by three temporally and neurotopically distinct ERP components (ELAN, N400, P600). The present study examined syntactic and semantic language comprehension processes by measuring ERPs in groups of dyslexic and matched control children. **Methods:** The ERPs to auditorily presented sentences were recorded in 13 dyslexic (ICD-10: F81.0, F 81.1, age 9-16 years, native German monolinguals) and 13 matched control children. Participants judged the correctness of syntactically incorrect, semantically incorrect, and correct sentences. **Results:** For semantically incorrect sentences, both dyslexic and control children showed an N400 with a similar amplitude. For syntactically incorrect sentences, control children elicited an ELAN, while dyslexic children did not. The P600, which for control children followed the ELAN, was observed for the dyslexic children as well, but with a clearly diminished amplitude. **Conclusion:** The N400 suggests no differences in the processing of semantic information in dyslexic and control children. The absence of the ELAN indicates that fast and automatic syntactic processes do not occur. Even the syntactic repair mechanism as reflected by the P600 seems to be less established in dyslexic children. Finally, the results support the conclusion that syntactic processing during language comprehension is not fully developed in this subgroup of dyslexic children even though, lexical-semantic language comprehension is not impaired.

P-004-068   Topic: 30, 82
Cognitive profiles and academic achievement in adolescents with specific learning disabilities: Comparison of two groups

Carlo Di Brina, University of Rome, Scienze
Neuropsichiatriche, Rome, Italy, cdibrina@tiscali.it
Nadia Tomassetti; Andrea Pagnacco; Flavia Capozzi;
Roberta Penge

Objective: Considerations of this work proceed from the hypothesis that profiles of subjects with childhood Learning Disabilities (LDs) persist in the adulthood in a stable way. **Methods:** We examined whether and how the two groups of adolescents with LD differed for neuropsychological profile and behavioural problems. Our sample is made up of 16 high school students, ages 13,7-15,6 years, 1) adolescents with LD followed by the Special Service of Neuropsychology, who practiced rehabilitation for at least 5 years 2) adolescents arrived from the high school, for the first time to our consultation. We assessed neuropsychologically academic achievement (reading, writing and computation) and valued cognitive and psychopathological characteristics. **Results:** For both groups the academic achievement differed from non-impaired: the most compromised variable is the reading speed; in computation tasks the two groups show significant deficits in "written calculation" and "time of execution", even if in the natural group appear less severe but more widespread deficits, less autonomous use of reading and writing as cognitive instruments. All participants have the Full Scale intelligence quotient higher than 90, the cognitive profiles show residual low rates in "Sequential" and "Conceptual" clusters. At the CBCL (Youth Self Report version), the two groups differ in social risk and thought functioning area. **Conclusion:** Data analysis illuminates how cognitive profiles and academic achievement in adolescents with LD persist in a stable way. It is interesting to note that even if adolescents that have received clinical support show a better control and compensation of their academic difficulties, persistency in time of the impairment influence the social competence and adaptive impairment in both groups.

P-004-069 Topic: 30, 81
Proposal for rehabilitation: A 'creative protocol' in learning disability and mental retardation

Fabio Bocci, Università La Sapienza Roma, Child & Adolescent Psychiatry, Rome, Italy, bocci.fabio@fastwebnet.it
Flavia Capozzi; Laura Cantonetti; Alessandra De Carlo; Barbara Scanferla; Teresa Sebastiani; Cristina Vagnoni

Objective: According to our clinical experience children with learning disabilities and childeren with mental retardation often present difficulty in the creativity areas. Founding on Treffinger, Feldhusen, Isaksen, and Urbans's human creativity representation model and on divergent thinking development procedures such as Brainstorming, CPS (Creative Problem Solving) and IEP (Instrumental Enrichment Program), the authors show a protocol suited for detection of creative capability as well as educational intervention and rehabilitation on LD and MR subjects. The experimental protocol shown is presently at use in a research environment. The aim of the study is to verify whether some methods and creative procedures can improve academic performances in LD and MR children. **Methods:** Such protocol consists in two parts, the first of which is aimed at child neuropsychological evaluation. Particularly, the following domains are evaluated: verbal and non-verbal creativity areas, both at therapy beginning and end, through the AECC's "Assessment fantasia"; cognitive level, through WISC-R and Raven Progressive Matrices scales; academical skills (educational profile), through maths and, for reading and comprehension, Cornoldi et al.'s MT tests. In our protocol's second part, tools are included which have to be used in recovery therapy: problem solving as well as planning activities, RAT, Calvi's expressions and EIP are used to increase creativity; language, maths and creative games to increase academical skills.

P-004-070 Topic: 28, 84
Association analysis between catechol-o-methyltransferase (COMT) gene and ADHD

Xueping Gao, Central South University, Dept. of Child Psychiatry, Changsha, China, xuepinggao@hotmail.com
Linyan Su; Yasong Du

Objective: To analysie the association between polymorphisms in human catechol-o-methyltransferase gene and ADHD, in order to find the disease-perdisposing alleles for ADHD. **Methods:** Genotypes and allele frequencies of the Val158Met polymorphism at the COMT gene in ADHD probands (n=54), their parents (n=82), and normal controls (n=30) were examined by PCR-RFLP techniques. Both case-control association study and family-based association study (HRR and TDT analysis) were used. **Results:** No differences in the genotype and allele frequencies of the Val158Met polymorphism at the COMT gene were observed between the ADHD group and control group (p>0.05), and in the nuclear families (p>0.05). The frequencies of G/G genotype and G allele of the Val158Met polymorphism at the COMT gene in the ADHD predominantly inattention subtype, were significantly higher than those in the combined subtype (p<0.05). The G/A frequency in the combined subtype was significantly increased (p<0.05). "A" allele was associated with certain clinical manifestations (attention problems, delinquent behavior and aggressive behavior). **Conclusion:** The COMT gene was not associated with ADHD in this study. The COMT gene was probably associated with clinical subtypes and clinical manifestations of ADHD.

P-004-071 Topic: 30, 81
Creativity – A bridge on academic failure.
An experience with learning disabled and mentally retarded children

Fabio Bocci, Università La Sapienza Roma, Child & Adolescent Psychiatry, Rome, Italy, bocci.fabio@fastwebnet.it
Flavia Capozzi; Laura Cantonetti; Alessandra De Carlo; Fabio Lorenzetti; Teresa Sebastiani; Cristina Vagnoni

Objective: In the last 50 years, creativity has been variously studied and interpreted. The main issues arisen in the discussion about creativity are: nature (talent) vs culture (achievement); intelligence (I.Q.) vs creativity; creativity outcome vs creativity process (the act itself). Nowadays, these dichotomies don't apply anymore, as creativity is seen as a transversal strategy affecting a large number of skills and domains. According to our clinical experience children with learning disabilities and childeren with mental retardation often present difficulty in the creativity areas. The authors present the outcomes of a study on LD and MR children, in order to show how some creative methods and procedures can improve a child's creative performances and academical achievement. **Methods:** Subject: five 8–9 years LD students; five 12–13 years MR students matched by mental age. Tools: AECC's Assessment Fantasia, Osborne's Brainstorming, Murdock's Guided Imagery, Mednick's Remote Association Test, Calvi's Test Espressioni, and other linguistic and mathematical creative games. **Results:** Data analysis is now in progress. **Conclusion:** At present, the authors notice that an affective involvement appears to increase children's time on task. Above all, the authors are keen to underline the importance of learning by doing and enjoying learning.

P-004-072 Topic: 30, 58
Development of spatial number representations and numerical abilities in children

Michael von Aster, St. Joseph-Krankenhaus Berlin, Kinder- und Jugendpsychiatrie, Berlin, Germany, vonaster@kjpd.unizh.ch
Martin Schweiter

Objective: The existence of spatial representations of number has been convincingly demonstrated in adults by associations between number size and response preference with faster left- than right-hand response for small numbers and faster right- than left hand response for larger numbers (Spatial Numerical Association of Response Codes: SNARC-effect). The current study investigates the questions (i) to which extent SNARC-effects are present in 2nd grade children, indicating an internal visual-spatial number representation (left to right oriented number line) and (ii) if the presence of SNARC-effects is related to numerical test performance in preschool age and at the end of the second school year. **Methods:** 113 children that have been administered to a number processing and calculation test battery (ZAREKI-K) during the preschool year and have been retested at the end of the second school grade with ZAREKI-R and a computerised SNARC-paradigm. **Results:** Concerning the presence of SNARC-effects we found considerable variance with N = 40 (22 boys) children showing SNARC-effects and N = 73 (35 boys) children showing not at all such effects. Analysis of ZAREKI (K, R) test performance revealed gender differences with boys performing better than girls. Oneway ANOVA confirmed significant effects of gender but no significant effects of SNARC-effect on ZAREKI test performance. However, we found a significant interaction of gender and SNARC-effect on test performance. SNARC-effects were positively correlated with test performance in boys but negatively in girls. In children that did not show SNARC-effects no gender differences were observed. **Conclusion:** To conclude, it seems that the development of abstract visual-spatial number representations indicated by SNARC-effects has different effects on math performance in boys and girls. This may be due to differences in attitudes and thinking strategies (verbal-analytical vs. visual-spatial) between boys and girls that develop in early childhood.

P-004-072A   Topic: 35
Development of neural networks for mental rotation

Karin Kucian, Universität Zürich, Kinderhospital, Zürich, Switzerland, karin.kucian@kispi.unizh.ch
Thomas Loenneker; Thomas Dietrich; Ernst Martin-Fiori; Michael von Aster

Objective: The dramatic changes in cognitive ability observed throughout childhood mirror corresponding changes in the developing brain. **Methods:** Using fMRI, we measured cortical activity in 20 healthy adults and 20 normally achieving school children (10 3rd grade, 10 6th grade) during trials of mental rotation tasks. Mental rotation is a complex cognitive skill, that produce the most consistent gender differences. **Results:** Although the activated network during mental rotation in adults and children looks quite similar, calculated contrasts revealed some differences. Adults show more activation in the left intraparietal sulcus (IPS). And children show more bilateral activation in the posterior cingulate gyrus and precuneus. We did not find gender differences in brain activation of children as we did in adults. **Conclusion:** Adults are more trained in visual manipulation resulting in faster performance and bilateral parietal activation. During development, active areas seem to shift from right to left due to automation of skills. This results in a bilateral activation pattern with stronger activation of the left IPS in adults. Dedicated visual attention load and learning in children is higher which is indicated by increased bilateral cingulate activation. Gender differences in cerebral representation of mental rotation seem to develop between childhood and adulthood and might be a consequence of different cognitive strategies.

P-004-072B   Topic: 35
Children's brains learn to calculate approximately

Karin Kucian, Universität Zürich, Kinderhospital, Zürich, Switzerland, karin.kucian@kispi.unizh.ch
Thomas Loenneker; Thomas Dietrich; Ernst Martin; Michael von Aster

Objective: The parietal lobe has been suggested as a potential substrate for a domain-specific representation of quantities in adults. The current study addresses the question, if this pattern of cortical specialization is already established in school children. **Methods:** Using fMRI, the cortical activity has been measured in 20 healthy adults and 21 normally achieving school children (10 3rd grade, 11 6th grade) during trials of approximate calculation tasks. **Results:** Adults activated most significantly the inferior parietal lobe (IPL, BA 40) bilaterally during approximate number processing. A functional ROI (Region Of Interest) analysis of the region showed that children use parietal regions as well, but much less intensive compared to adults. Children showed significant activation of the anterior cingulate gyrus (AC) bilaterally. A region that reflects attentional and working memory demands due to task difficulty. A ROI analysis of that region showed that brain activation decreases with age during approximate calculation. **Conclusion:** Comparing brain activation of 3rd and 6th grade school children and adults led us to draw the following conclusion: Children and adults use a similar parietal lobe network to determine the quantity of a number. However, this domain-specific parietal network seem to develop and to automatize during primary school years, indicated by decreasing activity in AC and increasing activity in IPL with age. Children's brains obviously have to learn to handle approximate calculation problems which results in better and faster performance.

P-005
Scientific disciplines/approaches II

P-005-073   Topic: 44, 52
The relation between aggression and depressive and obsessive symptoms among a sample of Alazhar University students

Hesham Abuhegazy, Alazhar Faculty of Medicin, Dept. of Psychiatry, Cairo, Egypt, abuhegazi@hotmail.com
Hashem Bahary

Objective: The overall purpose of this work is to study the relation between aggression, the depressive and obsessive symptoms, on a sample of Al-Azhar University Students **Methods:** The total sample of this study was 409 students selected in stratified random manner from Al Azhar University Student House for Males. The study was a cross sectional, Multistage type, all participants subjected to the following: Administration of Hand Test. Administration of symptoms check lest (the questions specific for depressive and obsessive symptoms). Semistructured clinical psychiatric interview a general and neurological Medical examination for all of these students fall under the upper quadratile and lower quadrantile ranges on hand test. **Results:** And the study has revealed that: There is no clear relation between aggressive behavior and sociodemographic variants of the participants such, age, residency, type of study, father work and family size. There is strong positive correlation between the aggression and depressive symptoms meanwhile there are no relation between it and the obsessive symptoms. And from the clinical interview study: prevalence of psychiatric morbidity was 27.11% prevalence of O.C.D. was 3.01% prevalence of depressive disorders was 7.23% distributed as following: 1.2% for major depressive disorder – single episode. 1.2% for major depressive disorder recurrent episodes. 1.2% for major depressive disorder. 1.8% for brief recurrent depression. 1.8% for dysthmia. There is no relation between aggressive behavior and the type of disorder. However more than third of disordered students was having Premorbid neurotic personality traits, past history, and family history of psychiatric disorders. **Conclusion:** There is strong positive correlation between the aggression and depressive symptoms meanwhile there are no relation between it and the obsessive symptoms.

P-005-074   Topic: 44, 96
Relationship between adolescent internet addiction and depression, impulsivity and obsessive-compulsivity

Dae-Hwan Lee, Seoul Nat. University Hospital, Dept. of Neuropsychiatry, Seoul, Republic of Korea, ener2@mdhouse.com
Bong-Seog Kim; Seong-Ill Jeon; Sun-Ju Chung

Objective: The aims of this study were to investigate the prevalence of the internet addiction and to examine the relations of internet addiction to depresssion, impulsivity, and obsessive-compulsivity in Korean high school students. **Methods:** Subjects were high school students in Namyangju city (N = 1413). The questionnaire consisted of items on demographic characteristics and internet use pattern. We assessed the level of internet addiction and depressive symptoms of adolescents using Young internet addiction scale and the Beck Depression Inventory (BDI), respectively. Barratt impulsiveness scale (BIS) and Maudsley obsessive compulsive inventory (MOCI) were also self rated. **Results:** In this study, the prevalence of internet addiction is 4%. Addicted group showed significantly higher mean scores of depression (F = 64.76, p < 0.001), impulsivity (F = 60.00, p < 0.001) and obsessive-compulsivity (F = 32.00, p < 0.001) than over-use group and non-addicted group. Among the subscales of impulsivity, addicted group showed significantly higher mean scores of non-planning

impulsivity (F = 22.25, p < 0.001), motor impulsivity (F = 96.11, p < 0.001), and cognitive impulsivity (F = 20.26, p < 0.001) than other two groups. Among the subscales of obsessive-compulsivity, subjects with internet addiction showed significantly higher mean scores of doubting (F = 9.64, p < 0.001), checking (F = 9.39, p < 0.001), slowness (F = 34.04, p < 0.001) and cleaning (F = 27.49, p < 0.001) than other two groups. **Conclusion:** In this study, the prevalence of internet addiction is relatively similar with the result of previous domestic studys. These results suggest that internet addicted adolescents are more depressive, impulsive, obssessive and compulsive than non-addicts. It is required to investigate the psychopathology of the internet addiction.

P-005-075   Topic: 42
Are teachers' ratings of early behavioural problems good predictors for substance abuse in adolescence?

Maria da Conceicao Taborda Simoes, Universidade de Coimbra, Faculdade de Psicologia, Coimbra, Portugal, mctabordas@fpce.uc.pt
Maria da Luz Vale Dias

Objective: The relevance of teachers' ratings for the identification of young students at risk for behavioural disorders and emotional difficulties is well demonstrated in a growing number of studies. The usefulness of "teachers as tests" (Lane, 2003) has been highlighted, also in the development of several instruments for assessing children's behaviour (e.g. Achenbach; Conners).The purpose of this paper was to know the efficacy of teachers' ratings of children's behavioural problems as predictors for substance abuse (including alcohol and tobacco) during adolescence. **Methods:** Data were collected from a large random sample of boys and girls who attended public schools in a municipality of Coimbra (Portugal). In this context teachers filled in several questionnaires (e.g. Achenbach's and Conners' checklists) to assess children's behaviour, at the initial assessment (time 1). Several years later the same pupils were assessed again in various domains including substance abuse. **Results:** Results showed that teachers' ratings in elementary schools were only very modest predictors of substance abuse at the end of adolescence. **Conclusion:** Several theoretical and practical implications are drawn from these findings.

P-005-076   Topic: 42, 93
Deaths and suicides among former child and adolescent psychiatric patients

Ulf Engqvist, Karolinska Institutet, Women and Child Health, Stockholm, Sweden, ulf.engqvist@mh.se
Per-Anders Rydelius

Objective: This study has two questions, whether CAP-patients still have an elevated risk of early death despite the important social changes and improvement of overall health that have occurred over the recent decades, and if so, what kind of information may predict later suicides. **Methods:** A sample of 1420 former CAP-patients (born 1957–76, treated 1975–1990) were followed up until Jan 1st 2003 by examination of hospital and criminal records and linkage to the National Cause of Death Registry. **Results:** The death rate was 2.7%, 24 males and 14 females (1.7 : 1.0) had died by the end of 2002. The SMRs was significantly increased in both genders. Behavioral problems,

	Non-addicted (N=558) Mean (SD)	Over-use (N=798) Mean (SD)	Addicted (N=57) Mean (SD)	F
BDI†	12.10 (7.18)	15.50 (7.88)	22.51 (9.35)	64.76
MOCI†	8.69 (4.57)	10.56 (4.98)	12.36 (5.55)	32
Doubting	2.87 (1.63)	3.22 (1.65)	3.52 (1.60)	9.64
Checking	2.66 (1.59)	3.01 (1.75)	3.38 (1.75)	9.39
Slowness	1.50 (1.21)	2.05 (1.39)	2.42 (1.52)	34.04
Cleaning	1.65 (1.69)	2.27 (1.87)	3.03 (2.15)	27.49
BIS†	34.43 (11.40)	40.48 (10.44)	44.70 (13.28)	60
Non-planning imp	16.31 (5.62)	18.18 (4.91)	18.59 (5.83)	22.25
Motor imp	7.76 (4.42)	10.95 (5.07)	14.38 (6.18)	96.11
Cog imp	11.61 (4.15)	12.98 (3.95)	13.47 (5.36)	20.26

†: p < 0.001
imp: impulsivity

Table 1. Comparison of the BDI, MOCI, and BIS among 3 groups

problems at school and criminality were occurring more frequently among the deceased. Suicide was the most common cause of death. However, only 2/19 that committed suicide had initially been admitted from attempted suicides. **Conclusion:** Behavioral problems, problems at school and co morbid alcohol/drug abuse and criminality (including alcohol related criminality) were found to be of prognostic importance. Maybe the prevention of suicide among adolescents and young adults is not just a question for psychiatry, but has to do with the society's interest in child social welfare work and the prevention of juvenile delinquency?

P-005-077   Topic: 42
Retention in primary school and anti-social behavior in adolescence
Maria da Conceicao Taborda Simoes, Universidade de Coimbra, Faculdade de Psicologia, Coimbra, Portugal, mctabordas@fpce.uc.pt
Maria das Dores Formosinho; Ana Monica Pinto

Objective: In this study, we aim to shed light on the relationship between early retention and anti-social behaviour in adolescence. **Methods:** The data were obtained from a large sample of portuguese students who have been assessed in a longitudinal study since 1992–1993. **Results:** Results showed that pupils with retentions in Primary School reveal later higher levels of anti-social behaviour than the non repeaters. **Conclusion:** Based on these data the authors make some considerations on the consequences of early retention and present some suggestions for future studies.

P-005-078   Topic: 42, 85
Identifying young students at risk for antisocial behaviour and school dropout:
The predictive power of teachers' ratings
Maria da Luz Vale Dias, Universidade de Coimbra, Faculdade de Psicologia, Coimbra, Portugal, valedias@fpce.uc.pt
Maria da Conceicao Taborda Simoes; Luiza Nobre Lima

Objective: The aim of this research was to examine the predictive power of teachers' ratings on antisocial behaviour and early school dropout. **Methods:** The sample consisted of a large number of first-grade students (boys and girls) from several public schools in Coimbra (in the centre of Portugal). Data were collected at two points in time: when they were in 4th grade (time 1) and 8 years later (time 2). At the initial assessment teachers completed several questions regarding their pupils emotional problems, antisocial behaviours and learning difficulties. **Results:** Results showed that: 1. Teachers' ratings of children behavioural and emotional problems provide only very modest predictions of antisocial behaviour and dropout on adolescence; 2. However, teachers' ratings of learning difficulties were good predictors of early school dropout. **Conclusion:** No good predictor was found for antisocial behaviour on adolescence or juvenile delinquency. There was a good predictive power of teachers' ratings of learning difficulties on early school dropout. These findings support the belief that an adequate assessment of children and adolescents difficulties (problems) requires the information from several sources and instruments. Several implications can be drawn from these data for the development of subsequent intervention programmes.

P-005-079   Topic: 42, 84
Attention Deficit Hyperactivity Disorder (ADHD) and self-concept: A 5 year follow-up of twins
Tobias Edbom, Karolinska Institutet, Dept. of Child Psychiatry, Stockholm, Sweden, tobias.edbom@kbh.ki.se
Jan-Olov Larsson; Paul Lichtenstein

Objective: It is from clinical experience assumed that Attention Deficit/Hyperactive Disorder (AD/HD) is related to low self-concept in children. However, relatively few studies have systematically studied the long-term relationship between ADHD symptoms and self-concept. The aim is to study the association between ADHD at 8–9 years of age and self-concept five years later using a case control study with co-twin design. **Methods:** Data were derived from the Young Twin Study which includes all twin pairs born in Sweden between May 1985 and December 1986. The first wave took place in 1994 where parents of all twin pairs received a mailed questionnaire regarding ADHD symptoms. The second wave took place in 1999 with questionnaires regarding self-concept. To test the association between ADHD and self-concept a General Linear Model analysis (GLM) where each twin contributed with one observation (n = 1746) using ADHD as a dependent variable and self-concept as an outcome. Secondly we used t-test to test the association between ADHD and self-concept. In the co-twin analysis we extracted all same-sexed twins, within pair discordant for a ADHD from the cohort (n = 37). The association between cases and their co-twin control were tested using paired t-test. Secondly performed the same analysis with monozygotic (MZ) twins (n = 16) and dizygotic (DZ) twins (n = 20). **Results:** In the GLM analysis ADHD symptoms were statistical significant related to self-concept. In the co-twin control analysis, there was statistical significant differences in all same sexed and DZ twin pairs. No statistical significant difference was found in MZ twins. **Conclusion:** The results show that children with ADHD symptoms at 8-9 years of age had lower self-concept att a five year follow up compared to their controls.

P-005-080   Topic: 44
Psychiatry, culture and symptoms
Bernardo Perez, Janssen Cilag Lab, Psychiatry, Madrid, Spain, amex.c.viajes@aexp.com
Macarena Marin

Objective: The focus on this review is analysing the prevalence of psychiatric symptoms and the socio-demographic characteristics of immigrant children, considering their singular adaptation to our country, compared with the indigenous population. **Methods:** Migration is nowadays a complex and raising issue. Therefore, is very important to be aware of the effect of migration on different aspects, such as on the relationships, social environment and family. Furthermore, the acknowledge of differences in each culture is necessary to make a proper clinical approach of the immigrants patients. Our geographic area, where live together people from different countries of Europe, South America and Africa, is a privileged place to study the influence of this phenomenon in the development of mental problems. Cross-transverse study. We analysed 30 immigrant patients and a control group of 60 indigenous. Subjects were selected randomly from 1341 patients, who received treatment during five years in our centre (from 1998–2003). Socio-demographic (age, sex, origin country, parents marital status, years living in Spain) and clinical factors were considered (type of referral, diagnosis, type of treatment and discharge). Statistic descriptive and univariate analyses of the above information were estimate. **Results:** Age and sex were similar in both populations. Regarding the type of referral, the most common was behaviour disturbance, but this problem was definitely confirm as a formal diagnosis in a meaningful percentage of the immigrants patients in comparison with the control group. About the diagnosis, the most frequent was adjustment disorders in the context of family problems, although, there were a higher level of separated or divorced parents between the immigrant group. **Conclusion:** This review try to detect the cultural, social and family factors, which lead to mental health problems in the immigrant children, thinking that it could be the best way to know the protective factors in the psychiatric disorders of this population.

P-005-081   Topic: 45, 47
Perceptual characteristics of Korean depressed mothers on children's behavior and the impacts on their perception

Su-Jin Yang, Chonnam General Hospital,
Dept. of Neuropsychiatry, Kwangju, Republic of Korea,
sj7512@lycos.co.kr
Helen Lee; Kyung-Sun Noh

Objective: The purpose of the study was to evaluate the perceptual characteristics of Korean depressed mothers on children's behavior and variables impacting on their perception. **Methods:** Fifty mothers were divided into two gorups, who were diagnosed as depressed and non-depressed. One child and adolescent psychiatrist, one psychiatrist, and one clinical psychologist were involved in the diagnostic process. Psychological tests battery including Korean Wechsler Adult Intelligence Scale (K-WAIS) were administered to all mothers. Mothers completed Korean version of Achenbach Child Behavior Checklist (CBCL), and teachers completed Korean version of Teacher's Report Form (TRF). **Results:** The results were as follows: 1) Depressed mothers scored significantly higher in somatic complaints, thought problems, aggressive behaviors, externalizing problems, and total problematic behaviors of CBCL in their children. 2) Depressed mother who had only one child, reported lower scores in school and total social competence than depressed mother who had two or more children. 3) After controlled for the scores of teacher's form, depressed mothers scored higher in aggressive behaviors and externalizing problems of CBCL in their children. **Conclusion:** Korean depressed mothers tend to perceive their child more negatvely than non-depressed mothers, especially in externalizing problems. Presence of sibling may impact on depressed mother's perception.

P-005-081A   Topic: 42, 37
Consumer satisfaction trajectories of adolescents during in-patient psychiatric treatment

Ferdinand Keller, Universitätsklinik Ulm,
Kinder- und Jugendpsychiatrie, Ulm, Germany,
ferdinand.keller@medizin.uni-ulm.de
Lutz Goldbeck; Alexander Naumann; Jörg M. Fegert

Objective: As most studies assess patient satisfaction and other aspects of process quality cross-sectionally (i.e. key date survey, or at discharge), little is known about change of satisfaction during the treatment period. This study describes the course of consumer satisfaction and related issues such as participation and motivation assessed twice weekly at wards of adolescent psychiatry. **Methods:** The study group consists of 88 adolescents (48 female, 40 male; age between 13 and 18 years) who delivered altogether 1003 time points (median per person is 8). The questionnaire consisted of 21 items that were asked by computer-assisted methods. Statistical analysis was done using hierarchical linear modeling (growth curve models) that is well suited for the analysis of data with different number of time points and missing data. **Results:** Person-specific levels (intercepts) of the different items are very heterogeneous, but the trends (slope of the growth curves) are around 0, i.e. in general the adolescents remain on their different levels during the treatment period. Exceptions are participation that increases during stay, and satisfaction with hospital staff that decreases, but of initially high values. Further analyses concerning group differences are currently going on. **Conclusion:** Evaluation of process characteristics has turned out to be feasible in clinical routine and promising for further insights into process quality. Theoretical explanations are discussed.

P-006   Topic: 83
Pervasive developmental disorders I
Track: Pervasive developmental disorders (PDD)

P-006-082   Topic: 83
Recognition of facial expression of emotions in children with Asperger syndrome: A case study

Ghizlane Benjelloun, Paris, France, benjelloung@yahoo.fr

Methods: Among theories of social impairment in Asperger syndrome, the hypothesis of a very early failure to coordinate affective perspectives has been explored. Hobson argues that in normally developing children the emotional relatedness is the basis of social understanding. It has been suggested that specific abnormalities in recognition of facial expression of emotions dissociated from preserved recognition of facial identity may distinguish children with Asperger syndrome from control subjects of equivalent verbal ability. **Results:** In our case study we compared a nine years old child with Asperger syndrome with a child with a pervasive development disorder and a control child concerning recognition of facial expression of emotions, of facial identity, and the ability to use these criteria in a sorting task, which may reflect the value devoted to emotional information by these children. We present our results and discuss them.

P-006-083   Topic: 83
Could ECT be effective in autism?

Dirk Dhossche, University of Mississippi,
Dept. of Psychiatry, Jackson, USA, dr6340451@pol.net
Sara Stanfill

Objective: Autism is increasingly diagnosed, but therapeutic options are limited in many children. The potential, risk, and feasibility of ECT in autistic children are discussed. **Methods:** Selected literature review. **Results:** The use of ECT in autism has not been systematically assessed. ECT is a safe and effective treatment for affective disorders, acute psychosis, and catatonia in people of all ages. Catatonic symptoms are common in autism. There are also speculations that certain types of autism may be the early expression of catatonia and that both disorders have identical (genetic) risk factors (Dhossche, 2004). Therefore, ECT may improve autism and, if started early enough, may prevent further development of autistic symptoms in some children. Two large ECT studies in children were done in the 1940's. Autism was not diagnosed because the autistic syndrome was just then being recognized as a separate entity. Findings from these studies attest to the safety of ECT in children but add little to the hypothesis that ECT may be effective in autistic children. Since then, ECT techniques have greatly improved. Widespread anti-ECT sentiment not only among the public but also within the medical community may well be the greatest deterrent to use ECT in autism at present times. Further studies on the relations between autism, catatonia, ECT, and central GABA function may support the hypothesis that ECT is effective in autism. **Conclusion:** The hypothesis that ECT can effectively treat autism and even arrest further autistic development, if started early enough, is the corollary of speculations about an intricate link between autism and catatonia. Early ECT studies attest to the safety of ECT in children. Unless anti-ECT prejudice can be overcome, it is unlikely that any ECT trial in autism will be done.

P-006-084   Topic: 83, 9
Psychodrama in children and adults with autistic disorders and with Asperger's disorder

Akiko Takahara, Kumamoto University, Faculty of Education, Kumamoto, Japan, kougen@educ.kumamoto-u.ac.jp
Minemitsu Kusu; Sumiko Watanabe; Tatsuya Matsui; Kengo Ikeda; Hiroe Matsuda

Objective: The aim of this study is to examine the effect of psychodrama in children and adults with autistic disorders and with Asperger's disorders. **Methods:** The subjects were 37 autistics and patients will Asperger's disorder aged 6-40 years old. Our psychodrama sessions have been conducted twice a month for 12 years. The therapeutic effect of the program were examined about people who took part in this program of psychodrama more than 2 years. **Results:** Results that were all recorded on VTR, were analyzed by 1. age level and 2. intellectual level. Analysis of the results showed that after the Psychodrama, they came to understand other's thinking better, came to be more interested in other's and expressed their own thoughts. Furthermore, psychodrama plays the role of a peer-counselor by providing the opportunity to discuss and to share their feeling with their peers under a controlled yet open environment. Finally, the effect mechanism of psychodrama was showed by the illustration. **Conclusion:** Psychodrama is an effective method for supporting life-span development of children and adults with autistic disorders and with Asperger's disorders.

P-006-085   Topic: 83
Sleep patterns of children with Asperger Syndrome or high-functioning autism

Hiie Allik, Karolinska Institutet, Dept of Woman and Child Health, Stockholm, Sweden, hiie.allik@kbh.ki.se
Jan-Olov Larsson; Hans Smedje

Objective: The aim was to explore if childhood Asperger Syndrome (AS) and high-functioning autism (HFA) are as-

sociated with abnormal sleep patterns. **Methods:** The study group was thirty-two school-aged children with either AS or HFA matched with thirty-two children without developmental disabilities. Pairwise comparisons were made between cases and controls. The sleep patterns were monitored over the course of one week using both parental reports to a sleep diary and actigraphy, computerised movement-based sleep-wake detection. Repeated measures ANOVA were used for the statistical analyses. **Results:** Diary and actigraphy recordings showed that children in the AS/HFA group spent a longer time awake in bed before falling asleep than the controls. However, the groups did not differ with respect to timing of sleep on school days, and the children in the AS/HFA group fell asleep earlier on weekends. Sleep duration and number of nighttime arousals did not differ between the groups. When comparing childen with AS and those with HFA, no differences in sleep patterns were found. **Conclusion:** Difficulties in falling asleep, possibly related to earlier bedtimes, were more common in children with AS/HFA compared with the controls. Other essential aspects of sleep patterns did not differ.

P-006-086   Topic: 83
Self-understanding and self-isolation in adolescents with High-functioning Pervasive Developmental Disorders (HFPDD)

Sadaaki Shirataki, Mukogawa Women's University, Dept. of Human Sciences, Nishinomiya, Japan, shiratak@kobe-u.ac.jp
Bonko Murakami

Objective: The objective of this study is to delineate the characteristics of self-understanding and self-isolation in adolescents with HFPDD. **Methods:** Our subjects were, 1) 29 healthy, junior-high school students as a control group, and 2) had 10 HFPDD adolescents as a clinical group. Among 10 HFPDD adolescents, 6 Asperger syndrome (AS), and 4 High-Functioning Autsim (HFA). Self-understanding was studied by using semi-structured questionnaires according to the Damon & Hart (1988) model of self-consciousness. This model divides the self-as-object and the self-as-subject, with the items self-definition, self-evaluation, self-projection in past and future, self-interest; self-continuity, self-agency, self-distinctness. Evaluation was done according to the category classification (physical, active, social and psychological), and level classification (early childhood, late childhood, early adolescent, and late adolescent). Self-isolation was studied by the modified Rubenstein and Shaver (1980)'s questionnaire. **Results:** HFPDD subjects found out that they responded more(by three times) toward questions for self-as-objects than for self-as-subject. If all answers within the self-as-object were calculated, the active and psychological self were the top (40%) and the social (13%), and the physical (7%) was the least. As to the level classification, the responses were most in level 2, level 1, level 4, and level 3 in order. As to the category classification, the responses were evenly distributed among 3 categorization for the questions toward the self-as-subject. There were some subjects with HFPDD who could not respond in any way to the questions asking for the self-isolation. Responses classified as psychological were the most, the next was active-self, social was the least, and there was no response in the physical-self category. The great majority of the responses in the level classification was in the level 1. HFPDD subjects responded to questions asking for self-as-object by answering more psychological catgegorization than in Healthy JHS group subjects. HFPDD subjects were also characterized by lower level of responses in psychological categorization. HFPDD subjects responded by answering more in psychological categorization and less in active categorization than the Healthy JHS group. **Conclusion:** We could clarify the differences in the way of self-understanding and self-isolation both in HFPDD subjects and healthy JHS subjects by means of semi-structured questionnaires developed by Damon & Hart (1988). HFPDD subjects found to be experiencing the self-isolation situation in terms of psychological feeling and furthermore in terms of negative subjective feelings. But, their way to express their feeling in the isolated situation is at least not sufficient enough to warrant the surroundings to be sympathetic. The relative weakness in looking at self from the viewpoint of self-as-subject can of course explain the poverty of subject consciousness, concerning behavior feelings, and emotions. We believe these findings would certainly to help us to guide the proper supporting ways for the HFPDD subjects.

P-006-087   Topic: 83
Speech characteristics for autistic children

Rawheya Ahmad Mohamed, Phonetics, Alexandria, Egypt, dr_rawhia@hotmail.com

Objective: To investigate the speech characteristic of autistic children. To correlate the speech features of autistic children compared to normal children. To analyze their type of speech with its relation to their perception and understanding speech or language. **Methods:** Experimental analysis will be done by using computerised program for speech. This will include some of acoustic parameters to investigate three main groups with different developmental ages and sex (n=26). A controled group of matched age and sex will be represented,t o assess the different characteristic features of speech. **Results:** The resulting data will support and display the general agreement about their speech which descibed as; monotonus, unpleasant, stereotyped, ecolalic speech with repetition of sounds, syllables and words. The specific characteristic of chanting or singsong speech that accompanied by staccato speech will be demonstrated. **Conclusion:** Phonetic diagnosis of autistic children can be implemented in assessment of their speech.

P-006-088   Topic: 83, 12
Efficacy and safety of risperidone in the treatment of children with autistic and other pervasive developmental disorders (PDD): A randomized, double-blind, placebo controlled trial

Fiona Dunbar, Janssen-Ortho Inc., C.P. Clinical Affairs, Toronto, Canada, fdunbar1@joica.jnj.com
Sarah Shea

Objective: This trial was designed to assess the efficacy and safety of risperidone in the treatment of behavioral symptoms in children with autistic and other PDD. **Methods:** During this eight-week, randomized, double-blind, multicenter trial 80 children aged 5 to 12 years with PDD received oral risperidone (0.01–0.06 mg/kg/day) or placebo. Efficacy was measured with the Aberrant Behavior Checklist (ABC), clinical global impression scale and the Nisonger Child Behavior Rating Form (N-CBRF). **Results:** At endpoint, patients receiving risperidone (mean dose 0.04 mg/kg/day) showed a significantly greater decrease from baseline on the ABC irritability subscale compared with placebo recipients (12.1 vs.

6.5, p<0.001, primary outcome). Additionally, significant improvements were recorded on all other ABC subscales. Significant differences favoring risperidone were also observed on the conduct-problem subscale of the N-CBRF (p<=0.01). Risperidone-treated subjects also showed statistically significantly greater mean decreases on the insecure/anxious (p=0.039), hyperactive (p=0.035), and overly sensitive (p=0.038) subscales of the N-CBRF. Decreases on the 'most troublesome symptom' visual analogue scale were significantly greater in the risperidone group (38.4 vs. 26.2, p<=0.05). Improvements on the Clinical Global Impression scale were observed in 87.2% of risperidone and 39.5% of placebo recipients (p<=0.01). Risperidone was well tolerated. Somnolence (72.5%) was the most frequently observed adverse event, but seems to be manageable in the majority of the subjects with dose and dose schedule modification. There were no significant differences in mean total score from baseline on the Extrapyramidal Symptom Rating Scale to any timepoints between the two treatment groups. Body weight increased more in risperidone compared with placebo recipients (2.7 vs. 1.0 kg). **Conclusion:** Risperidone significantly improves behavioral symptoms of autism and other PDDs (primary and secondary outcomes) and is well tolerated by patients 5 to 12 years of age.

P-006-089   Topic: 83
Early signs of autism based on home movies

Mariko Atsumi, Tokai University, Dept. of Psychiatry, Yokohama City, Japan, atumimari2000@yahoo.yco.jp
Hideo Matsumoto; Akitoshi Ooya; Seiji Koishi; Yutaka Aoki; Youichi Enseki; Yuri Nakamura

Objective: Objective was to identify early signs of autism and to find the difference of signs before and after 12 months. **Methods:** Ratings of behaviors in home movies of 18 infants who were later diagnosed as autistic and matched 19 healthy infants (age of 7–18 months) were performed by two diagnosis-blind psychologists with the evaluation scale. This scale was modified from the Infant Behavioral Summarized Evaluation by Adrien et al. The items of evaluation were classified to 6 fields (Socialization, Communication, Adaptation to environment, Motility, Emotional and instinctual reactions, Attention-perception). Intraclass correlation was used for the examination of interrater reliability. Mann-Whitney U test was used for comparisons between behaviors of healthy and autistic groups. Wilconsean T test was used for the longitudinal analysis of behaviors. **Results:** Results showed that the behaviors related to socialization, communication, adaptation to environment, and emotional reactions significantly differentiated autistic and healthy groups during the first year of age. The same behaviors had been observed even more during the second year in the autistic groups. **Conclusion:** Early signs of autism were identified during the first year of age, and observed even more during the second year.

P-006-090   Topic: 83, 10
Early intervention for autism:
The NAS earlybird programme in Greece

Kostas Francis, PDD Clinic, Athens, Greece, kostas.francis@psychiatry.oxford.ac.uk
Vassilis Kazaridis; Panagiota Kirillidou; Sofia Koukouvinou

Objective: Although early intervention cannot cure autism, it can minimize the build up of secondary behavioural problems and help the child to develop fully its potential. The UK National Autistic Society (NAS) set up the Early-Bird Programme, a three-month autism-specific programme, which combines 8 three-hour group training sessions for parents with 5 individual home visits (using video feedback). An efficacy study evaluated this programme in UK families with positive results (Autism. 2001 5(1):49-56). We evaluated the programme in 15 Greek families of preschoolers with Autism. Data related to parents psychosocial functioning is reported herein. **Methods:** Children with autism were identified using the ADI-R and ADOS. Two people (parents or other caregivers) from each family were then invited to participate. Parents were administered, both at the beginning and the end of the program, questionnaires used by the EarlyBird programme, as well as the Parent Stress Index (PSI). **Results:** 27 people participated (15 mothers, 11 fathers and 1 caregiver). The probands were 13 children with Autistic Disorder (2 HFA) and 1 child with Asperger's syndrome (mean age = 4 yrs (range 2,7 5,7)). At the end of the program, parents reported a 17% increase in the amount of time spent in play with their child, combined with a significant decrease in scores across all subscales within the parent domain of the PSI, with the exception of the depression subscale. **Conclusion:** The EarlyBird programme was found to be very effective in empowering parents to meet their child's psychoeducational needs and in reducing their own stress. The opportunities of improving parental psychological well-being will be further discussed.

P-006-091   Topic: 83, 26
Rising incidence of Autistic Spectrum Disorders
Sobharani Paliwal, Parkview Clinic,
Child & Adolescent Psychiatry, Birmingham,
United Kingdom, reenapaliwal@onetel.net.uk
William Whitehouse; Margo Edwards; Ayliffe Edwards;
Sunita Pandit; Judith Powell

Objective: The incidence and prevalence of autistic spectrum disorders (ASDs)seems to be rising. We therefore measured incidence and prevalence, in pre-school children, in two discrete, geographically defined populations in the UK. **Methods:** Children diagnosed with ASD aged 1 year to 4 years 11 months were ascertained from the Child Development Centres serving South Birmingham (population aged 1-4 years: 25,000) and Tamworth (population aged 1-4 years: 4,000), and a regional specialist psychiatry clinic, resident and diagnosed from 1.1.91 to 31.12.96 DSM-IIIR, DSM-IV and ICD10 categories were used. **Results:** The age-specific incidence for ASD was the same in both populations despite differences in social deprivation and the proportion of ethnic minorities and rose from 3.5/10,000/year in 1991-92 to 13.1/10,000/year in 1995-96. Even the incidence of the more narrowly defined 'Childhood Autism' rose: from 2.7 to 4.3/10,000/year. The incidence of ASDs increased on average by 37% per year. The annual period prevalence for 1996 was 34.0/10,000 and the cumulative incidence to 5th birthday for the 1991 birth cohort was 42/10,000. **Conclusion:** This study confirms the increasing incidence of ASDs. This may be due to a real biological increase or to increased willingness by professionals to use these diagnoses, especially for children without narrowly defined 'Childhood Autism', or a combination of both.

P-006-092   Topic: 83
Executive functions in children with Attention Deficit Hyperactivity Disorder (ADHD)
Mehdi Tehrani-Doost, Roozbeh Psychiatric Hospital,
Child & Adolescent Psychiatry, Tehran,
Islamic Republic of Iran, tehranid@sina.tums.ac.ir
Mitra Sepasi; Javad Alaghband-Rad; Reza Rad Goodarzi

Objective: The purpose of this study was to compare the executive functions in children with attention deficit hyperactivity disorder to normal children. **Methods:** Twenty children which were diagnosed as having ADHD according to DSM-IV were compared with 19 healthy children in terms of executive functions using the computerised version of Tower of London (Morris, 1993), Continious Performance Test (CPT), and Stroop Color Test. **Results:** In the "Tower of London" task, the performance of ADHD children was worse than that in normal children, which was significant at level 3 of the "Tower of London" task (p < 0.05). In the Continious Performance Test, the commission errors – which are an index of impulsivity – in ADHD children were significantly more than that in normal group (p < 0.01). The omission errors – which are an index of inattention – in ADHD children were higher (not significant). In the Stroop Color Test, there was no significant difference betwen two groups in terms of difference index (which is the subtraction of dots time of colors time although the length of time in color part was longer). **Conclusion:** Some aspects of executive functions such as planning and inhibition were impaired in ADHD children compared to normal children. In this study we did not find any significant difference in attention index in CPT.

P-006-094   Topic: 83, 9
Effectiveness of group psychotherapy and inpatient treatment in an adolescent with High-functioning Pervasive Developmental Disorder (HFPDD): A case report
Masaki Kodaira, Kohnodai Hospital, Child & Adolescent
Psychiatry, Ichikawa Chiba, Japan, masakik@xk9.
so-net.ne.jp

Objective: Because adolescents have ego function that is not mature enough to observe or verbalize their inner experiences, there are needs to modify psychotherapeutic strategies for their approach. This problem may be more remarkable on adolescents with pervasive developmental disorder (PDD). Their inability to communicate with others often makes it very difficult for them to develop mutual relationship with friends of the same generation. We will describe a case and comment on the importance and efficacy of group psychotherapy and hospitalization for adolescents with high-functioning PDD (HFPDD). **Methods:** We will describe a case of a 13-year-old boy with HFPDD, named K. K admitted to our child and adolescent psychiatry ward and received an inpatient treatment for 1year and 6 months. K has been socially withdrawn and has not been attending school for 5 years. He was brought up by his grandmother and was not recognized of having HFPDD until he was hospitalized. At the beginning of hospitalization, he showed little interest towards his peers and seemed to be easily irritated and excited. **Results:** He gradually learned to communicate with others through group psychotherapy sessions, as the other members started to accept him. Also, he received individual psychotherapy and started to verbalize his feelings, which lead him to spend his ward life without being irritated. **Conclusion:** This case illustrates the importance and efficacy of both hospitalization and group psychotherapy for adolescents with HFPDD.

P-006-095 Topic: 83, 27

The Asperger's disorder during adolescence and early adulthood – Some problems of differential diagnosis

Andrea Viertler, KJPP, Rostock, Germany,
caspermond@yahoo.com
Katja Elpel; Olaf Reis; Frank Haessler

Objective: This study discusses some problems that may occur with the diagnosis and prognosis of this pervasive developmental disorder. The concept of Asperger-autism disorder is still nosologically developing and not focussing yet on a coherent concept of psychiatric disorder. **Methods:** The study discusses the cases of two patients recently diagnosed as having an Asperger's disorder. Both cases of Asperger's disorder we report had a long history of psychiatric misclassifications before they were diagnosed as not being capable of taking responsibilities while having social deficits in adolescence. However, deficits in social functioning were going back to early childhood for both individuals. One patient was diagnosed with Asperger's disorder while being a patient in a forensic hospital, the other one being an out-patient of our hospital. **Conclusion:** Asperger's disorder appears as having a wide range of comorbid symptoms that may lead to misclassifications, such as obsessive compulsive disorder, reading disabilities, or schizoaffective disorder. During their childhood both patients were classified as having externalizing disorders. The diagnose of Asperger's disorder might be impaired by exceptional developmental qualities of the disorder during adolescence. These developmental qualities can be interpreted as a heterotypic continuity that starts early in childhood and leads to long-lasting inpatient careers. One problem is that standardized diagnostic instruments for this disorder are hard to obtain which increases the probability of misclassifications.

P-006-096 Topic: 83, 27

The comparison of the diagnostic subgroups of Pervasive Developmental Disorder (PDD) according to demographic variables and clinical characteristics

Melda Ayse Akçakýn, Medical School of Ankara, Dept. of Child Psychiatry, Ankara, Turkey, erdenmgul@yahoo.com
Gulsen Erden; Efser Kerimoglu

Objective: The aim of this study is to compare demographic and some clinical characteristics of children who were diagnosed as the autistic, autistic + R, PDD-NOS and relationship disorder (RD). **Methods:** The sample was obtained from Ankara University School of Medicine, Department of Child Psychiatry And The Research, Diagnostic and Treatment Center for Autistic Children. The Autistic, Autistic + R, PDD-NOS, Disintegrative Disorder, Rett, Asperger and RD children were selected from 738 case diagnosed with Pervasive Developmental Disorder who were assessed between the years 1976–2000. The children who were 3 years old and older at the admission were evaluated according to DSM-III-R and DSM-IV criteria. The children who were under the age of three at the admission were evaluated by the Diagnostic Criteria for 0–3. All children were diagnosed and assessed using a semistructured interview. The children were grouped based on their diagnosis, as the autistic group (N=274), the autistic + mental retardation group (N=129), PDD-NOS (150) and RD group (138). The children who were diagnosed as the Asperger (N=8), Rett (N=5) and Disintegrative Disorder (N=34) were excluded from comparison statistics because they were very few in number. The data was analysed with One way ANOVA. **Results:** The findings showed that the mean age and the education levels of parents of the RD group were significantly different from the other 3 groups. It was found that parents in the RD group have less number of children when compared to other groups. Data regarding to age of walking implied that children in autism and RD groups had walked earlier than others. Among the four groups, the earliest use of 'first words' was seen in the RD group. It was found that, among the four groups, parents in of the RD group had noticed the symptoms in their children earlier; they were followed by parents in the autism+MR group and then parents in the PDD-NOS group. Regarding the DSM III-R and additional symptoms total scores, the mean score of autism group was higher than the others. **Conclusion:** It is important to separately consider the diagnostic subgroups under the broad diagnosis of PDD and to make between-group comparisons. It is also suggested that it is necessary to compare subgroups regarding the variable of intelligence.

P-006-097 Topic: 83, 11

Play with other: A new approach in autism

Eric Lemonnier, Centre Hospitalier, Pédopsychiatrie, Bohars, France, eric.lemonnier@chu-brest.fr

Objective: Our experience with autistic children, as well as numerous studies (Wetherby 84, Loveland 86, Sigman 92, Baron-Cohen 96, Hobson 00) show that autistic children are impaired in triadic social functioning. J.M. Vidal has envisaged a therapeutic approach with the aim to help these children to tackle with these triadic situations better. This involves ten meetings with a child and one other person, and alternative meetings with or without a third person. The child has the possibility to accept or refuse the third person during these triadic meetings. We ask what benefits are accrued from this approach. **Methods:** Our study is made with 6 autistic children (F84.0 of ICD10) according to ADI-R. Evaluation is made by CARS and VINELAND before the therapy and then after 30 sessions. For the statistical analysis we used Wilcoxon test in SPSS 11.5. **Results:** The result show a significant difference before and after the therapy, for all of the three subdomain of the VINELAND (communication, daily living skills, socialization) and for the score of CARS. **Conclusion:** We discuss some methodological limits. The first is the absence of a control population. We also discuss the psychocognitive point of view. Autistic children might have cognitive difficulties and they sometime use bypassing strategies in advance. Our approach could help them in this.

P-006-098   Topic: 83, 26
Estimated prevalence of High-functioning Pervasive Developmental Disorders (HFPDD) in the psychiatric outpatient setting of an university hospital

Toshio Munesue, Kanazawa University,
Psychiatry and Neurobiology, Kanazawa, Japan,
munesue@med.kanazawa-u.ac.jp
Kouhei Mutoh; Kazunori Shimoda; Hideo Nakatani;
Yoshifumi Koshino

Objective: To estimate the prevalence of high-functioning pervasive developmental disorders (HPDD), mainly Asperger disorder and high-functioning autistic disorder, in the psychiatric outpatient setting of an university hospital. Adolescents and adults with HPDD showed various chief complaints such as difficulties in adjustment in their environment, impulse control difficulties, interpersonal conflict, and some psychotic-like symptoms. Consequently, they tend to be misdiagnosed as schizophrenia, personality disorder, or adjustment disorder. Clinicians seldom examine HPDD in their daily clinical work, and they are less likely to precisely diagnose HPDD. Therefore, estimated prevalence of HPDD is a useful and important clinical information. **Methods:** Medical records of all psychiatric outpatients in Kanazawa university hospital from January 1, 1977 to December 31, 2003 were reviewed. Two categories of HPDD were defined: definite HPDD were the diagnosis HPDD coincided with clinical descriptive records, and possible HPDD were the diagnosis was not-HPDD, but clinical records indicated HPDD symptoms based on DSM-criteria. **Results:** During seven years, 7,249 patients visited the psychiatric outpatient setting. There were 68 patients with definite HPDD (0.9%) and 17 patients with possible HPDD (0.2%). **Conclusion:** About one percent of psychiatric outpatients seemed to suffer from HPDD. Although stigma still attaches psychiatric disorders, patients with those conditions are more likely to visit Kanazawa university hospital with or without a letter of reference. The university hospital is located in the center of Kanazawa city, and carries two roles: one is the leading hospital, and the other is general hospital. Estimated prevalence of HPDD would be one out of 100 among psychiatric outpatients.

P-006-099   Topic: 83, 37
The Marburg rating scale for Asperger's Syndrome (MBAS)

Isabell Germerott, Universität Marburg,
Kinder- und Jugendpsychiatrie, Marburg, Germany,
iheinema@med.uni-marburg.de
Helmut Remschmidt

Objective: According to DSM-IV Asperger's syndrome (AS) is a pervasive developmental disorder, characterized by distinctive abnormalities in communication, qualitative abnormalities in reciprocal social interaction, poor social empathy, and circumscribed (intense) interests. An often observed associated feature is motor clumsiness. The etiology and validation of the AS is unclear. In the german language area there is no screening instrument for AS available. The purpose of this study is to present a screening instrument (MBAS) which is sensitive for this disorder. **Methods:** The instrument was offered a group of patients with AS, childhood autism and without the diagnosis autism. The psychometric properties of the instruments were investigated: Examinations for item difficulty, internal con-

sistency, reliability, validity, sensitivity and specificity were made. A factor analysis was carried out in order to analyze the structure of the instrument. **Results:** The difficulty of the items were mostly in average range as well as the all item-total correlations. It has an internal consistency of Cronbach's alpha = 0.91 and the convergent validity of the MBAS and the ADI-R reached r = 0.61 (p = 0.001). The total score of the questionaire discriminated highly significantly between the autism group and the non-autism group. With a sensitivity of 95.5% and a specifity of 95.7% only a few misclassifications were observed (mainly in young children). A 5 factor solution was found, with reasonable arrangement of the items. **Conclusion:** The MBAS can be looked upon as a reliable and valid instrument for screening children and adolescents for Asperger's syndrome.

P-007
Scientific disciplines/approaches III

P-007-100   Topic: 38
New nitrodibenzodiazepine as vasodilator

Eman Galal Sadek, Faculty of Science, Dept. of Chemistry,
Mansoura, Egypt, scimussaoffice@mans.edu.eg

Objective: New nitrodibenzodiazepine has been synthesized. Work was done to observe the effects of the new compound, selctive reverse mode NCX inhibitory, on changes in cytoplasmic calcium ion concentration and ventricular contactility during ischemia-reperfussion in perfused beating hearts. **Methods:** The hearts of rats were perfused and loaded with fura-2 to measure the fluorescence ratio as an index of calcium ion. Left ventricular pressure and ECG were recorded. **Results:** Per-ischemic diastolic flurosence ratio will not be affected by the new compound. Treatment of the new compound (10 yM) suppressed the increase in calcium ion induced by low-sodium ion exposure and the increase in diastolic calcium ion during ischemia. After reperfusion, the normalization of diastolic calcium ion was faster in the new compound in untreated hearts. **Conclusion:** In hibition of reverse mode NCX shows decrease of calcium ion overloaded and myocardial protection during ischemia and reperfusion in while heart model. A comparion study between the new compound and aldomet at different intervals has been done.

P-007-101   Topic: 37, 23
Estimation of a quality of life of adolescents with psychosomatic disorders

A. G. Litvinov, Center for Mental Health,
RussiaTatjana Dmitrieva

Objective: An estimation of different parameters of quality of life in adolescents with psychosomatic disorders. **Methods:** The instrument ILK (Inventar zur Erfassung der Lebensqualitat bei Kindern und Jugendlichen), designed by F. Mattejat and H. Remschmidt (1998) (an inventory to assess the quality of life in children and adolescents) was used. 151 adolescents aged from 12 to 17 years (97 girls, 54 boys) with psychosomatic disorders were investigated. **Results:** First, the highest (negative) average value were detected in areas: pressure of problems/disease, health, nerve/mood. The most positively estimated scales were: social contacts and family. Estimations of the adolescents

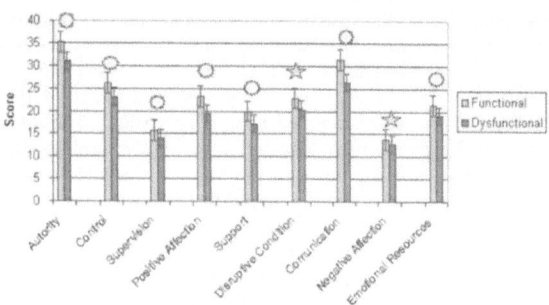

Functional-Dysfunctional Comparison for several factors

Comparison of the values average obtained in each one of the areas that explores the "scale of functional evaluation", in each one of the groups.

(Very significant difference) = ○

(Not very significant difference) = ☆

and their parents did not reveal essential qualitative distinctions. During psychotherapy we found a marked improvement of all indices of quality of life from the point of view of the adolescents and their parents. **Conclusion:** The instrument ILK represents a useful and practical inventory for quality of life research. It is expedient to use this instrument as a method of an evaluation of efficacy of therapy.

P-007-102   Topic: 37
Functional evaluation of families with a handicapped member

Froylan Calderón-Castañeda, Centro Nacional de, Rehabilitación Laboral, Mexico City, Mexico, froilanenrique@yahoo.com.mx
Alberto Enrique Nuno-Licona; Efren Alatorre-Miguel

Objective: To apply the scale to the families with a handicapped patient that have been assisted in the service of Family Therapy of the National Center of Rehabilitation (CNR), from November 2001, to March, 2003. Specific objectives to determine: a) If all the families present dynamic functional alterations or not. b) If there are relations between the patient's age and the scale's result, as well as between gender and scale's result. c) Which areas of the scale influence the family dynamic function. **Methods:** An interviewer applied the scale that consists of 40 questions, to 50 families. The values obtained for each one of the explored areas made arranged in charts and the averages and variances were analyzed with the statistical program InStat3. **Results:** About 54% of the families was functional, with a global score of 140.3 ± 6.4, and the dysfunctional families, 46%, with global score of 123.3 ± 6.4, the difference between both groups were significant ($P < 0.05$; t, Student). The areas that showed a significant difference ($P < 0.05$; t, Student) among groups were: disruptive behavior and negative affection. **Conclusion:** Not any family with a patient/disabled person is disfunctional. The scale and their analysis allow us to know the more affected areas in the family dynamics, which in turn will allow to design our therapeutic approach better.

P-007-103   Topic: 37, 24
Parent-rated assessment of personality for preschool and primary-school children – The German JTCI/3 and JTCI/7-11

Kirstin Goth, Universität Frankfurt, Kinder- und Jugendpsychiatrie, Frankfurt, Germany, c.goth@em.uni-frankfurt.de
Klaus Schmeck

Objective: According to Cloninger's psychobiological theory of personality and on the basis of the Preschool TCI (Constantino et al., 2002) we constructed specific german questionnaires for Preschool (JTCI/3-6) and Primary-School Children (JTCI/7-11) to provide a parent-rated assessment of the seven factor model of personality appropriate to these ages. Psychometric properties of both inventories and aspects of validity are presented. **Methods:** JTCI/3-6 was tested on the parents of 332 children from 30 Kindergarten, JTCI/7-11 on 277 parents from three Primary Schools in Germany. 108 and 105 respectively of this parents were enrolled in a longitudinal study and were retested after two months with JTCI and the Strength and Difficulties Questionnaire (SDQ; Woerner et al., 2002) to check retest-reliability and diagnostic validity. To evaluate Psychometric Properties we used item-difficulties (between 5 and 95% symptomatic answers), item-total-correlations (>0.30) and effect of sex and age on item-response (effect-size <0.50). Scale reliability was assessed with Cronbachs Alpha (>0.70). Factorial structure was checked with Exploratory Factor Analyses. **Results:** For both Inventories we selected each 86 five-point-scale items which fully met the described criteria. They showed satisfying scale-reliabilities ranging from 0.71 to 0.87, good retest-reliabilities from 0.75 to 0.87. and the assumed factorial structure. Correlations with psychopathology (SDQ) are in line with the predictions of Cloninger's diagnostic concept. The character-dimensions Self Directedness and Cooperativeness are negatively correlated with all SDQ-scales reflecting problematic behaviour, temperament-dimensions Novelty Seeking and Harm Avoidance are positively correlated with specific problematic behaviour (HA with emotional symptoms, NS with conduct problems). **Conclusion:** JTCI/3-6 and JTCI/7-11 provide a reliable assessment of Cloninger's model of personality, that shows to be applicable to Preschool and Primary-School Children whose development of personality is not yet completed.

P-007-104   Topic: 37
A new instrument for therapy evaluation of children and adolescents

Sibylle Winter, Charité Berlin, Kinder- und Jugendpsychiatrie, Berlin, Germany, sibylle.winter@charite.de
Anja Wiegard

Objective: Few instruments exist that evaluate psychotherapy for children and adolescents. This study shows the development of a new instrument for therapy evaluation of children and adolescents: The "Psychotherapie Basisdokumentation für Kinder und Jugendliche" (Psy – BaDo – KJ). Patients, parents and therapists name individual goals and problematic fields of life. Furthermore the therapy outcome is evaluated. **Methods:** At first we used a questionnaire originally developped for adults: the "Psychotherapie Basisdokumentation": Psy – BaDo (Heuft, Senf, 1998). For the development of the new instrument especially for children and adolescents we made an expert rating. This rating was analyzed qualitatively with the method of the Grounded Theory. The new questionnaire (Psy – BaDo – KJ) was tested in our clinic from Februrary 2002 to November 2003. Finally 62 inpatients (>=12 years) were included in this study (63,9% girls/36,1% boys). **Results:** The results of the expert rating led to the development of the new questionnaire for children and adolescents. We modified problematic items and changed the layout, also we developed a parallel parent report. Quantitative analyses show following results: According to the therapy goals patients, parents and therapists show a significant agreement. They formulate at first intrapsychic goals, most frequent the self-efficiency. As well they agree in naming the same problematic fields of life. Furthermore patients, parents and therapists evaluate consistently the therapy outcome. As a trend, patients are more content than their parents and therapists. In opinion of therapists the therapy outcome is significantly correlated with the length of therapy. **Conclusion:** The new instrument for children and adolescents (Psy BaDo KJ) can be used efficiently for therapy evaluation as a model for quality assurance.

P-007-105 Topic: 37, 57

On the psychological distress of young inmates – measured by the Brief-Symptom-Inventory (BSI)

Günter Hinrichs, Universität Kiel,
Kinder- und Jugendpsychiatrie, Kiel, Germany,
schuetze@kiju-psych.uni-kiel.de
Denis Köhler

Objective: The BSI - as a short version of the SCL-90-R (Symptom-Checklist Revised) - is a psychological status self-report symptom inventory of 53 items. The answers are combined in nine primary symptom dimensions, in addition the Global Severity Index (GSI) provides a measure of over all psychological distress. Until now standard measures for the general population are available, not so for forensic samples, especially incarcerated delinquents. **Methods:** In the present study 200 young inmates were tested with the BSI. **Results:** All mean values of the nine subscales were significant higher in comparison with the general population. Internal consistency of the symptom dimensions can be described as moderate to good, as very good for the GSI. The primary symptom dimensions show high intercorrelations, therefore only one factor could be extracted. Concurrent validity can be demonstrated by significant association between the subscales and measures oft personality as well as psychological distress. **Conclusion:** The results oft the study are discussed by investigating, how useful the BSI can be as a screening-tool for psychological disorders in young inmates.

P-007-106 Topic: 37

The cold test: A methodology to study perinatal stress responses

Martin Kammerer, Rüschlikon, Switzerland,
makam1@bluewin.ch
Diana Adams; Brida von Castelberg; Alyx Taylor

Objective: The Hypothalamic-Pituitary-Adrenal HPA axis is known to be altered in pregnancy and the post partum period with a cortisol overdrive towards the end of pregnancy and a sharp fall after childbirth. However, the effect of these changes on stress reactivity of the HPA axis has not been tested with a natural stressor and the effects on the circadian rhythm of saliva cortisol still remains unclear. Furthermore, the effect of these physiologic changes of the HPA axis on different kinds of depressive episodes may contribute fundamental understanding of the nature of depression. **Methods:** Depressed pregnant and postpartum women and matched healthy controls participate in a physical stress test the cold hand test in which saliva is taken just before and 20 minutes after immersion of the non dominant hand in water at 4 °C. **Results:** Controls showed a diurnal effect in the cold test response, with a significantly greater rise in the afternoon than in the morning. Towards the end of pregnancy the saliva cortisol baseline was increased and the reactivity to the cold test decreased compared with non pregnant healthy controls. **Conclusion:** With both these results the rise in response to the cold test was related to the baseline value, the higher the baseline the lower the response.

P-007-107 Topic: 37, 83

Factor analysis of the high-functioning autism spectrum screening questionnaire

Maj-Britt Posserud, University of Bergen, Centre for CAMH,
Bergen, Norway, maj-britt.posserud@rbup.uib.no
Kjell Morten Stormark; Astri J. Lundervold;
Christopher Gillberg; Maaike Steijnen; Sophie Verhoeven

Objective: The purpose of the study was to do a factor analysis of the high-functioning Autism Spectrum Screening Questionnaire (ASSQ) and to compare the factors with the 2 social subscales (Peer Problems and Prosocial) in the Strengths and Difficulties Questionnaire (SDQ). **Methods:** The SDQ and the ASSQ were included in the Bergen Child Study, a total population study of 9430 children in 2–4th grade in Bergen in Oct. 2002. The analyses were performed on children whose parents gave informed consent to participate, N=7007 (74%). Principal axis factor analysis with Varimax rotation of the ASSQ was performed for parents and teachers separately. The ASSQ factors were then correlated using Pearson correlation with the SDQ Prosocial and Peer Problem scale. **Results:** With minimum loading of 0.4, three factors were identified, explaining 36.8% of the variation of the ASSQ for parents and 40.8% for teachers. Based on the items included we named the factors "social", "Asperger" and "tics/ocd". The factors were consistent between parents and teachers. The Social factor correlated strongly with Peer Problems and moderately with Prosocial score, whereas the Asperger factor correlated fairly with Peer Problems and not at all with the Prosocial score. The findings were consistent for parents and teachers, except that the parent factors correlated somewhat less than the teacher factors. **Conclusion:** Social difficulty is a general and common symptom of psychiatric disorders and other disabilities in children. The social factor of ASSQ and peer problems in the SDQ seem to be measuring the same phenomenon, whereas the Asperger factor could be more specific of autism, explaining the much lower correlation for this factor with the more general social disability as measured by SDQ peer problems and social factor of ASSQ.

P-007-108 Topic: 37, 92
Evaluation of visual-motor Bender-Gestalt perception test (Bender test) in diagnosis of childhood migraine

Ivana Francula, University of Rijeka, Children's Hospital "Kantrida", Rijeka, Croatia, ifrancul@inet.hr
Igor Prpic; Rena Volga

According to International Headache Society (HIS) 3 to 5 attacks of specific headache is required to fulfil criteria for migraine, which sometimes means a period of year or more. In order to speed up the diagnosing of migraine we have analyzed the results of Bender test. Retrospectively 24 children with definite migraine diagnosis (according HIS criteria) were separated and their results of the Bender test analyzed. There were 9 boys (mean = 9,8 age) and 15 girls (mean = 11,8 age). The boys were statistically significantly younger than girls with no difference between boys and girls regarding their general intelligence and social background. The children performed Bender test at an early phase of the headache (mean = 2 days, SD 1,5 day) and repeated it in a period without headache (mean = 6 days, SD 2,5). At an early stage after the headache, suspected or definite organic cerebral dysfunction was found at 20 children while 4 had normal results. Bender test performed in phase without headache revealed only 3 children with organic cerebral dysfunction, and the rest of the children had normal results. There was significant statistical difference between the results of first and the second Bender test measurement (Fisher test: 0,00015). Our results revealed that visual-motor capacity is disturbed at children with migraine in an early phase of headache and it is needed at least 6 day to normalize. These findings demonstrated that Bender test may be used as a rapid and useful diagnostic tool in migraine diagnosis. One can make rather safe conclusion of migraine after specific headache accompanied by disturbed visual-motor perception. Furthemore, it was shown that children with migrenous attack need 4 to 8 days to regain their visual-motor abilities which is an important information considering child's daily school obligations, particularly reading and writing skills.

P-007-109 Topic: 37, 49
The assessment of family drawings from children who have lost a caregiver

Stefania Di Biasi, Policlinico Umberto I, Child & Adolescent Psychiatry, Rome, Italy, stefaniadibiasi@yahoo.it
Francesca Piperno; Filomena Puleo; Sara Cerracchio; Roberta Giacchè

Objective: The aim of this study was to investigate the quality of family drawings of children who have experienced the lost of a caregiver. **Methods:** The Family Drawing by ten children who have mourned a caregiver, ten children of a control group, all aged between 4–11 years old; was assessed and compared. The drawings were analysed using a specific Screening Inventory. This Inventory takes into consideration such qualitative and quantitative variables as Graphically-expressive maturity; Omitted subjects; Body distorsions; Identification roles; Affective proximity. The Authors have also grouped together several graphic indicators concerning: the quality of feelings, either of the depressive of the relational anxiety/anguish type. **Results:** The results have shown significant differences between the children who have lost a caregiver and the control group. The clinical sample is more likely to draw distorted bodies (distorsion and schematization of the body, absence or deformity of the face), the human figure is usually represented devoid of details, their drawings generally show clear signals of trauma. On the other hand, both distortion and schematization are absent in the control group. **Conclusion:** The family Drawings of children who have lost a caregiver significantly evidence a greater emotional distress than the drawings of the control group.

P-007-110 Topic: 37
Validity of the 'Five Minute Speech Sample' in reference to the 'Camberwell Family Interview'

Zoé Rein, Institut Mutualiste Montsouris, Dept. of Psychiatry, Paris, France, zoe.rein@imm.fr
Nathalie Godart; Fabienne Perdereau; Florence Curt; Philippe Jeammet; Jacques Fermanian

Objective: The aim of our project is: To demonstrate that the FMSS's measure of the EE in families with an anorexic patient is valid comparatively to the CFI's measure. Our hypothesis is: The level of EE in families with an anorexic patient may be reliably measured by the FMSS in comparison to the gold standard, the CFI. **Methods:** We have undertaken a preliminary study on the validity of the "Five Minute Speech Sample" (FMSS) in reference to the "Camberwell Family Interview" (CFI) in anorexia nervosa. We will outline here this study and discuss the results. We included in this study the parents of Anorexia Nervosa patients participating in the prospective follow up study on the "family therapy in anorexia nervosa". The assessment was conducted at intake, after the end of a hospitalization for anorexia nervosa. The mothers and the fathers included (40 in total) have been assessed individually. The FMSS was conducted first, followed after a ten minutes coffee-break by the CFI. We chose to administrate the FMSS first because of the verbatim instructions (free speech) and the length of the assessment (5 minutes). **Results:** The preliminary results of this study support our hypothesis.

P-007-111 Topic: 37, 72
Reliability and validity analysis of the Children's Yale Brown Obsessive Compulsive Scale (CY-BOCS) symptom checklist in Turkey

Emine Ozgur Bayman, Uludag Universitesi Tip Fak., Biyoistatistik Anabilim Dali, Bursa, Turkey, yesimtaneli@uludag.edu.tr
Yesim Taneli; Neslim Guvendeger; Bulent Ediz; Suna Taneli; Ismet Kan

Objective: The aim of this study was to assess the reliability and validity of the Children's Yale Brown Obsessive Compulsive Scale (CY-BOCS) Symptom Checklist in Turkey. **Methods:** Data of an OCD-population study performed by the Dept. of Child and Adolescent Psychiatry/ Uludag University were used. In that study, questionnaires had been sent to parents of 1709 Grade 4–8 students at seven elementary schools in Bursa (1.7% of 4–8 Graders of city total; term 1997–1998). Return rate had been 91% (n: 1556; 1.5% of city total). With all 805 children, for whom at least one OCD symptom was stated by their parents (51.7% of 1556), face-to-face psychiatric interviews had been conducted by a child psychiatry resident (N.G.) and had been supervised by a child psychiatrist (S.T.). Based on the CY-BOCS severity score assessed in the interviews, three study groups had been defined for these 805 children: 1) OCD, 2) Sub-clinical OCD and 3) Controls without OCD. The dataset of the now presented reliability/validity study comprised all 805 children. The Analysis: Cronbach Alpha coefficients were determined for the following groups: 1) OCD (n: 80, 9.9% of 805); 2) Subclinical OCD (n: 80, 9.9% of 805); 3) Controls (n: 645, 80.2% of 805) and 4) the entire study group (n: 805, 100%). SPSS was used (significance value: p<0.05). **Results:** Reliability and validity analysis revealed the following Cronbach Alpha coefficients: 1) OCD:0.9031; 2) Sub-clinical OCD: 0.7919; 3) Controls without OCD: 0.7895 and 4) Entire study group 0.9410. **Conclusion:** Our study results suggest, that the Turkish form of the CY-BOCS Symptom Checklist is a reliable and valid tool to determine obsessive compulsive symptoms in Turkish children.

P-007-112   Topic: 37
Child Mania Rating Scale (CMRS): Development, reliability and validity

Mani Pavuluri, University of Illinois, Child Psychiatry, Chicago, USA, mpavuluri@psych.uic.edu
David B. Henry; Julie A. Carbray

Objective: To develop a reliable and valid parent report instrument to screen children for mania. **Methods:** A 21-item questionnaire was administered to 125 subjects (normal controls=50; bipolar disorder=50; attention deficit hyperactivity disorder=25). The mean age of the sample was 10.41 years (±3.06). The Washington University Kiddie Schedule for Affective Disorders and Schizophrenia (WASH-U-KSADS) and a clinical interview were used to determine DSM-IV diagnosis. The Young Mania Rating Scale (YMRS), Kiddie Schedule for Affective Disorders and Schizophrenia Mania Rating Scale (KSADS-MRS), Child Behavior Checklist (CBCL), and Child Depression Inventory (CDI) were completed to estimate the convergent and discriminant validity of the measure. **Results:** Confirmatory Factor Analysis demonstrated the excellent fit of a single-factor model indicating that the scale measures a single dimension. The internal consistency of the measure by Cronbach's alpha was 0.96. The one-week test re-test reliability was also 0.96. The measure correlated .84 with the Wash-U-KSADS Mania module, 0.79 with the KSADS-MRS, and 0.79 with the YMRS. The CDI correlated 0.44, the CBCL Anxious/Depressed subscale correlated 0.68 and the CBCL Conduct Problems subscale correlated 0.61 with the CMRS. Analysis of ROC curves showed that using a cutoff score of 35, the CMRS had sensitivity and specificity of 0.92 for differentiating subjects with mania from either normal controls or subjects diagnosed with attention deficit hyperactivity disorder. **Conclusion:** The CMRS is a promising parent-report scale for pediatric mania screening. Future studies are needed to replicate these findings and test the predictive validity of the measure for use in treatment studies.

P-007-113   Topic: 37, 86
German translation and validation of the Screen for Child Anxiety Related Emotional Disorders (SCARED) – First results

Angela Plaß, University Clinic of Hamburg, Child & Adolescent Psychiatry, Hamburg, Germany, plass@uke.uni-hamburg.de
Claus Barkmann; B. Mack; K. Mittenzwei; Peter Riedesser; Michael Schulte-Markwort

Objective: To do a German translation of the American Screen for Child Anxiety Related Emotional Disorders and to apply the instrument in a sample of children and adolescents referred to a university department. **Methods:** The German translation was done in a group of five child and adolescent psychiatrists. A native speaker did a retranslation into the original language. The German version was applied in a sample of 41 patients and their parents, at the same time the CBCL and the YSR were applied. **Results:** The quality of data was comparably good. As the English version, the German translation of the SCARED yielded five factors: somatic/pain, general anxiety, separation anxiety, social phobia and school phobia. For the total score and each of the five factors, both the the child and parent SCARED demonstrated good internal consistency (cronbach's alpha=0.72 to 0.97), parent-child agreement was higher than for the English version (r=0.56 to 0.64). **Conclusion:** The German translation of the SCARED seems to be well accepted and shows promise as a screening instrument for anxiety disorders.

P-007-115   Topic: 37
Evaluation of the self-reported SDQ in a clinical setting: I. Do self-reports tell us more than ratings

Veit Roessner, Universität Göttingen, Kinder- u. Jugendpsychiatrie, Göttingen, Germany, vroessn@gwdg.de
Andreas Becker; Nicola Hagenberg; Matthias Berking; Tobias Banaschewski; Aribert Rothenberger

Objective: The aim of this study was to evaluate the German self-reported Strengths and Difficulties Questionnaire (SDQ) in a clinical setting. We also investigated whether this additional information gathered directly from older children and adolescents improves the prediction of clinical status when external ratings from their parents and/or teachers are already available. **Methods:** SDQ self-reports were collected from 214 in- and outpatients (81 girls and 133 boys) aged 11 to 17 years who were seen at the Department of Child and Adolescent Psychiatry of the University of Göttingen. Results obtained with the self-rated questionnaire were compared with the parent SDQs and corresponding CBCL/YSR scores. Finally, the additional diagnostical benefits of the self-reports were examined. **Results:** The scales of the SDQ self-report proved to be sufficiently homogeneous, and the factorial structure of the English original was replicated in this clinical sample. Scores on the self-reported SDQ scales were strongly associated with the corresponding scales of the YSR. SDQ self-reports significantly contributed to the prediction of diagnostic status, specifically if only parent or teacher ratings were available. **Conclusion:** The self-rated version of the SDQ was shown to be a reliable and valid method for the assessment of behavioural problems in children and adolescents. In the absence of adult informant reports from parents and teachers, the diagnostical value of self-ratings was also demonstrated.

P-007-116　Topic: 37, 23

Use of the HONOSCA scale in the team work of in-patient child psychiatry unit

Sigita Lesinskiene, Vilnius University, Dept. of Clinic of Psychiatry, Vilnius, Lithuania, sigita.lesinskiene@vrc.vu.lt

Objective: The aim of the investigation was to introduce HoNOSCA into the clinical practice and to assess the possibilities to use HoNOSCA in the interdisciplinary team work of child psychiatry unit. **Methods:** Having permission HoNOSCA was translated and prepared for the clinical use in Lithuania. Team members of the unit were trained to use the scale during the two training seminars. The scale was filled in the beginning and at the end of in-patient treatment. Child psychiatrist and clinical psychologist rated the scale independently during the first tree days of the treatment being the first who handled the information about the child and family. Child psychiatrist, clinical psychologist, nurse and caretaker independently rated the scale at the end of in-patient treatment thinking that nurse and caretaker spended much time with the child in variuos situations of the dayly life and their rating could be of the potential value. Interrater agreement between various groups of specialists was calculated. Intraclass correlation was calculated for the each item of the scale. **Results:** HoNOSCA was filled for 55 children 7–18 years old (mean age 12.9, SD 2.7), 35 boys and 20 girls. Six persons for each child filled the scale during the time of hospitalisation. 12 people (3 child psychiatrists, 2 psychologists, 2 nurses, 5 caretakers) participated in this study. It appeared that nurses and caretakers had no relevant information about the family relationships of the 28 (50.9‰) children. **Conclusion:** All members of the team in the in-patient department (child psychiatrists, psychologists, nurses, caretakers) can rate HoNOSCA scale. Use of HoNOSCA scale is helpful planning and organising the team work, interdisciplinary cooperation, complex interventions. HoNOSCA scale is sensitive, shows effect of interventions, changes over time.

P-007-117　Topic: 37, 78

French adaptation of expressed emotion measure in anorexia nervosa

Fabienne Perdereau, Institut Mutualiste Montsouris, Dept. of Psychiatry, Paris, France, fabienne.perdereau@imm.fr
Zoé Rein; Florence Curt; Philippe Jeammet; Nathalie Godart

Objective: We chose to adapt for the first time in France a measuring instrument of the concept of "Expressed Emotions". The Expressed Emotions, which was described in the families of schizophrenics in the fifties, reflects the family emotional climate reigning towards a subject reached of chronic disease. We choose to use an evaluation of this dimension in rating 5 minutes speech samples. **Methods:** We have, with the agreement of the authors, translated then back-translated this tool and its handbook. We then used this evaluation in a study concerning anorexia nervosa. **Conclusion:** The advantage of this new French instrument available will be discussed.

P-007-118　Topic: 37, 83

Is head circumference a powerful tool in the autism early diagnosis?

Nathalie Coulon, Centre Hospitalier, Pédopsychiatrie, Bohars, France, sabine.dupont@chu-brest.fr

Objective: Early diagnosis in autism is a recent great advance. In particular, the potentiel use of macrocephaly is discussed. Objective of this is to compare head circumference between autistics and a standard population. Is there a close connection between autism and macrocephaly? **Methods:** Design: Retrospective study with geographical boundaries, from birth to two years old. Setting: Brest CIERA*, who is commissioned to Bretagne and Pays de Loire. Methods: CIERA data base on typical and atypical autism (ICD 10*: F 84.0 and F84.1), confirmed by ADIR*, from 2001 November to 2003 December. **Results:** 47 cases of autism. Sex ratio: 4,9. No relation between birth head circumference and autism. From birth to two years old, both populations (N typical = 32; N atypical = 15) are above the fiftieth percentile, and macrocephaly is around 15 %. Nevertheless, first, the growth is faster in the typical autism than the atypical and secondly, a break and an acceleration appears in both autistic populations between the fourth and the ninth month. **Conclusion:** Head circumference absolute value seems insufficient for an autism early diagnosis. However, head circumference growth between the fourth and the ninth month is an interesting marker associated with others clinical signs.

P-007-119　Topic: 37, 49

The assessment of playing from children who have lost a caregiver

Daniela Tardiola, Rome University, Children Neuropsychiatry, Rome, Italy, laura_74@libero.it
Stefano Balsamo; Stefania Di Biasi; Francesca Piperno; Nadia Capriotti

Objective: Aim of the study was to analyse the quality of playing in children who have lost a caregiver in order to: – Define specific themes related to the mourning; – Evaluate consequences of trauma from a developmental perspective; – Identify the psychopathological outcomes related to this kind of trauma **Methods:** The play of ten children (aged between 4 and 11 years old) who have experienced the loss of a caregiver was assessed and compared to that one from a control group (comparison between two children equally aged"). The two samples were divided in two different subgroups: 1)children aged between 4 and 6 years; 2) children aged between 8 and 10 years. Two playing observations (lasting 30 minutes each one) have been made for each child using the Scenotest (Von Staabs, 1964). These observations were evaluated through a re-adjustment of the CPTI of P. Kernberg (1998). **Results:** The comparison between the two samples allows to define specific characteristics of playing of children who have lost a caregiver. These characteristics concern: – the spectrum, the modulation and the pertinence of expressed feelings; – the coming out themes; – the global pleasure expressed by child; -the skill of child to organise alone his own play; – the social abilities of child; – the type of relationship represented through the different characters of playing. These elements are different in the considered developmental age. Specifically prescholar children seem to express more rage while older ones have a more inhibited play. **Conclusion:** The assessment of playing of children who have lost a caregiver allows to approach their inner world without becoming intrusive. Discovering the way in which these children represent own caregivers and themselves in playing helps to construct a specific therapeutic project.

P-008   Topic: 83
Pervasive developmental disorders II
Track: Pervasive developmental disorders (PDD)

P-008-120   Topic: 83, 78
A clinical case of severe atypical eating disorder in a PDD patient
Tanveer Sandhu, Tampere Univ. Hospital, Dept. of Child Psychiatry, Tampere, Finland, tanveer.sandhu@phshp.fi
Tuula Tamminen

Objective: To evaluate the results of psychopharmacological treatment in a severe atypical eating disorder of PDD patients through a clinical case experience. **Methods:** A clinical case is described with some literature review. The problems related to food and eating like selectivity and aversion are common in autistic spectrum disorders, but only few cases have been reported with moderate difficulties in eating, combining behavioural and psychopharmacological interventions, mainly Risperidone. A 12 years old Finnish white girl with diagnosed PDD, developed total refusal to eat within a course of few weeks, marked with recurrent profuse vomiting and rapid loss of weight, finally leading to the insertion of a NG tube. The patient had been admitted to paediatric ward and later on to child psychiatric ward with continued NG feeding. Communicative difficulties made the psychiatric assessment difficult, however she did not have typical AN (active weight losing tendencies) neither bulemic features, rather inabilty to eat and recurrent vomiting were the main symptoms. All other endocrinic, metabolic, neuroradiological, gastroenterological screening tests were normal. At beginning the girl received Risperidone (Risperdal) 1.5 mg/day for 4 months without clear results as far as the core symptoms were concerned. Behavioural methods were planned using visual tools in a step-wise fashion to achieve the goal using different motivators suitable for her. However even a small stress brought a setback with worsening of symptoms and aggravating her anxiety related to eating. Vomiting made it necessary to re-insert the NG tube sometimes even 8-10 times a day. Total enteral feeding through the NG tube was continued for 5 months and possibility of gastrostoma was considered. At that point Citalopram(Cipramil drops) was started and the dose increased to 20 mg in 2 weeks time. **Results:** A dramatic response was noted; the girl started to eat and NG tube could be taken out after 3 weeks of the start of Citalopram(Cipramil). Also communication with her improved and she was pleased to be again able to eat. Vomiting also stopped within that period. **Conclusion:** Children with PDD can develop potentially dangerous and severe eating disorders which could clinically vary from those without PDD. Evaluation of the PDD/autistic patients for other psychiatric disorders like depression or anxiety disorders could be difficult and may need more research to develop suitable assessment tools. Psychopharmacological treatment including SSRI is still a valuable and effective treatment in severe psychiatric disorders in juvenile population, and further research to find their special role in a particular group of patients like PDD could be very interesting.

P-008-121   Topic: 83, 69
Main principles of integration of children suffering from infantile autism and early child schizophrenia among healthy children
Nina Iovchuk, Ass. of Child Psychiatrists, and Psychologists, Moscow, Russia, acpp@online.ru

Objective: Children suffering from infantile autism and early child schizophrenia show introversion, emotional deficit, formality, rigidity, bad orientation in living conditions. Most favorable environment for correctional work with this children is collective of mentally healthy children. Present investigation is based on integration in Moscow kindergarten N 1465 of 16 children who showed autistic tendencies. **Methods:** Clinical observation, interdisciplinary correctional pedagogics, family therapy. **Results:** In group 15 healthy children it's possible to integrate one autistic child and one or two children suffering from deep delay of mental development. First condition for favorable integration is adaptation of parents of healthy children, tutors, parents of "special" child for integrative process with the aid of programs for elevation of parental competence, training for specialists of kindergarten, making of special attractiveness of kindergarten. Second condition is gradualness and dosage of connections of "special" child with healthy children. Autistic child needs also individual escort, specially first months of stay in kindergarten. Tactics of correctional work determines interdisciplinary medical-psychological-pedagogical consultation which includes all specialists who take part in correctional-rehabilitative process. The tasks of work with family of ill child are: producing for all members of unit, adequate principles of conduction; overcoming of indifference and apathy about a future of child; orientation to at most possible level of education and professional training; the use in domestic conditions of adequate educational methods; overcoming of isolation and conservatism in family structure; overcoming of negativism to psychotropic medicines for child; formation of emotional interaction and mutual aid among members of several families with children who have special needs. **Conclusion:** Realization of specified conditions enable to prepare ill children for education in conventional school.

P-008-122   Topic: 83, 84
Attention difficulties in children with Asperger Syndrome
Ivona Milacic, Inst. for Psychophysiological, Disorders and Speech Pathol., Belgrade, Serbia and Montenegro, olivido@ptt.yu
Oliver Vidojevic

Objective: Asperger syndrome (AS) is a term used to mark a subgroup of autism with no delay in language or cognitive development. Research reveal language and cognitive impairments in AS (uneven profile of abilities on Wechsler intelligence scales, pragmatic deficits, receptive speech, narrow attention and difficulty in shifting attention"). The objective of this study is to examine flexibility of attention of children with AS. 12 children with AS age from 7-16 years old, 11 males, 1 female participated in the study. All children had an IQ in the normal range. **Methods:** Trail Making Test (TMT-A, TMT-B) was used in the present study as a measure of attention flexibility. **Results:** Scores gained by the children with AS comparing to the scores of the normally developing children (prolonged response time, more errors) indicate difficulties in visual scanning, attention flexibility and complex conceptual tracking. **Conclusion:** Prolonged response time on TMT-A point to motor slowing and on TMT-B which examines working memory and shifting of cognitive set (executive functions) point to the deficit in reasoning.

P-008-123 Topic: 83, 30
Neuropsychological assessment of cases with Asperger's Disorder (AD)

Ayse Kilincaslan, Istanbul Medical Faculty, Dept. of Child Psychiatry, Istanbul, Turkey, aysekilincaslan@hotmail.com
Nahit Motavalli Mukaddes; Gokce Sozen; Ayla Umut

Objective: Several studies have investigated the neuropsychological features in autistic spectrum disorders. But there is lack of study on comprehensive evaluation and comparison between subjects with AD and normal controls. The objective of the present study was to compare the neuropsychological characteristics of AD with age, gender, and IQ matched controls on intellectual, visuospatial, memory and executive function domains. **Methods:** 16 AD patients (14 boys and 2 girls, aged 7 through 16 years, mean: 11.9 ± 0.7) attending to our clinic and 13 volunteer control subjects (11 boys and 2 girls, at the same age range, mean: 11.8 ± 0.7) from mainstream schools were evaluated. AD diagnoses were made by using DSM-IV criteria and by the consensus of two child psychiatrists. The neuropsychological evaluation included a) WISC-R b) Wisconsin Card Sorting Test (WCST) c) Stroop Test d) Continuous Performance Test (CPT) e) California Verbal Learning Test-children's version f) Benton's Judgement of Line Orientation Test (BLO) g) Benton Facial Recognition Test h) Rey-Osterrieth Complex Figure Copying Test (RCFT) i) Controlled Oral Word Association Test (COWAT) j) Category Naming Test. Statistical analysis was conducted by using Mann-Whitney U Test. **Results:** There were no statistically significant differences between groups concerning total, verbal and performance IQ scores. However, AD participants performed better on information ($p = 0.03$) and similarities ($p = 0.001$) subtests. Only in RCFT Immediate Recall Test AD the group showed poorer performance ($P < 0.05$). Although there was no statistical significance between two groups in CPT, WCST, BLO, RCFT, COWAT and Stroop tests, the mean score of AD cases was much lower than controls. **Conclusion:** The statistically significant difference in RCFT may indicate a deficit in visual memory in AD patients. Lack of statistically significant difference between groups may be interpereted as a result of limited number of participants.

P-008-124 Topic: 83, 28
Dopamine-related gene polymorphisms and autism

Kenji Yamamoto, Tokai University, Dept. of Psychiatry, Kanagawa, Japan, key@is.icc.u-tokai.ac.jp
Shinko Koishi; Seiji Koishi; Noriko Natsume; Kosuke Yamazaki; Hideo Matsumoto; Eiji Nanba

Objective: It has been reported that autism and schizophrenia share many clinical symptoms such as indifference in human relationships and behavioral eccentricity. Although they are now regarded as separate clinical entities, these facts point to possibility that the two diseases might share some causal factors. Several lines of evidences suggested that clinical symptoms of schizophrenia are associated with dopamine (DA) activities in human brain, and the dopamine-related gene were thought to be causative gene for schizophrenia. Recent reports of genetic association studies between schizophrenia and these genes are still complicated, however, these might be associated with phenotypic variability of schizophrenia. Based on these observations, we hypothesized that the dopamine-related gene may be associated with autism or its phenotypic variability. To test this hypothesis, we conducted family-based genetic association study between DRD4, DBH gene polymorphisms and autism. **Methods:** 104 trios, all ethnically Japanese, were examined using the transmission disequilibrium test. Diagnoses for autism were conducted by two experienced child psychiatrists independently, according to the ICD-10 DCR and DSM-IV Criteria. Two polymorphisms (DBH5'-ins/del and DBH 444g/a) of the DBH gene, and one (–521C/T) of the DRD4 gene were genotyped according to previous reports using PCR reaction. The project was approved by the Research Ethics Board of each participating institution. **Results:** No associations were observed between these polymorphisms and autism. **Conclusion:** Our data did not support the associations between the DBH, DRD4 gene polymorphisms and autism.

P-008-125 Topic: 83, 32
Autism, attachment and cortisol response

Fabienne Naber, UMC-Utrecht location AZU, Child & Adolescent psychiatry, Utrecht, Netherlands, F.naber@azu.nl
Emma van Daalen; Jan Buitelaar; Marinus van IJzendoorn; Sophie Willemsen-Swinkels; Marian J. Bakermans-Kranenburg; Herman van Engeland

Objective: Studies on adrenocortical responses found attachment security to be related with lessened cortisol response under stressful circumstances (Gunnar et al., 1996; Spangler & Grossmann, 1993) and higher increasement of cortisol in insecure, and especially disorganised children. These findings are based on research with 'normal' developing children (Hertsgaard, Gunnar, Erickson & Nachmias, 1995; Spangler & Grossmann, 1993). Children 'at risk' of all sorts of developing disorders also participated in attachment research. Higher percentages of disorganization were found in these groups, merely at the expense of secure attachment (van IJzendoorn et al., 1999). These studies, however, were not performed at the right age, due to diagnostic difficulties. Therefore, the cortisol response of young children with autism and other developing disorders are not yet studied before. **Methods:** About 30 children under the age of 36 months with the disorder autism (spectrum disorders), mental retardation and language disorder, participated in a study for cortisol responses during an attachment setting. Before the Stange Situation Procedure started, saliva cortisol was collected, as well as 25 minutes and 55 minutes after the first separation. The children all received an attachment classification by trained observers. Cortisol responses of the children were analyzed for differences in response between different psychiatric diagnoses and different attachment classifications. **Results:** Differences in cortisol responses appeared between the different attachment classifications and between the different groups of diagnoses. **Conclusion:** Children with autism do show cortisol responses, however, there are differences compared to children with other psychiatric disorders as well as compared with normal developing children.

P-008-126   Topic: 83, 30
Superior disembedding in individuals with autism and their parents: The need of subtile measures

Maretha de Jonge, UMC Utrecht, Child & Adolescent Psychiatry, Utrecht, Netherlands, m.v.jonge@azu.nl
Chantal Kemner; Herman van Engeland

Objective: In this study, we assessed visuo-spatial skills in autism and the broader phenotype of autism. Superior disembedding performance is often, but not consistently found in autism, especially not in samples including autism spectrum disorders. Since our group consists of multi-incidence families, therefore having a higher genetic liability for autism, we hypothese that an asset on this task will be found in our autism spectrum group and in their parents. We might, however, need more subtle measures to differentiate between subjects and controls. **Methods:** Disembedding performance was measured with the Embedded Figures Test (Witkin et al., 1971) in high-functioning subjects with autism and autism spectrum disorders from multi-incidence families. There performance was compared to the performance of a group of control subjects, matched on gender, age and IQ. In addition the parents of these subjects were assessed, as well as a group of matched control parents. All assesments were videotaped in order to make coding blind to subject status possible. Performance was measured by assessing accuracy, response time and the number of errors made before finding the right shape. **Results:** The individuals with autism spectrum disorders were significantly faster than matched controls in locating the shape. Their fathers or mothers were not found to be faster than control parents. However, both the individuals with autism spectrum disorders as well as their fathers made significantly less incorrect attempts before finding the right shape. **Conclusion:** These results indicate that the number of attempts, is a more subtle measure for assessing superior disembedding skills and therefore useful in the assessment of individuals with spectrum disorders and the broader phenotype of autism.

P-008-127   Topic: 83, 28
Asperger Syndrome in association with XYY chromosomal abnormality

Andrea Caby, Marienkrankenhaus,
Kinder- und Jugendpsychiatrie, Aschendorf, Germany,
andrea_caby@yahoo.de
Filip Caby; Stefan Bendt

Objective: The etiology of autism is thought to be a genetic disposition, with several chromosomes interacting. **Methods:** Molecular biological studies concentrate on different candidate genes likely to be relevant for autistic disorder. Otherwise, some small patient collectives have been reported with chromosome aberations and repeated autistic abnormalities. In our three case reports, three male adolescents present with a diagnosis of Asperger syndrome in combination with XYY chromosomal disorder. **Results:** We will give an update concerning actual publications reporting on autism, genetics and/or XYY syndrome, and look into the specific clinical aspects of both disorders. **Conclusion:** Genetic studies in patients with autism indicate a multilocus etiology. As a very rare observation, we present three young individuals with Asperger syndrome in association with XYY chomosomal abnormality.

P-008-128   Topic: 83, 34
The effect of complex psychopharmacotherapy (Cerebrolysin with typical neuroleptics) on autism severity in mild/moderate and severe childhood autism

Vera Bashina, Mental Health Research Centre, Childhood Autism Res. Group, Moscow, Russia,
bashina@mhrc.comcor.ru
Maria Krasnoperova

Objective: To evaluate the efficacy of complex neurotrophic and antipsychotic therapy in childhood autism treatment. **Methods:** 30 patients with childhood autism aged 2,5-7,0 years received complex neurotrophic and antipsychotic therapy in outpatient and inpatient clinics. Therapeutic course included 15 intramuscular injections of 1,0 ml Cerebrolysin every other day and basic antipsychotic therapy with aethaperazinum, sulpiride, levomepromazine every day. During 3 month after the end of the therapeutic course (follow-up period) patients received only basic neuroleptic therapy. The assessment was done by clinical and psychometric tests (Clinical Global Impression (CGI), Childhood Autism Rating Scale (CARS)) at 3 times: before (0 day) and after the therapeutic course (30th day) and 4 month later (120th day, at the end of the follow-up period). According to the severity of autism measured by CARS the patients were divided into 2 groups: with mild/moderate autism (the 1st group, N = 10) and with severe autism (the 2nd group, N = 20). **Results:** Positive effects (on CGI scale) were observed at the end of the therapeutic course in 80% patients of the 1st group and in 85% – of the 2nd. At the end of the follow-up period these patients remained improved. After the therapeutic course patients of the 2nd group showed a significant decrease of autism severity (3,4 points on CARS scale). During the follow-up period the mean score on CARS scale in the 2nd group continued to decrease (on 4,8 points in comparison to baseline; $p < 0,001$). **Conclusion:** The complex psychopharmacotherapy with Cerebrolysin and typical neuroleptics improved communicative functions in preschool patients with childhood autism. The most significant decrease of autism severity was seen in patients with severe autism. One half of the patients (15 of 30) displayed a reduced autism severity at the end of follow-up period.

P-008-129   Topic: 83, 31
Poly unsaturated fatty acids in autism

Jan Croonenberghs, University of Antwerp, AZ Middelheim, Antwerp, Belgium, jan.croonenberghs@ocmw.antwerpen.be
Sonja Sliwinski; Armand Christophe; Dirk Deboutte; Michael Maes

Objective: Research on the biological pathophysiology of autism has found some evidence that alterations in fatty acids may play a role in the pathophysiology of that disorder. As a consequence we expected to find that autism is accompanied by abnormalities in the poly unsaturated fatty acids (PUFA) composition in plasma phospholipids. **Methods:** This study examines the plasma phospholipid w3 and w6 PUFA fractions and the w3/w6 ratio in autism. 16 high-functioning male youngsters with autism (age 12–18) and 22 healthy volunteers participated in this study. Group mean differences were assessed by means of analysis of variance (ANOVA). **Results:** In autism there was a significant increase of the PL22:6 w3 (docosahexaenoic acid, DHA) fraction (mean score 3.40%, SD 0.8 in autism and 2.83%, SD 0.6 in normal controls; $F = 5.47$; $p = 0.02$")

and an increase in the total w3/w6 ratio (mean score 0.17, SD 0.03 in autism and 0.15, SD 0.02 in normal controls; F= 3.74; p=0.05"). **Conclusion:** The results of this study suggest that an increase of the plasma phospholipid w3 PUFA, in particular DHA, and of the total w3/w6 ratio may take part in the pathophysiology of autism. One hypothesis is that an increase of w3 PUFA may cause alterations in the serotonergic turnover and the immune response system, both known to be associated with autism. This finding is in contradiction to the findings of previous, very limited studies in other centers and means a warning against the dietary advice of w3 PUFA supplementation given by commercial companies nowadays.

P-008-130   Topic: 83, 30

Mental retardation and Pervasive Developmental Disorders (PDD): Comparison between linguistic, narrative and representation abilities

Nadia Tomassetti, University of Rome, Child & Adolescent Psychiatry, Rome, Italy, n.tomassetti@libero.it
Alessia Tosco; Emanuela Giorgi; Monica Lazzarini; M. Liliana Iorio; Mercedes Becciu; Flavia Capozzi

Objective: In this study we have examined and compared the cognitive, linguistic-narrative and representation abilities of two clinical groups: high functioning Pervasive Developmental Disorders (DGS) and Mild Mental Retardation (RM). **Methods:** A sample of 20 school-aged children was selected, by mental age and full intellective quotient (10 with high functioning DGS, 10 with mild RM, under DSM-IV standards). The following tests were given: WISC-R, with particular attention to Vocabulary, General Comprehension, and Cube Drawing sub-tests, and an oral story telling test. **Results:** The WISC-R cognitive profiles revealed differentiated highs and lows in the two groups: mild RM obtain better results in General Comprehension sub-tests, whereas the DGS gain better results in Vocabulary Tests and Cube Drawing. In oral story telling comprehension tests both groups gain below normal marks: results differ in that RM subjects gain higher marks in the descriptive and inferential questions, DGS subjects fail above all where questions require the ability to understand intuitively the psychic motives behind actions and reciprocal communicating (the theory of the mind deficit, Frith, 1996). **Conclusion:** All subjects reveal difficulties, which differ in the two groups, related to the comprehension of oral story. Therefore story telling proves an accurate instrument for highlighting intellective disabilities or for "the theory of the mind" deficit.

P-008-131   Topic: 83, 35

Regional cerebral perfusion abnormality in PDD: A SPECT study using statistical parametric mapping analysis

Bung-Nyun Kim, Seoul Nat. University Hospital, Child & Adol. Psychiatry, Seoul, Republic of Korea, kbn1@snu.ac.kr
Jeong In-Hyoung; Seong-Ill Jeon; Dong-Hyun Ahn; Boong-Nyun Kim; Yun-O Shin; Kang-E Hong

Objective: Pervasive Developmental Disorder is a well-known psychiatric disorder which has a neural base. To investigate the underlying neurofunctional abnormalities, we performed a voxel based imaging study of cerebral blood flow. **Methods:** 31 children with untreated pervasive developmental disorder were selected among the patients

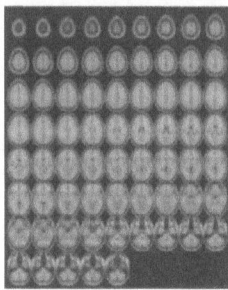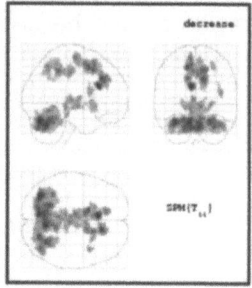

Figure 1. Brain areas with significantly decreased perfusion in PDD patients compared to normal controls (threshold. P=0.001, uncorrected)

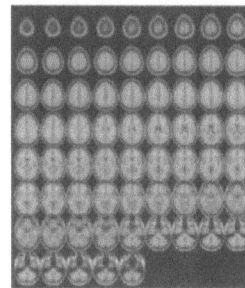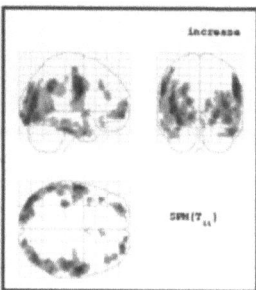

Figure 2. Brain areas with significantly increased perfusion in PDD patients compared to normal controls (threshold P=0.001, uncorrected)

visiting a child & adolescent psychiatric clinic of Seoul National University Hospital. They were assessed with DSM-IV criteria of pervasive developmental disorder and psychometric tools. Moreover, only when two psychiatrists independently agreed to the assessment, they were included in the patient group. All patients were examined by using 99mTC-HMPAO Brain SPECT. Using SPM analysis, we compared SPECT image of patients and Korean standardized SPECT image of normal children, that was developed by our team during 3 years, on a voxel by voxel basis using t-statistics. Voxels with a p-value of less than 0.01 were considered to be significantly different. **Results:** The autistic group had a significant decrease of cerebral blood flow in both medial frontal lobe, both cingulated gyrus, both cerebellum, both precuneus gyrus. In addition, they had a significant hyperperfusion in both inferior occipital and parietal lobes, both precentral gyrus, both fusiform gyrus. **Conclusion:** The results confirm the presence of functional defects in medial-frontal lobe, cingulated gyrus, cerebellum that have been already reported. So, they are compatible with earlier suggested disturbances in cerebro-cerebellar network.

P-008-132   Topic: 83, 35
Subtypes of autism by cluster analysis based on structural MRI Data

Michal Hrdlicka, Charles University,
Dept. of Child Psychiatry, Prague, Czech Republic,
michal.hrdlicka@lfmotol.cuni.cz
Jiri Neuwirth; Vladimir Komarek; Marketa Havlovicova;
Zdenek Sedlacek; Marek Blatny; Tomas Urbanek

Objective: Our study was an attempt to subcategorize autistic spectrum disorders using multidisciplinary approach. **Methods:** Sixty four autistic patients (mean age 9.4+5.6 years) entered the cluster analysis. Clustering was based on MRI data. **Results:** The clusters obtained did not differ significantly in overall severity of autistic symptomatology as measured by total score of Childhood Autism Rating Scale (CARS). The clusters could be characterized by following reciprocal significant differences: Cluster 1: Largest size of genu and splenium of corpus callosum (CC), lowest pregnancy order, lowest frequency of facial dysmorphic features. Cluster 2: Largest size of amygdala and hippocampus (HPC), least abnormal visual response in CARS, lowest frequency of epilepsy, least frequent abnormal psychomotor development during the first year of life. Cluster 3: Largest size of caput of nucleus caudatus (NC), lowest size of HPC, facial dysmorphic features always present. Cluster 4: Lowest size of genu and splenium of CC, amygdala, and caput of NC, most abnormal visual response in CARS, highest frequency of epilepsy, highest pregnancy order, abnormal psychomotor development during the first year of life always present, facial dysmorphic features always present. **Conclusion:** The multidisciplinary approach seems to be a promising method in subtyping autism. The methodological limitation of this study was only planimetric way of brain structures measurement. Further validation of our findings using volumetric measurement on a larger sample is needed. Longitudinal observation would also be helpful for assessing the prognostic value of identified clusters.

*P-008-133   Topic: 83, 42
Catatonia in adolescents and young adults with autism spectrum disorders: A long-term follow up

Masataka Ohta, Tokyo Gakugei University, Tokyo, Japan,
masataka@u-gakugei.ac.jp
Yukiko Kano; Yoko Nagai

Objective: Few published studies are available on the long term course of catatonia in patients with autism spectrum disorders. In this study, we diagnosed patients as having catatonia when we found that (1) in adolescence and early adult life they had abruptly stopped their movements and gotten locked into immobility or maintained bizarre posture and that (2) such a cataleptic state had continued for several minutes and appeared many times a day. **Methods:** Eleven patients (all male), most of whom have visited our outpatient clinic for more than ten years, were enrolled. The mean age was 27.6 years (SD: 5.5). The mean IQ was 27 (SD: 16.4). Information about their conditions was garnered from parents, case records and current examination. The parents consented to our publishing the results of the study. **Results:** Their morbid conditions at worst were congruent with the catatonic features specified by the DSM-IV. Catatonia was manifested in the subjects irrespective of the level of cognitive ability. In seven out of 11, the onset of catatonia was preceded by the appearance of slowness in movements accompanying the exacerbation of obsessive-compulsive-like

symptoms. In some of them it was found that catatonia manifested itself in association with freezing during an activity. Catatonia was also found to have some connection with Tourette syndrome (3 cases), adjustment disorders (1) and depressive mood disorders (1). In one case, the manifestations of catatonia had to be distinguished from those found in Parkinsonism caused by neuroleptic drugs. **Conclusion:** When we looked into the natural history of catatonia, there were cases in which the symptoms fluctuated during the day and continued to appear over a long period of time. In some cases, the symptoms disappeared in a relatively short period of time, while in others the manifestations returned after an interval of improvement.

P-008-134   Topic: 83, 47
Psychic life experience of siblings of children with Pervasive Developmental Disorders (PDD)

Anne Wintgens, Cliniques Univer. Saint-Luc, Child
Psychiatry Unit, Brussels, Belgium, a.wintgens@swing.be
Jean-Yves Hayez

Objective: To evaluate the psychic life-experience of siblings of children with PDD and to compare it to those of siblings without somatic or psychic disabilities. The authors made the hypothesis that they will find different sibling's psychic life experiences with two main thrusts: resiliency and mental health preoccupations (concerns). Between this both thrusts, they will find a wide of more or less successful adaptations. They also made the hypothesis that siblings of PDD children will be more affected by the communication's lack and by the social interactions disorders. **Methods:** Subjects: 25 siblings of children with PDD from 6 to 12 years and 25 siblings of children without somatic or psychic disabilities (control group) from 6 to 12 years, matched on sex, age, position and number of children in the family and socio-economic status. Instruments: All children take part in 6 Story-Stem completion Tasks centred on sibling's interactions and in semi-structured interviews. Statistical analysis are for instance in process. **Results:** Preliminary results: Inside the group of siblings of children with PDD, we find a part of siblings who developed self-sufficiency and resiliency and an other part who developed more preoccupied attitudes like adoption of a parental position, resignation, rivalry, domination... The relationship refusal entrains for the great majority of subjects a feeling of sadness and disappointment. Older is the child, more he is able to speak about the pathology of its brother or sister. The psychic life experiences are also relied on the parental attitudes and interventions in the sibling's relationships. We will now compare these results to the control group. **Conclusion:** The authors conclude preliminary about the importance to take in account the presence of brothers and sisters in all kind of therapeutic work of child with PDD.

P-008-135   Topic: 83, 47
Emotional and behavioral problems and parenting stress of parents in the patients of Rett syndrome

Seoung-Hu Lim, Dong-in Hospital, Dept. of Psychiatry,
Kangneung, Republic of Korea, psylim@hanmail.net
Ji-Hye Ha; Sung-Do David Hong; Jae-Won Yang; Hee-Jung
Byun; Ji-Hae Kim

Objective: The objective of this study was to examine emotional & behavioral problems and parenting stresses related to various clinical problems of Rett Syndrome (RS) patients. **Methods:** The subjects were 37 RS patients and their parents who belong to Korean Rett Syndrome Association. The control group were parents of 37 normal children who were matched by age with RS patients. We evaluated behavior problems, and analyzed parenting stresses and efficacy related to various areas of clinical problems, using Rett Syndrome Behavior Questionnaire (RSBQ), Parenting Stress Scale and other questionnaires regarding background informations and clinical features. **Results:** The clinical problem that were the most common and the most stressful to the parents were loss of skills using hand, problems in adaptive functions (daily living skills), and problems in communication. On self-abusive behavior, 21.6% of subjects were reported to show very frequently and 32.4% were very stressful and problematic in severity. In RSBQ, 3 items that were reported to be the most frequent were 'Hand movements uniform and monotonous', 'Has difficulty in breaking/stopping hand stereotypies', and 'Restricted repertoire of hand movement'. Three items that were reported to be the most stressful were 'Hand movements uniform and monotonous', 'Restricted repertoire of hand movement', and 'Has difficulty in breaking/stopping hand stereotypies'. Parents of RS subjects had lower parenting efficacy, more frustration and anxiety, and more parenting stress than parents of normal children. **Conclusion:** RS patients had various emotional and behavioral problems. Especially, problems that related to hand movement was the most stressful to parents. Although self-abusive behaviors was not prominent problem among various problems, it was substantially stressful problem to some parents.

P-009
Scientific disciplines/approaches IV

P-009-136   Topic: 41, 26
Behavioural and emotional disorders among Taiwanese adolescents: A cross-cultural comparative study
Rebecca Lee, Institute of Psychiatry, Child & Adolescent Psychiatry, London, United Kingdom, c.lee@iop.kcl.ac.uk
Eric Fombonne; Eric Taylor

Objective: The study compared the prevalence of DSM-IV psychiatric disorders and comorbidity between Taiwanese aboriginal and Han Chinese adolescents. The psychometric properties of the Youth Self Report (YSR) and Teacher Report Form (TRF) were also evaluated. **Methods:** A total of 307 adolescents aged between 13 and 15 (n = 158 aboriginal, n = 149 Han) were recruited from Eastern Taiwan using a multi-stratified sampling strategy. A one-phase design was used to identify disorders. The measure used was the semi-structured interview Schedule for Affective Disorders and Schizophrenia for School-Age Children (K-SADS-E). Final caseness was determined through the clinical judgement of raters after reviewing case vignettes. In addition, the adolescents and their class teachers completed the YSR and TRF respectively. **Results:** The one-year prevalence rate was higher for Aboriginal adolescents (27.2%) than their Han counterparts(15.4%). Specifically, Depressive disorders (7.6% vs 1.3% in the Han) and Alcohol use disorder (8.9% vs 3.4% in the Han) were more common within aboriginal adolescents. Thirty-six per cent of the cases suffered from more than one psychiatric disorder. The comorbidity between disruptive and substance use disorders was the most evident within both cultures. Re-

garding the psychometric properties of the YSR and TRF, the internal consistency and youth-teacher agreement were acceptable. Factor analysis provided some support for the validity of Achenbach's cross-informant syndromes. The area under the curve (AUC) was high which indicated a good screening detectability. **Conclusion:** The results accord with the majority of previous research in reporting higher levels of psychopathology among indigenous adolescents. The cross-cultural differences in adolescent psychopathology and the potential refinement of the YSR are discussed.

P-009-137   Topic: 41
Self-Image and identity development among adolescents
Füsun Çuhadaroğlu Çetin, Hacettepe University, Child & Adolescent Psychiatry, Ankara, Turkey, fusunc@hacettepe.edu.tr

Objective: Attention Deficit and Hyperactivity Disorder (ADHD) is one of the main developmental disorders of the childhood and adolescence. Social, cultural, familial as well as biological factors play important role in the development of secondary problems in these patients. When they reach adolescence, these children suffer from social and personal problems in addition to learning difficulties. In adolescence these problems are observed especially during the phase of identity and self-image development. Our observations pointed to an increased frequency of identity problems among adolescents with ADHD. The aim of this study is to inverstigate the development of identity and self-image in adolescents who were diagnosed as ADHD for the first time. **Methods:** Offer Self-Image Questionnaire and Sense of Identity Assessment Form were given to two groups of adolescents, one with diagnosis of ADHD, and the other having psychiatric problems other than ADHD. The age range of the research groups varied from 12 to 18. Groups are controlled for SES. **Results:** The two groups are compared for identity and self-image aspects. The results are discussed in respect of gender and age.

P-009-138   Topic: 41
Persistence of psychological problems in adolescents: A one year follow-up study
Deborah James, Regional Child & Family Centre, Dept. of Child Psychiatry, Drogheda, Ireland, deborah.james@nehb.ie
Maria Lawlor; Nick Sofroniou

Objective: To examine the prevalence and persistence of psychological problems in older adolescents **Methods:** This study is a one year follow-up of 110 adolescents, 64 girls and 46 boys attending three secondary schools in Ireland. All were 16 at initial testing. The Youth Self Report (YSR) was the measure used. **Results:** Over a fifth of adolescents have problems in the clinical range. These problems persisted from 16 to 17. Females reported more problems than males at both ages. Some females showed a slight reduction in internalising problems at 17. Both males and females showed an increase in externalising problems at 17. Odds ratios indicate that those in the clinical ranges of the YSR at 16, had increased risk of being in the clinical range at 17 compared to those in the no problem range at 16. In comparison to those with no suicidal feeling, those with suicidal feelings at 16 were at an increased risk of still feeling suicidal at 17.

More males remained Psychologically healthy than girls. **Conclusion:** A large proportion of adolescents in this sample have psychological problems and these appear to persist over a one year period. These problems impact substantially on the adolescents themselves, their families and society. Given the increasing suicide rate in young people and the persistence of suicidal feelings in this cohort, the inadequacy of mental health services in Ireland for adolescents, particularly those ages 16–18 is highlighted. The challenge of developing and providing adolescent friendly services is addressed.

P-009-139   Topic: 41, 49
Qualitative study on mourning work of adolescents bereaved of siblings by childhood cancer

Kiyoko Kamibeppu, University of Tokyo, Graduate School of Medicine, Tokyo, Japan, kkamibeppu-tky@umin.ac.jp
Iori Sato; Yasutaka Hoshi

Objective: The purpose of this study is to clarify the characteristics of mourning work of adolescents who were bereaved of siblings by childhood cancer. **Methods:** Three female and two male adolescents were interviewed and required to talk about how they experienced their bereavement of siblings. These interviews were recorded and transcribed verbatim. The transcripts were examined closely and the narratives of morning work were reconstituted. Plots were abstracted from each narrative and categorized. **Results:** Each adolescent lost his/her sibling from five to sixteen years before when he/she was at the age of four, six, nine, fourteen, and twenty-one. The core category which affected their mourning work was "the relation with their mothers". Not until their mothers psychologically returned to them from their deceased siblings did their mourning work start. **Conclusion:** The mourning work of adolescents who were bereaved of siblings by childhood cancer is characterized by not only their relation with the deceased siblings but the relation with their mothers as well.

P-009-140   Topic: 40, 90
Sexual dreams of students:
Influences of sexual instinct on sexual cognition

Miodrag Stankovic, Clinic for Mental Health,
Dept. of Child Neuropsychiatry, Belgrade,
Serbia and Montenegro, s-misa@eunet.yu
Jezdimir Zdravkovic; Petar Kostic; Sandra Stankovic

Objective: The aim of the study was to analyse the associations between sexual dreams as cognitive aspect of sexual behaviour and sexual instinct, in male and female adolescents. **Methods:** The sample consists of 656 participants, 245 males and 411 females, aged from 18-24 years, from Serbian language speaking area (Serbia, Montenegro, Republic of Srpska). The Sexual Behaviour questionnaire was used, which was specially designed for a National Study of Serbian Sexual Behaviour. For our research we used questions about the sexual history of examinee, ELNP personality questionnaire, Eysenck's questionnaire about sexual attitudes and a part on nocturnal sexual dreams that consisted of 5 questions. In statistical analyses we used parametric and nonparametric tests, as well as factor analysis of sexual attitudes. **Results:** Our findings showed that differences between genders were significant regarding the number of the dreams, more males had sexual dreams

than females (p < 0,01), dreamt more frequently sexually, (p < 0,01), often dreamt of strangers as sexual partners (0,001), often dreamt of coital activity and often had orgasmic experience in dreams (p < 0,01). Differences between genders were significantly influenced by personality and environmental factors. **Conclusion:** Sexual cognition was in a significant correlation with sex, personality and personality inhibitions, sexual stimulations, sexual abstinences and significantly corresponded with actual general sexual activity of examinees. On the basis of the data, we concluded that sexual dreams are cognitive aspect of sexual behaviour. Interrelationship between biological and environmental factors has been reflected to forms and content of the nocturnal sexual dreams.

P-009-141   Topic: 41, 93
Self-harm behaviour among child and adolescent indoor patients:
Frequency, comorbidity and treatment results

Khalid Murafi, WKKJPP Marl Sinsen, Haard Klinik,
Marl Sinsen, Germany, dr_murafi@hotmail.com
Michael Ries; Rainer Georg Siefen

Objective: The impact of experiences of sexual and physical abuse on self-harm behaviour (SHB) in inpatient treatment was investigated as well as the spectrum of related diagnoses. Another focus concerned the frequency of first manifestations of SHB during inpatient treatment and the treatment results concerning SHB. **Methods:** More than 1900 treatment records of 12–18 years old inpatients treated between 1999 and 2001 were re-examined in order to determine the frequency distributions related to the psychiatric diagnoses and the experience of sexual and physical abuse. In addition treatment results of patients with SHB prior to admission were compared to those of patients injuring themselves for the first time during the hospital stay. **Results:** Overall 36.24% of all patients showed SHB. Whereas 84.34% had injured themselves already before admission, 15.67% showed SHB for the first time during treatment (5.7% of all admissions). Of all patients ever showing SHB 76.84% were not suffering from that symptom anymore at the end of the treatment. Among the diagnoses most frequently related to SHB were: Disturbances of social behaviour, adjustment reactions and posttraumatic stress disorders. **Conclusion:** Obviously SHB is a symptom frequently found among 12 to 18 years old indoor patients. Traumatic experiences as well as specific diagnoses are significantly more frequent among patients who deliberately harm themselves. Regrettably almost every 5th patient still suffered from SHB at dismissal. Up to now the inpatient treatment does not seem to reduce self injurious behaviour sufficiently. More efficient therapeutic interventions ought to be developed and evaluated.

P-009-142   Topic: 41, 44
Life prospects of Czech adolescents:
Relations to personality and demographic variables

Martin Jelinek, Academy of Sciences, Institute of Psychology, Brno, Czech Republic, jelinek@psu.cas.cz
Marek Blatny; Helena Klimusova; Jaroslava Blizkovska

Objective: The aim of this study was to investigate relationships among life prospects, well-being, and selected personality and demographic variables in representative sample of Czech adolescents. **Methods:** A self-report survey using Life Events Schedule, Satisfaction with Life Scale, Rosenberg's Self-Esteem Scale, and personality inventory NEO-FFI was conducted in the total population of 779 students of various types of high/secondary schools (57% females; mean age 16.8). Research was performed in the regional capital and 4 municipalities in the administrative region of South Moravia. **Results:** Four clusters of adolescents according to perceived life prospects were identified: optimists, pessimists, realists with accent of professional self-confidence, and optimists without professional self-confidence accent. The strongest differences were found between optimists and pessimists. Optimists posit higher level of extraversion, emotional stability, consciousness, self-esteem, and life satisfaction than pessimists. As for demographic variables, significant differences were found in case of gender – approximately 1/3 of males were assigned to optimistic type in contrast to 1/5 of females – and also in the type of school – relatively small percentage of pessimists and higher percentage of optimists were found in gymnasium/high schools, which are aimed as a preparation for university studies. **Conclusion:** Our research revealed various views of life prospects in Czech adolescents with diverse associations to personality and demographic variables. Further analyses are needed with broader range of demographic variables.

P-009-143   Topic: 39, 69
Clinical peculiarities and therapy of childhood autism caused by early manifested endogenous psychosis

Maria Krasnoperova, Mental Health Research Center,
Dept. of Child Psychiatry, Moscow, Russia,
krasnoperova@mhrc.comcor.ru
Vera Bashina

Objective: To define the typology of early manifested endogenous psychosis, to reveal the correlations between the types of the psychosis and structure of deficit autistic state and to develop the favorable and non-favorable prediction criteria. **Methods:** Sixty-eight patients at the age of 2–8 years suffering from childhood autism manifesting with psychosis of different psychopathological structure aged up to 3 years have been observed. The clinical and psychopathological structure of manifesred psychosis, characteristic features of its course and the formation of mental developmental delay were investigated. The patients were assessed by clinical and psychometric tests – CGI scale and CARS (Childhood Autism Rating Scale). 25 patients of them received complex psychopharmacotherapy with typical neuroleptics (every day per os 30 days) and 15 intramuscular injections of 1.0 ml Cerebrolysin every other day. **Results:** Four types of manifested psychosis were specified and characterized – catatonic-regressive (19%), polymorphous-regressive (25%), catatonic (with breaks in mental development) (32%) and polymorphous (with breaks in mental development) (24%) varying in the psychotic condition severity, acuteness of autistic symptoms and level of mental developmental delay caused by the psychosis. Correlations between a structure of deficit autistic state and these psychoses were determined: 1) development of severe autistic state with pronounced mental developmental delay and a lack of speech in the most cases of catotonic-regressive psychoses; 2) autistic state of moderate severity with mental developmental delay of different severity and phrase speech formation in a less than half of the patients in polymorphous-regressive psychoses; 3) development of autistic state of moderate severity with mild mental devel-

opmental delay and phrase speech formation in the majority of the cases in catatonic psychoses; 4) formation of moderately pronounced autistic state in the absence of mental developmental delay or its mild degree and phrase speech acquirement after polymorphous psychoses. Positive effect was observed at the end of therapeutic course in 80% patients. The most improvement was seen in the subgroup of patients with catatonic psychosis (11 of 12 patients demonstrated significant or very significant improvement). **Conclusion:** Severe catatonic symptoms and regressive features are non-favorable prediction criteria. Patients with catatonic type of manifested psychosis have the best prognosis and demonstrate the positive therapeutics effects almost in all cases.

P-009-144   Topic: 39, 4
The change of day nursing system for disabled infants in Fukouks City

Minemitsu Kusu, Showagakuen, Munakata-gun, Japan,
syouwa@mocha.ocn.ne.jp

Objective: Determination of the factors influencing the Day Nursing System for Infants (D.N.S.D.I). **Methods:** Nursery School is a kind of social welfare institution and the local autonomous authority is primarily responsible for it's management. In Japan, caring for disabled children at nursery school means that the autonomous authority itself prepares staffs, methods of doing and especially, financial measure under certain regulation. Therefore, caring disabled children nursery is the same as keeping up DNSDI. **Results:** In 1997, Fukuoka City set up a Committee for directing the disabled infant in nursery school (C.D.D.N) as a consultative organization. The Committee has carried out various acts such as selecting the object of DNSDI, planning and operation on training and technical aid for nursery school teachers, exchanging information between staffs. The criterion of selection was made, based on clinical effect and developmental aid and also reserved school system in which were allowed to have a caring disabled. In 1997, many mothers with their disabled children the city assembly asked for the admittance of all disabled children in nursery school, and the city assemble was unanimous for this. In 2002, although there are some exceptions, every disabled children in Fukuoka City were able to enter every nursery school if they would like to.

P-009-145   Topic: 40, 2
Changing times: An audit of an patient child psychiatry unit over 3 year period in Ireland

Catherine McElearney, National Children's Hospital,
Child & Adolescent Psychiatry, Dublin 24, Ireland,
cjmulligan@eircom.net
C. Burke; B. Doody

Objective:. To audit the in-patient service to facilitate future service planning. – To obtain a profile of the patients admitted to the unit including basic socio-demographic information, mean length of stay and diagnostic categories. – To document the time between the referral and admission. – To evaluate the use of medication. **Methods:** This was a retrospective study of consecutive admissions to the unit over a 3 year period. Data collected included basic socio-demographic information, length of stay, number of admissions, diagnosis and medication prescribed. Information was taken from patient clinical files, drug kardex and the pin-point computer system. **Results:** A total of 100 children were admitted to the unit. A wide diagnostic group were identified. Children from all social classes were represented. **Conclusion:.** The service is offering a flexible assessment based in-patient stay. – The profile of patients admitted to the unit has changed with an emphasis on emotional disorders. A previous audit showed a prevalence of conduct disorders. – The median length of stay has decreased to 50.3 days. All social classes were represented. – 42.9% of children had no contact with their fathers. – 60% children were discharged on prescribed medication. Drugs were more frequently prescribed on a continuous basis with only 17 children requiring PRN medication. – Serotonin Reuptake inhibitors are the most frequently prescribed class of drug. – A documented history of familial mental health issues was identified in 51 cases. – The mean length of time waiting for admission was 43 days.

P-009-146   Topic: 39
Medical staff and parents confronted with a premature birth: The transition from infant care towards differentiated roles

Carole Müller Nix, Unité de Développement CHUV, Division de Néonatologie, Lausanne, Switzerland, carole.muller-nix@inst.hospvd.ch
Ayala Nicole

This work is part of a prospective longitudinal study entitled "Parental representation and outcomes of prematurity: a socio-emotional and neurodevelopmental approach". Using some of this data, we explored parents' subjective experiences and their relationships with medical staff. Semi-structured videotaped interviews (CLIP, Meyer 1993) were made at 42 weeks post-conception, and at 6 and 18 months (corrected age), with a population of 70 preterm and 30 full term parents. For the parents, having a premature baby appears to be a very stressful experience, with a direct effect on their view of themselves as parents. Most premature babies stay in the NICU for months. During this long hospital stay, the parents' relationship with their infant depends on a number of factors: the infant's health, the uncertainty of the outcome, as well as on their subjective experience. In particular, the investment into their role as parents, is challenged by the constant reference to the medical team and result in wide and complex range of feelings. Most parents have high praise for the skills, and support given by the medical team. However, parents may have difficulty affirming their position as parents, becoming either too dependant, or on the contrary too much in competition with the medical team. For example, parents may express feelings of being excluded or deprived of their parental role. Between these two extremes, it appears that a certain differentiation of the parental role as opposed to that of the medical team, is essential to the confidence and security of their relationship with their child at discharge. In light of this need for differentiation, occasional disagreements that emerge between parents and the NICU staff, are perhaps a significant part of this process. In this video presentation, we will see parent interviews which clearly illustrate the aforementioned difficulties, and ambivalent feelings.

P-009-148   Topic: 39
Tube weaning in early infancy

Markus Wilken, Universitäts-Kinderklinik Bonn, Abt. Neonatologie, Bonn, Germany, privat@markus-wilken.de
Marguerite Dunitz-Scheer; Alexandra Krasnovsky

Objective: We present an home based and inpatient tube weaning program. The program is interdisciplinary and focus on self regulation of feeding. The program based on psychodynamic psychotherapy. **Methods:** 207 children between 6 mon. and 7.7 years (M=29.7 mon.) of age were involved in the intervention program. Medical and psychosocial factors associated with tube weaning and the beginning of nutritional intake were recorded. The multiaxial ZTT-DC: 0–3 was used. **Results:** After intervention 96.3% of the whole sample were totally oral fed. The age at tube weaning, duration of tube feeding did not influence therapy success. **Conclusion:** The home based intervention for weaning tube feeding is an effective intervention program. Further evaluation has to be done. Prolonged tube feeding is often compromised by medical and psychological complications. Tube weaning after long-lasting tube feeding is based on therapeutic counselling. Therapeutic concepts for tube weaning are rarely developed and evaluated.

P-010
Disorders and other conditions I

P-010-149   Topic: 96, 81
Ocular anomalies, visuo-spatial skills and adaptive behaviour in Down syndrome

Anastasia Dressler, Universität Wien, Inst. für Kinderheilkunde, Wien, Austria, anastasiaflora@gmx.net
Valentina Perelli; Francesca Tinelli; Valentina Rafanelli; Stefania Bargagna

Objective: Little is known about the incidence of visual anomalies in individuals with DS in adulthood. Our aim was to investigate incidence and to study the relation between visuo-spatial skills, cognitive abilities and adaptive behaviour. **Methods:** We included 52 individuals and ascertained ocular abnormalities, as confirmed by recent ophthalmologic screening, tested Hirschberg's corneal reflex method, observed eye movements during fixation of a slowly moving object, assessed CPM, the figure of Rey, VMI, Street's completion test, agnosia and the Vineland Adaptive Behaviour scales. **Results:** We found bilateral cataract in 17.3%, hypermetropia in 19.2%, myopia in 28.8%, astigmatism in 17.3%, strabism in 48%, difficulties in the coordination of eye movements in 50%, and nystagm in 25%. Considering ID groups with mild and moderate ID, there are significant differences between age groups as cognitive abilities are concerned but not in adaptive behaviour nor in the incidence of ocular abnormalities. Cataract correlated significantly with IQ, figure of Rey, VMI, test of agnosia. On adaptive behaviour strabism correlated significantly with poorer performance in written and cataract with reception, written, communication, personal, domestic, and interpersonal relationships. A significantly higher presence of difficulties in eye movement coordination was found with increasing cognitive impairment and lower performance on VMI. **Conclusion:** We found a rather high incidence of ocular anomalies in adults DS not differing with age. The incidence of difficulties in ocular motor coordination is rather high and we suggest a global difficulty related to cognition in learning and applying of strategies of motor organisation. Adaptive behaviour is influenced to a smaller degree by the presence of ocular anomalies, only cataract and strabism seem to have a influence on adaptive skills. These findings suggest that the early training of visuo-motor skills, and early surgery for cataract and strabism may help in further acquisition of competences.

P-010-150   Topic: 95, 81

Psychopathological features, cognitive skills and adaptive behaviour in Down syndrome

Anastasia Dressler, Universität Wien, Inst. für Kinderheilkunde, Wien, Austria, anastasiaflora@gmx.net
Valentina Perelli; Valentina Rafanelli; Stefania Bargagna

Objective: Individuals with Down syndrome (DS) are at significant risk of psychiatric disorders when compared to their non-ID peers, but little is known about the variability of adaptive behaviour regarding different psychiatric co-morbidity. Our main goal was to assess the incidence and pattern of psychopathologic disorders in a population with DS and to identify the specificity of adaptive behaviour. **Methods:** We included 53 individuals from 19 to 52 years, took a detailed medical history, performed a non-structured psychiatric interview, assessed the Aberrant Behaviour Checklist (ABC), Raven's coloured progressive matrices (CPM), Dementia scale for Down syndrome (DSDS), the Vineland Adaptive Behaviour Scales (VABS) and Neuropsychiatric Inventory. **Results:** The incidence of psychiatric co-morbidity in our group is rather high (33,8%), autistic disorder NOS are followed by anxiety disorders and mood disorders, half of the individuals with depression also presented anxiety disorders. Adaptive abilities are significantly poorer in individuals with autistic disorder, in particular in expression, personal autonomy, socialisation and total score, whereas individuals with depressive symptoms do better than their peers. Adaptive behaviour is also significantly correlated to cognitive skills, individuals with mild ID perform better whereas moderate and severe ID do not differ. On the ABC, we find significantly higher scores for individuals with autistic features. The most frequent symptoms are in stereotypy and hyperactivity. There are no differences in years and age of schooling, rehabilitation programs, and teacher support between different psychiatric disorders, but they are significantly related to age. **Conclusion:** The incidence of psychiatric co-morbidity is quite high and autistic symptoms seem to be an important factor of vulnerability in adults with DS in adaptive behaviour as well as in cognitive abilities. It is crucial to consider early intervention programs in childhood to prevent the development of autistic symptomatology in Down syndrome and to maintain a higher level of competence.

P-010-151   Topic: 93, 12

Treatment options for self-injuring behaviour in adolescent females: Better acceptance of Ziprasidone (augmentation) due to lower weight gain

Gerhard Libal, Universitätsklinik Ulm, Kinder- und Jugendpsychiatrie, Ulm, Germany, gerhard.libal@medizin.uni-ulm.de
Paul Plener; Jörg M. Fegert

Objective: The use of atypical neuroleptics as a monotreatment or augmentation option in addition to SSRIs for re-ducing self-injuring behaviour in adolescent females with disruptive impulsivity is of increasing interest. One major limiting factor in this population for the use of atypicals is weight gain. We conducted a retrospective comparison in our inpatient population in order to evaluate symptom reduction and weight gain under various naturalistic treatment conditions. **Methods:** We report a retrospective chart review of 16 female inpatients (age range: 13.10–17.11, mean: 15.3), receiving psychopharmacotherapy to reduce self-injuring behaviour. We compared two groups, one with Ziprasidone alone or in addition to a SSRI and one with other atypicals alone or in addition to a SSRI. Assessments included symptom reduction of self injuring behaviour defined according to Favazza (1989) and Winchel (1991), adverse effects (ECG monitoring) and weight monitoring. **Results:** In the Ziprasidone group (n = 8) with a dose range 40–80 mg/d we found a 47.33% decrease in the rate of self-injuring behaviour measured as events of deliberate self-harm per day (range: 0.01–0.33 before ziprasidone vs. range: 0.00–0.18 after titration; p = 0.03) without weight change (mean: -0.11 kg; p = 0.78). In the group (n = 8) treated with Risperidone (n = 4), Olanzapine(n = 1), Chlorproxithen (n = 2) and Promethazine (n = 1) we found a statistically not significant lower symptom reduction rate of 17.82% (range: 0.02–0.27; before treatment vs. range 0.00–0.33 after full treatment dose; p = 0.53) and an average weight gain of 2.06 kg (p = 0.05). **Conclusion:** Ziprasidone may be a useful alternative in the treatment or in the augmentation of SSRI treatment of impulse control deficits with better effects on symptom reduction and less increase in weight.

P-010-152   Topic: 93

Psychopathology and comorbidity of psychiatric disorders in patients with wrist-cutting

Fumiko Enokido, Kanazawa Medical University, Dept. of Neuropsychiatry, Ishikawa, Japan, psychiat@kanazawa-med.ac.jp
Masako Higuchi; Istuki Jibiki

Objective: This study compared young patients (began to cut one's own arm first under 18 years of age) and elder patients (began to cut first over 19 years of age) with wrist-cutting behaviors on several key psychopathological dimensions. In addition, the comorbidity of axis 1 and axis 2 disorders in patients with wrist-cutting was examined. **Methods:** Fifty-seven patients who had received treatment with psychiatric complains and comorbid of wrist-cutting at our clinics between April 2001 and December 2003 were assessed for psychiatric and personality disorders according to DSM-4 criteria. A semistructured interview schedule and standardized questionnaires were used to investigate patients' background characteristics, the circumstances of family and school life, other self-injurious behaviors, their first informations about wrist-cutting and her/his purpose of those behaviors. **Results:** Young patients (26 female and 1 male) who cut first 15.8 years of age on average were associated with eating disorder (N = 11) and adjustment disorder (N = 9) and significantly high rates of borderline personality disorder (N = 15). Young group was characterized by female gender, lower full-IQ, many times cutting, higher proportions of impulsive attempt and positive psychiatric family histories and much other problem behaviors (e.g. shoplifting, school refusal, bulimia). Elder patients (21 female and 9 male) who cut first 26.2 years of age on average were associated with various disorders and significantly high rates of schizophrenia (N=6). Elder group was characterized by higher proportion of male, fewer attempts, more serious injuries and distinctively attempt for guilt as wrist-cutting. **Conclusion:** Recently there has been growing concern about youth self-harm. Young wrist-cutters had more symptoms of psychiatric and personality disorders compared to elder patients. These clinical characteristics suggested that stressful and unfortunate circumstances of growing-up play a great role in severer psychopathology.

P-010-153   Topic: 93, 58
Suicidal ideation among Slovene high school students
Martina Tomori, University Psychiatric Hosp., Medical Faculty, Ljubljana, Slovenia
Urša Mrevlje

Objective: The aim of the study was to assess the frequency of suicidal ideation and its correlation to other risk factors for suicide in the community population of adolescents. **Methods:** The study includes a representative sample of 4706 Slovene high school students in the age span from 14 to 19 years of age. We applied an structured questionnaire which was self-evaluative and included also self-assessment scales for measuring depression and self-esteem. The data collected were statistically processed by means of the computer program SPSS for Windows v.10. We used appropriate univariant statistical methods. **Results:** The prevalence of suicidal ideation was 44% at anytime in the respondent's life, more frequent in girls than boys (p=0.000). There were statistically significant differences between the adolescents with suicidal ideation and those without in: the family and peer support, health problems, experienced problems, non-functional abilities of reacting to stress, use of psychoactive drugs, suicidal behavior among close persons, level of depression and self-esteem. There were no differences in the religiosity found between the two groups. **Conclusion:** The findings of study have confirmed the high occurrence of suicidal thoughts among Slovenian adolescents. Suicidal ideation in adolescents is an important risk factor for suicide, especially when associated with other risk factors. This results provide important directions for prevention of the suicide risk among adolescents.

P-010-154   Topic: 96
Temperament and character profiles of internet addiction in Korean elementary school children
Hee-Jeong Yoo, Gyeongsang Nation. University, Dept. of Psychiatry, Jinju, Republic of Korea, neologue@hotmail.com
Su-Yeon Kim; In-Hee Cho; Sook-Kyeong Yune; In-Kyoon Lyoo; Ji-Hyun Ha

Objective: Internet addiction is one of the newly-developed, serious mental health problems in Korea. The objective of this study was to identify the temperament and character profiles of internet addiction in Korean elementary school children. We hypothesized that ADHD would be related novelty seeking in Junior Temperament and Character Inventory (JTCI), because internet provides one of the multi-modal, ever-changing stimuli for it's users. **Methods:** Four hundred fifty five elementary school students (male=299, female=226: mean age=11.05±0.98) in one city were participated in this study. The presence and severity of internet addiction were assessed by Young's in-

ternet addiction scale. Children and their parent did the Korean version of the child behavior checklist (CBCL) and JTCI. **Results:** 1) Sixty three children (13.9%) were classified as internet addiction group. Internet addiction group had a tendency to indulge on other activities like games, sports more severely than normal group. 2) Higher novelty seeking, harm avoidance and lower reward dependence, persistence were observed in internet addiction group than normal group. 3) In CBCL, Internet addiction group had higher score in withdrawal, somatic complaints, anxiety/depression, immaturity, thought problems, attention problems, delinquent behavior, aggressive behavior, internalizing problems, and externalizing problems than normal group. 4) CBCL subscales related with novelty seeking had significant positive correlation with severity of internet addiction. **Conclusion:** We found significant correlations between degree of novelty seeking and internet addiction in Korean elementary school children. Current findings suggest that there may be a biogenetic background associated with the novelty seeking in children with addictive behavior to internet. This results also suggest the possibility that internet addiction is related to the attention problem in children.

P-010-155   Topic: 93
Immediate functions of Self-injurious Behaviour (SIB): Construction of a questionnaire
Barbara Haas, Linz, Austria, barbara.haas@liwest.at

Objective: The aim of the study is the construction of a questionnaire that evaluates the immediate functions of SIB. **Methods:** SIB is defined as deliberate injuries on the skin such as burning, cutting or hitting. Suicidal attempts as well as self-injuries for an ideal of beauty were excluded. In a former study immediate functions of SIB have been collected in literature. According to them a questionnaire has been constructed. Via factor analysis (N=120) the functions 'self-punishment', 'coping with emotions', 'extreme rage', 'vivideness', 'dissociation', 'changed perception', 'body control', 'uniqueness', 'interaction', 'addiction', 'coping with sexuality' and 'expression of sexuality' were extracted. The Cronbach's Alpha of a first, shorted version was r=0.91 (N=120). Now the sample has been extended so that a new factor analysis will be computed. The immediate functions will be compared with diverse personality factors such as depressivity, negative attitude to ones body, aggressiveness and self-attention (N ~ 80). Furthermore differences between diagnoses an the intensity of the immediate functions will be expected (N ~ 60). **Results:** The study is still running, its results will be finished in june this year. **Conclusion:** According to the former study it is possible to evaluate the immediate functions of SIB via questionnaire. The comparisons with diverse personality factors will bring first aspects of its validity.

P-010-156   Topic: 93, 70
Typology of the suicides arising at depressive adolescents
Lyudmila Danilova, Ass. of Child Psychiatrists, and Psychologists, Moscow, Russia, acpp@online.ru

Studying of the adolescents, who have transferred nonpsychotic depressions, has revealed presence of suicidal tendencies at third surveyed, and suicidal attempts – in 16% of depressions. 2 types of suicidal actions – true suicides and parasuicidal behavior are allocated; parasuicides submit 3 subtypes. The interrelation of suicidal behavior with a typology of depressions is revealed. Parasuicidal behavior directed on restoration of social communications with associates was marked at melancholic, alarming, dysphoric depressions. Suicidal attempts arose after objectively insignificant psychotraumas, which played a role of the catalyst sharpened already available erased depressive experiences. The suicidal determination approached with acute affective reactions and was characterized by suddenness of occurrence and brevity of existence. More often parasuicides were made impulsively at height of affect in extra- or intropunitive type and have been deprived any struggle of motives. In other cases the adolescent was guided by desire to avoid searches of the resolution of conflict, "to be fenced off" from experienced situation without an adequate estimation of consequences. At the third subtype parasuicides had demonstrative character blackmail behavior with attempt to force surrounding to change the reference with the adolescent. The true suicidal behavior met seldom and was taped at monotonous apathy-adynamic depressions without connection with a psychogenia. Depression was accompanied by painted resonates on philosophical themes. Suicidal actions were consequence logic, frequently ridiculous conclusions about senselessness of existence. Suicidal reasoning was seldom poured out in actions, but suicidal acts were made is considered and as fiduciary from associates. This type of suicides represented the big danger since actions had steady motivation and were inclined to relapse. The classical form of suicides owing to depressive ideas of self-charge in researched group was not observed.

P-010-157 Topic: 94, 47
School phobia and parental psychopathology

Elisa Lapponi, Rome University, Childhood Neuropsychiatry, Rome, Italy, carla.sogos@uniroma1.it
Maria Carla Filipponi; Felicia Lauria; Carla Sogos

Objective: Recent reviewers have concluded that there is some evidence suggesting school refusal tends to occur in family contexts marked by dysfunction and emotional disturbance. Significant differences have been observed in familial aggregation considering the subgroups of school phobic children. The purpose of this study is to examine the relationship between parental psychopathology and the different clinical profiles shown by children with school phobia. **Methods:** We analyse a clinical sample of 25 children exhibiting school refusal behaviour (15 males and 10 females; range: 6–13; m.a.: 9.7 years; S.D.: 2) who referred to our Outpatient Service during the last 18 months. The subjects were submitted to the psychodiagnostic and neuropsychological protocol currently in use by our Centre (WISC-R, K-SADS PL, CDI, CDRS-R, Rorschach, CGI). The presence of a parental psychiatric disorder according to DSM-IV criteria was assessed by psychiatric interviews. **Results:** Data related to our clinical sample will be described (56% of the children have at least one parent who exhibits a psychiatric illness) and the relationship between parental psychopathology and subgroups of school phobic children will also be discussed. **Conclusion:** The results of this research confirm that there appears to be a high prevalence of psychiatric illness within the families of children with school phobia and suggest there might be a close association between parental psychiatric disorders and school refusal behaviour. Although further investigations

are required, we consider this kind of study a very helpful approach for gaining a better understanding of the pathogenesis of school phobia. Moreover, it may play an important role in identifying risk or vulnerability factors and in devising effective treatment programs.

P-010-158 Topic: 93, 68
Suicide behaviour and substance abuse

Daniele Giovanni Poggioli, Ospedale Maggiore, U.O. di psichiatria e psic. ee, Bologna, Italy, daniegio@libero.it
Giancarlo Rigon

Objective: Suicide behaviour represents a manifestation of serious psicological and social unease and many risk factors are involved. Substances abuse is one of the well known risk factors in the literature. **Methods:** We have verified substances abuse in a clinical group formed by 28 adolescents that had completed a suicide attempt and we have compared this group with a group of 26 adolescents who had declared a suicide attempt in a self report and also with a control group. The substances examined have been alcohol, cannabis, ecstasy, cocaine, heroin and amphetamine. **Results:** Statistics: the difference between the groups is confirmed by the Fischer's exact test for small samples. **Conclusion:** We can confirm that the substance abuse is more frequent in the group of suicide attempers than in the controll group. The difference regards both the group identified by self report and the clinical group. In the group of suicide attempers we have observed a subgroup of multiple substances abuse. In this group there are also adolescents who repeated suicide attempts.

P-010-159 Topic: 93, 45
Attitudes towards suicide in Hungarian and Austrian adolescents

Kanita Dervic, Medical University of Vienna, Child Neuropsychiatry, Wien, Austria, kanita.dervic@meduniwien.ac.at
Janos Csorba; Sandor Rozsa; Marjorie Kleinman; Laszlo Tringer; Max Friedrich; Madelyn Gould; Tuerkan Akkaya-Kalayci; Gerhard Lenz

Objective: The attitudes towards suicide of Central European secondary school pupils, whose suicide rates are concerning, have rarely been studied. Present study compared suicide attitudes of Hungarian and Austrian adolescents. **Methods:** 96 Hungarian (mean age 17.1 years) and 214 Austrian (mean age 15.5 years) secondary school pupils were surveyed using a self-report questionnaire to assess their suicide attitudes and prevalence of risk factors for suicide. **Results:** Secondary school pupils in the two countries did not differ significantly on the prevalence of suicide risk factors such as depression, substance use, exposure, suicidal ideation and suicide attempt, but they differed on gender and age. After controlling for confounders, significantly more Hungarian adolescents attributed an antidepressant effect to drugs and alcohol than their Austrian peers (24.0% vs. 10.7%, p < 0.001). The attitude that people who talk about suicide do not commit it, was also more prevalent in Hungary (76.0% vs. 44.9%, p < 0.001). Hungarian youth were also more likely to endorse suicide as a possible solution to problems than Austrian youth (24.0% vs. 19.6%, p < 0.05). As for help-seeking attitudes, Hungarian adolescents were less likely to advise a hypothetical suicidal friend to see a mental health professional

(47.9% vs. 68.7%, p<0.001) and call a hotline (15.6% vs. 26.2%, p<0.05), and more likely to talk to friend alone (75.0% vs. 50.5%, p<0.001). **Conclusion:** The results of this study show more undesirable and maladaptive suicide attitudes in Hungarian adolescents than in their Austrian peers, which may be attributed to cultural differences between two countries. However, the results in both countries highlight an obvious need for addressing adolescents' maladaptive attitudes towards suicide as a part of public health strategies in youth suicide prevention.

P-010-160   Topic: 93, 41
Incidence of wrist cutting among Japanese adolescents
Akihide Kitamura, Nara University of Education, Nara, Japan, kitamura@nara-edu.ac.jp

Objective: There are no reports about the incidence and actual conditions of wrist cutting among Japanese students in general. **Methods:** The investigation was conducted by giving 119 Yogo teachers (school nurse teachers) a questionnaire about actual conditions of wrist cutting among elementary school children and junior and senior high school students. **Results:** (1) 146 cases of wrist cutting by children and students were found. There were 136 females and 10 males. The ratio between female and male was 13.6 to 1. (2) The youngest children found to have cut their wrist began from 10 years old. (3) The chronological incidence change of the number of cases of wrist cutting, in the last four years, was markedly increased. (4) 11 cases (7.5%) had death wishes, and only one case succeeded in committing suicide. (5) As for the motives for wrist cutting, relief of stress was found most often. (6) As for the fundamental problems, parent-child relationships, divorced parents, physical and sexual abuse, influence of violent magazine, e-mail and internet friends were found relatively more often. (7) In the year 2002 alone, the incidence of wrist cutting among senior high school students (ages 16 to 18) was 0.6% among females and 0.05% among males. (8) 51 cases (34.9%) of the entire 146 cases could be psychiatrically diagnosed, but the other 95 cases (65.1%) could not be diagnosed. **Conclusion:** Recently in Japan, the incidence of wrist cutting among children and students is increasing. Of the entire 146 cases, 27% of the cases were cared for by the psychiatric medical institutions. Of the other 73% of cases, almost all of the students had cut their wrist in order to resolve their own conflict or frustration, therefore, it is hoped that students can be cared for or counseled at school too.

P-011   Topic: 84, 85
Attention-deficit/hyperactivity disorders (ADHD) I
Track: ADHD

P-011-161   Topic: 84
ADHD, ODD, ODD/CD:
An inhibition-deficit is what they have in common
Bjoern Albrecht, University of Göttingen, Child & Adolescent Psychiatry, Göttingen, Germany, balbrec@gwdg.de
Tobias Banaschewski; Aribert Rothenberger

Objective: Children with externalizing child psychiatric disorders may have difficulties in response inhibition. It is questioned whether these difficulties are specific for attention-deficit hyperactivity disorder (ADHD) or whether impaired response inhibition is also present in other externalizing disorders. **Methods:** In the study presented the stop-task was used to investigate response inhibitory control in 10 children with attention-deficit hyperactivity disorder (ADHD), 8 children with oppositional defiant disorder/conduct disorder (ODD/CD), 11 children with AD-HD+ODD/CD, and a group of 11 normal controls (aged 8–14 years). Event-related potentials and behavioural responses were recorded simultaneously. **Results:** Compared to normal controls, the clinical groups displayed longer stop-signal-reaction-times (SSRT) and a reduced N200-amplitude registered over frontal electrodes to the stop-signal. In normal controls this N200-amplitude was positively correlated with SSRT. Additional results did suggest, that different mechanisms may underlie inhibitory control in the groups investigated. **Conclusion:** Compared to normal controls, all examined groups with externalizing child psychiatric disorders display an inhibition deficit and abnormalities in an early stage of stop-signal processing. More research is needed to further clarify the relationship between electrophysiological parameters and performance measures.

P-011-162   Topic: 84
Association analysis between DBH Polymorphisms and Attention Deficit Hyperactivity Disorder (ADHD)
Xueping Gao, Central South University, Dept. of Child Psychiatry, Changsha, China, xuepinggao@hotmail.com
Linyan Su; Xianghui Zhang; Xuerong Li

Objective: To analyses the association between polymorphisms in human dopamineβ-hydroxylase gene and ADHD, and to explore the relationship between DβH activity in plasma and genotypes of DβH gene. To find the disease-predisposing genes of ADHD. **Methods:** Genotypes and allele frequencies of polymorphic (GT) n repeat at DβH gene in ADHD probands, their parents, and normal controls were examined by Amp-FLP techniques. Both case-control association study and family-based association study (HRR and TDT analysis) were used. Plasma DβH activity was photometrically assayed. **Results:** No differences in genotypes and allele frequencies of polymorphic (GT) n repeat at DβH gene were observed between ADHD group and control group (p>0.05), and in nuclear families (p>0.05). The frequency of DβH gene A4 allele in the subjects was very low. The frequency of A2 allele in "puried" ADHD group was significantly higher than that in comorbid group (p<0.05). The scores of social problems, attention problems, aggressive behavior and total behavior scores of CBCL in A2/A3 genotype in ADHD probands were significantly higher than that in A3/A3 genotype in ADHD probands (p<0.05). No difference was observed in the level of DβH activity in the plasma between ADHD group and control group (p>0.05). **Conclusion:** DβH gene was probably not associated with ADHD in this study. The frequency of A4 allele of DβH gene in the subjects was very low. The frequency of A2 allele was probably associated with "puried" ADHD. The polymorphic (GT) n repeat at DβH gene was somewhat associated with certain clinical manifestations in ADHD.

P-011-163   Topic: 84
ADHD-Problems with diagnostics

Vesna Hercigonja-Novkoviæ, Clinical Hospital Dubrava,
Psychotrauma National Centre, Zagreb, Croatia,
vesna.hercigonja@zg.htnet.hr
Dubravka Kocijan-Hercigonja

Objective: The objective of this study was to determine the factors that influence diagnistics for Attention Deficit Hyperactivity Disorder in school-aged children by parents, teachers and mental health professionals. **Methods:** Our target group comprised 80 pupils of the first grade from two preschools in Zagreb. The target groups were parents of the pupils parents, teachers of the pupils and mental health professionals (profesionals from our Organization: psychiatrist, psychologist, special educator) and the mental health profesionals from those two schools (school paedagogues and school psychologist). We have asked all of those parents and teachers to fill out the Conners scale for parents and teachers for all the children in those two first grades. Mental health professionals had to make diagnosis based on the DSM-IV diagnostic manual. **Results:** All together the results showed that aprox. 20% of pupils suffered from ADHD. However, there were many differences between parental diagnoses and many differences between teachers diagnoses. Therefore, their criteria differed greatly. Additionally we looked into the factors that played an important role in diagnosing for ADHD. **Conclusion:** In the parental group the prevailing factor when diagnosing for ADHD, was age. Younger parents who had less time to spend with their children and had longer working hours were more eager to diagnose ADHD that older parents with more patience and more flexible working hours. In the teachers group, age and experience were important factors as well. Younger and less experienced teachers have diagnosed more pupils with ADHD that older and more experienced teachers.

P-011-164   Topic: 84
Baseline information on the age of onset age of diagnosis and outcomes: Results from Attention Deficit Hyperactivity Disorder (ADHD) observational research in Europe

Stephen Ralston, Eli Lilly & Co Ltd., EHOR, Windlesham,
United Kingdom, ralston_stephen_j@lilly.com
Maria Lorenzo

Objective: To present the baseline information on age of onset, age of diagnosis and outcomes from the attention-deficit/hyperactivity disorder observational research in Europe (ADORE) study. **Methods:** ADORE is a 2-year, prospective, observational study of attention-deficit/hyperactivity disorder (ADHD). It is targeted to enrol 1500 patients from 10 European countries including Austria, Denmark, France, Germany, Iceland, Italy, The Netherlands, Norway, Switzerland, and the UK. Current enrolment stands at approximately 1214 patients. Enrolment for ADORE closes on April 9, 2004. **Results:** The full baseline dataset will be presented in the poster. Information will be reported from a Pan European and country-specific perspective. Data will be presented on the age that parents recognize that their child has ADHD symptoms, the age in which treatment was first sought, and the age of diagnosis. School outcomes will be presented including academic performance and behavior including the percentage exclusion

from normal school activities. Information on patient outcomes will be presented and include social activities and bullying. **Conclusion:** ADHD is a diagnosable, neurobiological disorder which may impact the child both at school and in social situations. From the data items above the impact of early symptom recognition and treatment will be described for school and social performance.

P-011-165   Topic: 84, 26
Prevalence of Attention Deficit Hyperactivity Disorder (ADHD) in Egyptian school children

Asmaa Amin Abdel Aziz, Neuropsychiatry Ain Shams,
University, Egypt, asmaamin@yahoo.com

Objective: Attention Deficit hyperactivity (ADHD) is one of the overt behavioral problems that starts as early as three years and peaks at school entrance. It is now being recognized in the Arab world with increasing speed much as it has been the diagnosis of decade for almost ten years. **Methods:** A survey of ADHD in childhood was conducted in a sample of 973 Egyptian school children 4–10 years old. A two stage design was used in order to achieve our aim, at first screening phase of all children by means of Conner's scale of ADHD, then a second phase of design, the diagnosed cases were subjected to Rutter scale for detection of abnormal psychosocial situation. **Results:** Only 786 of the paper was answered by both the parents and teachers. About 112 (14.24%) of children were diagnosed as ADHD by Conner's scale either in school or home. **Conclusion:** From the above data, it seems that we need a system to reduce and to cope with such ADHD in order to reduce it's prevalence and to counteract its deleterious effect on the child's psychological health.

P-011-166   Topic: 84
Comparison of parents' and teachers' reports of Attention Deficit Hyperactivity Disorder (ADHD) symptoms

Joseph Biederman, Massachusetts General Hosp.,
Dept. of Psychiatry, Boston, MA, USA,
biederman@helix.mgh.harvard.edu
Thomas Spencer; Rodney Moore; Haitao Gao

Objective: The validity of parent reports of children's attention-deficit/hyperactivity disorder (ADHD) symptoms has been questioned. This analysis compared the ability of parent and teacher reports to document change in symptoms during clinical trials. **Methods:** Data were pooled from 2 placebo-controlled clinical trials of atomoxetine using different versions (Parent vs. Teacher) of the same rating scale (the Attention-Deficit/Hyperactivity Disorder Rating Scale-IV- [Parent or Teacher] Version: Investigator-Administered and Scored). Exclusion criteria included history of bipolar disorder, psychosis, seizures, alcohol abuse, or positive drug screen. Patients (6–16 years old) who met entry criteria were treated with atomoxetine (titrated to a maximum dose of 1.8 mg/kg/day) administered once daily in the morning for up to 7 weeks. Parent and Teacher ratings were compared using an ANCOVA model. **Results:** The pooled analysis (N=318) revealed that treatment effects (mean change, baseline to endpoint) were similar between parent and teacher ratings (Total, p=0.762, Inattention, p=0.519; Hyperactive/Impulsive p=0.955). Effect sizes were also similar based on total scores (parent ratings=0.69; teacher ratings=0.63). **Conclusion:** These results extend to atomoxetine previously published results of a similar finding with long-acting stimulants and suggest that parent reports are as informative as teacher reports during treatment of children with ADHD when using long-acting compounds.

P-011-167   Topic: 84
ADD-treatment in parents and grandparents – empirical data from a transgenerational out-patient project in a swiss hospital

Oliver Bilke, Humboldt-Klinikum, Kinder- und Jugendpsychiatrie, Berlin, Germany, oliver.bilke@vivantes.de

Objective: To assess the effect of usual multi-dimensional treatment of ADD in parents and grand-parents of affected families we established an out-patient project in Eastern Switzerland in cooperation with pediatricians and regional psychiatric hospitals. **Methods:** As most relatives of ADD-children do not seek help for themselves spontaneously we coordinated our approach with the regional psychiatric hospitals and two well known pediatric out-patients centers. There was an open invitation for parents and particular grand-parents of diagnosed ADD-children to be assessed and treated themselves due to guidelines for adult ADD-patients. We used structured history taking, concentration tests and clinical and social measures. We took 21 consecutive cases from the age of 30 to the age of 61 and treated them with methylphenidate, individual ADD-coaching and transference focused psychotherapy. **Results:** All referrals met the ICD-10-criteria of ADD due to being screened by experienced pediatricians and psychiatrists before. There was a huge personal need for treatment having seen the positive impact of methylphenidate on children and grand-children. As pharmacotherapy and individual coaching including bibliotherapy worked very well, there were 9 cases in which a psychodynamic psychotherapy had to be added, as narcissistic personality disorder and dysthymia emerged. In particular three grandfathers at the age of 55–61 needed intensive support to stand the idea of having been a theoretically treatable individual, whose subjective suffering had never been seen by the relatives. Quality of life improved significantly in all cases. **Conclusion:** A multidimensional approach in ADD-treatment should include a routine assesssment and if indicated treatment not only of parents but of grandparents as well. Usual therapy schemes can be easily administered and the overall stress level in these families can be lowered. Systematic research would help these families.

P-011-168   Topic: 84
Attention Deficit Disorder (ADD) in adolescents

Josep Cornellà, Girona, Spain, cornella@comg.es
Àlex Llusent

Objective: To describe and identify the presentation forms, the comorbidity, and the treatment of the Attention Deficit Disorder (ADD) in adolescents. **Methods:** The study includes on 70 adolescents (aged between 14 25 years) with a diagnosis of ADD in an Adolescent Unit over a period of 48 months. The diagnosis is based on: clinical history, DSM IV criteria, and physical, neurological and psychological evaluations. **Results:** Prevalence: 17% of first visits during the indicated period. Mean age: 16.55 (SD: 2.83) years; 87.1% of them were males. Consultation reason: poor school performance (34.3%), school failure (12.9%),

emotional disorders (8.6%), conduct disorders associated to school failure (8.6%), attention and concentration problems (7.1%), conduct disorder (5.7%), organic discomfort (4.3%) and hyperactivity (4.3%). Treatment: Family and school orientation in all the cases. Pharmacological treatment (90%): Methylphenidate (MFD) (45.7%), MFD + fluoxetine (7.1%), nortriptyline (17.1%). 6% of the cases didn't accept the recommended treatment. Evolution: Globally favorable in 68.6%, bad evolution in 4.3%, and lost to follow-up in 27%. Comorbidity: Toxic habits (23%), depressive disorders (10%), speaking difficulties (5.7%), negativist defiant disorder (5.7%), impulsivity (5.7%), learning disabilities (4.3%). **Conclusion:** ADD in adolescents can come up as school failure, but it can debut as any comorbid form. The clinical history is especially important and so are the psychological and neurological exams. The treatment must be based on family, teachers and patient orientation and support, and medication.

P-011-169   Topic: 84
Hyperkinetic disorders: The possibility of earlier diagnosis

Natasa Potocnik Dajcman, Mental Health Service, Child & Adolescent Psychiatry, Maribor, Slovenia, davorin.dajcman@slon.net
Rok Holnthaner

Objective: We wanted to find out if it is possible to get data for early detection (at the age of 3 years) of hyperkinetic disorders and consequently enlarge the possibility of preventive activities. **Methods:** The retrograde study includes 40 accidentally selected children (ages 3 to 12 years) with the diagnosis of hyperkinetic disorders treated in our Center. The control group represents the equal number of children of the same age without any diagnosis. In our research we took the answers of parents on the questionnaire Spp 3/2 which is a part of a standardized psychological survey for early detection of children whose mental or personal development is at risk and is filled out at the child's age of 3. It includes 21 questions referring to different areas of the child's adaptation. The answers graduate from 1 to 3 (1 – the described sign does not occur, 2 – it occurs now and then, 3 – it occurs regularly). With some signs the increase is not possible, and there the only estimation is 1 or 3. We took the answers for five signs which are later significant for hyperkinetic disorders: hyperactivity, stubbornness, outbursts of temper, aggression, poor concentration and disability of bladder control. We compared both groups according to each variable with Chi square test. **Results:** We find out statistically significant differences between the groups for five variables: hyperactivity, outbursts of temper, aggression, concentration and bladder control. No differences were found for stubbornness. **Conclusion:** Parents of three years old children who get the diagnosis of hyperkinetic disorders later in life will estimate them significantly different compared with parents of three year olds who later don't get the diagnosis at all. These differences can be seen in the following areas: hyperactivity, outbursts of temper, expressed aggression toward other children, poor concentration and insufficient bladder control.

P-011-170   Topic: 84

Comparison of Serum 5-HT level in Attention Deficit Hyperactivity Disorder (ADHD) with or without Oppositional Defiant Disorder (ODD)

Xueping Gao, Central South University, Dept. of Child Psychiatry, Changsha, China, xuepinggao@hotmail.com
Linyan Su; Guangrong Xie

Objective: Oppositional defiant disorder (ODD) is usually comorbid with attention deficit hyperactivity disorder (ADHD). ADHD children with ODD have more extensive impairments than those with ADHD alone. Some authors considered that decreased central serotonergic (5-HT) activity was related to aggressive behavior in ADHD. This study examines the differences of serum 5-HT level between attention deficit hyperactivity disorder (ADHD) with or without oppositional defiant disorder (ODD). **Methods:** The sample include 61 children aged 7–14 years, divided into two groups based on DSM-IV Criteria: the ADHD group (n=33) and ADHD+ODD group (n=28). Serum 5-HT levels were assayed by high performance liquid chromatography (HPLC). Behavior of both groups was evaluated by Child behavior checklist (CBCL) and Teacher's Report Form (TRF). Intelligence was assessed with the China Wechsler Intelligence Scale for Children (C-WISC). Visual and auditory attention were measured with finger windows test in Children Memory Test, continuous test and rhythm test in the Halstead-Reitan Battery of Neuropsychological test for Children. **Results:** Levels of serum 5-HT in ADHD+ODD group were lower (327.01 ± 164.84 ng/ml) than that in ADHD group (451.11 ± 250.89 ng/ml) (p=0.02). Moreover, ADHD+ODD group showed poorer ratings on all variables including externalizing, internalizing problems, adjustment variables in CBCL and TRF, and impairment in attention test. **Conclusion:** This study explored the relationships between serum 5-HT level and attention deficit hyperactivity disorder children with and without oppositional defiant disorder in China, which suggested that the lower serum 5-HT level may be a potential biological marker of impulsive behavior in ADHD+ODD children.

P-011-171   Topic: 84

EEG-Differences in a visual and an acoustic Go-No-Go paradigm in children with ADHD compared to a sex and age matched control group

Ulrike Sühlfleisch-Thurau, Rostock, Germany,
Ulrike.Suehlfleisch-Thurau@ggp-hro.de
Wolfgang Gierow; Johannes Buchmann; Frank Häßler

Objective: EEG frequency analysis allows the examination of mental processes such as attention or information processing [1]. While such processes have already been well examined in adults, research into children is rare. In this study, using a Continuous Performance Test (CPT), EEG differences were examined in 15 children with ADHD and compared to a clinical control group. A CPT (Go-NoGo paradigm) is well suited for the examination of attention [2]. **Methods:** 30 Children aged 7.1 to 13.7 (mean age 11.9 maximal deviation 4.8) performed a visual and an acoustic CPT. 15 of them had been diagnosed with ADHS (DSM IV Predominantly Hyperactive-Impulsive Type or Combined Type, IQ>85, Score of the Conners Rating Scale short form>15). 15 sex and age matched children – patients of our department – formed the control group. For matched pair comparisons, age differences were less than 6 months.

In each CPT task 500 stimuli were presented randomly and in a constant time interval of 1.65 sec, 115 attention (yellow light/low tone) and 75 target (target, Go=red light follows yellow light/high tone follows low tone) stimuli. 40 were NoGo stimuli and the rest random stimuli (green light/middle tone). After the combination "attention – target", children should press a key as quickly as possible. Derived from 25 active electrodes and using a complex demodulation, the oscillations of the brain in the theta and alpha band of EEG were investigated within a time range of 650 ms. **Results:** In the acoustic test, children with ADHD showed higher frontal Alpha activation (F7, F3) in both, attention and target condition. Higher activation was also shown in Theta frequency band in parieto-occipital regions (P3, Pz, O1) in both conditions in acoustic tests; additionally in C3 and P4 in the attention condition. No differences were found when children performed the visual task. **Conclusion:** The Theta frequency band is discussed in connection with information processing, while Alpha frequency band is associated with attention processing. The higher activity in Theta band in children with ADHD maybe reflects that they need more effort to perform the task; that means we discuss a "processing automation deficit" in these children. Alpha band is connected with attention processes [3], and we discuss that higher activity in this band illustrate that children with ADHD had to pay more attention to the stimuli and for the task performance. This finding corresponds with an analysis of the reaction times (Horn et al. 2004) of these children.

P-011-172   Topic: 84

Time reproduction in finger tapping tasks by children with Attention Deficit Hyperactivity Disorder (ADHD) and/or Dyslexia

Margaret Tiffin-Richards, Universität Göttingen,
Kinder- und Jugendpsychiatrie, Göttingen, Germany,
mtiffin@gwdg.de
Michael Richards; Marcus Hasselhorn;
Tobias Banaschewski; Aribert Rothenberger

Objective: Deficits in timing and sequencing behaviour in children with dyslexia and with attention-deficit hyperactivity disorder have been investigated. However, many studies have not controlled for comorbidity between dyslexia and ADHD. This study investigated the timing and sequencing performance of children with either dyslexia, or ADHD, or co-occurring ADHD+dyslexia, and unaffected children using a finger-tapping paradigm. **Methods:** Four groups of children (ADHD×Dyslexia) with a total of 68 children were compared using a four factorial design with two between-subject factors (ADHD (yes/no), Dyslexia (yes/no)) and two within-subject factors, inter-stimulus interval (263 ms, 500 ms, 625 ms, 750 ms, 875 ms and 1000 ms) and tapping condition (free tapping, synchronous tapping, and unpaced tapping). In addition the complexity of rhythm reproduction pattern (unpaced tapping) was varied (simple/complex). **Results:** No significant differences were found either in the ability of the ADHD or the dyslexia groups to sustain a self-chosen free tapping rate or to generate a stable inter-response interval either by synchronising to the signal or in reproducing the interval without the previous pacing signal. Response averages showed the expected asynchrony and variability. This replicates results from studies using an auditory stimulus mode in a uni-manual finger-tapping task. In rhythm pattern reproduction the groups did not differ significantly in their ability to reproduce rhythms. However, a significant interaction effect between the factors dyslexia and complexity was apparent indicating that the difference in levels of performance for simple versus complex rhythms was more pronounced for the dyslexic groups. **Conclusion:** The results indicate that motor timing ability in the millisecond range below 1000 ms is intact in children with ADHD and/or dyslexia. The comorbid group showed similar performance to single disorder groups and the dyslexia disorder was affected by increased task complexity.

P-011-173   Topic: 84
Psychosocial factors affecting parents and teachers in their assessment of ADHD in children grades 1 to 5
Alper Bayrak, Uludag University, Child & Adolescent Psychiatry, Bursa, Turkey, yesimtaneli@uludag.edu.tr
Yesim Taneli; Suna Taneli

Objective: This study aimed to determine psychosocial factors affecting parents and teachers in their assessment of ADHD in children. **Methods:** Parents and 78 teachers of 2923 Grade 1–5 pupils from 8 elementary schools in Bursa and of 32 ADHD out-patients from the Dept. Child & Adolescent Psychiatry/Uludag University filled out an ADHD/DSM-IV symptom checklist for each child. Teachers additionally filled out the Ankara Conners Questionnaire (cut-off=16). For the ADHD group and matched controls (same school, classroom and sex) teachers and parents filled out the Parent Attitude Research Instrument (PARI) and psychosocial questionnaires designed for this study. Teachers additionally filled out the Maslach Burn-Out Inventory. School surveys were carried out in May and June 2003. Teachers knew the children for at least 8 months. **Results:** – Return rate was 87.2% for schools (2549 children; 775 valid cases – f/m: 352/423) and 100% for patients (n: 32; f/m: 10/22). – ADHD was described for 14.7% of the children by their parents and for 22.1% by their teachers. Only 4% overlapped. – M/F ratio was 2.0 in schools and 2.2 in outpatients. Mean scores did not differ by sex for Attention deficit (girls: 3.5 vs boys: 3.5; p>0.05) or Hyperactivity (girls: 3.3 vs boys: 3.6; p>0.05). – Parents' report of ADHD differed by sex of child, success, medical problems, sleep duration, school changes, play area, parent answering the questionnaire being of opposite sex as the child, less educated parent, parenting attitude, parents preferring reward or punishment and living district (p<0.05). – Teachers' with overprotective parenting attitude gave higher ADHD scores (p<0.05). Reported ADHD severity did not differ by age, degree of burn-out, sex, being married or not, having children, someone else looking after the kids, years of teaching and info-source about ADHD (p>0.05). **Conclusion:** Professionals using ADHD screening instruments should be aware of the fact that psychosocial factors may have sigificant impact on the assessment of children by their parents and teachers.

P-011-174   Topic: 84
Preliminary findings from Attention Deficit Hyperactivity Disorder (ADHD) Observational research in Europe (ADORE) Netherlands: Symptom severity and treatment prescribed
Stephen Ralston, Eli Lilly & Co Ltd., EHOR, Windlesham, United Kingdom, ralston_stephen_j@lilly.com
R. Rodrigues Pereira; W. Brussel; L. Vlasveld; H.G. Tuynman-Qua; M J Lorenzo

Objective: To present preliminary findings on Dutch patients from the ADORE study on symptom severity, comorbidities, and treatment regimen prescribed. **Methods:** ADORE is a 2-year, prospective, observational study in attention-deficit/hyperactivity disorder (ADHD) with data collected by paediatricians and child-psychiatrists. To date, 67 patients from the Netherlands have been included in the database and this information is reported. A full Netherlands dataset will be presented in the poster. **Results:** The dataset consisted primarily of boys 59 (89%) and the mean age for all patients was 8.7 years (SD 2.9). The mean ADHD rating scale score was 35.6 (SD 8.1), with a mean inattentiveness score of 17.5 (SD 4.5), and a mean hyperactivity/impulsivity score of 18.1 (SD 5.2). A diagnosis utilizing the DSM-IV diagnostic criteria alone was given most frequently (94%) followed by a combination of the DSM-IV and ICD-10 (2%). The mean Clinical Global Impression-Severity score was 4.1 (SD 0.9, scores ranging 1–7), and the mean Child Global Assessment Scale score was 57.5 (SD 17.0). Comorbid disorders included oppositional defiant disorder (36 [55%]), anxiety (29 [44%]), learning disorders (40 [61%]), depression (13 [20%]), conduct disorder (40 [61%]) and coordination problems (23 [35%]). Of other reported patient health problems, sleep was reported in 32 (48%) cases with 18 (27%) cases reporting significant interference. At baseline in 27 cases (42%), patients received some form of pharmacotherapy and in 24 cases (37%), a combination of pharmacotherapy and psychotherapy. Psychotherapy was not prescribed in isolation. The remainder of the patients either received "other" treatment (3 [5%]) or no treatment (11 [17%]). **Conclusion:** Reported information suggests that ADHD is recognised and treated in the Netherlands. The patients enrolled in ADORE are largely boys who have a moderate – severe symptom severity, comorbid disorders are prevalent, and that at baseline, over 75% of patients received pharmacotherapy treatment.

P-011-175   Topic: 84, 6
Effects of cognitive-behavioral treatments in children with Attention Deficit Hyperactivity Disorder (ADHD) taking Methylphenidate
Dong-Ho Song, Yonsei University, Dept. of Child Psychiatry, Seoul, Republic of Korea, dhsong@yumc.yonsei.ac.kr
Eun-Hye Ha; Eun-Sik Lee; Young-Min Yu

Objective: This study aimed at evaluating the effects of cognitive-behavioral treatment (CBT) in children with attention-deficit hyperactivity disorder (ADHD), taking methylphenidate. **Methods:** Subjects were 30 children with DSM-IV ADHD, assigned to MED or COMB group. MED group were 15 children treated with methylphenidate only, and COMB group were 15 children treated with methylphenidate and CBT. CBT were based on 'Think Aloud Program': Cognitive modeling, self-instruction training, and interpersonal problem solving. CBT were 15 group therapy sessions, twice a week for 8 weeks (45 mins/session), and each group consisted of 4–5 children. Pre- and post-treatment (8 weeks) measurement were conducted in both groups using computerized CPT, ADHD Diagnosis System (ADS), and following scales: Self Perception Profile for Children (SPPC), Conners Rating Scale (CRS), Home Situation Questionnaire (HSQ), and the Korean version of Child Behavior Checklist (K-CBCL). Methylphenidate was administered to all subjects during this study, and titrated up to 60 mg/day based on the patient's tolerability and clinical response. Follow-up post-treatment measurement was performed in COMB group 2 months later. **Results:** COMB group showed significant improvements of ADS variables (decreases of inattention, impulsivity and variance of response time; increase of sensitivity), CRS score, and SPPC scale score in post-treatment compared to pre-treatment measurements. MED group revealed significant improvements in impulsivity and sensitivity of ADS, School competence and Inattention subscales of K-CBCL, and CRS score. The follow-up post-treatment showed that the cognitive and behavioral improvements of COMB group were maintained in ADS and K-CBCL scores. **Conclusion:** Both MED and COMB group showed significant improvements of pre- and post-treatment comparative measurements in cognitive and behavioral aspects in children with ADHD. Combined treatments of CBT and methylphenidate were more effective in attentional functions in treating ADHD children, and those effects of CBT were maintained during the follow-up periods after the treatment.

P-011-176 Topic: 84
Development of executive functions in healthy and ADHD children and adolescents

Hans-Theo Weiler, Elisabeth-Klinik, Dortmund, Germany, t.weiler@elisabeth-klinik-do.de
Heike Hellrung; Caro Grünling; Stephan Overmeyer; Markus Ligges; Bernhard Blanz

Objective: Morphological and physiological changes have long been described during development. Therefore, children (8–12 y) and adolescents (13–17 y) should show clear differences in an executive function paradigm. **Methods:** Performance parameters of a go-nogo paradigm and related fMRI activation patterns in 25 children, representing the maturational pruning phase, were compared with those of 22 adolescents. The results were presented in the context with data from ADHD subjects (30 children and 20 adolescents). **Results:** The four groups differed not regarding omission errors (failing responses on go-stimuli). Adolescents (healthy subjects: 7.8, ADHD: 9.9) showed generally less commission errors (responses on nogo-stimuli) than children (healthy subjects: 12.3, ADHD: 19.0; healthy subjects: $p = 0.02$; ADHD subjects: $p < 0.0001$). Whereas healthy children showed less commission errors than ADHD children ($p = 0.01$), healthy adolescents did not show less than ADHD adolescents. ADHD children's responses showed also a larger variability compared to other groups ($p = 0.001–0.01$). There was a distinct large network which was activated by the go-nogo-paradigm. That network showed developmental changes, since it was differently active in children and adolescents. For behavioural inhibition the anterior cingulate cortex (ACC) and the dorsolateral prefrontal cortex (DLPFC) are essential as the findings of the ADHD subjects confirm. Moreover, there

seems to be a developmental order, in which the ACC activation has to precede the DLPFC activation. **Conclusion:** Therefore, in investigations regarding executive functions groups of children and adolescents, especially when considering ADHD, should not be confounded.

P-011-177 Topic: 84
Baseline information on symptom severity, diagnosis and treatment prescribed: Results from Attention Deficit Hyperactivity Disorder observational research in Europe (ADORE)

Stephen Ralston, Eli Lilly & Co Ltd., EHOR, Windlesham, United Kingdom, ralston_stephen_j@lilly.com
Maria Lorenzo

Objective: To present the study methods and baseline information on symptom severity, diagnosis, and treatment prescribed from the attention-deficit/hyperactivity disorder observational research in Europe (ADORE) study. **Methods:** ADORE is a 2-year, prospective, observational study in attention-deficit/hyperactivity disorder (ADHD). It is targeted to enrol 1500 patients from 10 European countries including Austria, Denmark, France, Germany, Iceland, Italy, The Netherlands, Norway, Switzerland, and the UK. Current enrolment stands at approx. 1214 patients. The primary objective is to describe the relationship between treatment regimen prescribed and the quality of life of patients with ADHD in different countries over a 2-year period. Additionally, ADORE will identify the relationship between diagnosis and ratings of ADHD symptom severity, and how treatment may vary depending on time, severity of symptoms, comorbidities, and different medical specialities. Data will be collected at baseline, first return to the physician, 3, 6, 12, 18, and 24 months. Enrolment for ADORE closes on April 9, 2004. **Results:** The full baseline dataset will be utilized to present information on symptom severity, diagnosis, and treatment prescribed. Information will be reported from a Pan European and country-specific perspective. Data will be presented on the age and gender of those enrolled, as well as the severity of illness at diagnosis. The frequency of comorbid disorders will be presented and include oppositional defiant disorder, learning disorders, conduct disorder, anxiety, coordination problems, and depression. We will also examine what factors may influence treatment choice including age, symptom severity, comorbidities and country of origin. **Conclusion:** ADHD is a diagnosable, neurobiological disorder treated in Europe. From the data items above we will be able to describe the predominant characteristics of ADHD patients in Europe.

P-011-178 Topic: 84
Ropinirole in the treatment of Attention Deficit Hyperactivity Disorder (ADHD) in children: A prospective open-label study

Armin Claus, Universität Würzburg, Kinder- und Jugendpsychiatrie, Würzburg, Germany, claus@kjp.uni-wuerzburg.de
Susanne Walitza; Peter Scheuerpflug; Christoph Wewetzer; Manfred Gerlach; Andreas Warnke

Objective: Attention deficit hyperactivity disorder (ADHD) is a relatively common childhood disorder characterised by inattention, hyperactivity and impulsivity. There is strong evidence implicating abnormal dopaminergic function in ADHD. Ropinirole, a non-ergot receptor agonist with preference for the D3 receptor, has been developed for the symptomatic treatment of Parkinson's disease. Theoretical considerations suggest, however, that dopamine agonists may also have beneficial effects in ADHD. Ropinirole may also have a longer lasting daytime efficacy and have no potential for abuse compared to methylphenidate. The aim of this ongoing prospective open-label study was to assess the efficacy and safety of Ropinirole in the treatment of children with ADHD. **Methods:** A total of six male children (age 8 to 13 years) with the combined type of ADHD as defined by DSM-IV were included in this trial. Ropinirole therapy was initiated at 0.25 mg once per day, and the maximal daily dose of 1 mg achieved after two weeks. Thereafter, there was a two week treatment period with methylphenidate. The efficacy assessments used were the Conners' ADHD/DSM-IV Scales for teachers and for parents. Attention and ability of impulse-control were assessed by using a variant of the Continous Performance Test (CPT). Adverse events were assessed throughout the trial using the Doses Record and Treatment Emergent Symptom Scale (DOTES). **Results:** Two of six children improved in attention and impulse control while receiving Ropinirole. In contrast, all children improved during the methylphenidate phase with a higher level of symptom reduction than Ropinirole. The most common side effects were nausea and headache. Daytime somnolence was reported in 2 cases. **Conclusion:** This preliminary result suggests that Ropinirole may not be beneficial in the treatment of ADHD. Whether the few patients improving under the therapy are a subgroup of ADHD needs further study.

P-012
Disorders and other conditions II

P-012-179   Topic: 78
The changes in the wishes to be thinner of adolescent women in recent 10 years

Mieko Aoki, Sanyo Gakuen Junior College,
Food and Nutrition, Okayama, Japan, myaoki@sguc.ac.jp
Shozo Aoki

Objective: As the wish to be thinner is very prevalent in adolescent females we studied how this wish changed during the last 10 years. **Methods:** We investigated 271 women in 1994, 191 women in 2000 and 133 women in 2003, in all 595 female adolescent college students by using the General Health Questionnaire (GHQ). Statistical analysis is done by Stat View. **Results:** Quantitatively the wishes to be thinner became more prevalent and qualitatively they appeared as smaller BMIs. **Conclusion:** The prevalent wishes to be thinner are observed. Why only young women have that wishes? It seemed there are social reasons.

P-012-180   Topic: 78, 92
Evaluation of renal function in Anorexia Nervosa (AN)

Shu Takakura, Kyushu University, Dept. Psychosomatic
Medicine, Fukuoka, Japan, stakakura2000@yahoo.co.jp
Nozaki Takehiro; Chikako Koreeda; Moriokaka Kayo;
Kawai Keisuke; Masato Takii; Chiharu Kubo

Objective: Renal dysfunction is sometimes seen in anorexia nervosa (AN) patients. In this study, we evaluated the renal function of AN patients and examined factors which influ-

encing to renal function. **Methods:** Data were from fourty five AN patients who had been hospitalized in our department during the eight years between 1995 and 2002. The patients were classified into three groups: the restricting (n = 18), the self-induced vomiting (n = 13), the laxative abuse (n = 14) types. In this study, we divided the binge eating/purging type into the self-induced vomiting and laxative abuse types. Twenty four hour-creatinine clearance (Ccr) was calculated within 2 weeks of hospitalization for comparison between the three groups. We also examined the serum potassium, the serum cloride, and the BUN. **Results:** Significant differences in Ccr among the three groups by ANOVA (p = 0.0062). Ccr of laxative abusers was significantly deteriorated compaired with restricters (65.8 ± 31.4 ml/min vs. restricting type: 104 ± 23.3 ml/min, p = 0.0016). No significant difference was found between Ccr of the laxative abusers and that of the self-induced vomiters (84.0 ± 41.1). No significant difference was found between Ccr of the restricters and that of the self-induced vomiters (p = 0.0903). Significant differences in the duration were found among the three groups (p = 0.0001). The laxative abuse type and the self-induced vomiting type had significantly longer duration of AN than the restricting type (p = 0.0188 and p < 0.0001). No significant difference was found between the duration of AN in the self-vomiting type and the laxative abuse type. Multiple regression analysis found the duration of AN to be a risk factor for the deterioration of Ccr in AN patients. **Conclusion:** The renal function of the laxative abuse type AN patients was more deteriorated than that of the restricting type. Duration of AN was a risk factor for impaired renal function in AN patients.

P-012-181   Topic: 78, 92
A comprehensive report of a treatment for type 1 diabetic females with eating disorders

Masato Takii, Kyushu University, Dept. Psychosomatic
Medicine, Fukuoka, Japan, takii@cephal.med.kyushu-u.ac.jp
Yasuko Uchigata; Takehiro Nozaki; Keisuke Kawai;
Shu Takakura; Chikako Koreeda; Chiharu Kubo

Objective: The purpose of this study was to show a comprehensive report of the treatment of type 1 diabetic females with various types of eating disorders and their outcomes. **Methods:** At the first visit to our outpatient clinic, type 1 diabetic females with eating disorders underwent a diagnostic interview based on DSM-IV criteria for eating disorders (SCID-P) and "Outpatient counseling at first visit". According to the eating disorder diagnosis and the presence/absence of inpatient therapy, patients with bulimia nervosa (BN) and binge-eating disorder (BED) were divided into four groups: BN-inpatients, BN-outpatients, BED-inpatients, and BED-outpatients. After a period of observation by the referring physician, patients without sufficient improvement were encouraged to undergo "Integrated inpatient therapy". Medical, psychological, and behavioral variables including glycosylated hemoglobin (HbA1c); BMI; psychological measures related to eating disorders (EDI), depressiveness (SDS), and anxiety (STAI); binge eating; and purging behavior were compared between baseline and follow-up. HbA1c and BMI were assessed every six months for at least three years. **Results:** In BED-outpatients, significantly lower HbA1c, SDS score, and frequency and amount of binge eating were seen at follow-up. In BN-inpatients, significantly lower HbA1c; EDI, SDS, and STAI scores; frequency and amount of binge eating; and rate of purging behaviors were seen at follow-up. **Conclusion:** The tested protocol led to a significant improvement of both the metabolic control and eating disorder of our type 1 diabetic females with BN and BED. BED patients were successfully treated on an outpatient basis, while BN patients needed "Integrated inpatient therapy". Since we also have experience treating other types of eating disorders, for example anorexia nervosa, we show a comprehensive report of the treatment of type 1 diabetic females with various types of eating disorders and their outcomes.

P-012-182   Topic: 78, 95
Duration of disease and the past minimum weight affect the severity of osteopenia in Anorexia Nervosa (AN)

Hitoshi Saino, Iwamizawa City Hospital, Dept. of Psychiatry, Iwamizawa, Japan, saino@ck9.so-net.ne.jp
Kenzo Denda; Kouichi Ito; Satoshi Asakura; Yukiya Sasaki; Fumi Sasaki; Seishiro Inoue

Objective: Osteopenia is known as a common complication of anorexia nervosa (AN). The mechanisms whereby osteopenia occurs in AN have been reported low nutrition intake, hypoestrogenaemia, hypercortisolaemia, and decreased mechanical stress on bones. We measured the lumber spine bone mineral density (LSBMD) of patients with variable duration of AN in order to investigate the long term prognosis of bone complication in AN. **Methods:** The LSBMD of fifteen patients with AN (two male and thirteen female) were measured by dual-energy X-ray absorptiometry. The correlation between BMD (age-matched value: Z score) and clinical factors were assessed using Pearson's correlation coefficients. **Results:** The mean age of the patients was 28 ± 15 (13–59) years and the mean duration of AN was 10 ± 11 (1–37) years. The weight at the time of the measure were 40.4 ± 5.6 (33.0–52.1) kg, which were 27.4 ± 9.8 (17.9–51.6) % below those expected. The past maximum and minimum weight were 49.1 ± 7.4 (40.0–64.0) kg and 31.6 ± 6.7 (21.0–40.0) kg, respectively. All female patients had amenorrhea which had continued for 5.6 ± 7.4 (1.0–22.0) years. The types of AN were five restricting and ten binge eating/purging. Seven patients had hyperactivity. As far as the bone condition, pathological fractures were observed in three patients and the LSBMD were decreased in fourteen patients compared with the same age (the average Z score were 81.9 ± 13.2 (64.0–109.0) %. LSBMD had a significant negative correlation between the duration of AN ($P<0.05$) and a significant positive correlation between the past minimum weight ($P<0.0001$). **Conclusion:** Ninety three percents of AN patients had a decreased LSBMD compared with the same age. The longer duration of AN and the lower past minimum weight affected the lower LSBMD and the risk of fracture.

P-012-183   Topic: 80, 30
The application of the psychobiological model of personality to an adolescent population: Is temperament a vulnerability factor?

Sonja Werneck-Rohrer, Medizin. Universität Wien, Kinder- und Jugendpsychiatrie, Wien, Austria, sonja.werneck-rohrer@meduniwien.ac.at
Susanne Ohmann; Ernst Eveline; Heidrun Eichberger; Carolin Prause; Bibiana Schuch

Objective: The aim of our study was to apply the psychobiological model of personality to a juvenile sample, part of whom suffering from various kinds of neuropsychiatric dis-

orders. The Psychobiological Model of Personality (Cloninger, 1987, 1993, 1996) describes temperament as a heritable variable of personality and character as being the concept of the self, with differences in aims and values emerging from the interaction between the individual and his/her environment. **Methods:** 293 juvenile patients from the University Clinic of Vienna and 582 healthy students from different schools in Vienna filled in the Juvenile Temperament and Character Inventory (JTCI). This questionnaire measures the temperamental factors and the dimensions of character, which are described in the Psychobiological Model of Personality. The clinical population also passed the Youth Self Report to evaluate behavior problems. Analyses of Variance were calculated for the group differences and correlations were calculated for the connections between behavior difficulties and temperamental factors. A hierarchical cluster analysis was conducted to separate different types of temperament. **Results:** The results show that adolescents with various psychiatric disorders differ in some aspects of personality. High novelty seeking is found in externalizing disorders, whereas high harm avoidance is found in internalizing disorders. Self-directedness also differs between the diagnosis groups. Gender differences are also found in our sample, as reward dependence is higher in girls than in boys. Differences between healthy youths and neuropsychiatric patients can be seen in some aspects of temperament and character. **Conclusion:** This study gives information about differences in temperamental factors found in psychiatric patients and healthy youths. It also indicates the importance of knowing about the patients' needs regarding intervention programs and therapy. Further studies are required to examine the development of temperament factors and character dimensions from childhood to adolescence.

P-012-184   Topic: 78, 26
Social class differences and obesity prevalence in a cross-sectional survey and a case-control study of preschoolers in Germany

Andreas Lamerz, Uni-Krankenhaus Aachen, Kinder- und Jugendpsychiatrie, Aachen, Germany, alamerz@ukaachen.de
Jutta Kuepper-Nybelen; Christine Wehle; Gabriele Trost-Brinkhues; Hermann Brenner; Johannes Hebebrand; Beate Herpertz-Dahlmann

Objective: To assess whether the socioeconomic status (SES) has a direct influence on childhood obesity and which factor in particular stands out in relation to obesity. **Methods:** When 2020 children attended their obligatory health exam prior to school entry in the City of Aachen, Germany, 1979 parents (97.9%) filled out a questionnaire on their child's weight development and on indicators of their family's SES in a cross-sectional survey. In addition, standardized measures of weight and height were taken. In a subsample all native German speaking children with a BMI greater or equal to the 85th percentile were defined as cases ($n=146$) and with a BMI between the 40th and 60th percentile as controls ($n=221$). More detailed information on several different SES variables was obtained by personal interviews. **Results:** The indicators of the parents' education were the variables most strongly associated with the children's obesity. Furthermore, there was a strong dose-response relationship between a composed index of social class and obesity. Children of the lowest social status had a more than threefold risk to be obese than children of the highest social status in the screening population (OR: 3.29, CI: 1.92–5.63). **Conclusion:** The findings established a strong relationship between parental years of education and childhood obesity. Prevention and treatment programs should endeavor to better target undereducated parents and their young children at high risk.

P-012-185   Topic: 78, 27
Dependencies between self images and images of mothers in women with Anorexia Nervosa (AN)

Beata Pawlowska, Medical Academy, Dept. of Psychiatry, Lublin, Poland, mkaczyn@oil.lublin.pl
Maria Chuchra; Marta Kaczynska-Haladyj

Objective: The aim of this work was to answer the following research issues: 1. What kind dependencies occur between actual self images and actual images of mothers in women with anorexia nervosa? 2. What kind of dependencies occur between ideal self images and ideal images of mothers in women with anorexia nervosa? The examined group consisted of 30 patients diagnosed with anorexia nervosa, undergoing a treatment at the Department of Psychiatry of the Medical Academy in Lublin. The average age of the examined females was 21 years. All patients had a secondary level education and came from full families. They were hospitalized for the first time. **Methods:** In order to carry out the test, the Gough and Heilbrun Adjective Check List (ACL) was used, which was completed by the examined patients four times following the instruction: "I am", "I would like to be", "my mum is", "I would like my mum to be". As a result actual and ideal images of patients and their mothers were obtained and then the r-Pearson correlation coefficients were calculated. **Results:** Significant statistical positive correlations were obtained between the actual images of patients and those of their mothers in 10 scales of the ACL test. Between the ideal images of the patients and those of their mothers significant statistical positive correlations occurred in 24 scales of the ACL test. **Conclusion:** 1. Negative autopresentation of women with anorexia is related to the negative assessment of their mothers. 2. Low sense of responsibility and autonomy, low self-reliance and the tendency to fulfill subordinate children's roles in women with anorexia co-occurs with discerning mothers as subordinate, irresponsible persons who avoid problems. 3. As regards the ideal images of patients and those of their mothers relationships between egocentrism, ambition, diligence, sense of loyalty, self control and striving at order were discerned. 4. The desire to establish positive interpersonal relationships, looking after other people, attracting the attention of the surrounding people, the desire for spontaneity in women with anorexia is connected with the desire for their mothers to possess these characteristics.

P-012-186   Topic: 78, 42
A follow-up investigation on bone mineral density and nutritionally dependent hormones in patients with early onset Anorexia Nervosa (AN)

Ulrike Margarete Elisabeth Schulze, Universitätsklinikum Ulm, Kinder- und Jugendpsychiatrie, Ulm, Germany, ulrike.schulze@medizin.uni-ulm.de
Simone Schuler; Dieter Schlamp; Peter Scheuerpflug; Peter Schneider; Christian Reiners; Andreas Warnke

Objective: Associations between bone mineral density and nutritionally dependent hormones in anorexia nervosa are described. Little is known about these correlations in pa-tients with onset of the eating disorder during childhood and adolescence. **Methods:** In a reinvestigation of 39 former patients, global outcome was assessed, bone mineral parameters and actual body composition were measured. At follow-up, we were also able to determine serum concentrations of leptin, insulin-like growth factor-I and II (IGF-I; IGF-II) and their binding proteins IGFBP-1, IGFBP-2 and IGFBP-3. **Results:** Correlations between eating disorder outcome and an improvement of bone mineral density were noted. Leptin levels seemed to reflect a relatively immediate response to the actual nutritional status, body composition and bone regain. In contrast to these findings, IGF subgroup values suggested a probably lasting disturbance of growth hormone (GH) secretion. Correlations between this hormone group and serum leptin concentrations or bone mineral parameters did not reach statistical significance. **Conclusion:** In conclusion, IGF related changes seemed to reflect the long-term effects of undernutrition on central endocrinologic pathways. They also differ from changes in adult and postmenopausal patients.

P-012-187   Topic: 78, 27
Psychopathological features of patients with prolonged Anorexia Nervosa (AN) as assessed by Minnesota Multiphasic Personality Inventory (MMPI)

Takehiro Nozaki, Kyushu University, Psychosomatic Medicine, Fukuoka, Japan, tnozaki@cephal.med.kyushu-u.ac.jp
Shu Takakura; Chikako Koreeda; Chihiro Morita; Keisuke Kawai; Masato Takii; Chiharu Kubo

Objective: The onset age of anorexia nervosa (AN) has recently extended to include younger and older patients. The duration of illness is lengthened in some AN patients. Patients with long term AN often are socially maladjusted and have physical problems because of sustained low body weight. Their treatments can be difficult because of their strong psychological defense and poor motivation for treatment. In the present study, we investigated the psychopathological features of patients with prolonged AN as assessed by the MMPI. **Methods:** Fifty-five AN patients completed the MMPI on admission to Kyushu University Hospital from 1999 to 2002. **Results:** 1) MMPI subscales, Hy (hysteria), VIII (family conflict), IX (problematic anger) and Lb (lumbago) showed a significant positive correlation and Si (social introversion) and SOC (social maladjustment) a significant negative correlation with the illness duration. Multiple regression analysis revealed that Hy, VIII and SOC were factors independently related to the duration of the illness. 2) The patients divided into three groups by illness duration: A, under 5 years (10 patients); B, over 5 and under 10 years (14 patients); and C, over 10 years (14 patients). The C group had significantly higher in Hy, VIIIand Lb scores than A group. 3) C group had significantly more mother-child problems than A+C groups. **Conclusion:** Patients with prolonged AN characteristically had more hysteria and family conflict. However, they also tended to be actively involved in society.

P-012-188 Topic: 79, 75

"COMPLEX" Psychopathology attached to functional somatic-vegetative disorders in children and adolescents

Anatoly Severny, Ass. of Child Psychiatrists, and Psychologists, Moscow, Russia, acpp@online.ru
Victor Brutman; Irina Kireeva

Objective: Child psychiatrists examined 285 children and adolescents of age from 1 to 15 years old suffering from functional febrility, functional disorders of heart rhythm, arterial hyper- and hypotension, vegetovascular dystonia. **Methods:** Psychopathological investigation. **Results:** Mental disorders of different intensity are revealed in 85–100% of cases: mono- and bipolar affective disorders are the most frequent, neurotic, psychopathic, psychoorganic, epileptiformic syndromes. Be-sides more or less "simple" syndromes, there are also very "complex" disturbances of subpsychotic level. 21 patients had pathologic conditions which gone out far from frameworks of neurotic or affective registers: 1) mild affective-delirium syndromes; 2) "hidden" paraphrenia; 3) rudimentary Kandinsky-Clerambault syndrome. 1st group is characterized by delirium phobias, dismorphomanic experiences, ideas of special relation, rudiments of delirium of special significance. 2nd group is characterized by the slow development of hardly hidden fantastic ideas of greatness, elect, prophetess, another origin, strange parents, etc. At initial stage as episodes are manifested short affective accesses with pseudohallucinational, polymorphic true hallucinational, sharp fantastic, derealisational and depersonalisational experiences with Kloos-accesses. Among the patients of 3d group there are showed dynamic spectrum of disorders in which structure mental automatisms have essential place. At the most mild conditions against the background of slight pathologic affect and neurotic-like symptoms manifest so-called small ideational automatisms (sper-rungs, mentism, uncontrolled withdraw of thoughts, etc.). At the more evident cases there are showed "sounding" thoughts, "echo"-thoughts, sudden appearance and rapid disappearance of "voices" in the head. At the full-scale picture there are pseudohallucinosis with delusional-like experiences including ideas of influence: "inner double", "possession", "space new-comers", etc. **Conclusion:** Children suffering from functional somatic-vegetative disorders need deep psychopathological investigation to reveal possible "complex" psychopathological syndromes.

P-012-190 Topic: 78, 27

Self-esteem and acceptance of mothers and fathers in girls with eating disorders

Beata Pawlowska, Medical Academy, Dept. of Psychiatry, Lublin, Poland, mkaczyn@oil.lublin.pl
Maria Chuchra; Marta Kaczynska-Haladyj

Objective: The aim of this work was to compare the level of self esteem, the level of acceptance of mothers and fathers in women with anorexia. **Methods:** The examined group consisted of 30 patients diagnosed with anorexia nervosa, undergoing a treatment at the Department of Psychiatry of the Medical Academy in Lublin. The average age of the examined females was 21 years and they were hospitalized for the first time. All patients had a secondary level education and came from full families. The test was carried out using the Gough and Heilbrun ACL Test, which was completed by the patients following the instructions: "I am", "I would like to be", "my mother is", "I would like my mother to be", "my father is", "I would like my father to be". First, actual self images as well as those of mothers and fathers were compared with ideal images (ANOVA), and then self acceptance rates as well as parents acceptance rates were determined and compared with the use of the t-Student test. **Results:** The self-esteem level is defined by the lack of significant differences in 10 scales, the level of acceptance of father also in 10 scales whereas the level of acceptance of mother in 22 scales out of 37 scales of the ACL Test. The acceptance rate of patents is 13.92, the acceptance rate of mothers – 11.63, whereas the acceptance rate of fathers – 16.86. **Conclusion:** 1. Patients accept their mothers in the highest degree, they accept themselves in a smaller degree and in the smallest degree they accept their fathers. 2. Patients' self-esteem is manifested by such characteristics as: self-control, looking after other people, passive resistance and verbal aggression. 3. Mothers are accepted by their daughters in the scope of characteristics conditioning the accomplishment of tasks and objectives in life. 4. In their fathers they accept striving for arousing interest, getting support and manipulating the surrounding people.

P-012-191 Topic: 80, 26

Prevalence of disorders of personality development in an inpatient adolescent psychiatry unit

Gerhard Libal, Universitätsklinik Ulm, Kinder- und Jugendpsychiatrie, Ulm, Germany, gerhard.libal@medizin.uni-ulm.de
Marc Schmid; Paul Plener; Antje Zander; Klaus Schmeck; Jörg M. Fegert

Objective: Only few studies are available about the prevalence of personality disorders in adolescence. Prevalence data for inpatient units differ between 5% for adolescents and 50% for adults. According to our clinical experience an increasing number of adolescent patients fulfill the DSM IV criteria for personality disorders. Many mental health professionals however avoid this diagnosis and suggest the concept of disorders of personality development instead, because patients have not yet completed their personality development in this developmental phase and diagnostic instruments are still insufficient. Our objective is to estimate the prevalence of disorders of personality development in an inpatient population at risk of developing a personality disorder. **Methods:** We report a retrospective chart analysis of diagnoses at discharge of all 132 inpatients with an age at admission between 14 and 18 (mean age 15.9) in the 2 years period from the opening of the inpatient unit in October 2001 until October 2003. We re-assessed the diagnoses at discharge for disorders of personality development by applying the DSM IV criteria for personality disorders and including the history before admission and the course of inpatient treatment. **Results:** In the 2 years period 38 (28 female, 10 male) of the 132 inpatients met the DSM IV criteria of a personality disorder (37 Cluster B- and 1 Cluster C-diagnosis). The estimated prevalence of a manifest disorder of personality development in our inpatient unit is 28.8%. **Conclusion:** The prevalence of disorders of personality development appears to be higher in adolescent inpatient units than published earlier. The possible increase of adolescents with disorders of personality development has to be evaluated in larger referred and non-referred samples.

P-012-192   Topic: 78, 27
Similarities and differences in self-image and the image of parents discerned by girls with anorexia

Beata Pawlowska, Medical Academy, Dept. of Psychiatry, Lublin, Poland, mkaczyn@oil.lublin.pl
Maria Chuchra; Marta Kaczynska-Haladyi

Objective: The aim of this work was to answer the posed research issue: within the scope of which personality characteristics do women with anorexia discern differences and similarities in themselves and in their mothers as well as in themselves and in their fathers? **Methods:** The examined group consisted of 30 patients diagnosed with anorexia nervosa, undergoing a treatment at the Department of Psychiatry of the Medical Academy in Lublin. The average age of the examined females was 21 years and they were hospitalized for the first time. All the patients had a secondary level education and came from full families. The test was carried out using the Gough and Heilbrun ACL Test, which was completed by the patients 3 times following the instructions: "I am", "my mother is", "my father is". Then the actual self images, the images of mothers and fathers were compared using ANOVA test. **Results:** Comparing self-images and pictures of mothers, 9 significant statistical differences were obtained (Ach, $p<0.05$; Dom, $p<0.01$, S-Cfd, $p<0.05$; Iss, $p<0.01$; Mas, $p<0.05$; NP, $p<0.05$, A, $p<0.001$; Ac, $p<0.05$; A-2, $p<0.05$) for 37 scales of the ACL Test. The same number of differences was obtained by comparing the images of patients and fathers, but within the range of other scales. Only within two scales (Dom – domination and Mas – masculinity) the girls discern differences both between themselves, their mothers and fathers. While comparing actual images of patients and mothers as well as actual images of patients and fathers, in both cases no differences were found within 28 scales. **Conclusion:** 1. Women with anorexia discern more similarities than differences in their self-images and the images of their mothers as well as self-images and the images of their fathers. 2. Patients discern a lot of similarities in self-images and those of their mothers as regards the majority of psychological needs (e.g. autonomy, disclosing themselves, humiliating, support, subordination), whereas as regards the above mentioned needs they are different from their fathers. 3. Similarities between patients and their fathers concern self-reliance, maturity, spontaneity and protectiveness, whereas in the same respect they are most different from their mothers.

P-012-193   Topic: 78, 26
Prevalence of obesity-related and non-related binge eating and night eating in a cross-sectional field survey of German preschoolers

Andreas Lamerz, Uni-Krankenhaus Aachen, Kinder- und Jugendpsychiatrie, Aachen, Germany, alamerz@ukaachen.de
Jutta Kuepper-Nybelen; Nicole Bruning; Gabriele Trost-Brinkhues; Hermann Brenner; Johannes Hebebrand; Beate Herpertz-Dahlmann

Objective: To assess the prevalence of obesity, obesity-related binge eating, non-obesity-related binge eating, and night eating in five to six year old children and to examine the impact of parental eating disturbances. **Methods:** When 2020 children attended their obligatory health exam prior to school entry in the city of Aachen, Germany, 1979 parents (97.9%) filled out a questionnaire on their child's eating habits and weight development in a cross-sectional survey. Anthropometric measurements were collected for all chil-

dren in a standardized form. **Results:** Episodes of binge eating were found in 2.0% of the children surveyed and night eating in 1.1%. There was a significant relationship between binge eating and obesity but not between night eating and the child's weight. Children's binge eating and night eating were strongly associated with eating disturbances on the part of their mothers (adjusted odds ratios [95% confidence intervals]: 6.1 [2.7–13.5] and 7.8 [2.1–29.4], respectively) and with a non-German native language (adjusted odds ratios [95% confidence intervals]: 2.6 [1.2–5.5] and 11.6 [3.5–38.7], respectively). **Conclusion:** In concurrence with studies on adulthood, binge eating is linked to obesity already in early childhood. Children of mothers with eating disorders and children of mothers with a non-German native language are at increased risk of developing eating disorders themselves. Future studies should focus on obesity and eating disorders in early childhood; prevention programs should seek to target young children at risk as early as possible.

P-012-194   Topic: 80, 37
The juvenile psychopathic personality – results of the validation of the German PCL-SV (Psychopathy checklist – screening version) in a population of incarcerated young delinquents

Denis Köhler, Universität Kiel, Kinder- und Jugendpsychiatrie, Kiel, Germany, schuetze@kiju-psych.uni-kiel.de
Günter Hinrichs

Objective: The PCL-SV is an international frequently used diagnostic instrument in the assessment of the personality and prognosis of delinquents. While there is a lot of research on validity of this instrument within the English speaking countries, we still habe a corresponding lack of it in Germany. **Methods:** In the present study 149 young male inmates were investigated with the PCL-SV and the structured clinical interview (SKID). Additionally psychological tests were administered and sociodemographic and forensic variables explored. **Results:** The results show according to expectation that the PCL-SV correlates significantly with the cluster B – personality disorders (DSM-IV). Factor analysis of the items of the questionnaire yielded four factors, which can entirely represent the juvenile psychopathic personality. This result is in contrast with the two factor-structure of the concept within the manual. **Conclusion:** Finally the findings of the study are discussed under the question, if psychopathic personality is a distinct disorder or can better be described by several personality disorders.

P-012-195   Topic: 78
Manual based cognitive behavioral group therapy (CBT) for adolescent girls with Anorexia Nervosa (AN) and their families

Susanne Ohmann, Medizin. Universität Wien, Inst. für Neuropsychiatrie, Wien, Austria, susanne.ohmann@meduniwien.ac.at
Christian Popow; Bibiana Schuch; Andreas Karwautz; M. Lanzenberger; H. Herzog; S. Miksch

Objective: AN in adolescent girls is a common, life threatening and difficult to treat disease. Prolonged ambulatory psychotherapy and familiar interventions are considered mandatory. Although treatment manuals offer important advantages for clinical practice, standardized therapy programs for adolescents are still lacking. The aim of our study was to develop and evaluate a manual for treating adolescent girls with AN and their families based on CBT principles. Therapy included psychoeducation, problem analysis, social skills training, communication training, problem solving strategies for interpersonal conflicts, cognitive schema therapy, hedonistic training and body therapeutic elements. **Methods:** 8 patients with AN (ICD-10 F 50.0, restrictive type) were assigned to one year of manual based group CBT (60 sessions) including family behavioral sessions. The therapeutic process was closely monitored by assessing psychopathologic symptoms (depression, social anxiety, alexithymia, eating and hedonistic behavior), schemas (cognitive, approach and avoidance schemas), family relations and treatment rating. These variables were assessed at baseline, during (3 monthly) and immediately and 6 months after therapy. BMI were controlled weekly. **Results:** The criteria for "good outcome" were met by 5 patients, 2 patients did not improve and continued single CBT, 1 patient dropped out after three months of therapy. **Conclusion:** Our manual based group CBT was effective in improving outcome and preventing relapse. To the authors knowledge these data empirically document for the first time the efficacy of CBT in adolescent patients with AN.

P-012-196   Topic: 78

A multi-centred study of 77 patients with Anorexia Nervosa (AN)

Sylvia Eimecke, Universitätsklinik Marburg, Kinder- und Jugendpsychiatrie, Marburg, Germany, eimecke@med.uni-marburg.de
Beate Herpertz-Dahlmann; Kristian Holtkamp; Eberhard Schulz; Christian Fleischhaker; Andreas Warnke; Fritz Mattejat; Helmut Remschmidt

Objective: To examine if 1) there is a change in quality of life for patients with anorexia nervosa during the clinical treatment and if 2) there is a relation between changes in quality of life and psychopathology. **Methods:** 77 patients (girls aged 12 to 19) with anorexia nervosa were assessed with several clinical instruments regarding clinical diagnosis, eating disorders, depression, quality of life, treatment issues and demographic data (ANIS, DIKJ, ILK, basis documentation) at the start and at the end of their clinical treatment. **Results:** 1) A significant improvement of quality of life was found, especially regarding the factors mental health and physical constitution. 2) Concerning the psychopathology a significant increase in weight (BMI) and a significant improvement of the psychosocial adjustment were found. Further, symptoms relating to eating behaviour (sickness, appetite etc.) displayed a significant reduction. Relations between outcome measures were analysed and presented. **Conclusion:** Besides narrow outcome measures related to symptomatology and psychopathology broadband measures including quality of life should be used in the evaluation of the treatment of eating disorders.

P-012-197   Topic: 78, 13

Treatment of binge eating disorder with Fluoxetine: A randomized controlled trial

Anna Capasso, University of Salerno, Pharmaceutical Sciences, Fisciano, Italy, annacap@unisa.it

Objective: Binge Eating Disorder (BED) is one of the most frequent eating disorders in industrialized societies. Re-

duced serotonin activity has been suggested to trigger some of the cognitive and mood disturbances associated with Bulimia Nervosa. Therefore, pharmacological treatment of BED is mainly based on the use of selective serotonin reuptake inhibitors, that have proved effective. At the present, the biological bases of this disorder are not yet completely clear. The aim of this randomized, controlled trial was to verify the efficacy of fluoxetine, a serotonin reuptake inhibitor, in a group of patients with a diagnosis of BED. **Methods:** Twenty female outpatients, with an age range of 24–36 years and diagnosis of BED-binge purging, as defined by the DSM IV, were assigned randomly to two treatment groups: the first group received 20 mg/day fluoxetine for 12 weeks, the second group received placebo. The study was conducted for 12 weeks with weekly clinical assessments. **Results:** At the end of the observation period, in the group treated with fluoxetine there was a statistical significant reduction in the number of binge eating crisis and purging with respect to the group who received placebo treatment. In no case, treatment was interrupted for emergency effects. **Conclusion:** This study confirms that fluoxetine is well tolerated and effective in reducing binge-eating crises and purging in patients with bulimia nervosa.

P-012-198   Topic: 78, 65

Law relating to compulsory treatment of patients with Anorexia Nervosa (AN)

Masaki Seki, Gifu University, Dept. of Psychopathology, Gifu-City, Japan, lollipop@mti.biglobe.ne.jp
Yu Wakabayashi; Ken Takaoka

Objective: Certain individuals with anorexia nervosa lack competence to make treatment decisions. Although recent studies conclude that involuntary admission is beneficial at least in the short term, the effects on treatments of legal protectors who consent to compulsory hospitalization have not been sufficiently investigated. The aims of the present study are to clarify problems, especially the influence of the legal protector on the patient's condition, under current Japanese law in comparison with relevant legislation in other countries. **Methods:** To that end, 8 involuntary patients were compared with 62 voluntary patients. To clarify intra-familial circumstances, a review of the involuntary patients' medical charts was also conducted. **Results:** The average length of admission of involuntary patients was significantly longer than that of voluntary patients. There were, however, no significant differences between the former and the latter in terms of either BMI on admission or outcome on discharge. The chart review revealed that intra-familial conflicts possibly lead to prolonged hospitalization in a direct and/or indirect way. **Conclusion:** In order to reduce the indirect effects of intra-familial conflicts on prolonged hospitalization, the definition of the legal protector should be expanded to include the local social services authority as a guardian.

P-012-199   Topic: 78, 9
A model of group therapy in Anorexia and Bulimia Nervosa of childhood and adolescence

Ulrike Margarete Elisabeth Schulze, Universitätsklinikum Ulm, Kinder- und Jugendpsychiatrie, Ulm, Germany, ulrike.schulze@medizin.uni-ulm.de
Marc G. Schmid; Claudia Zerahn-Hartung; Antje Zander; Jörg M. Fegert

Objective: Cognitive behavior group therapy for patients with eating disorders is described. The aim is to prevent an early relapse after hospital treatment, as Programmes for children and adolescents with anorexia and bulimia nervosa are still rare. **Methods:** We have started to develop a group therapy programm which includes patients from all units of our department (in- and outpatients, day clinic patients). In addition to individual care, two semi-open groups (two therapists, at most 8 patients), one 'motivation-group' and one 'main-group' are offered. They meet every two weeks. Parents' evenings are also offered. **Results:** While therapeutic work with the motivation-group patients mainly serves to acquire information and reasons for their eating disorder, the patients of our main-group have the opportunity to deal with defined congitive behavioral therapeutic modules. **Conclusion:** The division into two groups seems to be useful because of the different understanding of illness and its consequences for therapeutic work in individual patients.

P-012-200   Topic: 78, 32
The effects of plasma leptin and other factors on recovery from secondary amenorrhea in Anorexia Nervosa (AN)

Chikako Koreeda, Kyushu University, Dept. Psychosomatic Medicine, Fukuoka City, Japan, chikakok@d2.dion.ne.jp
Takehiro Nozaki; Shu Takakura; Kayo Morioka; Keisuke Kawai; Masato Takii; Chiharu Kubo

Objective: Amenorrhea is prolonged in some patients with anorexia nervosa (AN) after weight gain to within the normal range. In functional hypothalamic amenorrhea, the participation of leptin and thyroid gland-related hormones has been comfirmed, but mechanism of recovery from amenorrhea in AN is not clear. In this study, we investigated factors that might contribute to the resumption of menstruation in AN. **Methods:** Studied were nine AN patients who began to menstruate during treatment (Group A), thirteen AN patients with prolonged amenorrhea after treatment (Group B), and twelve healthy C). All AN patients had been admitted to Kyushu University Hospital. The testing points for Group A were on admission and after recovery from amenorrhea, for Group B on admission and just before discharge, and for Group C the follicular phase. At each test point, a fasting blood sample was taken early in the morning, and leptin, FSH, LH, prolactin, estrogen, TSH, freeT3, freeT4, GH, IGF-1 and cortisol were measured. We also measured weight and the percent of body fat. **Results:** The leptin level after recovery from amenorrhea of Group A was significantly higher than that after treatment of Group B. The TSH level of after recovery from amenorrhea of group A was significantly lower than that after treatment of Group B. The cortisol level on admission of Group B was significantly higher than that of Group A. In logistic-regression analysis, the factor most significantly related to resumption of menstruation was

leptin at the recovery of menstruation in Group A. **Conclusion:** It was suggested that leptin may be the most influencial factor in recovery from amenorrhea in AN.

P-012-201   Topic: 78
Internet communication for patients with eating disorders: www.hungrig-online.de, a virtual self-help group

Jan Nedoschill, Universitätsklinikum Erlangen, Child & Adolescent Psychiatry, Erlangen, Germany, mail@nedoschill.com
Peter Leiberich; Thomas Loew

Objective: The Internet serves as an outstanding facility for information about mental diseases and for communication with other affected people. The project www.hungrig-online.de is the largest german-speaking self-help website for eating disorders with over 13,000 participants, providing an informational content section, mailing list, discussion board and chat. The current study investigates demographic data, the patients' attitudes towards their disorder and the use of an internet self-help group. **Methods:** During the months June till October 2003 the users of www.hungrig-online.de were asked to take part in an online survey. They could fill out a self constructed questionnaire (73 questions concerning epidemiology, attitudes as a user of hungrig-online, and subjective use of hungrig-online) and four standardised questionnaires: Eating disorders inventory (EDI), Patient health questionnaire (PHQ), Fragebogen zum Befinden, Short Form (health questionnaire, SF36), Skalen zur Erfassung der Lebensqualität (quality of life assessment, SEL). **Results:** The survey was completed by 1006 participants. 15% were aged under 18 years, 25% were still attending school, 35% were still living at their parent's home. 39% suffered from anorexia nervosa, 35% from bulimia nervosa, 20% from bulimarexia. 47% of the long term users started psychotherapy since registration at hungrig-online, 41% acquired better coping strategies throug participating. 86% said to recommend hungrig-online. The results of the standardised questionnaires are explained during presentation. **Conclusion:** The internet-based self-help group www.hungrig-online.de cannot substitute psychotherapy, but plays an important role in gaining information, coping with the disorder and helping the patient to decide to start psychotherapy. A central factor is the attendance in and the support through a broad community of like-minded people. Further research is needed to compare web-based self-help groups with conventional ones and to describe the effect of attending an web-based self-help group during psychotherapy.

P-012-202   Topic: 78, 12
Recurrence or deterioration of eating disorders after initiation of clozapine/olanzapine treatment

Stefan Gebhardt, Universität Marburg, Klinik für Psychiatrie, Marburg, Germany, stefan.gebhardt@med.uni-marburg.de
Michael Haberhausen; Jürgen-Christian Krieg; Helmut Remschmidt; Johannes Hebebrand; Frank Theisen

Objective: The authors explored whether patients who suffered from an eating disorder (ED) prior to the use of antipsychotics may develop binge eating symptomatology or full-blown EDs after initiation of either clozapine or olanzapine treatment. **Methods:** Sixty-one consecutively admitted patients receiving clozapine or olanzapine were screened with the M-Composite International Diagnostic Interview (M-CIDI) for a lifetime history of an ED. The Questionnaire on Eating and Weight Patterns (QEWP) was used to identify ED symptoms under clozapine/olanzapine treatment. **Results:** Six subjects met DSM-IV criteria for a lifetime history of an ED (bulimia nervosa, n=2; anorexia nervosa, n=1; eating disorder not otherwise specified [ED-NOS], n=3); these EDs were present prior to the use of antipsychotics. Five of these patients reported onset of binge eating episodes immediately after initiation of cloza-pine/olanzapine. According to the QEWP 2 patients met DSM-IV criteria for binge eating disorder (BED) and 3 for EDNOS. An objective causality assessment using the Naranjo probability scale revealed a definite (n=1) or probable (n=4) relationship between these EDs and clozapine/olanzapine intake. **Conclusion:** These results suggest that clozapine/olanzapine may induce recurrence or deterioration of EDs.

P-013
Disorders and other conditions III

P-013-203   Topic: 87, 36
Regional cerebral perfusion abnormalities in Tic disorders: Statistical parametric mapping analysis

Bung-Nyun Kim, Seoul Nat. University Hospital, Child & Adol. Psychiatry, Seoul, Republic of Korea, kbn1@snu.ac.kr
Jae-Suk Jung; Young-Sik Lee; Sun-Ju Chung; Tae-Won Park

Objective: An investigation of cerebral blood flow using Tc-99m-HMPAO brain SPECT was conducted to identify functional abnormality of the brain of tic disorder. **Methods:** 21 patients with chronic tic or Tourette's disorder who had no previous treatment history were selected by using DSM-IV criteria (M:F=19:2, 9.73±2.11 y). After acquiring pretreatment Tc-99m-HMPAO Brain SPECT images from them, Statistical Parametric Mapping analysis was performed by using Korean standard template of child-adolescent normal control. **Results:** Decreased cerebral blood flow in both medial frontal gyrus, left paracentral lobule, left precuneus gyrus were found in tic disorder group compared to the controls (P<0.001). In addition, increased blood flow in both inferior, middle, superior frontal gyrus were found in tic disorder group (P<0.001). **Conclusion:** A significant cerebral blood flow abnormality in frontal lobe of tic disorder in our study suggests an association with the previously known abnormality in circuit of fronto-striato-thalamo-frontal area.

P-013-204   Topic: 92
The rigid spine syndrome: Is it a true syndrome?

Nadia Tomassetti, University of Rome, Child & Adolescent Psychiatry, Rome, Italy, n.tomassetti@libero.it
Carlo Di Brina; Paola D'Oto; Alessia Tosco;
Alba Sunshine Bettoschi; Pasquale Carboni

Objective: The purpose of this study has been to show that the rigid spine syndrome (RSS) is a syndrome and not a specific and distinct pathology. **Methods:** We assessed in a longitudinal design 202 children/adolescents (and parents in the cases with positive familiarity) affected of Duchenne muscular dystrophy (DMD, 15), Becker muscular dystrophy (25), motoric muscular dystrophy (10), congenital muscular dystrophy (negative merosine) (4), limb girdle

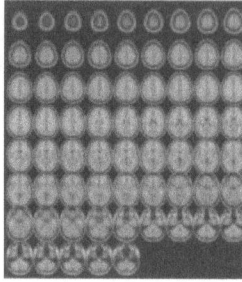
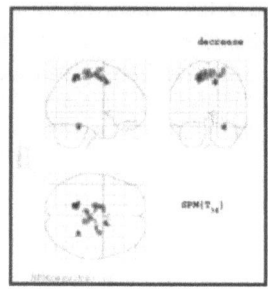

Figure 1. Brain areas with significantly decreased perfusion in tic disorder patients compared to normal controls (threshold P=0.001, uncorrected)

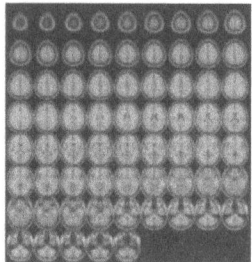
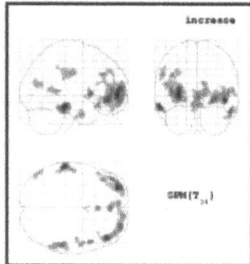

Figure 2. Brain areas with significantly increased perfusion in tic disorder patients compared to normal controls (threshold P=0.001, uncorrected)

muscular dystrophy (6), spinal muscular atrophy type III (30), peripheral neuropathy type Charcot-Marie-Tooth (15), congenital myopathies (7), congenital hypotonia with favourable outcome (CHFO 90). The sample underwent a detailed battery examination which included serum dosage of CPK and muscle biopsy. **Results:** The data available confirm that all subjects show a common substratum: hyperlaxity and hypotonic muscles. Previous studies (Goldspink et al. 1974), underlined that joints hyperlaxity may induce muscles working in shortening and so provide a sarcomeres number modification in muscle fiber. In our study we demonstrated that regular and specific physical training may represent a preventive and an efficacious remedy to avoid the observed shortening. The treatment effects are more significative in subjects with mild pathology. In fact treated CHFO subjects (12%) showed a better clinical course in comparison with not treated ones (31%). **Conclusion:** This work confirm the RSS to be, in our opinion, a syndrome. Moreover our study highlights the efficacy of movement and postures preventive treatment, particularly for CHFO subjects (11–18%).

P-013-205   Topic: 87, 12

Risperidone for children and adolescents with chronic Tic or Tourette's disorders in Korea

Soo-Churl Cho, Seoul Nat. University Hospital, Psychiatry, Seoul, Republic of Korea, soochurl@snu.ac.kr
Jeong-Mee Ahn; Young-Sik Lee; Dong-Hyun Ahn; Boong-Nyun Kim; Kang-E. Hong

Objective: The purpose of this study was to determine the short-term effects and safety of risperidone as an alternative for traditional antipsychotic drugs in the treatment of chronic tic disorder or Tourette's disorder in young children and adolescents through a 6-week open label design. **Methods:** The subjects were 15 young children and adolescents (the ratio of male: female subjects were 13:2 and the mean age was 10 ± 2.4 yrs). 7 subjects were diagnosed with Tourette's disorder and 8 with chronic tic disorder, and all subjects were administered risperidone without hospitalization. Of the 15 subjects, one had a comorbid disorder (obsessive-compulsive disorder) and all subjects had no previous history of psychiatric hospitalization. 10 out of 15 subjects were administered risperidone for the first time, and 5 subjects had been previously treated with traditional antipsychotics(haloperidol, pimozide). Clinical response was measured at baseline and at 1st, 3rd and 6th week after drug treatment by the Korean version of the Yale Global Tic Severity Scale and the Global Assessment of Functioning Scale. The side effects were carefully monitored using adverse event evaluation charts. **Results:** The mean dosage of risperidone was 0.53 ± 0.13 mg at 1st week, 0.90 ± 0.28 mg, at 3rd week, and 1.23 ± 0.37 mg at 6th week. Comparison between periods according to the Korean version of the Yale Global Tic Severity Scale showed significant difference ($t = 4.920$; df=14; p-value < 0.01) between 1st week and 3rd week period. At 6th week after administration the tic severity scale showed 36% of overall improvement. 13 out of 15 subjects showed significant improvement, 1 subject showed no difference in symptoms and for 1 subject the symptoms grew worse. Also the Global Assessment of Functioning scale score was mean 66.8 ± 10.8 at baseline which improved to mean 73.1 ± 10.1 in the 6th week after treatment. With respect to side effects, only one case of sedation was reported and drug administration was not stopped because of side effects. **Conclusion:** Risperidone, a potent combined serotonin (5-HT2) and dopamine (D2) receptor antagonist, was shown to be an effective and safe drug in the treatment for Tourette's disorder and chronic tic disorder in children and adolescents in Korea.

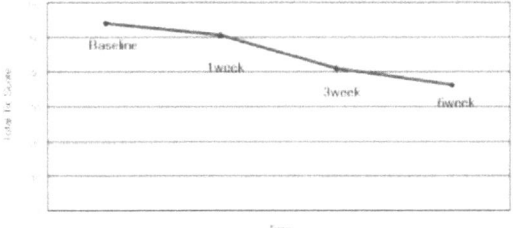

Fig. 1. Statistically significant change between 1st week and 3rd week
(t=4.920;df=14; p-value <0.01 in paired t-test and F=24.5, p<0.00 in repeated measure of ANOVA)

P-013-206   Topic: 87, 35

Striatal gray matter changes in children with Tourette's syndrome: A voxel-based morphometric analysis of 3-dimensional MRI

Andrea G. Ludolph, Universität Ulm, Kinder- und Jugendpsychiatrie, Ulm, Germany, andrea.ludolph@medizin.uni-ulm.de
Gerhard Libal; Jörg M. Fegert; Jan Kassubek

Objective: The Gilles de la Tourette Syndrome (TS) is a complex tic order. No specific diagnostic tests are available. There are some hints that the basal ganglia, especially the striatum, play an important role in the pathogenesis of TS. **Methods:** We enrolled 12 boys (mean age 12.5 years, SD 2.2, range 10–16 years) with TS diagnosed according to DSM-IV and ICD 10 Diagnostic Criteria in the study; 9 boys (mean age 13.4 years, SD 1.8, range 10–16 years) served as the control group. 3-D MRI data sets of the whole head were collected on a 1.5 Tesla clinical scanner (Siemens, Erlangen, Germany) using a T1-weighted magnetization-prepared rapid-acquisition gradient echo (MP-RAGE) sequence. The 3-D MRI data were analyzed by voxel-based morphometry (VBM) using Statistical Parametric Mapping (SPM99). The gray matter maps of the patients and the normal data base were compared statistically to detect whether each voxel had a greater or lesser gray matter density than the controls. **Results:** Significant structural changes, i.e. locally increased gray matter concentrations ($p < 0.001$, uncorrected), were found in the ventral nucleus caudatus in both hemispheres with right-sided predominance. Extrastriatal alterations were small and scattered. **Conclusion:** Morphometric changes in the basal ganglia may be a distinctive feature in TS.

P-013-207   Topic: 87, 34

Ondansetron augmentation in patients with medication refractory Gilles de la Tourette Syndrome in children and adolescents

Sylvia Quiner, University Hospital, Neuropsychiatry, Vienna, Austria, sylvia.quiner@meduniwien.ac.at
Heidrun Eichberger; Michaela Elena Seyering; Max H. Friedrich

Objective: Gilles de la Tourette Syndrom is a neuropsychiatric disorder with involuntary motoric and/or vocal tics, which begins in childhood and early adolescence. The first line treatment is neuroleptic medication. There is a group of some patients, who is resistant or don't respond efficaciously to neuroleptic treatment. The aim of our study was to investigate ondansetron, a selective 5HT3 antagonist, which may lower mesolimbic dopaminergic hyperactivity, as augmentation additional to current neuroleptic treatment. **Methods:** It is a double blind, placebo controlled cross over study with ondansetron. We planned to include altogether 12 patients between 8 and 18 years with the diagnosis of Tourette syndrom and who did not respond to neuroleptic medication within the last four weeks. Assessments included the Yale Global Tic Severity scale (YGTSS), the Children Yale Brown Obsessive and Compulsive Scale (CY-BOCS) and the Clinical Global Improvement (CGI). Furthermore we investigated neuropsychological changes of the executive functions with the Stroop test, the Wisconsin card sorting test and the trail making test. **Results:** Because the study is ongoing we have only preliminary data at this time. We have already examined 7 patients. One showed a definite response (Improvement score 60%), five patients showed a moderate or mild response mainly for the motoric tics (Improvement score 20–30%). One patient did not improve, the motoric and vocal tics worsened and the patient suffered from side-effects such as obstipation. **Conclusion:** Ondansetron appeared as a well tolerated medication. These preliminary findings show that there is some hope for patients who suffer from Tourette's syndrom and don't improve to neuroleptic medication efficaciously. But at this time we need further data to confirm our expectations.

P-013-208   Topic: 92
Cornelia de Lange Syndrome and developmental problems – case report

Milica Pejovic-Milovancevic, Institute of Mental Health, Dept. Children & Adolescents, Belgrade, Serbia and Montenegro, mpejovic@eunet.yu
Olivera Aleksic; Smiljka Popovic-Deusic; Ana Radojkovic; Ana Velimirovic

Objective: Cornelia de Lange Syndrome (CdLS) is characterized by low birth weight, delayed growth, small head size and small stature. Typical facial features include thin eyebrows which frequently meet at middle line, long eyelashes, short upturned nose and thin, down turned lips. **Methods:** In the paper we would present a case of six years old boy who is third child in a family of three children. He was hospitalize at Department for children and adolescents because of evident developmental delayed. **Results:** We would present all relevant developmental characteristic and we would discuss improvement in some aspects. The method of clinical observation, labaratory test and genetic findings would be discussed. **Conclusion:** CdLS is congenital syndrome and a child need not demonstrate each and every sign or symptom for a diagnosis to be made. Mental retardation usually ranging from mild to profound. Cause is not a clearly known although it is suspected that a gene may be responsible.

P-013-209   Topic: 89, 85
Investigation of attachment patterns in children and adolescents with disruptive behavior disorders versus other disorders

Sherese Ali, Queen's University, Dept. of Psychiatry, Kingston, ON, Canada, shereseali@hotmail.com
Kevin Parker

Objective: To measure attachment in children and adolescents with psychiatric disorders. To determine the extent to which attachment differs in patients with disruptive behaviour disorders (externalizing disorders) versus a comparison group (internalizing disorders). We tested the hypothesis that patients with externalizing disorders would show more Fearful attachment than the internalizing group. **Methods:** Three Attachment scales were administered to 26 adolescent inpatients: the Adult Attachment Questionnaire 4.0 (AAQ4.0), Experience in Close Relationships (ECL) and the Relationship Questionnaire (RQ). Externalizing diagnoses comprised DSM-IV Oppositional Defiant Disorder, Conduct Disorder, Attention Deficit Hyperactivity Disorder and Substance Use Disorders. Kappa statistic, Cramer's V and Chi-Square were used to determine concordance amongst the 3 scales. A consensus attachment rating was determined by choosing the rating that oc-

curred the majority of the time. When all scales disagreed, the RQ1991 was used as it had the best concordance with the other two scales. Chi-square was calculated to determine if there was a significant relationship between attachment and diagnosis. **Results:** The RQ was most strongly associated with the other two scales, while the ECL and the AAQ4.0 did not show significant correspondence. There was a basic pattern of more Secure attachment in the internalizing group and more Fearful attachment in the externalizing group, for ratings produced by each of the three scales, as well as the consensus rating. These differences did not achieve statistical significance. **Conclusion:** Our results although preliminary, show a non-significant trend towards Fearful attachment for patients with disruptive behaviour disorders compared to those with more internalizing disorders. Given that the effect size was medium or greater (Phi ≥ 0.3), the study was likely underpowered to capture the phenomenon. We intend to continue collecting data to determine if Fearful attachment is significantly associated with diagnoses of disruptive behaviour disorders versus the comparison group.

P-013-210   Topic: 91
Follow-up study: Presence of subclinical epileptiform activity (SEA) in a developmental period

Olivera Aleksic, Institute for Mental Health, Belgrade, Serbia and Montenegro, imz@imh.org.yu
Zarko Martinovic; Nadezda Krstic; Nevenka Buder; Veronika Ispanovic

Objective: 1. To examine cognitive, behavioural and emotional manifestation in these children. 2. To follow up EEG patterns and changes in the diagnosis through 5–7 year period. **Methods:** EEG registration, neurological, psychiatric, psychological and neuropsychological examination. **Results:** Children in experimental group were compared with children without SEA but with learning difficulties. The SEA group was statistically worse (Mann-Whitney-U) in verbal and executive functions and in respect to hyperactivity and impulsivity measured by Conners questionaire, which was pronounced in a subgroup with focal activity. **Conclusion:** Through follow-up period we have found no significant correlation between subclinical epileptiform activity and clinical picture of F8X-9X.

P-013-211   Topic: 91, 30
Formal aspects of emotional functioning of children and adolescents with epilepsy: A neuropsychological approach

Ewa Mojs, Univ. of Medical Sciences, Dept. of Health Sciences, Poznan, Poland, ewa.mojs@medscape.com
Maria Danuta Glowacka

Objective: Disturbances in emotional functioning in epilepsy are defined as multifactorial. They are connected with brain pathology, with parents' attitudes toward their children and with cultural and social influences. The aim of the study was to assess emotional functioning of children and adolescents with epilepsy. We concentrated on recognition and naming of emotion, mechanisms of external control of emotion. **Methods:** 30 patients were participated in the study. The patients aged 9–18 yrs with long term epilepsy. They were treated with novel and conventional antiepileptic drugs (AEDs) in bi- or polytherapy mode. The duration of the disease was 4.2 yrs. They were more than twice hospitalised on neurological ward. **Results:** Impulsivity was recognised as common trait in a group of children with epilepsy. The results showed the connection between term of lasting of the disease and lower control of emotion. Children with epilepsy had formal ability of naming emotion but there was noticed the negative influence of the level of making concepts on ability of naming emotions. **Conclusion:** The study is a part of bigger plan of estimation of emotional functioning of patients with epilepsy and shows significant differences between children with epilepsy and healthy persons.

P-013-212   Topic: 92
Mothers' adaptations to congenital gastrointestinal tract malformations in children

Junko Hayashi, Nagasaki, Japan, junko-hayashi@rio.odn.ne.jp
Syunichi Funakosi; Takamichi Kamiyama; Takashi Ueno; Tomohiro Ishii; Yutaka Hayashi; Hiroo Matsuoka

Objective: Congenital Gastrointestinal tract malformations are caused by anorectal anomalies or Hirschsprung's disease. Understanding the factors of mother adaptation to this disorder in the children will help practitioners enhance the ability of the child and family to cope with this stressful diagnosis. **Methods:** A qualitative descriptive case study methodology was used to explore the factors of mother adaptation to this disorder. Twenty two interviews were conducted with the mothers of children with anorectal anomalies or Hirschsprung's disease. Participant observations were made in the hospital. Psychological assessments by the SDS (Self-rating Depression Scale), STAI (State-Trait Anxiety Inventory) or CDI (Children's Depression Inventory) were included in the data analysis, along with the interview with the mothers. **Results:** The mothers noted that in the case of getting support from people close to them, they were able to better adapt to their children with congenital gastrointestinal tract malformations. This support was connected to the children's depression, assessed by CDI. **Conclusion:** Recognizing factors that may influence the mothers' adaptation to the congenital gastrointestinal tract malformations in the children will help the psychological stability of children and mothers.

P-013-213   Topic: 86, 25
Characteristics of pediatric 'internalizers' in primary care and factors associated with physician recognition

John Campo, Western Psychiatric Institute, Psychiatry, Pittsburgh, PA, USA, campojv@msx.upmc.edu
William Gardner; Amanda Lucas; David Kolko; Kelly Kelleher

Objective: To identify child and family factors associated with higher levels of internalizing psychiatric symptoms in children and adolescents in primary care and determine which of these factors increase the likelihood of recognition with a psychosocial problem by primary care clinicians (PCCs). **Methods:** Children aged 4 to 15 years participating in the Child Behavior Study (CBS) scoring greater than 4 on the internalizing subscale of an abbreviated version of the Pediatric Symptom Checklist (PSC) known as the PSC-17 (n=2.198; 10.4% of sample) were classified as "internalizers" and compared to lower scoring youth (n=18.865) on measures of demographics, school attendance and performance, attention and behavior problems, perceived physical health, service use, and insurance status. Univariate analysis was followed by logistic regression. Logistic regression was then used to explore relevant variables associated with clinician recognition of a psychosocial problem in internalizers. **Results:** Internalizers were older, had more attention and behavioral problems, used more mental health services, came from families perceived to be less supportive, and were more likely to complain of aches and pains, see the doctor with unexplained symptoms, and be perceived by parents to be in suboptimal physical health. Internalizers who were male, suffered from attention, behavior, or school problems, and who had previously used mental health services were more likely to be recognized with a psychosocial problem by PCCs. Physical health concerns did little to increase the likelihood of clinician recognition. **Conclusion:** Comorbid attention, behavior, and/or school problems increase the likelihood of children with high levels of internalizing psychiatric symptoms being recognized with a psychosocial problem in primary care, but potentially important clues related to physical health and functional somatic symptoms are under appreciated.

P-013-214   Topic: 86
Psychopathologic profile of inhibited children: A symptom based perspective

Maria Claustre Jané Ballabriga, U. Autonoma de Barcelona, Psicologia Salut i Social, Bellaterra, Spain, mjane@seneca.uab.es
Sergi Ballespi Sola; Montse Dorado; Natalia Diaz Reganon; Maite Gonzalez Alonso; Maria Dolores Riba; Edelmira Domenech Llaberia

Objective: The aim of this study is to compare internalizing and externalizing psychopathology between a group of extreme inhibited children and a group of control ones. Behavioral inhibition (BI) is the temperamental trait that predisposes to react with anxiety to unfamiliar persons, objects and situations. Although evidence suggests that BI is associated to internalizing psychopathology, and behavioral desinhibition predisposes to externalizing symptomatology, we found in previous investigations, an association between BI and both internalizing and externalizing disorders. **Methods:** Subjects: 526 preschool-age children (3 to 6 years old) were assessed through parents' and teachers' reports. Instruments: Early Child Inventory-4 (ECI-4; Sprafkin & Gadow, 1996) and Preschool Behavioral Inhibition Scales (PBIS; Ballespí, Jané, Riba & Domènech-Llaberia, 2003). Procedure: Inhibited group (IG) was defined as the 15% of boys and girls with the highest scores in Inhibition Scales, and the Control group (CG) as the 15% of children with the lowest scores in Inhibition Scales. **Results:** Teachers' reports showed that 20% of the IG and only 6% of the CG had inattention, forgetfulness and distractability symptoms. Parents' reports showed that IG had more predisposition to separation anxiety (30% IG–15% CG), oppositional symptoms (20% IG–10% CG), sleep problems (14% IG–1.2% CG), and enuresis (20% IG–10% CG). Parents and teachers agreed that the 25% of IG and only 5% of the CG showed excessive preoccupations and fears, elevated sensibility, easy cry and social phobia. All differences are statistically significative. **Conclusion:** These results evidence that BI is associated to both internalizing and externalizing symptomatology. As it has been suggested by Ballespí et al. (2003), it is possible that the temperamental trait called BI predisposes to react anxiously to unfamiliar situations and aggressively to familiar situations.

P-013-215　Topic: 87, 95

Comorbid obsessive-compulsive symptoms in children with Tic Disorders

Kayano Ishii, Tokyo Women's Med. Univ., Pediatrics, Shinjuku-ku, Tokyo, Japan, kayano@ff.iij4u.or.jp
Kayo Inoko; Aya Nishizono-Maher; Makiko Osawa; Mari Kasahara; Kazuhiko Saitou

Objective: The purpose of this study is to examine the relationship between severity of tics and severity of comorbid OC symptoms in the children referred to our clinic with tic disorders. **Methods:** Subjects were 32 children (23 boys and 9 girls), aged between 4 and 42 years (mean 11.3 years), with a diagnosis of Tourette's syndrome or other tic disorder. Tic symptom severity was rated using Yale Global Tic Severity Scale (YGTSS), which assessed motor tics, vocal tics, and impairment resulted from tics. The severity of OC symptoms was rated using the Children's Yale-Brown Obsessive Compulsive Scale (CY-BOCS). **Results:** The total scores of YGTSS were distributed between 10 and 84 (mean ± s.d.: 44.93 ± 19.95). The total scores of CY-BOCS were distributed between 0 and 33 (mean ± s.d.: 8.03 ± 8.54). There was a mild correlation between YGTSS and CY-BOCS total scores. (Pearson's correlation coefficient: 0.62). The severity of motor tics rated by motor tic score on YGTSS significantly correlated with the severity of compulsion rated by compulsion score on CY-BOCS (Pearson's correlation coefficient: 0.50, $p < 0.05$). **Conclusion:** Severity of tics and OC symptoms were correlated. In particular, motor tics and compulsive symptoms were strongly associated.

P-013-216　Topic: 92

A study of somatic complaints in a Japanese clinic sample

Satomi Murase, Nagoya University, School of Medicine, Nagoya, Japan, p47306a@nucc.cc.nagoya-u.ac.jp
Risa Oga; Takashi Murakami; Shuji Honjo; Hitoshi Kaneko; Shiori Arai

Objective: The most common somatic complaints in a clinic sample of child and adolescent school refusers were explored. Whether the days of absence, the levels of anxiety and/or depression are related to somatic complaints were also examined. **Methods:** Forty-seven school refusers, divided into complete refusers (CRs) and partial refusers (PRs) and 150 control group children were evaluated with clinical interviews and self-report questionnaires of somatic symptoms, depression as measured with CDI (Children's Depression Inventory) and trait anxiety as measured with STAIC (State and Trait Anxiety Inventory for Children). **Results:** School refusers complained more somatic symptoms and showed higher score on CDI and STAIC than control group. CRs were more likely to complain circulatory and sensory symptoms than PRs. **Conclusion:** Present study showed that both trait anxiety and depression independently contributed to the level of somatic complaints in a Japanese clinic sample of school refusers.

P-013-217　Topic: 91

Evaluation of neuropsychiatric status and clinical course of Unverricht-Lundborg progressive myoclonus epilepsy at 25 year old woman: A case report

Marta Kaczynska-Haladyj, Neuropsychiatric National, Health Service Lublin, Lublin, Poland, mkaczyn@oil.lublin.pl

Objective: The aim of the paper is to show long-term clinical course of progressive myoclonic epilepsy of Unverricht-Lundborg type PME-UL. The various psychiatric disorders occur frequently in PME. **Methods:** Case report included a longterm observation from infancy to adult time, the results of diagnostic and therapeutic procedures from in-patient and out-patient system care. **Results:** 25-year-old woman with onset of PME-UL at the age of 3, with severe myolonic seizures, which gave the troubles in eating and drinking and as with a typical EEG findings, with marked sensitivity to photic stimulation. At the school-age occurred frequent absence seizures and the girl presented the attention deficit hyperkinetic disorder ADHD with emotional and behavioral disorders. The patient's cognitive abilities were slightly affected. She was taken valproic acid (VPA) and other AEDs with good effect. In the puberty the tonic-clonic seizures with frequency one in a year developed. At this time the patient experienced an improvement in terms of decrease in frequency of myoclonus seizures and absence of seizures too. She was educated in the secondary therapeutic school. All time the patient and family actively participated in tailored comprehensive therapeutic management. The up-to-dated psychological test WISC-R showed the scores of intellectual capacities with dysharmonic profiles as II global = 67, II verbal = 75, II executive = 55. Independently from obtained results, she is open and spontaneus in personal and social interactions and as takes part in every day therapeutic workshops. **Conclusion:** A early diagnosis of PME-UL and as tailored comprehensive therapy are crucial for effective treatment, better prognosis and as for improvment of the quality of life. There is an increasing scientific interest in the relationship between psychopathology and clinical course of PME-UL.

P-013-218　Topic: 91, 30

Speech abilities of children with a benign partial epilepsy

Sabine Völkl-Kernstock, Medizinische Universität Wien, Inst. für Neuropsychiatrie, Wien, Austria, sabine.voelkl-kernstock@univie.ac.at
Sonja Bauch-Prater; Heidrun Eichberger; Martha Feucht

Objective: Manifestations of benign partial epilepsy with centrotemporal spikes, which occur quite frequently during childhood, are confined to ages of 3 to 12 years (Matthes & Schneble, 1992). From a topographical point of view the EEG typically shows unilateral or bilateral epileptogenic foci in the midtemporal region and/or above the Rolandic and/or the occipital regions. One important speech area – the Wernicke area – is localized in the planum temporale, the upper region of the temporal lobe (Deutsch, 1995). The present study investigates whether and to which extent children suffering from this type of benign partial epilepsy show deficiencies in the speech functions. **Methods:** 20 patients with diagnosed Rolandic epilepsy from 6 to 15 years of age and a control group of children corresponding in age and gender with average intellectual abilities and undisturbed sensory perception were tested at the Vienna University Clinic – Department of Neuropsychiatry for children and adolescents.

By means of a series of neuropsychological tests especially their speech abilities were investigated. **Results:** First results show that there is no significant difference between the patient group and the control group with regards to their basal functions of speech. But the patient group performed worse in finding and reminding words. **Conclusion:** The objective of the study is to indicate if and which measures are necessary for training speech abilities of children suffering from Rolandic epilepsy.

P-013-219   Topic: 92
Prevalence of psychiatric complications in children and adolescents with burns

Paula Vilariça, Hospital de Dona Estefânia, Pedopsiquiatria, Lisboa, Portugal, paulavg@sapo.pt
Isadora Pereira; Olivia Pastor; Susana Farinha; Pedro Caldeira; Maria Antónia Silva

Objective: To investigate the prevalence of psychiatric complications in a sample of children and adolescents with burn injury and to determine sub-groups of higher risk for psychiatric complications. **Methods:** The sample comprised all consecutive cases of children and adolescents with burn sequelae that were present for consultation in Psychiatry and/or Surgery in a 6-month period. Thirty children and adolescents with ages between 4 and 16 years, with burn injuries for more than 6 months were assessed. Personal interviews were conducted with the administration of Child Behaviour Check List (CBCL), the Youth Self Report (YSR) and a Checklist of Previous Problems (elaborated by the authors). The characteristics of the acident and the burn injury were assessed using a semi-structured interview elaborated by the authors. **Results:** The children and adolescents with burn sequelae are a population that was exposed to several traumatic experiences such as experience of pain, repeated admissions to the hospital, scarring and disfiguration. In our study there is a higher prevalence of boys that were burnt before the age of 3 years. The majority of the accidents occurred at home and the children were burnt in more than one area of the body. The parents refer the existence of 2 or more psychiatric problems before the acident. The more frequent were stubbornness, restlessness and distractability. In this sample the score for global problems was 30% in the clinical range (CBCL, YSR). There was a score in the clinical range for externalizing problems of 36% and of internalizing problems of 40% (CBCL, YSR). **Conclusion:** There is a high prevalence of psychiatric complications in the sample studied. The authors suggest that periodic psychiatric evaluation are indicated for many children and adolescents with burn sequelae.

P-014   Topic: 84, 85
Attention-deficit/hyperactivity disorders (ADHD) II
Track: ADHD

P-014-220   Topic: 84, 30
Inhibition of continuous reactions via implementation intentions in ADHD children

Caterina Gawrilow, Universität Konstanz, Psychologie und Motivation, Konstanz, Germany, gawrilow@soz.psychologie.uni-konstanz.de
Peter M. Gollwitzer

Objective: Children with an Attention-Deficit/Hyperactivity-Disorder (ADHD) are not able to inhibit a previously learned stimulus-reaction-association. Implementation intentions [Gollwitzer, Am. Psych., 54 (7), 493–503 (1999)] can counteract this negative influence of the previously described habituated action tendencies. Therefore, it is predicted that ADHD children benefit from forming implementation intentions. **Methods:** 30 ADHD children with an average age of 11.0 (SD = 1.4) and 28 control children without any psychiatric disorder and with an average age of 11.5 (SD = 1.1) participated in this study. The experimental setup followed classical experiments with a Stop-Task [Logan, Schachar & Tannock, Psychol. Sci., 8, 60–64 (1997)], in which participants were presented with a reaction time-paradigm. **Results:** As expected ADHD children with an implementation intention could inhibit there reactions significantly better than ADHD children without implementation intention ($p < 0.001$). Furthermore it seems that ADHD children benefit more from forming an implementation intention than control children do. **Conclusion:** Overall, the results of this experiment show that implementation intentions help ADHD children to make up for their deficits when working on exhausting and difficult tasks compared to the control children. This effect can be explained through released cognitive capacities via implementation intentions. Further studies in this line of research are planned and currently being conducted.

P-014-221   Topic: 84, 28
The homozygosity for 10-repeat allele at dopamine transporter gene and dopamine transporter density in basal ganglia: Relation to response to methylphenidate treatment in Attention Deficit Hyperactivity Disorder (ADHD)

Keun-Ah Cheon, Myong-Ji Hospital, Dept. of Psychiatry, Koyang, Republic of Korea, kacheon@dreamwiz.com
Young-Hoon Ryu; Jae-won Kim

Objective: The symptoms of attention-deficit/hyperactivity disorder (ADHD) can be treated with methylphenidate, a potent blocker of the dopamine transporter (DAT). The homozygosity of the 10-repeat allele at the dopamine transporter gene (DAT1) seems to be associated with a poor response to methylphenidate (MPH) in children with ADHD. In the present study, we investigated the association between DAT density using I-123N-(3-iodopropen-2-yl)-2β-carbomethoxy-3beta-(4-chlorophenyl)tropane ([I-123]IPT SPECT) and the homozygosity for 10-repeat allele at DAT1, and response to MPH in children with ADHD. **Methods:** Eleven drug-naive children with ADHD were included in the study and treated with MPH for about 8 weeks. After the genotyping and SPECT were performed, we compared DAT density between ADHD children with and without homozygosity for the 10-repeat allele at DAT1 and investigated the correlation between the homozygosity for the 10-repeat allele and response to MPH. **Results:** ADHD children with 10/10 genotype (n = 7) had a significantly greater increase of the DAT density in basal ganglia than the children without 10/10 genotype (n = 4) (Right: $z = -2.65$, p = 0.008; Left: $z = -2.65$, p=0.008). We found that while only 28.6% (2/7) of the subject with 10/10 genotype showed good response ($\geq$50% improvement) to MPH treatment, 100% (4/4) of the subjects without 10/10 genotype showed good response to MPH treatment (Pearson χ^2 value = 5.238, df = 1, p = 0.061). **Conclusion:** Our findings support an association between homozygosity for the 10-repeat allele at DAT1 and the DAT density assessed in vivo and correlation between the homozygosity for the 10-repeat allele and poor response to MPH.

P-014-222   Topic: 84, 12
Risperidone and Methylphenidate in reducing Attention Deficit Hyperactivity Disorder (ADHD) symptoms in children and adolescents with moderate mental retardation

Alceu Gomes Correia Filho, UFRGS, Child and Adolescent Psychiatry, Porto Alegre, Brazil, alcmed@brturbo.com
Luis Augusto Rohde; Tatiana Silva; Rafael Bodanese; Michael Aman

Objective: To evaluate the short-term efficacy and tolerability of risperidone and Methylphenidate in reducing symptoms related to Attention-Deficit/Hyperactivity disorder (ADHD) in children and adolescents with moderate mental retardation who fulfilled DSM-IV criteria for ADHD. **Methods:** In a 4-week, randomized, blind, parallel-group trial, 46 subjects with Moderate Mental Retardation and ADHD were assessed using objective rating scales (Swanson, Nolan, and Pelham scale-SNAP-IV, and Nisonger Child Behavior Rating Form) and side effects (Barkley's Side-Effects Rating Scale and Ugvald for Kliniske Undergelser). **Results:** Although ADHD symptoms were significantly reduced in both groups for all scales at the endpoint (intra-group analyses; $p < 0.005$; all effect sizes-ES > 0.80, except for the SNAP-IV hyperactivity score in the Methylphenidate group; ES = 0.64), there were no significant differences between the two groups in any scale at the end of the trial (all ES < 0.27). There were a significant weight reduction in Methylphenidate patients and a significant weight gain in risperidone group. **Conclusion:** Our preliminary findings suggest that both risperidone and methylphenidate might be effective in reducing ADHD symptoms in patients with moderate mental retardation. The profile of side effects of some importance in deciding wich medication should be chosen.

P-014-223   Topic: 84, 15
The efficacy of methylphenidate in children with epilepsy and ADHD: The role of dosage, epilepsy type

W. Boudewijn Gunning, Epilepsy Centre Kempenhaeghe, Dept. of Epileptology, Heeze, Netherlands, gunningb@kempenhaeghe.nl

Objective: Research on the effects of psychostimulants in hyperkinetic children with epilepsy has predominantly aimed at possible adverse effects on seizure frequency. In this study the aim was to look (in addition to safety) at the role of dosage, epilepsy type and psychiatric comorbidity. **Methods:** After thorough neurological and psychiatric assessment (and a DSM-IV diagnosis of ADHD) treatment targets were selected with the teacher, and then the child was treated with placebo and with methylphenidate in three dosages (high, moderate, and low, dependent on body weight) once a day at breakfast, evaluating behaviour during the first hours of the morning at school. Dosages were given doubleblind for four weeks, with each week another dosage. In our opinion, in children with epilepsy this is a safe way, still very close to the titration strategy of the MTA study (Greenhill et al., JAACAP 1996; 34: 1304–1313) and the European clinical guidelines for hyperkinetic disorder (Taylor et al., ECAP 1998; 7: 184–200). The study is a presentation of case histories from a cohort of patients who were referred to an epilepsy centre for their epilepsy and comorbid ADHD. **Results:** Roughly as many hyperkinetic children with epilepsy seem to benefit from methylphenidate as hyperkinetic children without epilepsy, and the optimal dosage is as diverse. Children with epilepsy benefit irrespective seizure type and epilepsy syndrome. In hyperkinetic children with autistic disorder the beneficial effect of methylphenidate can be disappointing, probably due to the fact that attention problems can be part of autism and epilepsy, and only mimic ADHD. In the cases that were studied no deterioration in seizure frequency was observed. **Conclusion:** A double-blind, placebo controlled way of testing the effects and titrating the dosage of methylphenidate (with one dosage a day) seems to be a safe method to improve clinical judgment with respect to clinical response.

P-014-224   Topic: 84, 16
Treatment of a 9 year old boy with severe disruptive behavior disorders with Atomoxetine after insufficient response to high dose methylphenidate: A case study

Gerhard Libal, Universitätsklinik Ulm, Kinder- und Jugendpsychiatrie, Ulm, Germany, gerhard.libal@medizin.uni-ulm.de
Klaus Schmeck

Objective: In 2002 the selective norepinephrine reuptake inhibitor atomoxetine was introduced as a non-stimulant alternative to methylphenidate for the treatment of ADHD. We present a case study of a 9 year old boy whose medication was changed from high dose methyphenidate to atomoxetine. **Methods:** This boy was treated with methylphenidate since the age of 5;10. Because of his severe disruptive behavior and lack of concentration the dosage was augmented to 80 mg (23 kg, i.e. 3.5 mg/kg) and desipramine was further added. A transient reduction to 40 mg per day led to a significant exacerbation so that the mother increased methylphenidate up to 160 mg per day (3.75 mg/kg). Temporarily haloperidol was added in low dosage. Despite this enormous amount of medication the treatment effect was still insufficient. We completely changed the medication to a combination of atomoxetine 50 mg/day (1.2 mg/kg) and risperidone 2 mg/day. **Results:** In the first weeks after the change of medication the boy was still disruptive with a low level of frustration but on a higher level of psychosocial functioning. At the time of discharge from day-care treatment however school-functioning and mother-child interactions were still severely disturbed. Getting along with other children and adults was difficult. About 8 months later the situation both at school and at home had changed in a very positive way. According to his mother the mother-child interaction was not impaired for the first time in his life. He was able to attend school (4th grade) in a regular way without severe academic or behavioral problems. **Conclusion:** In this case of a boy with severe ADHD and highly aggressive behavior the combination of atomoxetine and risperidone was the first medication that changed the behavioral and emotional problems in a substantial way. The long term course has to be followed up.

P-014-225   Topic: 84, 28
Is the dopamine D4 receptor gene exon III polymorphism associated with novelty-seeking in 15-year-old adolescents?

Katja Becker, Zentralinstitut für Seelische Gesundheit, Mannheim, Germany, kbecker@zi-mannheim.de
Manfred Laucht; Mahha El-Faddagh; Martin Schmidt

Objective: In recent years, studies focussing on an association between the dopamine D4 receptor (DRD4) gene exon III polymorphism and the personality trait of novelty-seeking (NS) have yielded inconsistent results. We therefore examined the association of the DRD4 exon III polymorphism with NS in a birth cohort of adolescents from a German high-risk community sample. Further, we investigated whether NS in adolescents is associated with ADHD diagnosis. Methods: 303 15-year-old adolescents (144 males, 159 females) from a high-risk community sample were examined. All participants were first-borns with singleton birth, had German-speaking parents and were neither mentally nor physically handicapped. To assess adolescent temperament, the Junior Temperament and Character Inventory (JTCI/12-18, Cloninger et al. 1993) was administered. Psychiatric diagnoses were derived from the highly structured Mannheim Parent Interview, which covers all symptoms related to major DSM-IV/DSM-III-R diagnoses including attention-deficit/hyperactivity disorder (ADHD). Genotypes were classified according to whether or not they contained allele 7r. Statistical analysis of group differences on JTCI scores was performed using two-way ANOVAs with the respective factors DRD4 group (7r vs. non-7r), gender and ADHD diagnosis. Results: At least one copy of the DRD4-7r allele was observed in 124 adolescents (61 males, 63 females), corresponding to 40.9% of the total sample. Males in the DRD4-7r allele group scored significantly higher on the NS (p = 0.002) scale than males without this allele. No association was observed in females. A significant effect of genotype (p = 0.002) was found, but no effect of either ADHD diagnosis or DRD4 by ADHD interaction. Conclusion: In male adolescents, individual differences in NS might be attributed to dopaminergic (genetic) factors, while in females non-dopaminergic factors appear to be more important. The association between the DRD4 polymorphism and NS in male adolescents is independent of any additional ADHD diagnosis.

P-014-226   Topic: 84, 24
Children's conceptions of ADHD

Jakob Nützel, Universität Ulm,
Kinder- und Jugendpsychiatrie, Ulm, Germany,
jakob.nuetzel@medizin.uni-ulm.de
Juliane Ball; Cornelia Elben; Jörg M. Fegert

Objective: The explorative study examines the conceptualization of ADHD in 17 boys with ADHD (8 boys actually under medication) and 24 age-matched boys without ADHD (age range 7 to 12 years). Methods: In a multiple-choice questionnaire the children were first asked five questions concerning the leading symptoms of ADHD to assess their knowledge about the disorder. The second part of the questionnaire was introduced by a short description of the behavior of a boy with ADHD. The children were then asked about their beliefs concerning the causes of the behavior and possible interventions to change the behavior. The children should rate the appropriateness of given causes/interventions in a five-step Likert scale. The catego-

ries of conceptualization were: medical, environment-related (parents/teacher), personal-motivational, therapeutically and not controllable. Data were calculated on a MANOVA. Results: We found no differences in the knowledge about the leading symptoms of ADHD but differences in the attribution of causes and interventions. The children without ADHD rated medical and personal-motivational causes of the ADHD-related behavior more often as being true. They obtained also general higher scores in the rating of appropriateness of all possible interventions. Conclusion: The results are discussed in the light of conceptualization of ADHD in the two groups, especially concerning the rating of medical causes and intervention for ADHD-related behavior in the ADHD-group. The general lower scores of children with ADHD concerning interventions are discussed as a more reserved estimation of the efficacy of interventions which is maybe linked to disappointing experiences in efforts of social adjustment.

P-014-227   Topic: 84, 11
Attention Deficit Hyperactivity Disorder (ADHD) in children: The role of psychoeducation

Halina Kadziela-Olech, University of Bialystok,
Psychosomatic Medicine, Bialystok, Poland
Janina Piotrowska-Jastrz

Objective: The main purpose of the therapy in ADHD is to increase the chances for proper psychosocial development of a child, and prevent the disordered behavior. The main goal of the research was the attempt to find the answer to the question whether the early diagnosis of ADHD children, and application of psychoeducation of parents and teachers has influence on the process of ascertained disorders. Methods: The subject of the research were 60 children (51 (85%) boys and 9 (15%) girls, aged 4–10 years with symptoms of ADHD. The ADHD was diagnosed according to the ICD-10 criteria, whereas the intensification of the disorder was measured using the modified scale according to Costello. The therapeutic procedure was conducted with psychoeducation of parents and teachers. The effects of the therapy were evaluated after 3.6 and 12 months of its duration. Results: The results were statistically using a computer program STATISTICA 5.0 (the Wilcoxon test was applied). Conclusion: Pvalues 0.05 were chosen as significant. Summing up the year-long phase of observation of children with ADHD, it was stated that psycho-education and the elements of behavioral therapy had influence on the reduction of intensification of ADHD symptoms in examined children.

P-014-228   Topic: 84, 28
A family-based and case-control association study of the dopamine D5 receptor gene and dopamine beta hydroxylase gene polymorphism in Attention Deficit Hyperactivity Disorder (ADHD)

Taewon Park, Chonbuk Nat. Univers. Hospital, Dept. of Psychiatry, Jeonju, Republic of Korea, ptaewon@yahoo.com
Boong-Nyun Kim; Myung Ho Im; Soo-Churl Cho; Daehee Kang; Hee Jeong Yoo

Objective: Attention deficit hyperactivity disorder (ADHD) is the most common childhood psychiatric disorder, affecting 3–5% of school age children. Although the biological basis of ADHD is unknown, family studies provide strong evidence that ADHD has a genetic basis. Recent genetic studies have suggested a preferential transmission of the D5 receptor gene (DRD5) 148bp marker allele and dopamine beta hydroxylase gene (DBH) Taq I A1 or A2 allele in ADHD. The aim of this study is to test for the association between DRD5 and DBH polymorphism and ADHD in Korean. **Methods:** We processed DNA extraction and PCR genotyping. 40 Korean children with ADHD and their parents were analyzed using the transmission disequilibrium test(TDT) and haplotype based haplotype relative risk (HHRR) methods. The ADHD children were also compared with 130 controls. **Results:** No significant evidence was found for an association between the allele of DBH Taq I polymorphism and ADHD. We did not observe significant evidence for an association of the 148-bp allele of DRD5 (CT/GT/GA)n dinucleotide repeat polymorphism, however we did observe biased transmission of the 144-bp allele in case control study. **Conclusion:** The number of informative transmissions for 144-bp allele was too small, therefore it would be premature to make any conclusions from our study concerning the role of DRD5 in ADHD. Further work is needed to support this new finding.

P-014-229   Topic: 84, 16

Developmental outcomes of long-term Atomoxetine treatment in juveniles with Attention Deficit Hyperactivity Disorder (ADHD)

David Michelson, Lilly Research Laboratories, Dept. of Neuroscience, Indianapolis, IN, USA, michelson@lilly.com
Thomas Spencer; Shuyu Zhang; Dustin Ruff; Peter Feldman

Objective: Attention-deficit/hyperactivity disorder (ADHD) is typically treated over extended periods during childhood and adolescence, but few studies have systematically assessed the effects of pharmacologic treatments on development. We review here data relevant to development from preclinical and long-term clinical studies conducted with atomoxetine. **Methods:** Growth, sexual development, and intellectual development were assessed in preclinical studies involving juvenile animals and in long-term clinical studies as part of the drug development process for atomoxetine. Juvenile animals were treated with atomoxetine from shortly after birth into adulthood to determine effects on prespecified sexual and neurodevelopmental landmarks. Developmental landmarks including growth, IQ, and Tanner stage were assessed in pediatric patients who received atomoxetine in studies lasting 1 or more years. **Results:** Studies in animals do not suggest clinically meaningful effects on growth, sexual development, or neurodevelopment. Clinical studies suggest that, on average, patients experience an initial modest decrease in growth velocity that normalizes during long-term treatment and is unlikely to significantly affect final stature. Long-term studies do not suggest atomoxetine affects sexual development, as judged by progression through puberty, or intellectual development, as judged by IQ scores. **Conclusion:** Preclinical and clinical studies support the safety of atomoxetine relative to development during long-term treatment. Research funded by Eli Lilly and Company, Indianapolis, Indiana, USA.

P-014-230   Topic: 84, 27

Psychometrics of an Attention Deficit Hyperactive Disorder (ADHD) problem scale developed from the Child Behavior Checklist

Niels Bilenberg, Odense University Hospital, Child & Adolescent Psychiatry, Odense C, Denmark, niels.bilenberg@ouh.fyns-amt.dk
Jørgen Jensen

Objective: To develop an Attention Deficit Hyperactive Disorder- (ADHD-) problem scale from the Child Behavior Checklist (CBCL) problem item pool and to evaluate its internal and external validity. **Methods:** Latent trait analysis and internal consistency analysis was performed on data from a community based sample (N=779) and a clinically based sample (N=146), all information was from children between the age of 4–16 years. Additionally, the ADHD problem scale was evaluated as a screening device and compared with thorough clinical assessment in another community based sample of nine-year-old children (N=135). **Results:** Twelve items were retained after exploratory and confirmatory analyses (smallest factor loading: 0.59). Internal consistency was high with a Cronbach alpha coefficient=0.87. Mean ADHD problem scale scores (range 0–12) for age and gender strata are presented. Best cutoff in screening was determined using Receiver Operating Characteristic- (ROC-) curve analysis. A scale score 6 was optimum, corresponding to a sensitivity of 0.93 and a correct classification rate of 0.84. **Conclusion:** The performance of the ADHD problem scale compares favorably with other similar questionnaire-based scales. The CBCL questionnaire is widely used and the proposed scale and scores are easily administrated and computed. The scale is utilized in a large Danish community study in progress.

P-014-231   Topic: 84, 26

Surveying the Attention Deficit Hyperactivity Disorder (ADHD) symptoms of preschool children based on their parents and teachers report at day care centers in Tabriz in 2003

Azar Moradi, Tabriz University, of Medical Sciences, Tabriz, Islamic Republic of Iran, chancellor@tbzmed.ac.ir
Vahed Alaey

Objective: ADHD is the most common behavioral problem in childhood. The studies identified the peak age of ADHD as occurring between three and four years of age, and two thirds of children in whom ADHD is later diagnosed would have been identifiable during the preschool years. However most studies on this disorder have been carried out in school age populations. Caring out such as this investigations in preschoolers is important from the view point of early detection, provision of help and prevention from complications. Pediatric nurses as health consultants or health visitors can apply screening services to identifying behavioral problems and safety issues, and/or can play important role as a liaisons to other health professionals. **Methods:** This research is a descriptive-comparative study with the aim of finding out ADHD symptoms of preschool children at day care centers in Tabriz based on their parents and teachers report. 273 children between the ages of three to five years of age were randomly chosen from 31 day care centers and the questionnaires were completed by their parents and teachers separately. The questionnaire of ADHD symptoms consist of 15 bulletins for parents

(ADHD-P) and 15 bulletins for teachers (ADHD-T). The items in ADHD questionnaire were based directly upon DSM-III-R criteria for ADHD. Howerer the criteria were modified slightly so that they would be more appropriate for preschool children. The questionnaire is based on 'not at all', 'just a little', 'pretty much' and 'very much' answers. The validity and reliablity of ADHD Scale were tested by means of content validity and test-retest respectively. The statistic tests of the Mcnemar, One-way anova, Chi-square and in dependent 'T' were used for information analysis. **Results:** Findings of research showed that 10.3 percent of children based on their parents report and 7.7 percent of them based on teachers report have ADHD symptoms. Although comparison of their reports in idicated that parents tend to report hyperactivity-impulsivity symptoms more than inattention symptoms. But there was no significant differences between parents and teachers report. **Conclusion:** Whereas there were no significant differences between parents and teachers report, using of each two group reports may be useful in behavioral screening of preschool children aimed to identifying ADHD symptoms. Also with regard to high percent of ADHD in preschool children, for nurses along careful evaluation of ADHD symptoms, families psychopathology is recommended.

P-014-232   Topic: 84, 16
Effects of long-term Atomoxetine treatment for young children with ADHD

Christopher Kratochvil, University of Nebraska, Psychiatry, Omaha, NE, USA, ckratoch@unmc.edu
Timothy Wilens; Laurence Greenhill; Haitao Gao; Douglas Gelowitz

Objective: To date, few clinical investigations of attention-deficit/hyperactivity disorder (ADHD) extend beyond a few months. The purpose of this presentation is to report on the long-term efficacy and tolerability of atomoxetine treatment among young children with ADHD. **Methods:** Data were pooled from 6- and 7-year old children (n = 192) enrolled in similarly designed clinical trials and who met the DSM-IV criteria for ADHD. The children had a minimum of 12 months of atomoxetine treatment and 97 (51%) received treatment for greater than 24 months. The mean modal dose (± SD) of atomoxetine was 1.55 mg/kg/day (0.32). The primary efficacy outcome measure was the mean change from baseline to endpoint in the parent-rated ADHD Rating Scale IV (ADHDRS). The Conners' Parent Rating Scale-Revised: Short Form (CPRS-R:S) was a secondary efficacy measure. **Results:** The pooled analysis revealed significant mean treatment effects from baseline to endpoint for ADHD RS scores and T-scores (p < 0.001 for Total, Inattention, Hyperactive/Impulsive) and for CPRS scores and T-scores (p < 0.001 for Index, Cognitive, Hyperactive, Oppositional). Analysis of ADHD RS total scores over time showed that after approximately 3 months of atomoxetine treatment, there was a marked improvement in ADHD symptoms, and this improvement was maintained throughout long-term treatment. Adverse events were clinically minor and transient, and only 1.6% of children discontinued due to adverse events. There were no clinically meaningful changes in laboratory tests, vital signs, or electrocardiography. **Conclusion:** Long-term atomoxetine treatment appears to be well-tolerated and effective in young children with ADHD.

P-014-233   Topic: 84, 19
Attention Deficit Hyperactivity Disorder (ADHD) and bipolar disorder association in youth: Differential diagnostic and treatment challenges

Leon Patrice Celestin, Hosp Poissy-St.Germain-En-Laye, CMP-Sector78I02-Psychiatry, Paris, France, celestinlp@aol.com
Smadar Celestin-Westreich

Objective: In recent years, an Attention Deficit/Hyperactivity Disorder (AD/HD) and Bipolar Disorder (BD) association in youth has attracted research attention. While AD/HD has become widely recognised, BD identification in youth is generally complicated by its polymorphous clinical manifestations. Moreover, AD/HD and BD may present overlapping phenomenology and comorbidty, such as psychomotor hyperactivity, as well as dysphoric mood or oppositional behaviour. Early recognition of Bipolar Disorder is especially crucial given its association with significant risk-taking behaviour and need for lifetime follow-up. The present paper aims to clarify the nature of this AD/HDBD association in youth. **Methods:** First, state-of-the art regarding the AD/HD – Bipolar Disorder association is reviewed. Second, a qualitative case series analysis systematically and identifies critical aspects of differential diagnosis & early therapeutic implementation within the context of Medical-Psychological Centre consultations in Paris' suburban regio. **Results:** Early BD manifestations tend to be mistaken for AD/HD symptoms. Detailed anamnestic interviewing and special attention for tapping specific family antecedents underlying the development of Bipolar Disorder are instrumental in guiding the differential diagnostic process. Effective identification of "real" AD/HD-BD comorbidity remains hampered so far by a lack of adequate differential criteria of childhood-onset BD manifestations, especially as regards (hypo)mania symptoms. For children receiving AD/HD diagnosis while presenting initial early BD signs, follow-up is needed to specify possible evolution of AD/HD-manifestations into BD at a later age. **Conclusion:** While it is currently thought that AD/HD-symptoms may constitute BD precursors as well as occur simultaneously, more systematic screening for BD in (AD/HD) children is needed to rule out methodological artefact of this association. Implementation of differential developmental and (family) background leads enforces adequate diagnostic identification along with contributing to adequate treatment follow-up.

P-014-234   Topic: 84, 15
Audit on use of methylphenidate in children with ADHD

Somnath Banerjee, School & Child Health, Ramsgate, Kent, United Kingdom, somnath.b@doctors.org.uk
M. Chandola; S. Venables

Objective: To audit the current practices in East Kent ADHD clinics against the UK national and local guidelines. **Methods:** A retrospective review of case notes of children diagnosed with ADHD between 1 October 2001 and 31 March 2002 and subsequently started on methylphenidate. **Results:** A total of 47 notes were audited. Conners' rating scales were used in 31 (66%) children. 2 (4%) children were below age 6 years while on methylphenidate. Major diagnosis criteria were used in 43 (92%) children. Schools, parents and GPs received written information respectively in 28 (60%), 30 (64%), and 42 (89%) cases about the start of methylphenidate and 25 (53%), 27 (57%), and 35 (75%) cases about the most recent visit. 44 (94%) children had their growth and 24 (51%) had their pulse and blood pressure recorded before start of medication. 26 (58%), 30 (71%), and 32 (86%) children due for review within specified time limit had first, second and subsequent review of medication respectively. 31 (89%) children had their growth and 28 (80%) had their blood pressure monitored over the next one year. 2 (4%) children were getting the repeat prescriptions from their GPs. A trial off medication was considered in 3 (16%) children. **Conclusion:** This audit identified some deficiencies. The areas for improvements are use of ADHD specific checklists and recognised diagnosis criteria in all children, regular monitoring of growth, pulse and blood pressure, communication to parents/carers and school, consideration of a trial off medication, and shared care arrangements with GPs. The audit demonstrates multidisciplinary working, carer involvement and improvements to patient care.

P-015   Topic: 84, 85
Attention-deficit/hyperactivity disorders (ADHD) III
Track: ADHD

P-015-236   Topic: 84, 36
Event-related potentials (ERPs) as auxiliary measures in the differential diagnosis of Attention Deficit Hyperactivity Disorder (AD/HD)

Hideki Negoro, Nara Medical University, Dept. of Psychiatry, Kashihara Nara, Japan, gorosan@naramed-u.ac.jp
Junzo Iida; Hidemi Iwasaka; Masanori Kyo; Tatsushi Nagano; Kanae Kishino; Toshihumi Kishimoto

Objective: Some disturbance of cognition and/or information processing might be involved in Attention Deficit/Hyperactivity Disorder (AD/HD). We studied Event-related potentials (ERPs) children with AD/HD. We measured P300 and the early negativity components which reflect attention function: negative difference (Nd) and mismatch negativity (MMN). We had observed children with AD/HD that a) in the AD/HD group, prolonged latency and reduced amplitude of P300 were observed more than in the normal control group, b) in the AD/HD group, reduced amplitude of Nde and MMN were observed more than in the normal control group. Then we investigated whether ERPs could be useful for differential diagnosis, and these biological abnormalities are specific to AD/HD. **Methods:** Subjects were child patients whose chief complaints were hyperkinetic and inattentive. Children with mental retardation were excluded. All subjects were naïve to medication. Subjects of this study consist of three groups: AD/HD group (n=25), PDD group (n=11) and adjustment disorder group (n=10). There was no significant difference on ADHD-RS points among three groups. Written informed consents were taken from all the children and all the parents. The examiners who were blind to diagnosis measured ERPs (P300, Nd, MMN). **Results:** The amplitudes of P300 and Nde were significantly smaller than in AD/HD group as compared with adjustment disorder group. The MMN latency and amplitudes in AD/HD group did not differ from another two groups. **Conclusion:** In the present study we distinguished the AD/HD group from the adjustment

disorder group whose patients were hyperkinetic and inattentive. These results suggested that ERPs might be useful auxiliary measures for differential diagnosis in child patients who were hyperkinetic and inattentive.

P-015-237   Topic: 84, 35
Regional cerebral perfusion abnormalities in ADHD – Statistical parametric mapping analysis

Soo-Churl Cho, Seoul Nat. University Hospital, Psychiatry, Seoul, Republic of Korea, soochurl@snu.ac.kr
Dong-Hyun Ahn; Yun-O Shin; Bong-Suk Kim; Jun-Won Hwang

Objective: An investigation of cerebral blood flow using Tc-99m-HMPAO brain SPECT was conducted to identify functional abnormality of the brain in boys with ADHD. **Methods:** 31 boys with ADHD (mean age 8.14±2.03) who had no previous treatment history were selected by using DSM-IV criteria. After acquiring a pretreatment Tc-99m-HMPAO Brain SPECT images from them, Statistical Parametric Mapping (SPM) analysis was performed by using Korean-standard template of child-adolescent normal control. **Results:** Decreased cerebral blood flow in Left Medial Frontal Gyrus, Right Medial Frontal Gyrus, Left Paracentral Lobule, Left Precuneus Gyrus, Left Thalamus, Both cerebellum was found in ADHD group compared to the controls (P < 0.001). In addition, increased blood flow in Both Inferior, Middle, and Superior Frontal Gyrus, Left inferior Temporal Gyrus, Left Fusiform Gyrus was found in tic disorder group (P < 0.001). **Conclusion:** A significant cerebral blood flow abnormality in frontal lobe of ADHD

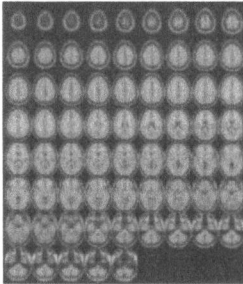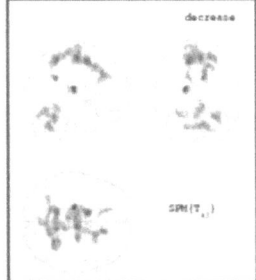

Figure 1. Brain areas with significantly decreased perfusion in ADHD patients compared to normal controls (threshold: *P*=0.001, uncorrected)

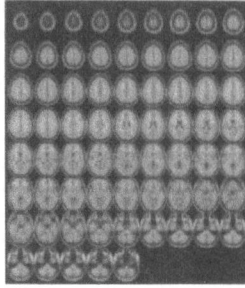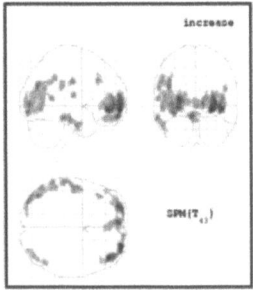

Figure 2. Brain areas with significantly increased perfusion in ADHD patients compared to normal controls (threshold: *P*=0.001, uncorrected)

boys in our study suggests an association with the previously known abnormality in circuit of cortico-striato-thalamo-cortical area.

P-015-238   Topic: 84, 36
Event-Related Potentials (ERPs) and severity of symptoms in children with Attention Deficit Hyperactivity Disorder (AD/HD)

Masanori Kyoh, Nara Medical University, Kashiwara Nara, Japan, kyoh@naramed-u.ac.jp
Iida Junzo; Negoro Hideki; Nagano Tatsushi; Kishino Kanae; Iwasaka Hidemi; Kishimoto Toshifumi

Objective: Some disturbance of cognition and/or information processing might be involved in Attention-Deficit/Hyperactivity Disorder (AD/HD). We studied Event-related potentials (ERPs) in the child AD/HD. We measured P300 and the early negativity components which reflect attention function: negative difference (Nd) and mismatch negativity (MMN). We had observed that a) in the AD/HD group, prolonged latency and reduced amplitude of P300 were observed more than in the normal control group, b) in the AD/HD group, reduced amplitude of Nd and MMN were observed more than in the normal control group. Then we investigated the relation between the Event-Related Potentials and the severity of symptoms in children with AD/HD. **Methods:** 20 children (mean age: 8.2 years) with AD/HD based on DSM-IV were studied. Subjects were the patients whose chief complaints were hyperkinetic and inattentive. Children with mental retardation were excluded. All subjects were naïve to medication. Written informed consents were taken from all the children and all the parents. The examiners were blind to diagnosis measured ERPs (P300, Nd, MMN). AD/HD-Rating Scale was used as the index of the severity of symptoms. **Results:** Significant positive correlation was found between AD/HD-RS and MMN latency, and significant negative correlation was found between AD/HD-RS and amplitudes of MMN. **Conclusion:** MMN might represent the automatic and precognitive processing of information. In this study, there were some difficulties in the automatic and precognitive processing of information in AD/HD patients, and it was suggested that MMN might be the objective index of the severity of symptoms.

P-015-239   Topic: 84, 30
Selective inattention deficits in patients with Attention Deficit Hyperactivity Disorder (ADHD)

Rael Strous, Beer Yaakov Men. Health Center, Dept. of Psychiatry, Beer Yaakov, Israel, raels@post.tau.ac.il
Simion Kertzman; Z. Ben Nachum; Moshe Kotler; Roni Hegesh

Objective: Poor performance in the Continuous Performance Test (CPT) (sustained attention) among children with ADHD remains a consistent finding. Another facet of attention, selective attention, is however less investigated in ADHD. Moreover, brain mechanisms describing aspects of these two subtypes of attention appear to be different in normal individuals. By means of a novel neurocognitive paradigm, in this study the intention was to investigate whether impairment in ADHD patients is restricted to sustained attention, or rather that selective attention is impaired as well. **Methods:** 77 young male patients suffering from ADHD (DSM-IV criteria) were included in the study

(mean age 11.0 ± 3.2 years). The control group consisted of 47 healthy children matched by age. The instrument used the computerized neuro-cognitive battery "CogScan"; from which 2 subtests were activated namely the Stroop test and Continuous Performance test by means of a novel method of computerized administration and analysis. Statistical analysis was performed using Pearson correlations, and univariate ANOVA wherein Stroop test results served as dependent variables and the CPT was used as a covariate. **Results:** While correlations between CPT results and Stroop results were non-significant in the control group, correlations between CPT and Stroop results in ADHD group were significant ($r = 0.426$–0.465, $p = 0.000$). ANOVA results yielded significant differences in Stroop results between ADHD group and control group, even after excluding CPT results from the variance (F $(1.121) = 10.69$, $p = 0.001$). **Conclusion:** Results suggest that ADHD patients are impaired not only in sustained attention, but also in selective attention. Moreover, unlike normal subjects, a relationship was found between these two components of attention in the ADHD subgroup. The association between the impairments on selective and sustained attention among ADHD subjects may be as a result of a defect in inhibition ability. Further neurobiological investigation is required in order to clarify these clinical neurocognitive findings.

P-015-240   Topic: 84, 56
Measuring quality of life in children with Attention Deficit Hyperactivity Disorder (ADHD) in the United Kingdom

David Coghill, The Centre for Child Health, Child & Adolescent Psychiatry, Dundee, United Kingdom, cyuen1@jacgb.jnj.com
Quentin Spender; Joanne Barton; Chris Hollis; Cammy Yuen; Irina Cleemput; Lieven Annemens

Objective: Health authorities conducting cost-effectiveness evaluations commonly use utility scales such as the EQ-5D. A utility scale is a type of quality of life measure that produces a utility score between 0 (death) and 1 (perfect health). Although utility values for children with various diseases have been derived using the EQ-5D for cost-effectiveness analysis, in the past these values were only estimations either by clinicians or health economists. Our aim was to derive 'real life' utility values for children with Attention-Deficit-Hyperactivity-Disorder (ADHD) and determine whether the EQ-5D is sufficiently sensitive to detect differences in the quality of life of these children. **Methods:** The EQ-5D questionnaires were completed as part of a non-interventional, cross-sectional study of 151 ADHD patients in the UK. Parents were used as proxy raters in the study. Where possible, parents completed the forms in consultation with their child. During the clinic visit, physicians assessed the change in the patient's ADHD symptom severity compared to the previous consultation. In order to determine if there was a relationship between the resulting utility scores and current symptom severity or symptom improvement since the last consultation, a multivariate regression analysis was performed. **Results:** Results of the regression analysis showed that patients with mild, moderate and severe disease, were associated with utility values 0.815, 0.782 and 0.749. Patients with improved symptom severity since the last consultation, ceteris paribus, had a utility value of 0.804. Those who did not improve, had a utility value of 0.739. **Conclusion:** This is the first attempt in measuring the real world utility values of children with ADHD, using the EQ-5D. These results suggest that the EQ-5D was able to differentiate between children with ADHD according to symptom severity or clinical improvement.

P-015-241   Topic: 84, 47
Family assessment in the context of ADHD:
A comparison of the perspectives of different family members

Susanne Eschmann, Universität Zürich, Kinder- und Jugendpsychiatrie, Zürich, Switzerland, s.eschmann@ppkj.unizh.ch
Karl Christoph Käppler; Maycoln M.L. Teodoro; Eva Stieger; Anouk Mugier; Stephanie Stüttler

Objective: In family assessment there are only a few studies which compare the multiple perspectives of family members. Thus, the aim of the present study is to investigate basic dimensions of family structures in families including one child with ADHD (Attention-Deficit-Hyperactivity-Disorder) from the viewpoint of at least four family members. **Methods:** Three recently developed devices in family assessment were applied. The Family-System-Test (FAST, Gehring, 1998), in the tradition of sculpture techniques, consists of wooden figures which symbolize the family members and allow analysis of the two basic dimensions of cohesion and power/-hierarchy in family relations. Subjective representations of the family should be given three times by the participant: in normal daily life, during a conflict and as an ideal constellation of the family. The Family-Identification-Test (FIT, Remschmidt & Mattejat, 1999) allows to describe different self-concepts (real, ideal...) and concepts from others (parents, peers...) by sorting 12 cards with attributes derived from common personality dimensions (intro-, extraversion; emotional stability/lability...). The correlations between these concepts indicate identification patterns (i.e. 'I'm like my mother', "I want to be like my father"...). The Familiogram (Teodoro & Käppler, 2003) is based on Moreno's Sociogram and modern network approaches from sociology. Family members have to rate subsequently how close the relations in all dyads from his/her family seem to them. Cohesion as one of the main dimension of family networks is measured by the standardized density of each dyad. With the dichotomization of the values a graph is created that represents the cohesion patterns in a given family. **Results:** Results indicating remarkable differences between family members will be presented, with special focus on the child with ADHD diagnosis. **Conclusion:** As a conclusion, the different perspectives of family members should be considered systematically in assessment procedures, intervention strategies and treatment evaluation.

P-015-242   Topic: 84, 37
Diagnostics of ADHD: Diagnostical assistance by the use of the parent version of the Strengths and Difficulties Questionnaire (SDQ)

Cord Alexander Heise, University of Göttingen, Child and Adolescent Psych., Goettingen, Germany, cheise@gwdg.de
Tobias Banaschewski; Andreas Becker; Henrik Uebel; Aribert Rothenberger

Objective: The aim of the study was to assess if the SDQ (Strengths and Difficulties Questionnaire) with its subscale hyperactivity/inattention qualifies as a useful tool to screen for ADHD. **Methods:** We investigated 314 male child psychiatric patients within the age range of 5–13 years whose parent SDQ (subscale hyperactivity/inattention; H/I) was either normal, borderline or abnormal. The registered values for the subscale were correlated with the clinical diagnosis of ADHD (n = 126 with ADHD; n = 188 with other or without any child psychiatric problems), in order to estimate the predictive value of the subscale for the diagnosis of ADHD. **Results:** It was shown that a normal value on the subscale H/I was associated with absence of clinical diagnosis of ADHD in 84% of the cases (true negatives). The relative percentage of true negative ADHD cases among children with normal H/I scores was similarly high (78–88%) throughout the investigated age range. In contrast, only 59% of the children with abnormal H/I values were clinically diagnosed ADHD cases (true positives). Thus, the prediction of positive ADHD cases by SDQ-H/I scores was only moderately good and better in younger (72%) than older (48%) children. **Conclusion:** Hence, the subscale H/I of the SDQ seems to be a helpful component to exclude ADHD within the scope of a multidimensional diagnosis. An abnormal value of this subscale has not to be considered as diagnostic evidence for an existing ADHD but calls for further steps of assessment.

P-015-243   Topic: 84, 30
Oculomotor inhibition in children with and without Attention Deficit Hyperactivity Disorder (ADHD)

Charlotte Hanisch, Universität Aachen, Kinder- und Jugendpsychiatrie, Aachen, Germany, chanisch@ukaachen.de
Kerstin Konrad; Ralph Radach; Beate Herpertz-Dahlmann

Objective: The aim of the present study was to examine oculomotor inhibition in children with attention-deficit hyperactivity disorder (ADHD). Compared to normal hand motor inhibition tasks, like the Go-No-Go or Stop-Signal task, oculomotor inhibition tasks may have the advantage that they escape the ancillary problems in motor and langugage development that often accompany ADHD. We were particularly interested if we could identify a specific inhibition deficit by using multiple oculomotor paradigms. **Methods:** 22 ADHD patients and 22 age- and gender-matched healthy children were compared in their performance on an oculomotor fixation task, a pro- and an antisaccade paradigm and a countermanding saccade task (an aculomotor adaptation of the Stop-Signal Task). **Results:** Two major results were obtained: First, our prosaccade task suggested similar saccadic response preparation and saccadic accuracy in the ADHD compared to the control children. Secondly, the fixation, the antisaccade and the countermanding saccade task indicated deficits on various measures of oculomotor inhibition in ADHD patients. Inhibition deficits were specifically pronounced in the countermanding saccade task, and here especially under the most difficult task condition. **Conclusion:** In line with previous work we found ADHD children to show normal oculomotor responses and to be specifically impaired in inhibitory functions. Deficits were particularly evident in a task that has been associated with activation of the anterior cingulate gyrus. This cortical structure is discussed to play a crucial role in the frontostriatal network that might be involved in the pathophysiology of ADHD.

P-015-244   Topic: 84, 30
Reaction time and number of errors in a visual and acoustic stimuli-reaction test in children with Attention Deficit Hyperactivity Disorder (ADHD) compared to a sex- and age matched control group

Ralf Nordbeck, Groß Kussewitz, Germany,
ralf.nordbeck@med.uni-rostock.de
Dagmar Horn; Wolfgang Gierow; Ulrike Sühlfleisch-Thurau;
Frank Häßler; Johannes Buchmann

Objective: Two most outstanding symptoms of children with ADHD are impulsivity and attention deficit. When confronted with tasks that demand sustained attention like a GoNoGo paradigm, they make more mistakes and need more reaction time [1]. Research in this field is rare. Only a few studies reflect whether number of failures and reaction time depends on acoustic or visual quality of the stimuli. This study compares reaction time and number of failures of ADHD children in a visual and acoustic GoNoGo paradigm to those of a clinical control group. **Methods:** 30 Children aged 7.1 to 13.7 years (mean age 10.4, maximal deviation 3.3 years) performed a visual and acoustic continuous performance test. 15 of them had been diagnosed with ADHD (based on research criteria of DSM IV, predominantly Hyperactive-Impulsive Type or Combined Type, IQ 85, Conners Rating Scale short form > 15). 15 sex and age matched children – patients of our department – formed the control group. For matched pair comparisons, age differences were less than 6 months. The visual and acoustic test was structured as follows: 500 stimuli were presented randomly and in constant intervals of 1.65 s. 115 of these stimuli were attention stimuli (yellow light, low tone), 75 target (Go = red light follows yellow light, high tone follows low tone), 40 NoGo stimuli (yellow/green light follows yellow light, middle/low tone follows low tone) and the rest were random stimuli (green light/middle tone). After the combination attention-target (Go) the children had to press a key as fast as possible. We measured reaction time and errors. **Results:** Children with ADHD made more errors of omission in both, the visual and the acoustic test. As a whole in both groups, the number of mistakes was higher in the acoustic test. In the acoustic paradigm, reaction times of the ADHD group were significantly longer than those of the control group (p = 0.05). No differences between the two groups were found in the visual paradigm. **Conclusion:** Sustained and focused attention is impaired in children with ADHD. Most studies mainly refer to visual stimuli [1]. Based on our findings we discuss, that longer reaction times and more errors of ADHD children in the acoustic paradigm can be interpreting as depended on stimulus modality.

P-015-245   Topic: 84, 30
Actigraph as an objective measure for diagnosis of Attention Deficit Hyperactivity Disorder (ADHD)

Noa Tsujii, Kinki University School, Dept. of
Neuropsychiatry, Osaka, Japan, noa@pop21.odn.ne.jp
Akira Okada; Noriko Kuriki; Junko Matsuo;
Kazushi Hanada; Takeshi Kusube; Kazuhiko Hitomi

Objective: To evaluate attention-deficit/hyperactivity disorder (AD/HD) using actigraph. **Methods:** 10 AD/HD (6–12 years old) children and 10 normal controls (6–12 years old) were examined using actigraphic monitoring in classroom structured in-seat situation. AD/HD children all were diagnosed mainly hyperactive or combined type according to the DSM-IV criteria. Mean 1-minute activity level (Zero crossing mode counts) and standard deviation for 30-minute in classroom were compared with AD/HD and controls. **Results:** There were no significant differences in Mean 1-minute activity level between AD/HD and controls. There were significant differences in standard deviation. **Conclusion:** We believe that the results show the characteristics of children with AD/HD and actigraph as an objective measure in diagnosis of AD/HD is useful.

P-015-246   Topic: 84, 55
ADHD predominantly inattentive type: A case-control study of maternal smoking during pregnancy and ADHD parental diagnosis

Marcelo Schmitz, Porto Alegre, Brazil,
mschmitz@orion.ufrgs.br
Daniel Denardin; Tatiana da Silva; Thiago Pianca;
Tatiana Roman; Mara Hutz; Luis Augusto Rohde

Objective: To assess the association between attention-deficit hyperactivity disorder predominantly inattentive type (ADHD-IT) and pre-natal exposure to maternal tobacco smoking, and parental ADHD diagnosis in a school sample of Brazilian children and adolescents (6 to 18 years of age). **Methods:** A case-control study was conducted with 35 ADHD-IT subjects and 35 non-ADHD controls of both genders. The sample of pupils were recruited from 12 state schools located in 3 poor neighborhoods in Porto Alegre, Brazil. The diagnoses of ADHD according to DSM-IV criteria were given using semi-structured (K-SADS-E) + clinical interviews with both the subjects and their parents. The associations between the disorder and maternal smoking, and the occurrence of ADHD in the parents were analysed by chi-square test. **Results:** We found that pre-natal exposure to nicotine was significantly higher in ADHD-IT cases (34.3%) than in non-ADHD controls (8.6%) (p = 0.02). In addition, a parental ADHD diagnosis was significantly more frequent in ADHD-IT subjects (45.7%) compared to non-ADHD controls (11.4%) (p < 0.01). **Conclusion:** Our results replicate for a non-referred sample of ADHD-IT subjects, previous findings suggesting an association between diagnosis of ADHD in probands and both maternal smoking and parental ADHD diagnosis in referred samples.

P-015-248   Topic: 84, 45
ADHD in a Tunisian clinical population

Asma Bouden, Hôpital Razi, Service de Pédopsychiatrie,
Manouba, Tunisia, claude.farhat@gnet.tn
Ines Dengezli; Mohamed Halayem

Objective: The aim of the study is to extract epidemiological and clinical characteristics of ADHD in a clinical population. **Methods:** It's a retrospective study. Our population was recruited among outpatients aged from 3 to 12 years, referred for hyperactivity and/or attention disorders during two years 1998 and 1999. Statistical analysis was carried out with EpiInfo6 software. **Results:** 43 children (21%) met the DSMIV criteria for ADHD. the sub-categories of the disorder were: 92% combined type, 4% predominantly inattentive type and 4% ADHD NOS. The sex ratio was 3 boys to one girl. The age at the first consultation varied between 9 and 12 years in 60% of cases. The disorder was isolated in 25% of cases. Comorbidity found: conduct disorder or disruptive behavior disorder in 44% of cases, elimination disorders in 25.5%, learning disorders in 22.9%, mood disorders in 11.75%, anxiety disorders in 14%, communication disorders in 16.25% and adjustment disorders in 4.75%. **Conclusion:** Results found in our population are closely related to those found in the literature. High rate of comorbidity (75% of cases) raise the problem of the homogeneity of ADHD.

P-015-249   Topic: 84, 42
Reboxetine treatment in ADHD: A 1-year longitudinal study
Óscar Herreros, Hospital Univ. de Canarias, Dept. of Psychiatry, La Laguna, Spain, oherreros@comtf.es
Francisco Sanchez; Belen Rubio; Ramon Gracia

Objective: Despite well-documented improvement in ADHD (attention-deficit hyperactivity disorder) with the available pharmacological treatments, a number of children are difficult to treat because of adverse events or non-response to usual agents. The aim of the study is to collect data assesing the safety, tolerability and efficacy of reboxetine, a non-stimulant inhibitor of norepinephrine reuptake potentially useful for treating ADHD. **Methods:** A cross-sectional design for assessing 29 children (from 5 to 12 years old) receiving clinical care in a specialized Child and Adolescent Psychiatry Unit, all of them treated with reboxetine for ADHD now or in the past, was made by the authors to evaluate its effects on core symptoms of ADHD, and also its safety and tolerability in children and adolescents. **Results:** Reboxetine was initiated at 1 mg per day and adjusted on a clinical basis depending on response and adverse effects, in one or two doses per day. Changes in ADHD symptoms, measured with the ADHD Rating Scale-IV (parent's version), was the efficacy measure. Adverse events were assessed each week at the beginning of treatment. An important improvement on ADHD symptoms was observed (70% of the patients were considered responders), with transient somnolence as the most frequently reported side effect (and all of them were transient, from one week to one month). **Conclusion:** This preliminary findings suggest that reboxetine is efficacious and well-tolerated in ADHD children, but further controlled studies are needed in order to assess its efficacy and safety with respect to standard ADHD pharmacological treatments.

P-015-250   Topic: 84, 36
Shortened latency and prolonged duration of transcallosally mediated motor inhibition in children with Attention Deficit Hyperactivity Disorder (ADHD) after medication with Methylphenidate (MPH)
Simone Henrike Weber, Rostock, Germany, simone_h_weber@gmx.de
Johannes Buchmann; Alex Wolters; Frank Häßler; Wolfgang Gierow

Objective: In a previous study we presented our findings of prolonged latency and reduced duration of the ipsilateral silent period (iSP) in ADHD children compared to control children [1]. Now we investigated latency and duration of iSP in children with ADHD before and after intake of methylphenidate (MPH). **Methods:** Using focal transcranial magnetic stimulation (MagStim Rapid 200, stimulation of left motor cortex, 100% stimulator output, target muscle: left

m. interosseus dorsalis I [ID-1], with standardized voluntary isometric contraction) we measured latency and duration of iSP. The 10 tested children with ADHD (9 male/1 female) had an average age of 130 months (130.2 ± 21.8). Diagnosis of ADHD was based on DSM-IV research criteria (hyperactive and combined type) and a Conners-Score (short form) of more than 15. The children took an average dose of 0.66106 mg/kg weight (SD: ± 0.31150 mg) of MPH. Neurophysiological investigation was repeated with children on medication at least on one week. **Results:** As principal clinical result MPH reduced the Conners Score of ADHD children significantly (21 ± 3.4 before MPH, after MPH 12 ± 6.3; p = 0.0001). Neurophysiologically, iSP latency was significantly shortened (mean: 41.2 msec, SD: ± 3.2 msec before MPH; after MPH $39,.2 \pm 2.8$ msec, p = 0,009) and its duration was significantly prolonged (14.8 ± 3.0 msec before MPH, after MPH 19.6 ± 4.1 msec, p = 0.007) after medication with MPH, with it approximately matching data obtained from control children in our previous study [1]. **Conclusion:** Prolongation of iSP-latency and reduction of iSP-duration in ADHD might be a result of a disturbed influence of transcallosally mediated inhibition on neuronal network between cortex layer III – the projection site of transcallosal motorcortical fibers – and layer V, the origin of the pyramidal tract [1]. MPH may improve the function of output neurons of transcallosal fibers and restore partially the supposed imbalance of this neuronal network. Literature: [1] J. Buchmann, A. Wolters, F. Haessler, S. Bohne, R. Nordbeck, and E. Kunesch, Disturbed transcallosally mediated motor inhibition in children with attention deficit hyperactivity disorder (ADHD). Clin Neurophysiol, 2003. 114(11): p. 2036–2042.

P-015-251   Topic: 84, 16
Atomoxetine treatment in children with Attention Deficit Hyperactivity Disorder (ADHD) and Comorbid Tic Disorders
Albert J. Allen, Eli Lilly and Company, Indianapolis, IN, USA, allenaj@lilly.com
Roger Kurlan; Donald Gilbert; David Dunn; F. Randy Sallee; Thomas Spencer

Objective: This study was designed to test the hypothesis that atomoxetine does not cause worsening of tic severity relative to placebo in children with attention-deficit/hyperactivity disorder (ADHD) and comorbid tic disorders. **Methods:** Study subjects were between 7 and 17 years old, met DSM-IV criteria for ADHD, and had concurrent Tourette Syndrome and/or chronic motor tic disorder. Patients were randomly assigned to double-blind treatment with placebo (n = 72) or atomoxetine (0.5–1.5 mg/kg/day, n = 76) for up to 18 weeks. **Results:** Atomoxetine treatment was associated with greater reduction of tic severity relative to placebo that approached significance on the Yale Global Tic Severity Scale (-5.5 ± 6.9 versus -3.0 ± 8.7, p = 0.063), and Tic Severity Self-Report (4.7 ± 6.5 versus -2.9 ± 5.2, p = 0.095) and achieved significance on the Clinical Global Impressions (CGI) tic/neurological severity scale (-0.7 ± 1.2 versus -0.1 ± 1.0, p = 0.002). Atomoxetine patients also showed significantly greater improvement on the Attention-Deficit/Hyperactivity Disorder Rating Scale total score (-10.9 ± 10.9 versus -4.9 ± 10.3, p = 0.002) and CGI severity of ADHD/psychiatric symptoms scale (-0.8 ± 1.1 versus -0.3 ± 1.0, p = 0.015). Atomoxetine patients had greater increases in heart rate ($+8.3 \pm 12.0$ versus -1.2 ± 12.7 bpm, p < 0.001) and decreases of body weight (-0.9 ± 1.9 versus $+1.6 \pm 2.3$ kg, p < 0.001), and rates of treatment-emergent decreased appetite and nausea were significantly higher. No other clinically relevant treatment differences were seen in any other vital sign or adverse event or electrocardiographic or laboratory parameters. **Conclusion:** Atomoxetine did not exacerbate tic symptoms. Rather, it appeared to decrease the severity of reported tics while reducing symptoms of ADHD. Treatment appeared to be safe and well tolerated. Research funded by Eli Lilly and Company, Indianapolis, Indiana, USA.

P-015-252   Topic: 84, 16
Atomoxetine's efficacy over time in children and adolescents with Attention Deficit Hyperactivity Disorder (ADHD)

Albert J. Allen, Eli Lilly and Company, Indianapolis, IN, USA, allenaj@lilly.com
Christine Thomason; Virginia Sutton; Denai Milton; Dustin Ruff

Objective: Atomoxetine has been shown to be efficacious for treating ADHD in children and adolescents. Onset of action is demonstrated in 1 to 2 weeks, and greater efficacy is evident beginning at 4 to 5 weeks. The pattern of treatment effect size over time across 5 trials is presented. **Methods:** Study design, except for dose administration, was similar across trials. Children and adolescents with ADHD were randomized into a 6- to 9-week, double-blind, placebo-controlled acute treatment period and received atomoxetine or placebo. Symptoms were assessed by the ADHD RS. Cohen's d was selected as the effect size statistic. **Results:** Nine hundred eighteen (918) children and adolescents were randomized (atomoxetine n = 560, placebo n = 358). Mean reductions in the ADHD RS total score were superior for patients randomized to atomoxetine compared to placebo ($p < 0.001$ in each study). Effect sizes from baseline to endpoint (LOCF) ranged from 0.6 to 0.8. For by-visit assessments, effect sizes at Week 1 ranged from 0.10 to 0.66 and at the final acute treatment visit ranged from 0.59 to 1.03. **Conclusion:** Response to atomoxetine increases with exposure to treatment, and may be more of a function of time.

P-016
Scientific disciplines/approaches V

P-016-253   Topic: 26, 40
Child psychiatric comorbidity in Danish 8–9-year old children

Dorthe Petersen, Odense University Hospital, Child & Adolescent Psychiatry, Odense C, Denmark, dorthe.petersen@ouh.fyns-amt.dk

Objective: Comorbidity is very common in child and adolescent psychiatry and in this study occurrence and patterns of comorbidity was examined. **Methods:** A two-step design was used with a parent questionnaire, the Child Behaviour Checklist (CBCL) in the first step. In second step was used a semistructured diagnostic interview, the Schedule for Affective Disorders and Schizophrenia for school-aged children, Present and Lifetime Version (K-SADA-PL), a global impairment scale, the Childrens Global Assessment Scale (C-GAS), and a cognitive test, the Wechsler Intelligence Scale for Children (WISC-III). A total of 751 was approached in the screening and a subsample of 188 was assessed further in the second step. The children was as-

sessed as a child psychiatric case according to the results from both the interview and the achieved C-GAS-score. **Results:** The average number of comorbid diagnoses in 61 children fulfilling criteria for caseness was 2.7 including the main diagnosis. The most frequent main diagnosis was Attention Deficit Hyperactivity Disorder (ADHD) (n = 24) and Pervasive Developmental Disorder (PDD) (n = 11). Seventy-five percent of children with ADHD and 82% of those with PDD had comorbid diagnoses. Thirty-three percent of children with ADHD as main diagnosis had Learning Disabilities (LD). **Conclusion:** The rate of comorbidity was high. Children with ADHD had comorbidity as found in other studies. LD and Developmental Coordination Disorder (DCD) was common in children with ADHD as expected from the literature. There was considerable comorbidity across Neuropsychiatric Disorders and Behavioural Disorders, LD, Emotional Disorders and Affective Disorders. There was a particularly high rate of comorbidity associated with PDD.

P-016-254   Topic: 26, 37
Danish standardization of the child behavior checklist for ages 1½–5 (CBCL/1½–5): Screening in a population based sample

Solvejg Kristensen, Odense University Hospital, Child & Adolescent Psychiatry, Odense, Denmark, solvejg.kristensen@ouh.fyns-amt.dk
Niels Bilenberg

Objective: This study was the first of a series of multi centre studies concerning validity and reliability of the CBCL/1½–5. The primary aim of the actual study was to assess parent and caregiver-reported behavior in a population-based sample of preschool children. **Methods:** Study information and the two checklists, Child Behavior Checklist (CBCL/1½–5) and Caregiver-Teacher Report Form (C-TRF) were mailed to 1250 families. For participating children prospective information on maternal characteristics, lifestyle factors and obstetric risk factors were available from the birth cohort at Aarhus University Hospital. The checklists have 100 items concerning aspects of behavioral, emotional and social functioning. Items are scored according to the categories; "Not True" = 0, "Somewhat or Sometimes True" = 1" or "Very True or Often True" = 2. Scores are obtained on a total problem scale and subscales. **Results:** A total number of 622 parents and 497 caregivers replied. Participation was equally distributed according to age and sex. Children with non-Danish background were underrepresented. Mean total problem score (TPS) of parent reported problems was 17.4 (16.3–18.6). In both sexes there was a decrease in TPS with increasing ages, in addition TPS was higher in boys than in girls. Children of Danish parents scored significantly lower than did children of non-Danish background ($p < 0.01$). Children of mothers who had smoked during pregnancy were rated significantly higher than children of non-smoking mothers ($p < 0.04$). Both parents and caregivers rated children using day care more than 35 hours per week significantly higher than children with a lesser need of day care ($p < 0.5$). **Conclusion:** In an easy and cost-effective way the CBCL/1½–5 enables users to obtain ratings and descriptive details of preschoolers. Until further clinical validation is obtained, the checklists can be used as a systematic way of collecting information about symptoms and psychopathology. A thorough validation of CBCL/1½–5 and C-TRF is going on in Denmark.

P-016-255   Topic: 26
Frequency of RLS symptoms in childhood

Jörg Kinkelbur, Gleichen, Germany,
joerg.kinkelbur@gmx.net
Juliane Hellwig; Martin Hellwig; Aribert Rothenberger;
Eckert Rüther

Objective: The prevalence of the restless legs syndrome (RLS) in adults is about 5–10%. Retrospec-tively, more than 30% of patients with RLS describe the onset of their symptoms before the age of 10 years. In fact, until now no studies have explicitly addressed epidemiological aspects of RLS in childhood. The prevalence of attention deficit hyperactivity disorder (ADHD), one of the major differential diagnosis of RLS in childhood, is about 4–6%. Piecchietti et al. (1998) demonstrated a frequency of 12% RLS among a sample of 69 children with ADHD. Generalizing these nonrepresentative data, a first estimation of RLS prevalence in children would be 0.5%. **Methods:** To further elucidate this topic, 1084 children (age 6–17 years) who presented sequentially in 12 paediatric practices were examined with an RLS questionnaire, additionally the mothers filled in the "strengths and difficulties questionnaire (SDQ)". The RLS questionnaire consisted of 9 questions regarding the severity of RLS symptoms according to established criteria. The symptom frequency (single and combined symptoms) was calculated. Further analyses were done for different age groups, boys and girls separated and in respect to associated psychopathology. **Results:** The frequency of RLS symptoms (seldom/frequent/most of the time, in %) was: Dysaesthesiae 14.5/3.1/0.4. Urge to move 21.1/13.2/4.7. Motor restlessness 19.5/13.9/4.6. Insomnia 24.6/15.0/9.0). When these symptoms were present, 55.8% of this children reported an alleviation by motor activity and 47.7% an aggravation by rest. Worsening of symptoms in the evening or at night was reported by 10.7%. The combination of dysaesthesiae, alleviation by motor activity and worsening in the evening was found in 14 (8 boys/6 girls) of 1084 children (1.3%). 6 (4 boys/2 girls) of these 14 children (43%) showed a pathologic SDQ score, compared with 12,8% in the whole sample of 1084 children. **Conclusion:** Our study examined the frequency of RLS symptoms in children, who visited a paediatric practice. This can be seen as a first step in the research of RLS epidemiology in children. The prevalence of single RLS symptoms in this sample was quite high; the frequency of the typical symptom combination was 1.3%. This reflects probably an estimate of RLS prevalence in childhood. The association with psychopathological abnormalities emphasizes the importance of the psychiatric differential diagnosis of children with RLS symptoms.

P-016-256   Topic: 26, 2
Depression, depressive and suicidal symptoms in adolescents in rural South Western Nigeria

Olayinka Omigbodun, University College Hospital,
Dept. of Psychiatry, Ibadan, Nigeria, 4yinkas@skannet.com
O. Esan; K. Bakare; B.O. Yusuf; F. Nuhu; A. Adesokan

Objective: To determine the prevalence of major depressive disorder and self reported depressive and suicidal symptoms in high school students in rural Southwest Nigeria. **Methods:** This study consisted of 484 randomly selected adolescents from two rural school districts in Southwestern Nigeria. Instruments used are the global school health questionnaire (GSHQ) and Youth DISC Predictive Scale (DPS). **Results:** There were 268 (55%) males and 212 (45%) females, with a mean age of 16.27 (SD: 2.33). 61 (12.6%) students met the criteria for major depressive disorder. On univariate analysis, factors associated with depression include polygamous home (2 = 3.4; p = 0.047: Fishers Exact Test), 'not living with grandparents' (2 = 7.011; p = 0.008), sexually active (2 = 4.55; p = 0.033), 'going hungry due to a lack of food at home' (2 = 11.547; p = 0.001), and 'physically attacked in the last year' (2 = 20.237; p < 0.001). On logistic regression, not living with grandparents and physical attack were retained as significant. In order of increasing frequency, depression symptoms ranged from 'tried to kill self' {49 (10.1%)}, 'thought seriously about killing self' {117 (24.2), 'feels cannot do anything well' {141 (29.1%); 'not interested in anything' {160 (33.1%)}, 'not thinking clearly' {169 (34.9)}, 'less energy than usual' {180 (37.2%)} and 'little things make feel tired' {185 (38.2%)}. All the individual depressive symptoms were significantly associated with 'physical attack' while 'going hungry' was associated with all symptoms except 'tried to kill self'. Sexual activity was associated with 'lack of interest', 'low energy' and thoughts of suicide. Having divorced parents was associated with 'thoughts of killing self'. **Conclusion:** This study reveals that depression, depressive symptoms and suicidal behaviour are prevalent among adolescents in rural Southwest Nigeria. Adolescents who have suffered physical violence, frequent hunger and who are sexually active need particular attention.

P-016-257   Topic: 25, 22
Evaluation of a training for doctor-child-parent communication

Marie Kopecky-Wenzel, Med. Universität München,
Inst. für Kinderpsychiatrie, München, Germany,
maru.kopecky-wenzel@med.uni-muenchen.de
Reiner Frank

Objective: We report on the long-term evaluation of a training course in communication skills for pediatricians in family consultations regarding the triad between doctor, mother and child. The aim of the training is an improvement of basic care of children. **Methods:** The course comprises 18 training hours in three sessions, four weeks apart, and a final meeting two months after. We offered a second version with a shorter duration. By means of videotaped role-plays of 5 minutes duration the physicians are expected to develop a sense of different partners in a more-than-one person consultation. They play different roles from own examples of consultations perceived as difficult, such as having discussions with demanding parents. The facilitators give a supportive feedback by analyzing the videotapes. The participants of three courses (n = 26) assessed the usefulness two months and ten months after the end of the training. **Results:** The course is well accepted by the physicians. Playing every role of child and parents gives doctors insights into the feelings of their patients. Feedback by video analysis of role-plays is the component regarded as most effective. Compared to the baseline an important immediate result is the improvement regarding sense of security of participants in consultations. Long-term assessments show a measurable effect even in the long-term range. **Conclusion:** Feedback from colleagues and facilitators can help bring about a change in attitude and behaviour. To incorporate communication skills in everyday work may be difficult and takes time. The participants regard the training after ten months still as useful for the work. But they wish to continue the course once a year on an ongoing basis.

P-016-258 Topic: 27, 59
Converting the Dutch version of the NIMH DISC IV into an internet version: Pilot study
Mark-Peter Steenhuis, Accare, Child and adolescent psychiatry, Groningen, Netherlands, m.p.steenhuis@accare.nl
Ruud Minderaa

Objective: Large epidemiological studies require cost-effective screening instruments. For this and other purposes the National Institute of Mental Health Diagnostic Interview Schedule for Children (NIMH DISC) was developed. Current version is the DISC IV. The NIMH DISC is strongly based on the DSM IV and the ICD-10. The NIMH DISC is a highly structured interview and can be adminstered by interviewers after a minimal training period. The questions in the DISC are short and simple. The DISC has 358 "stem" questions. There are almost 1300 "contingent" questions that are asked if a stem or previous question has been answered positively (Shaffer, Fisher, Lucas et al, 2000). One of the new DISC versions is the "VOICE DISC". The Voice DISC is a self-administration version using a computer with headphones or speakers. In the West of Scotland study (West, Sweeting, Barton, et al., 2003) the Voice DISC was used 1860 times, 97% completed the entire Voice DISC. Why not try an internet version? The internet is an interactive medium and perfect for collecting data. The Netherlands has more than 9.7 million internet connections, 65% of the population and this is still rising fast (world factbook 2002). The internet DISC will focus on the parent version first. The child version will be build later. The objectives of the pilot are [a] what do parents think of the internet version? [b] To compare the internet version with the oral interview version. **Methods:** There is a complete Dutch version of the DISC IV, the internet-DISC uses this text unchanged. For the internet version of the DISC a private website is created and the technology used is a web-based database and "server sided scripting". This latter method means that all the "decisions" are made at the server side. The only thing which is send through the internet is the text of the next question and the response of the parent. The entire DISC is at maximum 2800 questions long and for practical reasons and avoiding mistakes each question is a very short script. The interview DISC has separate modules and the website has it too. It is possible for the researchers to skip some modules like "drugs". Each question is immediately stored in the datase on the server, therefore a parent can fill out the internet DISC in multiple sessions. The University Center for Child and Adolescent Psychiatry (www.accare.nl) has about 1500 new outpatients each year and the DISC IV classification is a very welcome screening method or diagnostic method. Parents will be asked to participate in the pilot study and will be randomly selected into two conditions; [condition 1] first the interview version and a few days later the internet version. [condition 2] First the internet version and a few days later the interview version. **Results:** The internet DISC is in a test period. The pilot study will be started in july 2004. So far the technical part is functioning correctly. **Conclusion:** Hopefully the first results will be presented on the final version of the poster in Berlin 2004.

P-016-259 Topic: 27
Typical syndromes in girls with severe antisocial problems
Marie-Louise Körlof, Statens Institutionsstryreske, Research and Development, Stockholm, Sweden, mia.korlof@stat-inst.se
Margit Wångby; Lars R. Bergman

Objective: The development of severe antisocial adjustment problems in girls was long a neglected area. Even today much more is known about this type of problems in boys than in girls. The aim of the present study, which is still in progress, is to identify typical patterns of adjustment problems in girls with severe antisocial problems. **Methods:** A person-oriented approach is applied, with a focus on syndromes of problems in the individual. **Results:** A broad array of problems is hereby considered, including alcohol and drug abuse, criminality, psychological health and somatic complaints. Data are taken from a unique data base at the Swedish National Board of Institutional Care, which includes data from all girls who have been admitted to specially approved institutions in accordance with the Swedish Care of Young Persons Act (LVU) since 1997. The girls were interviewed at intake with the Adolescent Drug Abuse Diagnosis (ADAD). **Conclusion:** The data base covers almost the entire population of Swedish girls with the most severe antisocial problems.

P-016-260 Topic: 25
Comparative study of self-concept of school-age children in urban and rural areas
Xueping Gao, Central South University, Dept. of Child Psychiatry, Changsha, China, xuepinggao@hotmail.com
Suwei Yu; Linyan Su

Objective: To compare the difference of self-concept of school-age children in urban and rural areas. **Methods:** 842 students (aged 8–17 years old) were measured with Piers-Harris Children's self-concept Scale. **Results:** The factors "behavior" and "anxious" scores in country group were significantly higher than that of city group ($p < 0.01$). The scores on factors such as "behavior", "intelligence" and "self-body image and sexual identification" were relative to educational degrees of their parents. **Conclusion:** The school-age children in city in this sample considered that they had more "inconsiderable" behavior and emotional problems; Moreover, the difference of educational degrees of parents also influence their behavior, intelligence and self-body identification.

P-016-261 Topic: 27, 52
Classifying aggressive behaviour with latent class approaches
Ferdinand Keller, Universitätsklinik Ulm, Kinder- und Jugendpsychiatrie, Ulm, Germany, ferdinand.keller@medizin.uni-ulm.de
Klaus Schmeck

Objective: Aggressive behaviour can be differentiated in various subtypes according to clinical experience and to results of factor analytic studies. Probabilistic methods like latent class approaches have only rarely been used up to now. We use this approach to classify symptom patterns of aggressive behaviour in a large clinical sample. **Methods:**

The sample consisted of CBCL ratings of 3503 child and adolescent psychiatric patients (age 4–18; 2405 boys, 1098 girls). Two core items of each of the CBCL scales "aggressive behaviour", "delinquent behaviour", "attention problems" and "anxious/depressed" were used for classifying subtypes of aggressive behaviour. Latent class analyses were performed with the latent cluster option of Latent-GOLD 3.0. **Results:** According to Best Information Criterion (BIC), a solution with six latent classes was suggested. Inspection of the profile plots revealed that there were three types of symptom patterns, each with two different degrees of severity. These were one type "aggressive/delinquent/impulsive" (26%), a second type "hyperactive" with only a modest degree of aggressive behaviour (38%) and a third type "sad/anxious" without aggressive behaviour (36%). The more severe form of type one consists of about 5% of this clinical sample which is close to the prevalence of severe antisocial behaviour in the general adolescent population. Inclusion of the variable sex as an inactive covariate showed that the two aggressive subgroups have a 85:15 ratio (boys:girls). **Conclusion:** The use of latent class analysis reveals clinically meaningful results that we are going to further differentiate with more advanced probabilistic models (e.g., latent factor analysis).

P-016-262   Topic: 26, 25
Military fitness class of Finnish 18-year-old men: Prediction of military fitness class at call-up with the YASR and sociodemographic factors

Petteri Multimäki, Turku, Finland, petteri.multimaki@ecd.fi
Kai Parkkola; Andre Sourander; Georgios Nikolakaros; Hans Helenius

Objective: To examine psychosocial factors associated with military fitness class, classified as capability of service, vs. temporary or permanent exemption from service. **Methods:** Participants were 2,340 (80% of the original sample) Finnish 18-year-old men at call-up for obligatory military service who filled in the Young Adult Self-Report (the YASR) questionnaire. **Results:** Temporary exemption from military service was independently associated with the YASR total problem score, externalizing and internalizing problems, excessive alcohol use, drug use, problems with peers and family, and mental health service use. Permanent exemption was independently associated with problems with peers and family. **Conclusion:** The YASR is a potential selection tool to be used at call-up. Temporary exemption was more strongly associated with psychosocial problems than permanent exemption. Because of the high level of psychological problems among those temporarily exempted, the call-up situation offers a unique opportunity to identify those with problem behaviour and risk of marginalization. Key words: military psychiatry, personnel selection, questionnaires.

P-016-263   Topic: 26, 70
Depressive symptoms in preadolescents and adolescents in Funchal (Madeira Island/Portugal): A prevalence study

Carina Freitas, Hospital Dona Estefânia, Lisboa, Portugal, carinafreitas@mail.com
Assunção Rocha; Lídia Pocinho; Pedro Caldeira da Silva

Objective: The aim of this study is to estimate the prevalence of depressive symptoms in preadolescents and adolescents who attend 7th, 8th and 9th grades in 2003/2004 at state and private schools of Funchal. **Methods:** From a target population consisting of 4787 subjects: boys and girls, aged 11 to 17 years, a sample of 741 was randomly selected and stratified by school years (7th, 8th and 9th grades). To these, it was given a Portuguese version of Children Depression Inventory (CDI). The CDI, devised by Kovacs, is a self rating scale used for the assessment of depressive symptomatology in children. It consists of 27 items. Total scores range from 0 to 54. Kovacs indicates a 19 point cut-off as the ideal thresold discriminating children at risk of depression from non depressed children. After a written consent to participate in the study from parents, this questionnaire was given by teachers and school psychologists in classroom. **Results:** Results will estimate depressive symptoms prevalence. We expect that it will range from 5 to 20%, as reported by other epidemiological studies that used self report measures of depressive symptoms such as CDI. **Conclusion:** Results will enable the planning for the provision of care services for those at risk. Further investigations will be helpful to identify which of the children considered at risk of depression are really depressed.

P-016-264   Topic: 25, 26
A statistical study of new outpatients at a Japanese child and adolescent psychiatric hospital

Shinichi Arai, Tokyo Umegaoka Hospital, Dept. of Psychiatry, Tokyo, Japan, onmyouji@k05.itscom.net
Hironobu Ichikawa; Ikuko Hirosawa

Objective: Tokyo metropolitan Umegaoka hospital is one of the largest hospitals for child and adolescent patients with mental disorder in Japan. We studied the data of outpatients in order to clarify the clinical feature and trend of patients with mental disorder in Japan. **Methods:** We surveyed new outpatients visited us since April of 1992 until March of 2002. We examined each item (sex, age, chief complaint, diagnosis (by ICD-10), reference route, family history, past history, etc.). **Results:** Total number of new outpatients under 20 years old in 10 years was 10536 (female: 3600, male: 6936). The number of new outpatients increased gradually, especially in preschool age and primary school age. The patients diagnosed pervasive developmental disorder and hyperkinetic disorder increased, respectively in male. **Conclusion:** The class of child & adolescent patients visited our hospital was increasing and changing. So we concluded that we are needed to modify the service of our hospital.

P-016-265   Topic: 25
A clinical database in child and adolescent psychiatry

Niels Bilenberg, Odense University Hospital, Child & Adolescent Psychiatry, Odense C, Denmark, niels.bilenberg@ouh.fyns-amt.dk

Objective: In Denmark, hospital-based child and adolescent mental health services (CAMHS) have a total of about 8,000 referrals per year. In order to improve and evaluate assessment and treatment, an internet-based database is in process of implementation nationwide. **Methods:** For every single patient referred, a number of variables are registered at referral (t0), at the first meting with the patient and family (t1), and at the end of treatment or after six months (t2). As measures of change in symptom load the "Health of the Nation Outcome Scale for Children and Adolescent" (HoNOSCA) are completed at t1 and t2. In field trials, the sensitivity to change of HoNOSCA in comparison with a clinician rated global outcome measure and the clinical feasibility of HoNOSCA were evaluated. **Results:** A total of 173 patients were rated both at initial assessment and at follow-up. There was a highly significant association (ANOVA (F=25.4, P<0.001)) between change in HoNOSCA scores and global clinical ratings of change. Mean HoNOSCA scores varied between psychiatric diagnoses. **Conclusion:** Clinical databases and evidence based treatment are matters of great interest. HoNOSCA is a feasible, sensitive and valid measure of change in symptom load for children and adolescents attending CAMHS. We look forward to be able to present large-scale clinical outcome results in the future.

P-016-266   Topic: 24, 25

Poverty, home environment and social and academic adjustment in urban adolescents

María Elena Márquez-Caraveo, Child Psychiatric Hospital, Research Division, Mexico, marquezmalena@hotmail.com
Verónica Pérez-Barrón

Objective: To explore social competence and academic achievement as adolescent outcomes and their relation to proximal and distal contextual variables such as adolescent's perception of child rearing practices, home environment and socioeconomic status. **Methods:** Participants will be 100 preadolescents, and adolescents and their mothers living in Mexico City. After an informed consent is obtained, a school and a home visit will be done. Instruments will include: child's grade-average for academic achievement, and the sociogram for measurement of social competence. Adolescent's perception of child-rearing practices will be evaluated with the Child-rearing perception's scale (Jiménez-Ambriz, 2001), and the EA-HOME-SF (Bradley, 2001) will evaluate cognitive stimulation, emotional support and discipline at home. A questionaire taken from he National Register (INEGI) will inform about the socioeconomic status of these families on a multiple-indicator basis. A first exploratory study will confirm the psychometric viability of the EA-HOME-SF as a home environment measure for mexican adolescents. **Results:** Description of variables will include means and standard deviations. Data will have a process of validation through factor analysis and Cronbach's alpha. A bivariate correlation and a matrix correlation of all variables will be included. **Conclusion:** Preliminary analysis will confirm that competent conduct in school is a developmental outcome related to proximal and distal variables. Findings will be presented according to Developmental psychopathology as a framework for better understanding adolescent development under a perspective systems view. Implications for policy and intervention will be discussed.

P-016-267   Topic: 27, 40

DSM-IV or ICD-10 diagnoses in child and adolescent psychiatry – does it matter?

Merete Juul Sørensen, Child Psychiatric Hospital, Research Dept., Risskov, Denmark, mjs@buh.aaa.dk
Ole Mors; Per Hove Thomsen

Objective: While the DSM-IV is the most widely used diagnostic classification system in research the ICD-10 is more widely used in clinical diagnostic practise. Knowledge of discrepancies is essential when results from research are

implemented in daily clinical practise. The aim of this study was to determine the clinical importance of differences between the two diagnostic systems regarding three major child psychiatric diagnostic categories: major depressive disorder (MDD), attention deficit hyperactivity disorder (ADHD) and oppositional defiant disorder (ODD). **Methods:** One hundred ninety-nine consecutive child psychiatric patients were interviewed using a semi-structured diagnostic interview (K-SADS-PL) and additional questions covering specific ICD-10 criteria. The children were diagnosed according to both diagnostic systems and discrepancies described. **Results:** Disagreement between the diagnostic systems was analysed using strict diagnostic criteria. Disagreement was found in seven out of 27 cases (25.9%) regarding MDD. Four cases were diagnosed with MDD according to DSM-IV but not according to ICD-10, due to the demand of two core symptoms in ICD-10. Three cases were diagnosed with MDD according to ICD-10 but not according to DSM-IV, because only four depressive symptoms are necessary in ICD-10. Disagreement was found in 18 out of 70 cases (25.7%) regarding ADHD. Seventeen cases were diagnosed with ADHD primarily hyperactive/impulsive according to DSM-IV. This diagnosis is not available in ICD-10. Fifty-one children were diagnosed with ODD according to ICD-10. Of these children 50 also had a DSM-IV diagnosis of ODD. There was no effect of age or gender on the discrepancy. **Conclusion:** The disagreement between DSM-IV and ICD-10 regarding MDD and ADHD is extensive. DSM-IV includes more children in both MDD and ADHD categories. This must be taken into consideration when implementing results from DSM-IV studies in clinics using ICD-10 diagnostic criteria. The diagnosis ODD appears interchangeable between the two diagnostic systems.

P-016-268   Topic: 24

Associations between self- and other-reported psychopathological symptoms and peer relationships in kindergarten children

Kai von Klitzing, Universität Basel,
Kinder- und Jugendpsychiatrie, Basel, Switzerland,
kai.vonklitzing@unibas.ch
Sonja Perren; Agnes von Wyl; Dieter Bürgin

Objective: There is a clearly established link between peer relationship problems – such as victimisation or peer rejection – and the development of psychopathology. The quality of peer relations may be considered as indicator or result of emotional/psychopathological problems but also – in more complex models – as being a resource or a risk factor for children's well-being and mental health. Studies among school age children showed that internalising and externalising symptoms can be risk factors for peer rejection and victimisation. Until now, no study addressed this issue in kindergarten children. Our study among 4–6-year-old children from 16 kindergarten classes investigated the association between peer relationships and self- and other-reported psychopathological symptoms. **Methods:** All children of the kindergarten class (N=183) completed a peer nomination task on liking and disliking (peer rejection and popularity). Children also nominated their best friends and playmates. Children who were the first year in kindergarten (N=98) were interviewed using the symptoms and social scales of the Berkeley Puppet Interview (BPI, Measelle & Ablow). Moreover, parents and teachers completed the Strengths and Difficulties Questionnaire (SDQ, Goodman). In addition, teachers completed a questionnaire on bullying and victimisation. **Results:** Self-, parent- and teacher-reported psychopathological symptoms were associated with peer rejection and victimisation. Children with behavioural or emotional difficulties were disliked by their peers, had fewer friends and were frequently victimised. However, having a close friend served as a protective factor against peer victimisation. **Conclusion:** Our results showed that considering the quality of peer relationships as possible indicator or risk factor of psychopathological symptoms may contribute to a more holistic view of children's mental health. Furthermore, friendships seem to be important already in kindergarten children. Promoting close relationships with one or more peers may not only protect children from victimisation but may also increase children's well-being.

P-016-269   Topic: 25, 56
The relationship between hyperactive-impulsive behavior in children and parental rearing patterns

Xueping Gao, Central South University, Dept. of Child Psychiatry, Changsha, China, xuepinggao@hotmail.com
Linyan Su

Objective: To examine the relationship of hyperactive/impulsive behavior in children and parental rearing patterns. **Methods:** Hyperactive/impulsive group (n=47) and normal controls (n=795, aged 8~17 years old) were measured with Parent Symptom Questionnaire (PSQ) and Egna Minnen AV Barndoms Uppfostran (EMBU). **Results:** The factor "affect warmth" scores for the father and mother scale of EMBU in hyperactive/impulsive group were significantly lower than that of control group. The scores on factors such as "publishment", "refusal" of father and mother scale of EMBU in Hyperactive/impulsive group were found significantly higher than that of control group (p<0.01). Logistic analysis showed that the factors "publishment" of father and "affect warmth" of mother were affected to hyperactive/impulsive behavior in children. **Conclusion:** Parents of children with hyperactive/impulsive behavior have had rearing patterns, which may be one reason of causing hyperactive/impulsive behavior.

P-016-270   Topic: 26, 58
Psychiatric morbidity of the Early Primary School children in Korea: Using Korean version of K-SADS-PL

Han-Ik Yoo, Asan Medical Center, Dept. of Psychiatry, Seoul, Republic of Korea, hanny1@chol.com
Boong-Nyun Kim; Min-Sup Shin; Soo-Churl Cho; Kang E. Hong

Objective: This study aimed to identify the actual mental conditions of Korean early school children using objective diagnostic interview tool and to utilize these data for the objective and fundamental data equipment of childhood mental health. These outcomes can be useful for setting prevention and intervention plans for improving the elementary school mental heath in Korea. **Methods:** Data from 6,959 2nd and 3rd grade-schoolers were drawn from 28 elementary schools. Screening assessments using child problem-behavior screening test (28-items) 2) and K-CBCL, diagnostic individual interviews with K-SADS-PL-K were performed. All statistical analyses were carried out using SPSS 11.0 for Windows. **Results:** The psychiatric prevalence of 5,118 subjects in our study was 4.12%. And the prevalence of externalizing disorders, internalizing dis-

orders, neurotic disorders and developmental disorders were 2.17%, 0.73%, 0.81%, and 0.39% respectively. Boys were made 2.56 times more psychiatric diagnoses than girls and 34.4% of morbid juveniles were concluded as having comorbid psychiatric disorders concurrently. **Conclusion:** We could confirm that the prevalence rate of psychiatric disorders of Korean early elementary school children was similar to other countries.

P-016-271   Topic: 24, 26
Prevalence of emotional and behavioral disorders in children and adolescents in Germany: A systematic literature review

Claus Barkmann, UKE Hamburg-Eppendorf, Kinder- u. Jugendpsychosomatik, Hamburg, Germany, barkmann@uke.uni-hamburg.de
Michael Schulte-Markwort

Objective: Methods and results from empirical research carried out so far on the prevalence of psychopathology in children and adolescents in Germany are presented. **Methods:** The relevant studies (n=29) identified by systematic literature search are presented and compared in table form on the basis of important epidemiological key factors, and a descriptive analysis is provided. **Results:** The prevalence of emotional and behavioral disorders is 17.2±5.07% (M±SD). Determination of the prevalence rates is influenced by the study methods used. The results presented here do not indicate an increase or decrease in the prevalence of psychopathology in childhood and adolescence over the past decades. **Conclusion:** The results are discussed with respect to study quality, also in an international context, and recommendations are made for standardization of future studies.

P-016-272   Topic: 26
Pattern of referral and frequency of different disorders at a child psychiatric clinic at a university hospital in Pakistan

Ehsan Syed, Aga Khan University, Dept. of Psychiatry, Karachi, Pakistan, ehsan.syed@aku.edu
Sobia Haqqi

Objective: Child Psychiatry in Pakistan remains at its rudimentary stage.In a country of over 140 million people there is not a single child psychiatric ward, unit, department or clinic which could cater to the psychiatric needs of children exclusively. Children are mostly seen by either adult psychiatrist or paediatricians even at large tertiary care hospitals. Recently a child psychiatric clinic was setup at Aga Khan Univesity Hospital for children up to the age of 15 years, under the supervision of a child psychiatrist. The following presentation looks at the demographic, diagnostic and other profile of all the children referred to this clinic over a period of one year. **Methods:** All children (n=135) referred to the clinic in a one year period were included in this study. Data regarding their demographic characterstics, psychiatric history, sources of referral, diagnoses and treatment was collected and then analysed using SPSS 10.0. **Results:** Our data showed that majoity of our referrals were in the 6–10 age group (43.7%) and were mostly boys (69.6%). Academically 45.9% were at the primary school level i.e. class 1 to 5. 43% of fathers were professionals and 60% mothers were housewives and 85% of children belonged to married couples. The most frequent diagnosis overall was ADHD (26.7%)and depression at 11.9% was at second place. A whole spectrum of disorders was found including OCD, Autism and PDD, Developmental delays including Speech Delay (19.3%) and other mental retardation etc. Physical abuse was reported in 5.2% and vebal abuse in 7.4% of the cases with sexual abuse in only 1 case (0.7%). The medications most commonly pescribed were from the anti depressant group (TCAs & SSRIs) with Stimulants to follow. **Conclusion:** Our data is an initial attempt to find out some basic facts about our child psychiatric population. It does not indicate the pattern in our society but gives us some crude estimates of our clinical population. We thought that it was interesting that ADHD remains the commonest presentation to our clinic in Pakistan as is else where in the world.

P-016-273   Topic: 24
Psychological diagnosis as system-forming component of the work of the clinical psychologist

Michail Semago, University of Moscow, Dept. of Education, Moscow, Russia, intpsychol@mail.ru

Objective: The model of the analysis of development is examined, in basis of which the "concept-based components" (CBC) of psychical development is included. On the basis of the formed pattern within the framework of the proposed model is created the exceptionally psychological classification of the disontogeny. Thus the built psychological diagnosis becomes a system-forming component as diagnostic, so the psychologist's correction – determines the area of his activity. **Methods:** The system model of the child's development was proposed, called "three-component model of the analysis of development". The basis of model is the ideas about the main structural units of psyche, main components of child's psychical development. The CBC include: (1) the arbitrary regulation of mental activity; (2) spatial conception; (3) base affective regulation. **Results:** All three analyzed components possess the multilevel vertically organized structure. Analysis of the child's development from the point of view of this model, will made possible the development of the original psychological typology of the disontogeny. For each of the types is the specific pattern of CBC. The use of typology makes it possible to determine the meaningful sphere of action of psychologist. Isolation of the most essential indices of the mental development of child for each type, it is fixed in the name of this version, which gives the possibility to consider as it's psychological diagnosis. **Conclusion:** The use of the concept of base components (CBC) of development, for their formation and interrelations makes possible to create the original periodical system of child's development, to determine the main moments of development, to build the effective assistance for different kind of children.

P-016-274   Topic: 26, 38
Epidemiological study of child mental health in Lithuania: Overview of the screening phase

Sigita Lesinskiene, Vilnius University, Dept. of Clinic of Psychiatry, Vilnius, Lithuania, sigita.lesinskiene@vrc.vu.lt
Sigita Girdzijauskiene; Dainius Puras; Grazina Gintiliene; Dovile Cerniauskaite

Objective: The aim of the study is to assess prevalence of symptoms and disorders, functional impact, psychosocial background, service use. **Methods:** Study consist of two

stages: screening and clinical. The first stage consisted of a Stengths and Difficulties Questionnaire (SDQ, Goodman) and psychosocial background questionnaire for parents and teachers developed by the authors. In the second stage parents of all screen-positive and some screen-negative children will be invited to a structured interview (DAWBA, Goodman). **Results:** First stage of the first epidemiological survey of child mental health in our country is finished.Representing sample was randomly selected according 3 demographic characteristics: age, gender and living place. Questionnaires for 3334 children (1711 boys and 1623 girls) were distributed. Children aged 7–16 years old in selected classes of 15 urban, 10 town and 22 rural scools throughout the country were investigated. 3100 parents (93%) and 3319 teachers (99.6%) of children aged 7–16 years old filled in the questionnaires. 1987 (1017 boys and 970 girls) children aged 11–16 years filled in SDQ form for children. Data about 1854 children (921 boys and 933 girls) were obtained from all three sources of informants: parents, teachers, children. Parents of 78 children noticed that their child has diagnosed emotional or behavioral disorder. Lithuanian translation of SDQ was adapted for clinical use, SDQ norms, reliability and validity were calculated. More detailed analysis of the results will be presented. **Conclusion:** A high participation rate of teachers and parents was obtained in this epidemiological study. There was a relationship between emotional and behavioral symptoms of children and psychosocial risc factors in their families.

P-016-275   Topic: 24, 30
Outpatient diagnostic special service for preschool children with behaviour and/or developmental disorders

Christiane Bormann-Kischkel, Kinder- und Jugendpsychiatrie, Tagklinik, Regensburg, Germany, christiane.bormann@medbo.de
Rosemarie Schmoetzer; Diana Frischholz; Martin Linder

Objective: To present the aims, structure and methods of a special diagnostic service for preschool children with behavioural and/or developmental disorders in a group setting. **Methods:** Case descriptions of typical patients including diagnoses, therapeutic and psychosocial recommendations will be presented. **Results:** The issues raised by the patients ranged from psychosocial interventions, parent counselling and training, counselling other professionals to neuropsychiatric diagnostics. The full range of child psychiatric topics was evident. **Conclusion:** This setting provides intensive information on different aspects of children's problems. Observations in group settings and everyday situations add to information from standardized tests and thus help in a) seeing the entire child with his/her needs, b) providing appropriate counselling. Given the importance of early diagnosis and early intervention as well as prevention for many child psychiatric disorders the special service provides an appropriate format for children with special challenges.

P-016-276   Topic: 24, 42

Mental, motor and behavioral development of very low birthweight infants (<1500 g) at a corrected age of three years

Catharina Ganseforth, Universität zu Köln, Frauenklinik, Köln, Germany, cganseforth@web.de
Daniela Rödder; Angela Kribs; Frank Pillekamp; Alexander von Gontard; Bernhard Roth

Objective: Improved survival rates of very low birthweight (VLBW) infants have focused interest on the outcome of these infants. The objective of this study was to give a current picture of mental, motor and behavioral development of these high-risk infants in comparison to a full term control group at three years of age. **Methods:** Of 113 VLBW infants, born in 1999 in the NICU, Clinics of the University of Cologne, 85 consecutive infants were recruited in a prospective longitudinal study. 79 (92.9%) were seen for testing at a corrected age of three years and were compared with a control group of 23 full terms, born in 2000 at the same clinic. 72 (84.7%) were examined with the "Bayley-Scales of Infant Development-II" (BSID-II). **Results:** The mean gestational age of the preterms was $28+4$ $(23+3-34+1)$, the mean birthweight was 1028 g (380 1480), those of the controls $39+3$ $(37+0-42+0)$ and 3379 g (2400–4130). 54.4% of the preterms were girls (controls: 52.2%), 45.6% boys (controls: 47.8%), 44.3% were multiples (controls: 34.8%), 55.7% were singletons (controls: 65.2%). Sociodemographic data were comparable except for a higher educational level and only families of German nationality in the control group. On mental development 12% of the preterms were significantly and 6.7% mildly delayed (controls: 0% delayed). On motor development 16% significantly and 17.3% mildly delayed (controls: 0% significantly, 4.3% mildly). For behavior rating scale 9.9% of the preterms were classified as non-optimal and 21.1% als questionable (controls: 0% non-optimal, 21.7% questionable). **Conclusion:** Although there are improvements of postnatal care in the last decade VLBW infants are still at higher risk for developmental delays and need special aftercare.

P-016-277   Topic: 25, 47

Parental perception and attitude toward their primary school age children's hyperactivity problems

Tjhin Wiguna, University of Indonesia, Dept. of Psychiatry, Cengkareng, Jakarta-Barat, Indonesia, twigi00@yahoo.com

Objective: To explore how did parents perceived and their attitudinal reactions toward their primary school age children who were perceived as having hyperactivity problems by their class teacher, in terms of assessing the awareness of this issue in the community. **Methods:** This was a descriptive-qualitative study with cross sectional design. Class teachers using the Abbreviated Connors' Teacher/ Parent Rating Scale (ACTRS) randomly screened 600 students (grade one to three) from 30 elementary schools through out Central Jakarta. Parent of students with hyperactivity problem (defined by the class teacher's perception on the ACTRS score above or similar to 12) will be randomly in-depth interviewed. Interview will be done by using a questionnaire, which was made for this study. Socio-economic data was also obtained in this study. **Results:** In this study, by using randomization, we interviewed 20 parents. Most of parents (92 percent) in this study had a

negative perception, reactions and attitude toward their primary school children's hyperactivity problems. There was a clear difference in attitude toward their children from parents whose came from high education and socioeconomic level. They were more aware and positively approach toward their children's hyperactivity behavior. Consequently, they were more straightforward in acceptance our information according to their children hyperactivity problems, but they were more reluctant in receiving our suggestion for the treatment. **Conclusion:** Parental perception and attitude regarding their primary school children's hyperactivity problems were very awful. Developing and creating awareness program for parents, teachers, and others professionals is a must, in order to detect and to manage this kind of children as early as possible.

P-016-278   Topic: 25, 63

Working with primary care

Cristina Maria Ribeiro Marques, Hospital Dona Estefânia, Barcarena, Portugal, mmaiaesi@jnjpt.jnj.com
Teresa Goldschmidt; Teresa Cepeda

Objective: The authors are developing a child and adolescent Mental Health Training Programme for Primary Care staff. This was initiated in order to fulfil a need felt by Primary Care staff in acquiring skills in the appropriate assessment, management and referral of children and adolescents with mental health problems. Child psychiatrists are also eager for a more effective collaboration of Primary Care as partners in a joint intervention. Nevertheless and although many feel this need, only a reduced number of staff (GPs included) does in fact attend the child mental health training programmes implemented so far. A questionnaire was then created by the authors and applied in several Community Health Centres with the aim of evaluating training needs so that successful training programmes may be implemented in future. **Methods:** Questionnaires were distributed to 200 Primary Care staff (GPs, nurses, social workers, psychologists) from several Community Health Centres throughout the country. The questionnaire evaluates areas such as: confidence on dealing with children and adolescents suffering from mental health problems, symptoms more frequently found, main difficulties, type of training programmes and specific training needs, availability for different training programmes. **Results:** Data on the several areas mentioned above were statistically analysed with the purpose of creating a cost effective training programme. Questionnaire results on main difficulties, training needs, availability and subject's suggestions were especially accounted for. **Conclusion:** Primary Care staff's training in Mental Health issues is of an unquestionable importance but training programmes should be planned according to staff's objective needs in order to be successful.

P-016-279   Topic: 24, 82

Language development of very low birthweight preterms (<1500 g) at a corrected age of three years

Daniela Rödder, Universität zu Köln, Kinderpsychiatrie, Köln, Germany, droedder@web.de
Catharina Ganseforth; Angela Kribs; Frank Pillekamp; Alexander von Gontard; Bernhard Roth

Objective: Improvements in neonatal care have been associated with decreased mortality, and the focus now has shifted to concern with developmental outcome. Very low birthweight (VLBW) preterms have been consistently identified as deficient in receptive and expressive language as in speech abilities, especially during preschool years. The objective of this study was to investigate language comprehension and production of VLBW preterms in comparison to a control group of term born infants at 3 years of age. **Methods:** Of 113 VLBW preterms, born in 1999 and treated in the NICU, Children's Hospital, University of Cologne, 85 infants could be recruited consecutively in a prospective longitudinal study. At a corrected age of 3 years 79 were seen. They were compared with a control group of 23 three-year-old term born infants, born at the same Hospital (Department of Gynecology and Obstectrics, Faculty of Medicine, University of Cologne). All 102 infants were examined with the 'Sprachentwicklungstest für zweijährige Kinder' (SETK-2) and the 'Reynell Developmental Language Scales III' (RDLS-III). A complete language assessment was possible in all term born and in 41 preterm infants, partly possible in 31 preterms, and impossible in 7 of the preterm infants. 6 preterms were not able to be tested because of major neurological disabilities (e.g. cerebral palsy, severe visual and hearing impairment). **Results:** Results showed that VLBW preterms in comparison with term born infants were significantly delayed in receptive as well as in expressive language development. Regarding the severity of language delay receptive language was below the average for one fourth and expressive language even for more than half of the VLBW infants. **Conclusion:** In Conclusion one can say that VLBW preterms are at greater risk for a delay in language development especially a delay in language production and thus are at greater risk for later developmental problems.

P-016-280   Topic: 26, 84

Symptoms of inattention and hyperactivity in habitual snorers vs. controls in primary school children: Evidence from an epidemiological study in Istanbul

Ayse Arman, Marmara University, Dept. of Child Psychiatry, Istanbul, Turkey, aarman@marmara.edu.tr
Refika Ersu; Dilsad Save; Goksin Karaman;
Koray Karabekiroglu; Bulent Karadag; Meral Berkem

Objective: In 2002, a survey was carried out to determine the prevalence of habitual snoring (HS) and related symptoms in 2147 primary school children in Istanbul. The prevalence of HS was estimated to be 7% in this study. After one year, children with HS and 2 age and sex matched control children for each HS were studied. The aim of this study was to examine the differences for hyperactivity/attentional measures among 151 HS and 302 controls. **Methods:** Parents and teachers completed two common behavioral measures, an inattention/hyperactivity scale (IHS-P and IHS-T, respectively for parents and teachers) derived from DSM-IV, and Conners' Rating Scales (CONNERS-P and CONNERS-T, respectively for parents and teachers). Data were summarized with means and standard deviations and t- test was applied for comparision of the groups. Parents were also asked whether they believed their child to be hyperactive (from never to almost always in a 4-point scale), results were analyzed by Pearson Chi square test. The level of significance was set at P < 0.5. **Results:** Response rate was 85.9% (105 HS vs. 201 controls). 16% of control children started to snore and 4.5% of HS did not snore any longer. 24% HS vs. 11.4% controls described mild hyperactivity (p: 0.002) and trend

analysis showed that there were increasing rates of HS among hyperactivity scale (p: 0.001). T-test results were significant for CONNERS-P (27.0 ± 16.7 vs. 17.7 ± 12.6; p: 0.001) and IHS-P (0.7 ± 0.5 vs. 0.4 ± 0.4; p: 0.007) in HS vs. controls. There was no statistical difference for CONNERS-T and IHS-T. **Conclusion:** HS does not resolve spontaneously in majority of children and is related to significant attentional/hyperactivity problems when compared to controls. Increasing rates of HS among 4-point hyperactivity scale might reflect a negative impact on overall neurobehavioral health of these children that is likely to be described by parents rather than teachers.

P-016-281   Topic: 27, 26

Use of the ICD-10 classification in Danish child and adolescent psychiatry – have diagnoses changed after the introduction of ICD-10?

Lene Ruge Møller, Psychiatry Hospital for, Child & Adolescent, Risskov, Denmark, lene.ruge@dadlnet.dk
Merete Juul Sørensen; Per Hove Thomsen

Objective: A greater specification of diagnoses was expected with the introduction of the 10th version of the International Classification of Diseases (ICD-10). Reflecting the time trend more neuropsychiatric diagnoses are expected. The aim of this study is a nationwide test of these hypotheses on diagnoses used in child and adolescents psychiatry in Denmark. **Methods:** From the nationwide Danish Psychiatric Central Register data were drawn on clinical discharge diagnoses. All patients aged 0 to 15 years examined at psychiatric hospitals from 1995–2002 in the whole country were included. From the register-data a description of diagnoses, changes over time, age and gender was made. **Results:** During the study period 22,469 children and adolescents with a first contact (96% outpatients) were registered. The most frequent discharge diagnoses were pervasive developmental disorder (PPD) (11.9%), adjustment disorders (10.6%) conduct disorder (9.5%), emotional and anxiety disorders (7.6%) hyperkinetic disorders (7.3%) and specific developmental disorders (7.3%). During the study period the use of diagnoses for neuropsychiatric and affective disorders increased. 45% of the 22.469 diagnoses were only partly specified according to ICD-10, distributed on Z-diagnoses (11%), F88, F89, F99 (4%) and 'not specified' on the four-character level (Fxx.9) (30%). A subgroup of 4.153 became inpatients. The distribution of the most frequent discharge diagnoses after the first admission as inpatient was PPD (15.1%), conduct disorders (7.3%), hyperkinetic disorders (8.5%), adjustment disorders (7.3%), eating disorders (6.0%), psychotic disorders (5.0%). 34% of the inpatients had diagnoses only partly specified. **Conclusion:** This was a nationwide study with a complete inclusion of all children and adolescents seen in psychiatric hospitals in Denmark. A specification of diagnoses and an increase in the use of neuropsychiatric diagnoses were seen after the introduction of ICD-10. The subdivision 'unspecified' was used in 30% of the cases, consequently a more detailed specification of the ICD-10 is still required.

P-017
Disorders and other conditions IV

P-017-282   Topic: 69
A comparative study on Schizophrenia with onset in childhood, adolescence and adulthood:
A developmental perspective

Parathasarathy Biswas, Inst. of Medical Education, Dept. of Psychiatry, Chandigarh, India, savitam@sancharnet.in
Savita Malhotra; Anil Malhotra; Nitin Gupta

Objective: To compare clinical features, genetic loading, pre-schizophrenic symptoms, neuropsychological and neurobiological functioning, course and outcome of COS with AdOS and AOS groups. **Methods:** Sample was chosen from patients attending the Department of Psychiatry at a tertiary care center in North India. The COS group had 15 patients while AdOS and AOS groups had 20 patients each who fulfilled ICD-10 DCR criteria for schizophrenia; were matched on gender and duration of illness. The assessment was done on Instrument for the retrospective assessment for onset of schizophrenia (IRAOS), PANSS, FIGS, Condensed neuropsychiatric examination for the examination of soft neurological signs (SNS), Neuropsychological test battery and WHO life chart schedule. Analysis of variance (ANOVA) and chi-square test was used. **Results:** The study was based on the theoretical paradigm of "Neurodevelopmental hypothesis" of schizophrenia. Significantly greater number of patients in COS group showed preschizophrenic symptoms (p<0.01), during 1 year before the psychotic breakdown. COS patients continued to show significantly higher scores on PANSS. COS patients were characterized by greater frequency of obsessions, magical thinking and other non-psychotic symptoms. COS group had relatively low family history of schizophrenia and spectrum disorders. The COS group showed overall presence of more SNS; maximum dysfunction being in temporal and frontal lobes. COS group also had significantly poorer scores on all subtests of IQ, overall memory and perceptuomotor functioning. COS group had a significantly poorer course and outcome and poor response to typical antipsychotics. **Conclusion:** Deficits on neuropsychological tests and scores of SNS and preschizophrenic symptoms were maximum in the COS group with AOS group having the least scores and AdOS groups falling in between these two extremes. These results show that onset of schizophrenia in childhood has serious repercussions on the developing brain leading onto most severe brain dysfunction and a more virulent form of illness as compared to the later onset types of schizophrenia. In COS patients there was significant cognitive arrest but not cognitive decline, which is more in keeping with the "Neurodevelopmental hypothesis" of schizophrenia.

P-017-283   Topic: 70, 37
The Children's Depression Inventory (CDI)
as measure of depression in Swedish adolescents.
A normative study

Tord Ivarsson, OCD-Anxiety Program, Child & Adolescent Psychiatry, Göteborg, Sweden, tord.ivarsson@vgregion.se
Oeystein Litlere; Per Svalander

Objective: Self-Rating Scales are an economical and practical aid in diagnostic evaluation, given that the measures are reliable and valid and that normative data from the general population are available to interpret the scores. The study aims to evaluate and to obtain normative data for the Children's Depression Inventory (CDI) in Swedish adolescents. **Methods:** 405 adolescents selected to be fairly representative of the general population (both ethnical Swedes and born abroad) filled in a questionnaire containing the Children's Depression Inventory (CDI), the Multidimensional Anxiety Scale for Children (MASC) and background data (including Socioeconomic status (SES), weight and height). **Results:** The CDI was reliable in terms of internal consistency (0.86) with a mean inter-item correlation of 0.18 and item-total score correlations ranging from 0.26 to 0.57. The CDI sub-scales ('Negative Mood', 'Ineffectiveness', 'Anhedonia' and 'Negative Self-Esteem') had good internal consistency values slightly above 0.60, except for sub-scale 'Interpersonal Problems' with poor internal consistency (0.36). The 90th and 95th percentiles respectively were defined by scores 15 and 18 for boys and by scores 20 and 23 for girls. Common correlates of high scores were female gender, broken family but not SES, nor ethnicity. An interesting finding was an U-shaped distribution of CDI scores for girls around the ideal Body Mass Index (BMI) (for age and gender) with the lowest CDI scores ±1 SD. This distribution was accentuated when estimating marginal means controlling for other factors influencing CDI scores. Also, some estimates of the concurrent validity of the CDI were found in a Pearson correlation of 0.40 with the MASC total score and in the capacity of the CDI (predictive validity) (OR=1.1) in predicting suicidal ideation. **Conclusion:** The CDI is a valid and reliable measure of depression in adolescence. The relationship between BMI and depression needs further study.

P-017-284   Topic: 70
Behavioural and cognitive therapy in complex treatment for depressions

Yelena Yelikova, Kirov State Medical Academy, Dept. of Psychiatry, Kirov, Russia, golovin_vladimir@list.ru

Objective: To investigate dynamics of depressive disorders due to combination of drug therapy and psychotherapy. **Methods:** Biochemical, clinical therapeutic, clinical psychopathological methods as well as Hamilton's anxiety and depression scale were used. Female patients were studied. They had a depression pattern according to ICD-10 criteria for recurrent depressive disorder. The treatment program included behavioural and cognitive psychotherapies. The control group received only routine drug therapy. **Results:** All the patients had melancholic signs of depression. In 47% of patients, depressions were accompanied by anxiety. It was revealed that changes in total lipids in the blood serum, lipoproteins of low density, triglycerides, cholesterol and its fractions in lipoproteins of low and high density mostly correlated with clinical evidence of depressions. These biochemical criteria of lipid metabolism were recommended to evaluate courses of depressive disorders. 88% of patients showed positive dynamics in treatment for depressions. Use of behavioural and cognitive therapies allowed to use drug therapy more effectively and to improve remissions. 21% of patients demonstrated complete improvement of depressions. 79% of patients showed partial remissions. This correlated with the tendency to normalization of biochemical parameters of lipid metabolism in the blood serum and oxidant antioxidant system of the organism. **Conclusion:** Investigation of biochemical criteria of lipid metabolism in combination with analysis of clinical and psychopathological peculiarities of depressive syndrome is recommended to control of treatment efficacy and prediction in case of complex cognitive behavioural therapy for depressions.

P-017-285   Topic: 68
Comparison between male and female alcoholics in regard to child neglect/abuse in the family

Petar Nastasic, Institute of Mental Health, Department of Alcoholism, Belgrade, Serbia and Montenegro, nastasic@verat.net
Snezana Filipovic; Roza Panoski; Goran Lazetic

Objective: Purpose of this study is to establish differences, according to sex and type of neglect/abuse maltreatment in parent's alcoholics of both sexes, who were treated at the Institute of mental health. Methods: Study is made in the period 2002–2003 at the Department of alcoholism. Total sample was N = 298 (79 female, 217 male). Into account were taken: demographic data (age, education, employment, marriage status); family history of alcohol abuse; family history of neglect/abuse; numbers, sex and age of children. Demographic data are obtained from the registration data and anamnesis, while the data on neglect/abuse were taken from Risk factor matrix and interview. Results: It was found that, in both primary and own family, there is higher rate of physical and emotional neglect/abuse in fathers, aggressive alcoholics, than mothers. Conclusion: In order to estimate more exact data on higher rate of physical and emotional neglect/abuse of children by father's alcoholics, it is necessary to follow further functioning of these children in their families.

P-017-286   Topic: 69, 30
Disharmony as a specific feature of cognitive activity on Schizophrenia in childhood (Psychological Investigation)

Nataliya Zvereva, Ass. of Child Psychiatrists, and Psychologists, Moscow, Russia, acpp@online.ru

Objective: To conduct the comparative experimental psychological study of age dynamic of certain aspects of cognitive activity with schizophrenic and normal children. Methods: 3 groups of schizophrenic and normal children (from 7 to 14 years) had been examined by experimental blocs of methods of clinical psychology, authorized and modified: 1. 106 schizophrenic children (66 boys and 40 girls); 2. 86 schizophrenic children (56 boys and 30 girls); 3. 34 schizophrenic children and 34 normal ones (23 boys and 11 girls). Results: (1) Above 60% of patients have development dissociation of certain aspects of cognitive activity (operational, social-oriented, selective) in thinking and in visual perception. 2. Above half examinees in the group of 86 schizophrenic children showed the prevalence of thinking operational aspect in comparison with the perceptional one (3). Dissociation of the modal-specific memory types was found. Arbitrary memory was studied, namely, audio verbal, visual, tactile (texture and haptic), as well as the conditional competition of modalities (tactile haptic and visual). showed varying proportions between the effectiveness of memorizing in different modalities. Conclusion: Schizophrenic children showed development type distinguished from normal, characterized by disharmony and dissociation, i.e. normal and surpassing development of the operational aspects under the condi-

tions of development retardation of the selectivity and subject-oriented aspects. The study of development dissociation of operational aspect of thinking and perception showed that by schizophrenic children thinking is better developed in comparison with perception The dynamics of the obtained indices by age groups also permitted to distinguish among schizophrenic and normal children. We consider the obtained cognitive activity features as a variant of cognitive dizontogenesis by schizophrenic children.

P-017-287   Topic: 69, 32
A severe form of PMDD or cycloid psychosis triggered by hormonal imbalance during adolescence?

Monika Strauss, KJPD, St. Gallen, St. Gallen, Switzerland, monika.strauss@kjpd-sg.ch
A. Graf; R. Zollinger

Objective: To discuss the differential diagnosis and introduce different treatment options including antipsychotic, hormonal as well as psychotherapeutic aspects of treatment. Methods: Case-report of a 14-year old girl suffering from recurrent severe states of confusion and unspecific psychotic symptoms, which were associated with the menstrual cycle. The case has been in our follow- up screening for 4 years now and a first conclusive evaluation can be drawn. Results: The outcome is quite favourable. The patient has been free of psychotic episodes for 3 years now and is without any medication. Conclusion: More research data is necessary to differentiate severe psychological states associated with the menstrual cycle in young girls. In certain cases favourable outcomes seem to be possible even though the psychopathology at onset was severe. The role of the development of the female hormonal cycle as well as the system of neurotransmitters and their interdependence with each other is yet to be studied more precisely.

P-017-288   Topic: 70, 26
Affective disorders in adolescence: Etiological pathways

Tanja Brückl, MPI of Psychiatry, Clinical Psych./ Epidemiology, München, Germany, brueckl@mpipsykl.mpg.de
Michael Höfler; Lena Schwender; Hans-Ulrich Wittchen; Roselind Lieb

Objective: To model etiological pathways leading to affective disorders in adolescence by considering pregnancy/birth factors and childhood disorders. Methods: Data stem from the Early Developmental Stages of Psychopathology Study (EDSP), a prospective-longitudinal study conducted in a representative sample of originally 3021 subjects aged 14–24. Statistical analyses are restricted to a subsample of the younger cohort (birth cohorts 1977–81; aged 14–17 at baseline) for whom parental information on childhood is available and who did not report any affective disorder in childhood (N = 942). Affective disorders in adolescence were assessed with the Munich-Composite-International-Diagnostic-Interview (M-CIDI) according to DSM-IV criteria. Childhood and pregnancy/birth conditions were assessed from the mothers in a separate parent investigation. A graphical model based on logistic regressions was used to analyse different factors and subsequent onset of affective disorders. This method also investigates the links between the covariates by controlling for prior and concurrent factors and thus, allows for separating direct from indirect pathways. Two temporally ordered groups of factors were included in the model: (1) pregnancy/birth and (2) childhood conditions. The results were adjusted for age and sex and visualized with so-called association chain graphs (ACGs). **Results:** Childhood separation anxiety (OR = 5.2) and affect lability (OR = 2.0) were directly linked to onset of affective disorders in adolescence. Childhood Conduct disorder/Oppositional defiant disorder were indirectly related to affective disorders via their association with affect lability. Several indirect pathways were identified via mother's mental stress during pregnancy: This factor e.g. was associated with an elevated risk for Attention-Deficit/Hyperactivity disorder (OR = 5.3), what, in turn, was linked to affect lability (OR = 7.6). **Conclusion:** Childhood separation anxiety and affect lability seem to play a key role in the development of adolescent affective disorders. Pregnancy factors were associated with onset of affective disorders in adolescence via mediating childhood factors.

P-017-289   Topic: 69, 11

A remediation program of facial-affect recognition in adolescents with First-Episode-Schizophrenia: A pilot study

Sonja Werneck-Rohrer, Medizin. Universität Wien, Kinder- und Jugendpsychiatrie, Wien, Austria, sonja.werneck-rohrer@meduniwien.ac.at
Angelika Schweitzer; Jane Edwards; Monika Schlögelhofer; Paul G. Amminger

Objective: Recognizing facial affects is important for the social functioning of the individual. Individuals with schizophrenia show problems in the perception of emotional expression. Frommann, Streit and Wölwer (2003) developed a training program for the remediation of facial-affect recognition (TAR). The TAR is a 12-session program which uses restitution and compensation strategies and the principles of errorless learning. The TAR shows good feasibility in adults with schizophrenia and our purpose was to examine its applicability in adolescents with first-episode schizophrenia. **Methods:** Training occurred in pairs. The intervention utilised a detailed treatment manual provided by Frommann. For evaluating the training effects assessments were undertaken at baseline end-of-treatment and three months post treatment with two multiple-choice labelling tasks. **Results:** Eight juvenile patients have passed the training by now. The pattern of results generally suggests improvement between baseline and end-of-treatment and stabilisation between end-of-treatment and three months post intervention. **Conclusion:** the TAR appears suitable for use with adolescents with first-episode schizophrenia with minor modifications. Evaluation of the effectiveness requires further investigation.

P-017-290   Topic: 69, 12

Treatment of schizophrenic spectrum disorders in adolescence: A long term comparison between antipsychotics

Maria Giuseppina Ledda, University of Cagliari, Child & Adolescent Psychiatry, Cagliari, Italy, emmegielle@yahoo.com
A. Zuddas; T. Piroddi; M. Abis; A. Mereu; Carlo Cianchetti

Objective: This is a retrospective study of the effect of drug treatment in adolescents with schizophrenia (SPh)

and schizoaffective (SA) disorders. **Methods:** The study concern 29 subjects (18 with SPh and 11 SA) followed for a period ranging from 3 to 10 years. In the course of their disorder they were treated with different antipsychotics in subsequent. periods. The therapeutic efficacy in relation to adverse effects was evaluated using the Efficacy Index (EI), according the Clinical Global Impression. The EI was calculated in relation to treatments with haloperidol (HAL), risperidone (RISP) and clozapine (CLZ), in patients which were treated with 2 or more of them. **Results:** All subjects were treated initially with HAL or RISP. After initial HAL, 5 cases were given RISP and 7 CLZ. After RISP, 8 were given CLZ. All these changes were due to insufficient efficacy of treatment. Changes from CLZ to RISP occurred in 3 cases, due to leukopenia in 2 and convulsions in 1. Six patients (2 SPh and 4 SA) responded well since onset with RISP (in the 4 SA in combination with mood stabilizers). At present, 15 patients are under treatment with CLO from 2 to 10 years, and 8 with RISP from 1 to 9 years, without relevant adverse effects. In the subjects treated with HAL and subsequently with RISP, the EI was 1.1 for HAL and 1.6 for RISP, with a significant difference (P < 0.05); in those treated with RISP and subsequently with CLZ, the EI was 1.6 for RISP and 2.8 for CLZ, with a significant difference (P < 0.01). **Conclusion:** Our data show the higher efficacy of CLZ compared to RISP and HAL, with a limited number of drop outs, and the safety of a long-term treatment.

P-017-291   Topic: 69, 35

Disturbed gyrification in the prefrontal region in adolescents suffering from Schizophrenia

Fabian Härtling, Universität Frankfurt, Kinder- und Jugendpsychiatrie, Frankfurt, Germany, f.haertling@em.uni-frankfurt.de
Ralf Tepest; Tanja Goncharova; David E.D. Linden; Peter Falkei; Kai Vogeley; Fritz Poustka

Objective: Gyrification is an early neurodevelopmental phenomenon that takes place during pregnancy and approximately the first year of childhood. A longitudinal study has shown that the gyrification is robust thereafter and can be taken as a measure for the relative convolutedness of the outer brain surface. The purpose of this study was to assess gyrification in patients with early onset schizophrenia (EOS) compared with healthy controls, by employing a gyrification index (GI) as the ratio of inner contour (corresponding to the pial surface) and outer contour (corresponding to the connecting line of gyri crests). As studied earlier, the GI is significantly increased in the frontal lobe in schizophrenia in adults. **Methods:** To examine whether frontal lobe hypergyria can also be detected in early onset schizophrenia, the mean frontal as well as parieto-occipital GI (left and right) was determined in the MRI scans of 14 patients (mean ± SD age, 17.0 ± 1.2 years; range 13 to 18 years with the ICD-10 diagnosis of schizophrenia or schizoaffective disorder (6 females, 8 males) and 16 normal controls (matched for age, sex, handedness, IQ, height and weight). T1 weighted high-resolution MR-images were acquired on a 1.5 Tesla scanner. All images were processed by Analyze. Contour outlining was performed with the software Optimas. **Results:** The mean frontal, but not parieto-occipital GI showed a significant bilateral increase in schizophrenic patients as compared to control subjects (mean GI: F = 4.73, p < 0.05). **Conclusion:** The result of this study corroborates earlier findings of frontal hypergyria in adult schizophrenia and support the view that the frontal hypergyria is acquired already during pregnancy and early childhood and indicates neurobiological changes that predispose for the acquisition of schizophrenia during adolescence.

P-017-292 Topic: 70, 32
Prevalence of Thyroid antibodies in affective disorder with psychosis: Onset in adolescence (13–19)

Miriam Spinner, McMaster University, Faculty of Health Sciences, Hamilton, ON, Canada, mspinner@mcmaster.ca
Julian Dobranowski; Duncan MacCrimmon; Jim Gibson; Susan Fawcett; Margarita Criollo

Objective: Abnormalities of thyroid antibodies have been described in psychiatric patients with bipolar disorder and depressive disorder. In addition, Kupka et al. (2002) suggest thyroid antibodies were more prevalent in bipolar patients (28%) than in psychiatric controls (3–18%) and were not associated with Lithium exposure. In adolescent cases having affective disorder with psychoses, antithyroid perioxidase antibody (TPO-Abs) was evaluated at the onset of illness prior to treatment. We hypothesize that thyroid antibodies will be abnormal prior to treatment. **Methods:** Patients were recruited from consecutively admitted adolescents (age 13–19) from an adolescent inpatient program at St. Joseph's Healthcare, Hamilton, Ontario. Inclusion criteria were a DSM-IV diagnoses of first episode psychosis: bipolar disorder, manic episode with psychotic features; bipolar disorder, mixed episode with psychotic features; bipolar disorder, depressed episode with psychotic features; and major depressive disorder with psychotic features. TPO-Abs was measured by quantitative Elisa technology. **Results:** Forty-one subjects; 23 males and 18 females and mean age of 16.7 (±1.6); had antithyroid antibodies assessed. None were treated with Lithium prior to enrollment in the study. Thyroid antibodies were present in 22% (9 cases) of this population. **Conclusion:** Our data are consistent with Kupka and suggest an increased prevalence of thyroid antibodies at the onset of first episode affective disorder with psychosis in adolescents. The presence of thyroid antibodies may reflect underlying pathophysiology in a subset of affective disorders. Studies including controls would further clarify the significance of these findings. References: Kupka RW et al. High rate of autoimmune thyroiditis in bipolar disorder: lack of association with lithium exposure. Biol Psychiatry 15; 51(4):305–311, 2002.

P-017-293 Topic: 69, 70
Peculiarity of creative giftedness by adolescents suffering from endogenous affective psychoses

Nina Iovchuk, Ass. of Child Psychiatrists and Psychologists, Moscow, Russia, acpp@online.ru

Objective: We observed 59 children suffering from circular schizophrenia who showed anticipating development with intellectual giftedness, high productivity in premorbid period. **Methods:** Psychopathologic and follow-up investigation. **Results:** The illness manifested in early school age or in adolescents mainly as depressive and maniac symptoms. During active period of illness decreased the rate of intellectual development, appeared pseudo-regressive disturbances, difficulties of thinking. After 2–7 years has come longtime remission with emotional deficit and with former or slight reduced activity. After period of active appearances of ill-ness and longtime social (school) disadap-

tation was restored fully abilities of sick persons but they relaxed noticeably or lost the possibility of its realization owing to several causes: 1) reduction of emotions or its disproportionality with surplus sensibility, suspiciousness, shyness, or reduction of motivation; 2) light reduction of activity with lack of energy for realization of wide interests; 3) high attention to own health and wish to avoid long emotional and intellectual efforts because of misgiving of exacerbation; 4) mental rigidity leads to stable structure of life, to hard daily time-table, and to impossibility to determine the main line of life; 5) special daily rhythm with low activity in first half of day, and with increasing of activity, improvement of self-filling in second half of day; 6) a lack of normal adolescents, harsh distortion of maturing of social adaptation, social skills, and social connections. **Conclusion:** To preserve the possibility of realization of giftedness of mentally ill children and adolescents it is necessary well-founded interdisciplinary approach. This system can't confine itself to medical help, and must unite efforts of many specialists including psychologists, pedagogues and especially hilly skilled in the field of giftedness of ill child.

P-017-294 Topic: 69, 47
Expressed Emotion (EE) and head position behaviour of schizophrenic adolescents and close relatives: A study of mutual emotional action tendencies in communication

Brigitte Ramsauer, UKE Hamburg-Eppendorf, Kinder- und Jugendpsychiatrie, Hamburg, Germany, b.ramsauer@uke.uni-hamburg.de
Nina Janke; Peter Riedesser

Objective: Little research has been done on Expressed Emotion (EE)-level and emotional communication in interaction of schizophrenic adolescents and close relatives. The EE-level (high-EE, low-EE) is defined as part of the relative's emotional attitude towards the patient. Changes in head position are seen as an important relational action tendency of emotional communication. **Methods:** Therefore, the head positions of inclination and disinclination have been examined during 10 minutes of contact at the time of discharge of the adolescent patient. The relative's EE-level was rated by the Five-Minute-Speech-Sample (FMSS). The head position changes of 10 schizophrenic adolescents and their close relatives were coded by the Berner System of Nonverbal Interaction. The respective head positions showing inclination or disinclination were examined in relation to relative's EE-level. **Results:** Schizophrenic adolescent patients communicating with low-EE relatives have a higher rate of head position changes compared with adolescent patients communicating with high-EE-relatives. In low-EE dyads, there is a higher tendency of mutuality, both in synchronous with and in series of head positions, compared with high-EE dyads. At the same time, low-EE dyads show more often head position series of indirect inclination followed by direct inclination or disinclination compared with high-EE dyads. Low-EE dyads differ significantly in their head position changes of indirect inclination compared with high-EE dyads. **Conclusion:** This communication study reveals significant differences in emotional behaviour of adolescent schizophrenic patients depending on the relative's EE-level. Further studies are necessary, e.g. to confirm the relevance of these results in the course of schizophrenia in adolescence.

P-017-295   Topic: 68
The prevalence of substance abuse in period 2002–2004 at a department for children and adolescents

Petar Nastasic, Institute of Mental Health, Department of Alcoholism, Belgrade, Serbia and Montenegro, nastasic@verat.net
Milica Pejovic-Milovancevic; Snezana Filipovic

Objective: Purpose of this article is to survey, for children and adolescents who are treated at the Institute of mental health, if it is, for early assessment and treatment of substance abuse, more significant co-morbidity for insufficient knowledge of patterns of behavior problems of young abusers. **Methods:** Research is conveyed with clinical population of children and adolescent who were treated at the Department for children and adolescents in the period 2002–2004 (27 months). Reqruited are patients, total 279, all with psychiatry problems. Following clinical and other instruments are used: CAST 6, Test of urine drugs and structured diagnostic interview. **Results:** The total number of 279 children and adolescents, 42 of them have abuse substances. Co-morbidity assessed for: behavior disorders, family problems and psychotic symptoms. **Conclusion:** In order to make evaluation and therapeutically process, there is need for specific program for children and adolescents who are both psychiatrically ill and abuse substances.

P-017-296   Topic: 68
Abuse in families of alcoholics: Multiple addictions

Vera Trbic, Institute of Mental Health,
Dept. Substance Abuse, Belgrade, Serbia and Montenegro, danicica@eunet.yu
Danica Boskovic Djukic

In alcoholic family systems coexist at least two addictions: emotional neglect and abuse, with the existing alcohol addction. Physical abuse happens very often; therefore, every member is a victim and abuser, only the roles change in specific way: It begins by being a victim in childhood, later on, a vistim becomes an abuser by growing up. In this way pathological spiral of addiction doubles: alcholism and abuse go hand in hand by taking both children and alderly in their nest. Violence becomes a drug without which it is imposible to live; alcohol serves as an alibi. By sistematic understanding we concluded that this process could be stoped by cooperation of a number of antites: legal, social, cultural, heltose, repressive and so on. In their works the authors showed a family where alcohol and abuse in different aspects lasted for many generations. By explaining diagnostic and therapeutical processes they showed possibilities of the stated entities of local community insoliving both aspects of addiction.

P-017-297   Topic: 69
Early onset schizophrenic spectrum: Between premorbid and adolescent development

Ignazio Ardizzone, Rome, Italy, ignazio.ardizzone@fastwebnet.it
Nadia Tomassetti; Fabiola Napoli; Raffaella Valente; Valeria Neri; Mauro Ferrara

Objective: From the point of view of the Vulnerability-Stress-Coping model, the authors try to analyse, define and characterize features, development and transformation of the EOSS psychopathological core. **Methods:** Review of international literature about premorbid development and the Bio-Psycho-Social features of adolescent development. The relational premorbid and clinical history a fifteen schizophrenic adolescent subjects has been compared with an OCD Sample and healthy group age-matched (SCID, PAS, premorbid adjustment scale). **Results:** According to the international literature finding the premorbid development in EOSS is characterized by a peculiar psychopathological core that provokes an extreme neuropsychological and affective vulnerability. The adolescent development represents a crucial stress factor. **Conclusion:** Behind the negative symptomatology that characterizes the premorbid development of EOSS it's possible to recognize the presence and the funtioning of a psychopathological core.

P-017-298   Topic: 70
Childhood depression: Modification of symptoms in preschool and school age

Nadia Capriotti, Institute of Mental Health, Dept. of NPI, Rome, Italy, pollon_75_1999@yahoo.it
Carla D'Agostini Costa; Christian Veronesi; Carla Sogos

Objective: The purpose of this study is to evaluate two characteristic depressive symptoms of adult depression in patients in preschool and school age and to assess the quantity and the quality of these symptoms in the two groups. **Methods:** Eigthy children consecutively referred to our out-patient service for psychopathological developmental disorders during the last 2 years, were retrospectively analysed. The sample was composed of: a) 30 prescholar depressed children (mean age 4.4 ys); b) 50 scholar depressed children (mean age 9.5 ys). From the clinical charts, data regarding psychodiagnostic and neuropsychological assessment were derived. In the clinical charts, a section was devoted to sleep behavior and disturbances, another one investigated eating behavior and disorders. The analysis has provided data regarding the presence and the clinical types of these two depressive symptoms. The prevalence of different types of sleep and eating disorders was analysed between the two groups. **Results:** The prevalence of sleep disorder in prescholars was 81%, while in scholars was 64%. Intragroup analysis showed that night and early morning awakenings in prescholar children (87% vs 37%; $2 = 10.75$; $p = 0.001$) and parasomnias in scholar children (54%) were the most prevalent sleep abnormalities. In prescholars the prevalence of eating disorder was 86%, while in scholars was 34%. The analysis of clinical types didn't show any difference between the two groups; the appetite loss resulted the most prevalent clinical type in the two samples. **Conclusion:** Sleep and eating disturbances are frequent in depressed children, but their clinical manifestations seem to be unspecific. Nevertheless it is important to note that the prevalence of this two depressive symptoms is higher in the prescholar than the scholar depressed children.

P-017-299   Topic: 70
Symbolic organization in depressed school age children

Roberta Giacchè, Rome University, Childhood Neuropsychiatry, Rome, Italy, carla.sogos@uniroma1.it
Sergio Melogno; Achille Gigliotti; Bruna Mazzoncini

Objective: In this study the authors attempt to highlight characteristics of symbolic organization and affective development in depressed children through the technique of play observation. **Methods:** The clinical sample (group A) consists of 21 subjects (15 males and 6 females; range: 6–12 years; m.a.: 8.9; S.D.: 2 years) randomly selected among the depressed children consecutively and spontaneously referred to our outpatient service. The sample was assessed with the diagnostic and neuropsychological protocol used by our Centre (WISC-R, K-SADS PL, CDI, CDRS-R, Rorschach, CGI). The group A was compared to two control groups: the group B consists of 21 nonclinical children, while the group C consists of 21 nondepressed clinical peers. The three groups were submitted to a play session (Sceno-Test) during which some important aspects were examined (play structure, contents and emotions) and inserted in a checklist made by the authors. The data were analysed using Fishers Exact Test. **Results:** The play in depressed children shows particular features compared to the play in the control groups. The authors underline some particular aspects in depressed children play: their way of playing and the correspondence between representations and emotions. **Conclusion:** The results of this study suggest that the play is a very helpful tool for investigating the symbolic organization and the emotional development of children. These findings need to be confirmed by a larger sample and longitudinal studies.

P-017-300   Topic: 68
Hyperactivity, aggression and substance abuse in children and adolescents

António Fonseca, University of Coimbra, Faculty of Psychology, Coimbra, Portugal, acfonseca@fpce.uc.pt

Objective: This paper is aimed at assessing the relationship between hyperactivity, aggression and substance abuse in a large community sample of children, including boys and girls. Specifically the following questions were set for analysis: 1) How common are these problems in Portuguese population? 2) How does the relationship between them evolve with age for both genders? 3) Do children who display both hyperactivity and aggression are at higher risk of substance abuse in adolescence? **Methods:** Several hundreds of children from public schools in the Municipality of Coimbra, were assessed three times between the age of 7 and 17 years. Information was collected from parents, teachers and pupils themselves. Questionnaires and interviews were used for this purpose. **Results:** The findings only partially support the idea that children with both disruptive problems are at higher risk of substance abuse. The patterns of relationship among these variables were rather similar for boys and girls. **Conclusion:** Our results are discussed in the light of the conclusions of previous studies on these issues.

P-017-301   Topic: 70, 37
Depressive symptoms in a school sample of children and adolescents: Using the Birleson Depression Self-rating Scale for Children (DSRS-C)

Kenzo Denda, Hokkaido University, Dept. of Psychiatry, Sapporo, Japan, kdenda@med.hokudai.ac.jp

Objective: The aim of this study was to examine the prevalence of self-reported depressive symptoms in a Japanese school sample of children and adolescents using the Birleson Depression Self-Rating Scale for Children (DSRS-C). **Methods:** The participants consisted of 3331 students (1535 boys and 1796 girls; 6 to 15 years old) coming from three different cities, Sapporo, Chitose and Iwamizawa in Hokkaido, northern Japan. **Results:** The DSRS-C mean score in our sample (9.02±5.81) was higher than that previously reported findings. There were significant differences in gender and age with regard to the DSRS-C score. Girls scored higher than boys, and the total score rose with age. There was not the significant difference in an area. The prevalence of depressive risk in this sample was 13.0%, when the DSRS-C cutoff score of 16 was taken as threshold. This figure was higher than that reported by other studies. Factorial analysis yielded two factors, lack of enjoyment and depressive mood or sadness. Our findings indicated that 18.8% of the students reported thoughts of death, and 4.0% showed explicit suicidal ideation. **Conclusion:** Our data suggested that the prevalence of self-reported depressive symptoms in a Japanese school sample was relatively high, and therefore that the prevalence of Major Depressive Disorder in children and adolescents could be possibly similar to that reported by other epidemiologic studies of Western countries.

P-017-302   Topic: 69, 42
Childhood onset schizophrenia (30 y follow up study)

Eva Malá, Charles University, Child & Adolescents Psychiatry, Praha 5, Czech Republic, eva.mala@fnmotol.cz

Objective: 1. What is the hereditary loading of child-onset schizophrenia (COS)? 2. What is the prognosis of COS? 3. What is the mortality of COS? **Methods:** During a 30-year follow-up study 120 patients were hospitalized between 1964–1994 with COS in the Psychiatric Clinic Prague. There were 28 children 10–13 years (age of 1st symptoms)=23% and 92 children 13–15 years=77%. Sex ratio male:female=68:52=57%:43%. **Results:** The literature followed by our results in italics are presented. 1. Most schizophrenics born during the 1st trimester of the year: 34% patients were born in January to March. 2. Broken homes are frequent: 40% had a broken home. 3. Frequent experience with death: 8% experienced the death of one parent before age of 15 y (3% mother 5% father). 4. Frequent complications in pregnancy: 30% of our patients (in comparison to 10% of the general population). 5. No increases of pathological births: 16% in the schizophrenic (as compared to 25–33% in the general population). 6. No increased premature birth rate. The same result. 7. Poor peer relationships: Poor sociability 43% preschool, 47% school. 8. Depressive symptoms occur at the onset of the disorder: 63% depressive symptoms (including tentamen suicide in 13% of the cases). 9. Neurological soft sign (including abnormal EEG): found in 66% patients. Data will also be presented on genetics and mortality. **Conclusion:** In patients with COS there is a poor prognosis, a high mortality rate, and a high hereditary loading.

P-017-303   Topic: 68, 41
Predictors of smoking in early adolescence

Erika Hohm, Zentralinstitut für Seelische Gesundheit, Mannheim, Germany, hohm@zi-mannheim.de
Manfred Laucht; Katja Becker; Martin H. Schmidt

Objective: Early tobacco use during infancy and adolescence is considered to be a risk factor for developing a later dependence. Many factors for the onset of tobacco use are being discussed. The influence of the social environment is thought to be most important. The present investigation examines the role of smoking-associated expectations and how peers' and parents smoking behaviour contributes to the beginning of tobacco consumption. **Methods:** Participants were from a longitudinal study of a birth cohort of 384 children at risk for later psychopathology. The initiation and use of tobacco were assessed at the age of 15 years with the substance use questionnaire (SUQ). Assessments of smoking-related instrumentality (INSSMOK), smoking-related self-efficacy (SWSMOK), parental and peers' smoking behaviour together with measures of social context, were obtained by using standardized interviews (MEI). **Results:** Approximately 60% of 15-year-olds reported lifetime cigarette use. Among those who had ever smoked, nearly 25% were current daily users. One's tobacco consumption is linked to smoking-related expectations (self-efficacy and instrumentality), and peers' and parental smoking practices. Smoking behaviour of close friends causes both directly and indirectly whether non-smoking adolescents start to smoke or not, whereas the role of the parenting model has only a direct affect. The lower the self-efficacy, the higher the smoking rate. **Conclusion:** These findings allocate the influence of social and personal factors for the onset of tobacco use. Recognizing the importance of the smoking environment, especially peers' smoking behaviour, seems to be critical to the prevention of adolescent smoking.

P-017-304 Topic: 69, 28
Mitochondrial complex I expression: A peripheral marker of Schizophrenia?

Claudia Mehler-Wex, Universität Würzburg,
Kinder- und Jugendpsychiatrie, Würzburg, Germany,
mehler@kjp.uni-wuerzburg.de
J. Catharina Duvigneau; Romana T. Hartl;
Dorit Ben-Shachar; Andreas Warnke; Manfred Gerlach

Objective: Schizophrenia is one of the most severe psychiatric disorders. Since diagnosis depends on descriptive behavioral and symptomatic aspects only, it is important to develop biological tests for confirmation of diagnosis and follow-up. Previous studies of Ilani and Dror (PNAS 2001, 98:625–628; Mol Psychiatry 2002, 7:995–1001) suggested the D3-receptor mRNA on blood lymphocytes and the platelet mitochondrial complex I activity as a peripheral marker of schizophrenia in adults. In the present study we assessed these parameters in the peripheral blood cells of early-onset schizophrenia patients in order to confirm potential markers of this disorder. **Methods:** According to ICD-10 and DSM-IV criteria, 10 first-onset child and adolescent schizophrenic in-patients (age at admission 11.6 to 17;2 years) were recruited. Healthy controls were matched for age and gender. 15 ml blood were drawn every 4 weeks, RNA was isolated and DNAse-treated. After reverse transcription cDNA was analysed by real-time PCR using SYBR Green and iTaq polymerase; primer sequences were designed by the Beacon Designer Software. Statistical evaluation was done by Mann-Whitney Test for comparison between patients and controls and by Wilcoxon Test for comparison of the patients' follow-up data. **Results:** We found a significant increase of the 75 kDa-subunit expression of the mitochondrial complex I in the peripheral blood cells of schizophrenic patients compared to controls ($p = 0.007$ **). Interestingly, using the same procedures and primer sequences as Ilani et al. (2001), the D3-receptor-mRNA was not traceable in our young patients. The data of the four-months-follow-up investigations did not signifi-

cantly change. **Conclusion:** Taken together our results on the mitochondrial complex I in early-onset schizophrenic children and adolescents confirm the data of a previous study on adult schizophrenics. Therefore, these results suggest the platelet mitochondrial complex I as a potential peripheral marker of schizophrenia.

P-017-305 Topic: 69, 12
Clozapine: Impact on aggressive behavior in children and adolescents with treatment refractory Schizophrenia

Harvey Kranzler, Albert Einstein College,
Child & Adolescent Psychiatry, Bronx, NY, USA,
bcmdhnk@omh.state.ny.us
Sanjiv Kumra; Ginny Gerbino-Rosen; David Roofeh;
Courtney DeThomas; Carolyn Dombrowski;
Marjorie McMeniman

Objective: To evaluate the effectivenss of clozapine on aggressive behavior for treatment-refractory children and adolescents with schizophrenia (295.×) at Bronx Children's Psychiatric Center/Albert Einstein College of Medicine, Division of Child Psychiatry. **Methods:** Clozapine treatment was administered in an open label fashion using a flexible titration schedule. The frequency of administration of emergency oral and injectable medications and the frequency of seclusion events secondary to aggressive behavior three months immediately prior to the initiation of clozapine and from 12 to 24 weeks after the initiation of clozapine treatment (when optimal clozapine blood levels were achieved) were compared. **Results:** Twenty Clozapine treated children and adolescents (mean dose at week 24, $476\,mg \pm 119\,mg$) were included. A statistically significant decrease in the frequency of the administration of emergency oral medications, the administration of emergency injectable medications, and seclusion events was found in children and adolescents during week 12 to 24 of clozapine treatment compared to their baseline condition prior to clozapine initiation. **Conclusion:** These preliminary data indicate the benefits of clozapine treatment in children and adolescents with treatment-refractory schizophrenia for aggressive behaviors. Although open data limit conclusions from this study, it is important that there was a clinically significant improvement in aggressive behaviors that enabled patients to be discharged to a less restrictive setting. Controlled clinical trials of clozapine are needed and are presently ongoing in treatment-refractory children and adolescents.

P-017-306 Topic: 68
Tridimensional theory of personality: Applications to substance abuse disorders in adolescents

Hsueh-Ling Chang, Chang Gung Children Hospital,
Dept. of Child Psychiatry, Tao-Yuan, Taiwan,
chang0687@adm.cgmh.org.tw
Sue-Huei Chen; Keh-Chiang Yu

Objective: This study intended to examine Cloninger's temperamental dimensions in a sample of young male juvenile offenders with drug use history. We aimed to examine temperament, behavioral problems and psychiatric disorders in relation to delinquency and substance use. **Methods:** 60 subjects were recruited from a juvenile correction facility in northern Taiwan. All subjects were interviewed with the Chinese version of Schedule for Affective Disorders and Schizophrenia.Self rated questionnaires including Cloninger's Tridimensional Personality Questionnaire and Drug use history were completed by the subjects. **Results:** Adolescents with history of drug abuse showed more novelty seeking behavior, lower harm avoidance and reward dependence in their personality profile. Novelty seeking is positively correlated with the age of onset of alcohol consumption. **Conclusion:** Our findings replicate previous studies showing higher Novelty Seeking behavior among adolescents with substance use.

P-017-307   Topic: 70, 13
Is St. John's wort an evidence based treatment-alternative for depressed Minors? Facts and prescribing trends in Germany

Michael Kölch, Universitätsklinikum Ulm, Kinder- und Jugendpsychiatrie, Ulm, Germany, michael.koelch@medizin.uni-ulm.de
Reinhild Bücheler; Christoph H. Gleiter; Jörg M. Fegert

Objective: The FDA Public Health Advisory of spring 2004 about side effects of antidepressant medication in adolescence emphasises the need of pharmacotherapeutic alternatives to SSRI. In traditional medicine in Asia and, based on ecological movement, in Germany, herbal medicine is considered as a therapeutic alternative without side effects. The best examined herbal medicine against mood disorder is St. John's wort. As a first step to investigate safety and effectiveness of St. John's wort, we examined the presciping patterns for outpatient children. **Methods:** We performed a retrospective analysis of 1.74 million prescriptions, written in January through March 1999 for 27% of all children aged 0 to 16 years in Baden-Wuerttemberg by 6886 paractitioners of general, internal and pediatric medicine at the expense of the Allgemeine Ortskrankenkasse Baden-Wuerttemberg. Prescriptions for St. John's wort were categorised in terms of their licence-status for age groups and Anatomical Therapeutical Chemical Classification groups. **Results:** In the sample, 268 prescriptions of St. John's wort and 96 prescriptions of compound preparations were found. Overall 54.9% of the prescriptions of St. John's wort and 26.0% of compound preparations were off-label. **Conclusion:** These prescribing-data suggest a small but relevant off-label use of St. John's wort in minors. Composed products may have more side effects than pure extracts of St. John's wort. They are prescribed even for very young children.

P-017-308   Topic: 69, 12
Clinical observations on psychopharmacological therapy of Schizophrenia in adolescents with main focus on Amisulpride

Stephanie P. Bohne, Universität Rostock, Kinder- und Jugendpsychiatrie, Rostock, Germany, stephanie.bohne@med.uni-rostock.de
Frank M. Häßler; Bärbel Gierow

Objective: This investigation reports about effects and drug safety of the atypical neuroleptic Amisulpride used for children and adolescents. Adding to the sparse literature we report on six adolescents presenting with a first episode of schizophrenia and one adolescent suffering from a schizo- affective disorder. **Methods:** Amisulpride was adminstered to three boys and four girls so far. On average the sample was 15.4 years old. We evaluated the

course of disease in regards to efficacy, assessed with the BPRS (Brief Psychiatric Rating Scale) and the PANSS (Positive and Negative Symptom Scale). Drug safety was assessed by clinical judgement along with efficacy. Besides Amisulpride, all patients received other neuroleptics (levomepromazine, risperidone, haloperidol), anxiolytics (lorazepame), or antidepressives (citalopram, clomipramine). The maximal daily dosage administered was between 400–1200 mg. Observations covered a period of 32 days. **Results:** Efficacy: Three patients showed a pronounced clinical improvement with a decrease of particularily positive but also negative symptoms. (mean scores: BPRS: 63–30; PANSS, positive: 25–9; PANSS, negative: 19–13). Drug safety: In two cases an increase of negative symptoms was found. Extrapyramidal symptoms were to be seen in six out of seven patients. Distinct increases of prolactine were assessed in all patients reaching clinical salience in one patient. Laboratory results, ECG and EEG findings stayed in normal range. However, patients gained in weight for 3,2 kg in average. **Conclusion:** Contradictory to previous findings patients with predominantly positive symptoms benefied more than those with distinct negative symptoms from neuroleptic therapy. As typical neuroleptics, amisulpride provoked EPS. Despite an increase of prolactine concentration in all patients only one patient showed clinical symptoms during the observation. To evaluate long- term efficacy and a favourable risk-reward-ratio, we need as well a longer investigation period as a larger sample.

P-017-309   Topic: 70, 14
Risperidone augmentation of Lithium in preschool: Onset bipolar disorder

Mani Pavuluri, University of Illinois, Child Psychiatry, Chicago, USA, mpavuluri@psych.uic.edu
David B. Henry; Julie Carbray; Sampson Gwen; Michael Naylor; Philip G. Janicak

Objective: To determine the safety and efficacy with risperidone augmentation of lithium in preschool-onset bipolar disorder. **Methods:** Thirty eight (38) subjects between the ages of 4 and 17 years (mean age = 9.6 ± 3.8 years) with a manic or mixed episode entered the trial. They were treated for 8 weeks with lithium monotherapy with the option of subsequent risperidone augmentation in nonresponders for up to 12 months. The Young Mania Rating Scale (YMRS) was the primary outcome measure. Additional data was collected on diagnostic comorbidity, family history, number of hospitalizations, perinatal risk factors, history of physical or sexual abuse, Child Depression Rating Scale Revised (CDRS-R), Clinical Global Impression Scale for Bipolar Disorder (CGI-BP), Clinical Global Assessment Scale (C-GAS) and adverse effects. **Results:** Twenty-one subjects required risperidone augmentation. Comorbid attention deficit hyperactivity disorder (ADHD) and a history of sexual or physical abuse predicted the need for augmentation. Response was defined as 50% change from baseline and a total score of 12 on the YMRS. This was achieved in 84.2% of the entire sample. The response rate among those requiring risperidone augmentation was 85.7%. Similar responses were noted on CDRS-R (entire sample: 30.14 ± 9.72; augmented group: 29.47 ± 9.91), CGI-BP severity (entire sample: 1.78 ± 0.78; augmented group: 1.89 ± 0.76) and C-GAS (entire sample: 56.26 ± 6.94; augmented group: 55.14 ± 6.03). **Conclusion:** Augmentation with risperidone was efficacious and safe for preschoolonset pediatric bipolar unresponsive to lithium monotherapy.

P-017-310   Topic: 70, 14

Divalproex monotherapy for pediatric mixed mania: A six-month open-label trial

Mani Pavuluri, University of Illinois, Child Psychiatry, Chicago, USA, mpavuluri@psych.uic.edu
David B. Henry; Julie A. Carbray; Michael W. Naylor; Philip G. Janicak

Objective: To examine the safety and efficacy of divalproex sodium (DVPX) in pediatric mixed mania. **Methods:** Thirty-four subjects with a mean age of 12.3 (SD = 3.7) years. A DSM- IV diagnosis of a current mixed episode and a baseline Young Mania Rating Scale (YMRS) score 20 were treated with DVPX in a 6-month, prospective open-label trial. Outcome measures included the YMRS, Clinical Global Impression Scale for Bipolar Disorder (CGI-BP), Child Depression Rating Scale-Revised (CDRS-R) as well as measures of safety and tolerability. **Results:** The effect size (Cohen's d) based on change scores from baseline was 2.9 for the YMRS and 1.23 for the CDRS-R. Response rate (50% change from baseline YMRS score and 40 score on CDRS-R at the end of the study) was 73.5%. Significant improvements ($p < 0.001$) from baseline were seen for mean scores on all efficacy measures (YMRS, CGI-BP and CDRS-R). DVPX was safe and well tolerated with no serious adverse events during the 6-month trial. **Conclusion:** This study provides evidence for the safety and efficacy of DVPX for the treatment of pediatric mixed mania over a 6 month period.

P-018

Disorders and other conditions V

P-018-311   Topic: 82, 40

Learning difficulties and psychiatric disorders among 8-year-old children

Anja Taanila, University of Oulu, Dept. of Public Health Science, Oulu, Finland, anja.taanila@oulu.fi
Katri Hautala; Päivi Kemppainen; Arto Kotimaa; Hanna Ebeling; Irma Moilanen

Objective: To study the association between learning difficulties and symptoms of externalizing, internalizing and hyperactive disorders among 8-year-old children in the Northern Finland 1985/86 Birth Cohort (N = 9432). **Methods:** Teachers assessed children's psychiatric disorders using the Rutter scale and evaluated their learning difficulties in reading, writing and mathematics. The association between learning difficulties and children's psychiatric disorders were analyzed in relation to children's age, gender, family structure, social class, maternal education. Children with intellectual disability were excluded. **Results:** 21.4% of children had learning difficulties and they were more common among boys than girls. 17.5% of boys and 8.4% of girls had verbal (reading and writing) difficulties, but girls (3.7%) had more difficulties in mathematics than boys (2.6%). Only 1.4% of the children had all three (combined) learning difficulties. Younger children had a significantly higher risk for learning difficulties than older ones. An always two-parent family, a family's higher social status and a mother's higher education were the protective factors against children's learning difficulties. Children with learning difficulties had statistically significant risks for externalising, internalizing and hyperactive disorders, but the risk for internalizing disorders was highest (for girls OR 6.0 and for boys OR 3.9). Verbal difficulties were significantly associated with externalizing, internalizing and hyperactive disorders both among boys and girls (ORs ranged from 2.3 to 3.9). A mathematical learning difficulty was most frequently associated with hyperactivity in boys (OR 4.3, 95% CI 2.8–6.6) and internalizing disorder in girls (OR 7.1, 95% CI 4.2–12.1). The association was strongest between combined learning difficulties and externalizing, internalizing and hyperactive disorders. **Conclusion:** In our study we found a remarkable association between learning difficulties and internalizing disorders. This association needs further study to improve these children's possibilities for normal learning and mental development.

P-018-312   Topic: 82, 30

Neuropsychological correlations in dyslexic children

Monica Biscaldi, Universitätsklinikum Freiburg, Kinder- und Jugendpsychiatrie, Freiburg, Germany, biscaldi@psyallg.ukl.uni-freiburg.de
Bettina Wagner; Klaus Hennighausen; Eberhard Schulz

Objective: It is controversially discussed in dyslexia whether deficits in low sensory/motor information processing correlate with phonological and/or language developmental disorders. One concern of this study was to investigate the relationship between neuropsychological functions (K-ABC), saccadic eye movements and reading/spelling performances of dyslexic children. **Methods:** We measured the saccadic eye movement performance (prosaccade overlap task and antisaccade gap task) of 32 dyslexic children (8–12 y.) previously assessed by the Kaufman Assessment Battery for Children (K-ABC) and by standardised reading (reading speed and errors) and spelling tests. Pearson correlation and the principal components factor analysis were used for statistical analysis. **Results:** First, reading speed was hardly associated with neuropsychological functions. We found a significant positive correlation between spelling and visual-spatial skills. Lexical reading (errors) and visual-spatial skills positively loaded on the same factor. Slower reaction times of prosaccades were correlated with a poorer performance in text reading. On the other hand, lower visual-spatial abilities were associated with slower saccadic reaction times of prosaccades and with a higher error rate in the antisaccade task. **Conclusion:** These results suggest that visual-spatial abilities could play a role in compensating reading and spelling deficits of dyslexics. Although the results encourages the usage of visual-spatial training in dyslexia remedy programs, its effect on reading and spelling performance should be further investigated.

P-018-313   Topic: 82

Eye movement patterns of dyslexic and nondyslexic German speaking children

Ute Dürrwächter, Universitätsklinikum Tübingen, Kinder- und Jugendpsychiatrie, Tübingen, Germany, ute.duerrwaechter@med.uni-tuebingen.de
Susanne Trauzettel-Klosinski; Jens Reinhard; Gunther Klosinski

Objective: Central point of interest of the study was to investigate, whether difficulties in the cognitive processes of word recognition are reflected in the eye movement pattern of dyslexic children. **Methods:** Eye fixation patterns of 16 dyslexic and 16 age-matched, nondyslexic, German-speaking children were compared when reading loudly words of different length and frequency. The eye movements were registered using a Scanning Laser Ophthalmoscope (SLO), which allows a high accurate recording and minimizes interfering artifacts. **Results:** The results show a highly significant word-frequency effect for central parameters of the analysis, like the percentage of regressions, the number of fixations and the fixation duration. Furthermore, the results indicate that the regularity of the graphem-phonem-correspondence leads to differences in eye movement parameters, and the outcome of the word-frequency and word-length effect between the German and English written language. **Conclusion:** Overall, the results support the hypothesis, that the eye movement patterns of dyslexic children reflect their difficulties in word recognition and are not merely caused by an oculomotor deficit.

P-018-314   Topic: 82, 30
Memory deficits in German children with spelling disorders

Ellen Plume, Universität Würzburg,
Kinder- und Jugendpsychiatrie, Würzburg, Germany,
plume@kjp.uni-wuerzburg.de
Gerd Schulte-Körne; Helmut Remschmidt; Andreas Warnke

Objective: A German family genetic study assesses neurobiological, neurophysiological and psychological aspects of spelling disorders. Parts of this study examine the role of working memory, phonological recoding and speed of lexical access in children with spelling disorders. **Methods:** 51 children with spelling disorders at the age of 9 to 14 years (experimental group) were compared with their 31 non affected siblings (control group) according several variables. A pseudoword reading test was administered to assess phonological recoding and rapid naming tasks measured the speed of lexical access. Working memory capacity was assessed by digit span. **Results:** Children with spelling disorders were significantly inferior in phonological recoding and lexical access in comparison to their non affected siblings. No group differences were found in digit span. **Conclusion:** German children with spelling disorders do have specific memory deficits.

P-018-315   Topic: 82, 37
Screening for emotional disturbances in children with specific learning disabilities:
A pilot study with Conners Questionnaire for parents

Nadezda Krstic, Institute for Mental Health, Belgrade,
Serbia and Montenegro, imz@imh.org.yu
Olivera Aleksic; Branko Aleksic; Ana Velimirovic

Objective: Despite well recognized vulnerability of children with specific learning disabilities to emotional disturbances, such problems in this population, unless quite pronounced, seem to be easily neglected in standard procedures of diagnostic and treatment of learning disabled child, mostly due to (professionals' and parents') overfocussing child's outstanding neurocognitive deficit. **Methods:** To examine usability of Conners Parent Symptom Checklist (PSC) – often routinely used in screening of child psychiatric population – in enlightening possible emotional difficulties of a minor scale in our patients, we have analyzed PSC scores in five groups of younger school age children (specific learning disabilities, ADHD, epilepsy, emotional & behavioral disturbances, healthy controls; n = 15–20, N = 87). **Results:** Although LD children, as well

as all other 'clinical' groups, scored significantly higher than controls in respect of total PSC points, none of special scores derived from the questionnaire appeared characteristic for this group. However, statistical discriminant analysis of individual items of the questionnaire has offered two discriminant variables able to classify correctly 76% of children with LD, ADHD and emotional & behavioral disturbances, where dimensions related to LD group appeared to encompass primarily a certain trend towards internalizing behavior and social withdrawal together with signs of behavioral immaturity. **Conclusion:** These data suggest possibility to make use of other 'markers' beside 'psychopathology scores' on Conners Questionnaire, as well to employ even shorter forms of the instrument in selected clinical population.

P-018-316   Topic: 82, 3
Long-term outcome of a preschool training in phonological awareness in the prevention of Dyslexia

Regula Blaser, Univer.-Psychiatrische Dienste, Kinder- und Jugendpsychiatrie, Bern, Switzerland, regulablaser@web.de
Ulrich Preuss

Objective: The Bern Study of child development was designed to test the possibilities to prevent dyslexia on the basis of early competencies in phonological information processing in a sample of Swiss children. **Methods:** The study started in autumn 1999 with a sample of 260 kindergarten children. After the baseline visit, half of the sample was trained with a Swiss adaptation of a training program in phonological awareness and in letter-sound correspondence for 20 weeks. Meanwhile the control group followed the regular kindergarten program. All children were reassessed several times after the training to gain a detailed picture of their course of development and to be able to determine the effectiveness of the training program in the prevention of dyslexia. **Results:** Results showed that the training had a great short term effect on the development of the phonological awareness of the children. However, long term effects (four years follow up) on the acquisition of reading and writing competencies could not be demonstrated as impressive as in other studies. **Conclusion:** There are several hypotheses which could explain the present results. One is that the training groups were too big to really reach the children with the greatest deficits in phonological awareness. An other is that the children had difficulties to transfer from the contents of the training program, which were presented in dialect, to standard German that is taught in school. Several other hypotheses will be discussed as well and a perspective for the daily work of the kindergarten nurses will be given.

P-018-317   Topic: 82, 1
Needs of families with language impaired children

Claudia Meusel, Universität München,
Kinder- und Jugendpsychiatrie, München, Germany,
suchodoletz@lrz.uni-muenchen.de
Waldemar von Suchodoletz

Objective: Speech and language therapists usually involve parents in the intervention process. Little is however known about the special needs of parents of language impaired children. The aim of the study was to determine the needs, wishes and expectations of families with language disturbed children and to develop a questionnaire for the use in intervention practice. **Methods:** A questionnaire for families with language impaired children was constructed on the basis of the "Family Needs Survey" for parents with mentally retarded children (Bailey et al. 1992). The questionnaire items were validated by means of an experts rating and checked in a pre-study. The final questionnaire, consisting of 24 items in five dimensions, was sent to families (n = 1892) with language impaired children via language therapists or teachers of special language preschool units or schools. 45% (n = 858) of the families completed the questionnaire. **Results:** 77% of the parents expressed the wish for more information about their child's condition or disability, 51% for more counselling by experts and support in finding a special care institution, 51% expressed the wish for financial support for the participation on intervention programmes and 46% for assistance with social integration. The parents of children with combined disabilities (language disorders combined with conduct or attention deficit disorders) expressed more needs than those of children without co-morbidity. **Conclusion:** The results suggest that parents expect more from specialists than the improvement of their children's language ability. The evaluated questionnaire proved to be suitable as an efficient means to obtain information about the special needs of families with language impaired children. The application of the questionnaire can therefore be recommended to improve the planning of intervention programmes for the care of language impaired children.

P-018-318 Topic: 82, 61

Stigmatisation of language impaired children and their families

Georg Macharey, Universität München,
Kinder- und Jugendpsychiatrie, München, Germany,
suchodoletz@lrz.uni-muenchen.de
Waldemar von Suchodoletz

Objective: It is generally assumed that conduct and emotional disorders in language impaired children result at least in part from stigmatisation. The aim of this study was to examine to what extent parents of language impaired children experience stigmatisation or support of either their child or themselves, and which areas of their lives are affected. **Methods:** The "Perceive Stigma Questionnaire" (Link 1985) was adapted for use with language impaired children. To improve the validity, a rating by experts was performed. The final version of the questionnaire consisted of 58 items for the stigmatisation and support scales. The questionnaires were sent (n = 877) to parents of children who either received speech and language therapy or attended preschool language units or special language schools. 44% of the questionnaires were returned. **Results:** The results show that parents observe support more often (20–40%) than stigmatisation (5–15%) from relatives and neighbours. Based on the parents' rating, 20–30% of language impaired children experience rejection, teasing and bullying in peer groups as a result of their disability. The extent of stigmatisation was related to the severity of the language impairment and to the occurrence of conduct disorders. No correlation with age, sex or socio-economic status was found. **Conclusion:** The findings suggest that most adults accept language impairment in children. They express sympathy and consideration more frequently than rejection. Stigmatisation is particularly observed in peer groups. The results show that language impaired children need support with the integration in groups of children.

P-018-319 Topic: 81, 34

Pharmacological treatment of psychiatric disorders in individuals with intellectual disability: A study on adaptive behaviour

Anastasia Dressler, Universität Wien,
Inst. für Kinderheilkunde, Wien, Austria,
anastasiaflora@gmx.net
Valentina Perelli; Valentina Rafanelli; Stefania Bargagna

Objective: Individuals with intellectual disability (ID) are at a significant high risk of psychiatric disorders when compared to their non-ID peers, as ID constitutes a factor of vulnerability. Our main aim was to assess the efficacy psychopharmacological treatment in a population with Down syndrome (DS) and to define the relationship of treatment effect and adaptive behaviour. **Methods:** We included 55 individuals from 15 to 52 years, performed a non-structured psychiatric interview, assessed the Aberrant Behaviour Checklist (ABC), Raven's coloured progressive matrices (CPM), Dementia scale for Down syndrome (DSDS), and the Vineland Adaptive Behaviour Scales (VABS). **Results:** The incidence of psychiatric co-morbidity in our group is rather high (36.6%), anxiety disorders are the most frequent, followed by PDD-NOS and mood disorders, half of the individuals with depression also presented and anxiety disorder. Adaptive abilities are significantly poorer in individuals with the presence of a psychiatric disorder. Individuals with psychiatric co-morbidity and psychopharmacological medication obtain overall higher scores. On the ABC, there are no significant differences between both groups, but we find overall higher scores on symptoms in the treatment group. Their most frequent symptoms are in the area irritability and hyperactivity. **Conclusion:** The persistence of positive psychopathologic features such as irritability and hyperactivity seems to reflect in the treated group a more obvious symptomatology even before treatment and the necessity of treatment if more psychopathological features are present. Negative symptoms, such as lethargy do not differ on mean score. It seems important to consider psychopharmacological medication in a population ID together with other rehabilitative and occupational treatment to improve adaptive skills and as a consequence quality of life. Psychiatric co-morbidity impairs adaptive behaviour, however psychopharmacological treatment may be a useful support.

P-018-320 Topic: 82, 21

Effects of temporal resolution training at the sound and phoneme levels in addition to school-based reading training as usual

Ulrich Strehlow, Klinik an der Lindenhöhe,
Kinder- und Jugendpsychiatrie, Offenburg, Germany,
strehlow@ortenau.mediclin.de
Johann Haffner; Jürgen Bischof; Volker Gratzka;
Peter Parzer; Franz Resch

Objective: This study examines the effects of temporal resolution training at the sound and phoneme levels for 8 year old children with reading disabilities. **Methods:** Data are reported from three samples of children. Sample A (N = 37) is used to test the reliability of the sound and phoneme discrimination tasks. Sample B (N = 51) consists of a group of normal children to determine the range of normal performance on the sound and phoneme discrimination task. Sample C (N = 44) consists of three groups of children with readings disabilities who participated in one of three training programs: (1) sound discrimination and reading training; (2) phoneme discrimination and reading training; (3) reading training only. The sound discrimination task involved reporting the sequence of two dynamic tones changing in pitch and interval. The phoneme discrimination task involved CV syllables with stops and/a/varying length and intensity of the consonant. The training was given daily for four weeks. **Results:** Sample A showed appropriate test-retest reliability for both tasks. Sample B showed that normal children performed better than children with reading disabilities. Results from the training groups of sample C showed that sound discrimination training improved performance in sound discrimination but these gains were not maintained at follow-up. Phoneme discrimination training improved performance in phoneme discrimination. Gains were maintained at 6 months follow-up but no more at 12 months. There was no transfer of improved sound discrimination performance on phoneme discrimination performance and vice-versa. At follow-up at 6 months the sound discrimination group showed improvements in spelling, but this was not maintained over 12 months. All three groups showed significant improving in reading with no differences between the groups. **Conclusion:** There is a marked improvement of sound and phoneme discrimination performance after an intensive training for four weeks. However, a stable transfer on reading and spelling could not be demonstrated. Due to the limited power of the study, it is not possible to exclude that an effect of training on reading or spelling might be overseen. As an auxiliary result we can confirm the effect of the school-based reading training.

P-018-321   Topic: 82, 37
Comparability of language test results in two year old children
Steffi Sachse, Universität München,
Kinder- und Jugendpsychiatrie, München, Germany,
steffi.sachse@lrz.uni-muenchen.de
Beatrice Anke; Waldemar von Suchodoletz

Objective: Language tests with different types of material (pictures vs. toys) and parent-report questionnaires are used to diagnose language retardation in young children. The aim of the study was to determine the comparability of the test results. **Methods:** The expressive language abilities of 34 children aged from 24 to 28 months were evaluated by means of a parent-report questionnaire (German version of the McArthur Communicative Development Inventory – ELFRA2), a language test mainly based on pictures (Sprachentwicklungstest für zweijährige Kinder, SETK-2) and a language test predominantly based on toys (German translation of the Reynell Developmental Language Scales, RDLS III). **Results:** All children who were classified as late talkers by means of the ELFRA2 (n=22) were also labelled as language delayed by the SETK-2. Only 81% of these children showed subnormal scores on the Reynell Scales. Children with normal expressive language abilities based on the results of the ELFRA2 (n=12) were all also classified as normal by using the Reynell Scales. 82% of these children reached scores within the normal range by means of the SETK2. The intercorrelation between the test results was high and significant and ranged between 0.75 and 0.93. **Conclusion:** The findings of this study indicate that the results of the evaluated language tests are comparable. However, the SETK-2 and the

ELFRA2 classified more children as late talkers than the Reynell Scales. The parent-report questionnaire ELFRA2 proved to be a valid instrument for diagnosis of late talkers. The questionnaire can be used economically and without great effort and can therefore be recommended to paediatricians as a screening method. Children who have been determined through the parent-report questionnaire to be late talkers should be carefully assessed by means of language tests to obtain information not only on language production but also on language comprehension.

P-018-322   Topic: 82, 37
Prognostic validity of the German version of the McArthur Communicative Development Inventories
Steffi Sachse, Universität München,
Kinder- und Jugendpsychiatrie, München, Germany,
steffi.sachse@lrz.uni-muenchen.de
Monika Adamski; Angelika Pecha;
Waldemar von Suchodoletz

Objective: ELFRA1 and ELFRA2 (German versions of the McArthur Communicative Development Inventories) are parent-report questionnaires for the detection of language delay at the ages of 12 and 24 months. The aim of the study was to determine the predictive value of these screening instruments. **Methods:** To evaluate the ELFRA1 parents of 12 months old children were sent the questionnaire (n=238). 61% of the parents returned it and were sent a further questionnaire one year later. The final sample of monolingual German speaking children for whom data for both points in time could be collected contains 121 subjects. For the evaluation of ELFRA2 we assessed children at the age of 24 months (n=251, return rate: 74%) and 36 months. The final sample contains 149 subjects. **Results:** 38% of the 121 one year old children and 13% of the 149 two year old children were classified as language delayed after the first screening. After taking into account the children's language abilities at the second screening, we found for ELFRA1 a sensitivity of 52% and a specificity of 65%, whereas the prognostic validity of ELFRA2 was significantly higher (sensitivity 69%, specificity 92 %). The gender of the child and the educational background of the mother proved to be predictors. **Conclusion:** The predictive value of the ELFRA1 at the age of 12 months is too low for identifying children at risk for later language impairment. The ELFRA2 at the age of 24 months, however, seems to be a useful parent-report screening instrument. Most of the three year old children with developmental language disorders can be identified at the age of 24 months. The number of false positives is, however, high: the language abilities of 50% of the two year old late talkers turned out to be within the normal range at the age of three.

P-018-323   Topic: 81
Conceptual functioning of mild mentally retarded children
Dragana Macesic-Petrovic, University of Belgrade,
Faculty for Special Education, Belgrade, Serbia and
Montenegro, macesicd@yahoo.com
Svetlana Slavnic

Objective: The basic aim of this investigation was to determine the level and the quality of the cognitive functioning of mild mentally retarded school age children. **Methods:**

The sample of 124 mild mentally retarded children, aged 8–13.6 years, attending special schools in Belgrade, were tested by the Test of Concept Utilization (Crager & Lane). **Results:** The results of research indicate the poor cognitive efficiency of mild mentally retarded children in cognitive fields and both global conceptual categories, which were tested at the investigated sample. The achievement on the implemented test has shown up the 31.5% successfully children and 68.5% children whose achievement is unsuccessful at the implemented test. **Conclusion:** The cognitive problems of the investigated sample indicate that there is marked weakness of rehabilitation treatment of the mentally retarded children tested in this investigation.

P-018-324   Topic: 82
Intellectual factors which affect the writing and reading disorders in Japanese

Chie Hatagaki, Nagaoya-City, Japan,
kamonegima@yahoo.co.jp

Objective: To examine some intellectual facter which affect Writing and Reading Japanese (HIRAGANA, KATAKANA and Chinese character) in the Child. **Methods:** 47 patients (35 boys and 12 girls, from 6 to 15 ys. old, M = 10.21 ys.) who had consulted the child psychiatry. They under go WISC-3 (Wechsler Intelligence Scale for Children-Third Edition), Test for Writing Japanese (HIRAGANA, KATAKANA and Chinese character), Test for Reading Japanese (HIRAGANA, KATAKANA and Chinese Character) and Test for apprehension of abstraction. **Results:** 1) Ability of reading Chinese Character have correlations with [Knowledge] (r = 0.52) and [Similarity] (0.55). 2) Ability of writing Chinese Character have correlation with [Apprehension of obstraction].

P-018-325   Topic: 81, 30
Neuropsychological underpinning of social problems in Klinefelter Syndrome, compared to PDD and ADHD

Hanna Swaab, University Medical Center,
Child & Adolescent Psychiatry, Utrecht, Netherlands,
h.swaab@azu.nl
P. Cohen-Kettenis; Herman van Engeland

Objective: To examine the relation between social problems and neuropsychological functioning; or the search for the endophenotype of social disfunctioning. **Methods:** 35 boys with 47, xxy are compared to 41 boys with PDD, to 51 boys with ADHD and to 50 normal control boys with respect to (1) pragmatic language use, (2) recognition of faces, (3) recognition of facial emotions and (4) regulation of attention. The social problems were measured with several standardized methods. **Results:** Boys with 47, xxy show severe problems in social functioning in comparison to the other patient groups. These problems appear to be correlated with pragmatic language disabilities, difficulty in recognition of faces and identification of facial emotions and to attention problems. These children especially show problems in selection of relevant information during information processing. **Conclusion:** In 47,xxy an extra X-chromosome is appearantly responsible for social problems that present themselves in a way that is common to the problems in children with pervasive developmental disorders. Problems in pragmatic language use, in recognition of faces and emotions and in regulation of attention appear to be the underlying endophenotype of these social problems.

P-018-326   Topic: 82
Multiple-problematical families and compliance to therapy in early development disorders

Roberta Di Scipio, Rome, Italy, r.discipio@tiscali.it
Ester Patruno; Alessia Tosco; Anna Fabrizi

Objective: The aim of our study was to evaluate how family's problems could influence the development of children with Early Development Disorders. **Methods:** We studied two groups of children. Each group was composed of 20 children matched for age, type an severity of the disorder. The two group was divided according on the presence/absence of familiar risk factors (at least 3 of the following items: severe parents conflictuality, divorced parents, absence of one parent, parents psychopathology, adoption) and on the presence/absence of index of neglet (at least 2 of the following items: severe parents amnesia about development data, multiple caregiver, inadeguate cares, ipo or iper stymolations). Both groups were evaluate, after a 12 month follow-up, according to development of the disorder, the answer after therapy and according to the compliance to the therapy. **Results:** Children coming from the multiple-problematical families showed significant differences compared to the control group, without risk factors, about the compliance and the answer to the therapy. These data shows how the risk factors that we studied could be considered as negative prognostic index in the development of the disorder. **Conclusion:** The data examined seems to show a correlation between familiar risk factors and the low compliance and the worst outcome after treatment in children with Early Development Disorders.

P-018-327   Topic: 82, 23
'I can stutter – I can speak': Psychological evaluations of a group speech therapy for stuttering adolescents

Sabine Völkl-Kernstock, Medizinische Universität Wien,
Inst. für Neuropsychiatrie, Wien, Austria,
sabine.voelkl-kernstock@univie.ac.at
Sylvia Reinelt-Straka; Liselotte Hoffmann; Max H. Friedrich

Objective: Of all disorders of speech, stuttering is one of the most intensively researched (Natke, 2000). In the course of their speech development, 5% of all children display some symptoms of stuttering, 1% of whom develop long-term, chronic stuttering. The primary symptoms of stuttering comprise the involuntary repetition of sounds, syllables and words, extention of sounds and blockages before or during a word. Secondary symptoms can develop in reaction to the primary ones (Bloodstein, 1995). **Methods:** Based on Van Riper's concept (1973, 1984), this group speech therapy was divided into four phases, namely: (1) identification, (2) desensitization, (3) modification and (4) stabilization. The group therapy sessions took place on 9 weekends. Two sessions were always held on consecutive weekends and the following two took place after a therapy-free time of 5 to 6 weeks, in which the new input could be applied and tried out in everyday life. The psychological and speech therapeutical diagnoses were undertaken at three different stages: at the beginning and end of the group therapy, and half a year later. Various research tools were used, including SSI, SSMP, CBCL, YSR and J-TCI. To reflect the distribution of stuttering in the population on the whole, 5 boys and 1 girl, from 12 to 16 years of age took part in the group therapy. **Results:** The results of the first two test stages have been made available so far. The measurements at the second occasion give evidence of significant reductions in the secondary symptoms as well as the quantity of stuttering on the whole. All adolescents were also able to actively modify their core stuttering behaviour and, thus, regain control over their speaking. A further significant result became apparent in the adolescents' self-evaluations with regard to their qualitative and quantitative stuttering symptoms. At the same time, their self-assuredness in their speaking abilities increased significantly, especially for public occasions. **Conclusion:** This pilot study has shown so far that this patient group learned to get a grip on their stuttering symptoms and that two relevant factors are their personal attitudes to stuttering and increased self-esteem.

P-018-328   Topic: 81
Cognitive rehabilitation of mild mentally retarded children at the education treatment

Dragana Macesic-Petrovic, University of Belgrade, Faculty for Special Education, Belgrade, Serbia and Montenegro, macesicd@yahoo.com
Svetlana Slavnic

Objective: The research deals with the scientific study of the successes of the rehabilitation of the cognitive and motor functioning of mild mentally retarded children. The analysis represents the basis for assessment of applied treatment with respect to education of this population of children. The analysis of quality of cognitive and motor development is based on observation of the degree of development of gnostic, praxic and conceptual-verbal functioning as compared to learning process and adaptive ability of the mild mentally retarded children. **Methods:** The sample of 124 mild mentally retarded children, aged 8–13,6 years, attending special schools in Belgrade, were tested by the following tests: – Luria/Nebraska Neuropsychological Battery Children's Revision (Golden) – Trial Making Test for Children (Reitan) – Stick Test (Benson & Barton) – Token test (Boller & Vignolo) – Conners Rating Scales (Conners). Statistical analysis implemented in this investigation is based on chi square test and coefficient of correlation and contingency. **Results:** The results of investigation point up the significance of the rehabilitation procedures in the investigated sample. This sample's marked disorder is in the area of the learning processes and behavior. More than 30% of investigated sample have developmental problems in the tested developmental areas. **Conclusion:** The poor cognitive efficiency of the investigated sample defined as disorder of development and learning process indicates that there is a weakness of education and reeducation of psychomotor activity treatment.

P-018-329   Topic: 81, 6
The development and pilot of an intervention for teenage siblings of children with an intellectual disability in Western Australia

Monique Nesa, Curtin University, School of Psychology, Perth, Australia, m.nesa@curtin.edu.au
David Hay; Clare Roberts; Mairead McCoy

Objective: Intellectual disability is a significant issue in the world today. While the effects of disability on the individual, their parents and their family as a whole have been extensively researched, the specific effects on siblings have gone relatively unrecognised. Consequently, few services have been available for siblings and very few have been provided for teenagers. The present research is concerned with the development and pilot of a novel intervention to assist the positive adjustment of teenage siblings of children with an intellectual disability. **Methods:** Information gained from focus groups along with recent literature, provided an outline for the intervention. The result was a 6-week program, consisting of 90-minute groups covering "Sharing My Story", "Exploring Differences and Disabilities", "Exploring and Communicating Feelings", "Problem Solving", "Relaxation Skills" and "Finding Meaning". The intervention was piloted with two groups, aged 12–17 years. Paired samples t-tests were conducted to determine whether the "perceived effect of disability" of participants' significantly changed from pre to post-test. **Results:** Participants' perception of "Family Differences", "Worry About What Others Think" and "Lack of Time with Others" improved significantly. These quantitative results along with extensive qualitative data provide strong evidence for the importance of such an intervention. **Conclusion:** These results will overall assist in providing a more permanent service for teenage siblings in Western Australia and aid awareness of the effects of disability on this particular group.

P-018-329 A   Topic: 82, 95
Psychiatric comorbidity in children with dyslexia

Harriet Salbach, Charité, Child and Adolescent Psych., Berlin, Germany, harriet.salbach@charite.de
Uta Klopfer; Swantje Hagen; Bürger Arne; Ulrike Lehmkuhl

Objective: While extensive research has been dedicated to the relation between externalizing disorders and dyslexia, there is only few literature on the relation of dyslexia and internalizing disorders. This study investigates the comorbidity of internalizing and externalizing psychopathology respectively, in association with dyslexia. **Methods:** Within a case control design 70 children (39 with dyslexia; 31 without dyslexia) were recruited systematically. Participants were clinic-referred outpatients aged 8 to 13 years (mean age of the dyslexia group 10.6 ± 1.5 years and 10.3 ± 1.4 for the non-dyslexia group), their IQ was within the normal range. Both groups did not differ in gender and socioeconomic status. We assessed children's psychiatric diagnoses after a broad clinical diagnostic phase including neurological as well as psychological examination, and extensive interviews with parents and children. Data were analyzed by chi-square statistic. **Results:** Both groups did not differ significantly in terms of their comorbidity relating to internalizing and externalizing categories. However, sub-analyses showed more ADHD and less oppositional defiant or conduct disorders in the dyslexia group compared to the non-dyslexia group. Furthermore, internalizing disorders were equally represented in both groups. **Conclusion:** This study emphasizes not only the association between dyslexia and ADHD but also the connection between dyslexia and internalizing disorders, which is often disregarded. The high rate of psychiatric comorbidity in children with dyslexia shows a great demand for psychotherapeutic intervention.

P-019-330   Topic: 84, 58

Therapeutic after-school programs for young adolescents with Attention Deficit Hyperactivity Disorder (ADHD)

*Bradley Smith, University of South Carolina,
Dept. of Psychology, Columbia, SC, USA, smithbrad@sc.edu*

Objective: To examine the effectiveness of an after school treatment program for young adolescents with Attention-Deficit/Hyperactivity Disorder. **Methods:** Participants are 60 students aged 11 to 14 enrolled in grades 6 to 8. Referrals were solicited through teachers, school staff, and informational flyers to parents. Diagnoses were made by program staff on the basis of ratings and structured interviews. Participants attend the program 2 to 3 days a week for 2 hours a day. Each day in the program, students receive about 45 minutes of individualized counseling focussing on organization skills and school to home communication. Students also participate in 45 minutes of group and individual academic skills training and 45 minutes of therapeutic recreation. Primary counselors have weekly contact with parents and teachers. Many families participate in parent training or family therapy. Program effects are assessed via quarterly school grades, the Behavioral Assessment System for Children (BASC), and impairment ratings. The BASC and impairment ratings were completed by parents and two classroom teachers on three occasions. **Results:** Results in this poster submission are preliminary, as study completion is set for May 2004. In two separate pilot studies, moderate to large treatment effect sizes (i.e., Cohen's d of 0.5 or greater) were seen on measures of inattention, classroom behavior, and grade point average. **Conclusion:** It was feasible to implement the program in American middle schools with modest funding (i.e., less then $ 1,000 USD per student). Preliminary evaluation of program effectiveness are promising. Research on after-school programming for adolescents with ADHD is warranted given 1) the dearth of research on psychosocial treatments for ADHD in adolescents, 2) promising results in a few psychosocial treatment studies suggesting improvements in multiple domains of functioning in these youth, and 3) limitations associated with reliance on psychoactive medications as the sole treatment for adolescents with ADHD.

P-019-331   Topic: 85, 12

Case Series: Ziprasidone as a treatment option for improving impulse control in prepubertal boys at risk for weight gain

*Michael Kölch, Universitätsklinikum Ulm,
Kinder- und Jugendpsychiatrie, Ulm, Germany,
michael.koelch@medizin.uni-ulm.de
Gerhard Libal; Paul Plener; Jörg M. Fegert*

Objective: The use of atypical neuroleptics for treating disruptive behavior and impulsivity in school children with ADHD is well established in child psychiatry today. One major limiting factor is weight gain. We used Ziprasidone as a weight neutral alternative to the well established Risperidone treatment **Methods:** We report a retrospective chart review of 4 male patients (age range 9–13) who were treated in an off label condition with Ziprasidone (dose range 40–60 mg/d). Selection criterion for the use of Ziprasidone was pre-existing obesity or excessive weight gain under Risperidone. Assessments included psychometric questionnaires, adverse effects (ECG) and weight monitoring. **Results:** Ziprasidone led to an improvement in the clinical impression and in ratings for impulsivity. Weight gain measured by BMI was moderate (mean BMI 0.91, range 0.47–1.7) in the first 4–6 month. One nine year old boy showed a transient increase of irritability and anxiety. **Conclusion:** Even though Risperidone is labelled in Germany for the treatment of disruptive behaviour disorders for children aged six and older Ziprasidone may be a useful alternative. In a high risk group of four obese boys we found similar clinical effects and less weight gain even in long-term treatment.

P-019-332   Topic: 84, 91

Absences as differential diagnosis in child and adolescent psychiatric patients

*Judith Sinzig, University of Cologne, Child & Adolescent Psychiatry, Köln, Germany, ju.k.sinzig@web.de
Martin Holtmann; Alexander von Gontard*

Objective: Absences are regarded as one of the most important differential diagnoses of attention-deficit/hyperactivity disorder (ADHD) and resulting school-problems. Attention deficit-symptoms might develop through absences, even though there is no diagnosis of ADHD. Routine EEG-wavings are made, in order to exclude epilepsy as a reason for attention-deficits. **Methods:** In this paper the EEGs of 8132 male and female children and adolescents from two clinics for child and adolescent psychiatry in Germany were analyzed retrospectively. The aim of the study was to assess how many patients were concerned by abscences and whether they presented a specific psychopathology. **Results:** In summary for the first time diagnosed absences occured in 0.44% (N = 12) of the patients in the first centre and in none of the patients in the second centre. The average age was 9.5 years. 50% of the patients were diagnosed with ADHD. A specific psychopathology of the patients was not found. **Conclusion:** There is a minimal occurrence of absences in child and adolescent patients. Therefore it is not a main differential diagnosis that has to be considered in children with attention-deficit problems. Due to the late age at the time of diagnosis and the possible good treatability with antiepileptics, it is nevertheless important to regard absences as a rare differential diagnosis.

P-019-333   Topic: 85, 59

Television game experience and children's aggression: An attempt to clarify the link in Japanese elementary school children

Takayo Mukai, University of the Sacred Heart, Psychology, Tokyo, Japan, mukai@silk.plala.or.jp

Objective: While Japanese television games (TV games) are widespread, there have been few empirical investigations regarding their possible influence upon children's attitudes and behavior. The present study aimed at examining the link between the extent of TV game experience and the level of aggression in Japanese 5th graders, using questionnaire and projective, picture-drawing methods. The TV game experience was expected to be related to children's aggression. **Methods:** A total of 200 5th graders

(Mean age = 11.4 years-old) responded to a questionnaire, assessing the level of aggression, self-efficacy, as well as the past and current exposure to TV games. In this study, aggression was assessed mostly in terms of aggressive attitudes, such as irritation and competitiveness, rather than physical violence. The respondents were also administered with the structured HTP (House-Tree-Person), a picture-drawing technique, to assess their aggression and reality-testing ability. Children were divided into 2 groups based on their level of exposure to TV games. The children in the High exposure group reported, on the average, to play TV games 5 or more days per week, spending 2.5 hours or more each time, and had started to play as early as in pre-school or in the 1st grade. The children in the Low exposure group either had no experience or had started to play in the 3rd or 4th grade, spending less than 1 hour at a time. **Results:** According to the one-way ANOVAs, the children in the High exposure group showed significantly greater aggression and less self-efficacy than children in the Low exposure group. In addition, the children in the High exposure group were more likely to draw unrealistic and aggressive pictures in HTP. **Conclusion:** The present results suggest that TV game experience seem to increase children's some form of aggression. Future attempts are needed to study mechanisms underlying the association.

P-019-334   Topic: 85
Callous-unemotional traits are associated with clinical severity in referred boys with conduct problems
Pia Enebrink, Karolinska Institutet, Div. of Forensic Psychiatry, Huddinge, Sweden, pia.enebrink@neurotec.ki.se
Niklas Långström; Henrik Andershed

Objective: Children that present with conduct problems constitute a heterogeneous group that may benefit from improved formats for diagnostic subtyping. We investigated whether high levels of callous-unemotional traits (i.e., lack of empathy, remorselessness, and shallow affects) would differentiate clinic-referred conduct-problem boys from those low on such traits. **Methods:** A consecutive series of 41 boys with conduct problems (6–13 years, mean age = 9.60 years) referred to public child psychiatric units in Sweden were studied with data elicited from caregivers. Parent-ratings of the APSD (Antisocial Process Screening Device) were used to divide the boys into subgroups of high (13 boys) or low (28 boys) on callous-unemotional traits. These subgroups were then compared regarding type and frequency of aggressive or conduct-disordered behaviour, psychiatric diagnoses (DSM IV), circumstances in the family, school performance, and responsivity for treatment. **Results:** Conduct-problem boys with many callous-unemotional traits had significantly more pervasive, varied and aggressive disruptive behavioural problems than boys low on these traits had. Higher levels of conduct problems in subjects with callous-unemotional traits were not explained by confounding presence of DSM-IV AD/HD and ODD/CD symptoms. Boys with callous-unemotional traits also experienced poorer household circumstances and lived in families under high stress. Interestingly, they less often received help in school from special teachers but were more often diagnosed with Dysthymia than boys low on callous-unemotional traits. **Conclusion:** Callous-unemotional traits might designate a subgroup of boys with different etiology to their conduct problems and possibly with specific treatment needs. However, the present findings need to be replicated with larger samples.

P-019-335   Topic: 85, 73
Psychological, neuropsychological and physiological evaluation of delinquent adolescents with and without Post-Traumatic Stress Disorder (PTSD)
Louis Richer, UQAC, Dept. of Psychology, Chicoutimi, QC, Canada, louis_richer@uqac.ca
Lise Lachance; Claude Dubé; Serge Saintonge

Objective: Delinquents are at risk of developing physical and mental health problems. They show adaptation problems during a critical developmental period: conduct disorder, violence, suicidal behavior, etc. Posttraumatic stress disorder (PTSD) may contribute to clinical manifestations of these problems. It can also alter social functioning and modify hypothalamic-pituitary-adrenal axis functioning. This axis controls cortisol secretion, a physiological indicator of stress. Prolonged alteration of cortisol level may produce health problems and affect cognitive functions. PTSD victims manifest a variety of symptoms and require a multidimensional evaluation approach. This research estimates PTSD prevalence among adolescents in a youth centre with a multidimensional protocol and examines the relationship between PTSD diagnosis, cortisol level and some cognitive functions (IQ, attention, memory). **Methods:** Twenty-nine male neuroleptic free delinquents (14–17 years old) completed the Trauma Symptom Checklist for Children, the Parental Bonding Instrument and the Adolescent Dissociative Experiences Scale. They were also evaluated with the Diagnostic Interview Schedule for Children-Revised to establish hyperanxiety, major depression, ADHD, oppositional defiant disorder and conduct disorder symptoms. A brief neuropsychological evaluation was done (WISC-III subtests, d2, Rey Auditory-Verbal Learning Test). Saliva samples (3 times/day) were obtained for cortisol level evaluation 2 days before and after the diagnosis of PTSD with the Clinical-Administered PTSD Scale. **Results:** Descriptive analyses indicate that 14% of the delinquents present chronic PTSD and that 68% show conduct disorder symptoms. ANOVAs reveal significant differences between chronic PTSD adolescents and others on many scales: anxiety, depression, posttraumatic stress, sexual distress, dissociation and paternal care. No significant difference was found on anger, maternal bonding, paternal overprotection, cortisol level, estimated IQ, attention and memory. Significant results concern more direct aspects associated to PTSD. **Conclusion:** Lack of power and the fact that the subjects are too young to manifest long term physiological and consequently cognitive effects of PTSD may explain nonsignificant results.

P-019-336   Topic: 85
Free plasma cortisol and brain tryptophan availability levels in physically aggressive adolescent subjects with conduct disorder
Hanna Ebeling, University Hospital of Oulu, Dept. of Child Psychiatry, Oulu, Finland, hanna.ebeling@ppshp.fi
Irma Moilunen; Matti Virkkunen; Jyrki Liesivuori; Risto Bloigu; Jari Tiihonen

Objective: Previous studies suggest that children with conduct disorder (CD) have low cortisol levels and that habitually violent offenders with antisocial personality disorder (ASP) and alcohol abuse may have high brain tryptophan availability when compared with control subjects. The aim of this study was to test the hypothesis that physical aggression in adolescents with CD (which precedes ASP in adulthood) is associated with low cortisol and high brain tryptophan availability levels. **Methods:** Free plasma cortisol and free tryptophan/competing amino acid levels were measured in 14 physically aggressive reform school subjects and 20 non-aggressive control subjects aged 14 to 18 years. Aggressive behavior was assessed with Child Behavior Checklist. The differences in cortisol and free tryphan levels between aggressive probands and non-aggressive controls were tested in both genders separately by Mann Whitney U-test. The final analyses were made by Univariate analysis of variance. **Results:** Physical aggression was associated with low free cortisol levels, high brain tryptophan availability and tryptophan/cortisol availability ratio. Low cortisol levels were seen in aggressive girls and high tryptophan levels were more obvious in girls than in boys. **Conclusion:** Physical aggressive behavior with CD especially in adolescent girls is associated with low free cortisol and high brain tryptophan availability. The gender difference may reflect consistency and seriousness of female aggressive behavior, whereas male aggression in this age group is more common and its predictability still more diffuse.

P-019-337   Topic: 85, 95
Oppositional defiant patterns of behaviour in primary school age children with ADHD, combined type: What drives them?

Alasdair Vance, Royal Children's Hospital,
Dept. of Paediatrics, Melbourne, Vic., Australia,
avance@unimelb.edu.au
Chidambaram Prakash

Objective: The association of oppositional defiant disorder with increased rates of ADHD, combined type (ADHD-CT), anxiety disorders and depressive disorders are replicated findings. However, to date, the specific associations between oppositional defiant disorder, ADHD-CT, anxiety disorders and dysthymic disorder symptoms have not been studied in primary school age children with ADHD-CT. **Methods:** Data from a standard multiple regression analysis of ADHD-CT, dysthymic disorder and anxiety disorders symptoms on oppositional defiant disorder symptoms in 189 stimulant medication naive primary school children with ADHD-CT are presented. **Results:** Altogether 44% (adjusted $R2 = 0.44$) of the variance in oppositional defiant disorder symptoms was predicted by knowing scores on these three variables. However, only ADHD-CT (15% of the variance) and dysthymic disorder (8% of the variance) symptoms made a unique contribution. **Conclusion:** Dysthymic disorder is important to recognise in primary school age children with ADHD-CT. Then specific psychological and/or medication treatments can be investigated for this comorbid group. Secondly, the nature of the association between dysthymic disorder, anxiety disorders, oppositional defiant disorder and ADHD-CT needs to be systematically studied both within this developmental period and across developmental periods: for example, pre- and post-adrenarche and pre- and post-pubarche.

P-019-338   Topic: 85, 12
Long-term efficacy and safety of Risperidone in children with DBDs

Magali Reyes-Harde, Johnson & Johnson, Titusville, NJ,
USA, mharde@prdus.jnj.com
Krisztina Csaba; Marielle Eerdekens; Roza Olah

Objective: This two year extension study assessed the long-term safety and efficacy of risperidone in children with conduct (CD), oppositional defiant (ODD) and disruptive behavior disorder not otherwise specified (DBD-NOS), comorbid ADHD and below-average intelligence (IQ 35–84) who previously completed a one year risperidone trial. **Methods:** This trial followed 35 children, aged 515 years, who received risperidone for an additional 24 months. Safety was assessed by the Extrapyramidal Symptom Rating Scale (ESRS), adverse events, clinical laboratory tests, vital signs, changes in body mass index (BMI), and electrocardiogram (ECG). Efficacy was measured by the Clinical Global Impression Severity (CGI-S) score. **Results:** The mean dose of risperidone was 0.048 mg/kg/day (range 0.01–0.07). Symptoms continued to be well controlled in these children as measured on the CGI-S (mean 3.1 decreased from 5.6). Risperidone was well tolerated during long-term administration. Few extrapyramidal side effects occurred as assessed by the ESRS. The children showed a modest increase in BMI, which may be due to normal growth. **Conclusion:** Continuing low dose risperidone during three years appeared to be safe and effective in children with disruptive behavior disorders.

P-019-339   Topic: 84, 82
Comparison of memory function between Attention Deficit Hyperactivity Disorder and learning disorder children

Min-Sup Shin, Seoul Nat. University Hospital,
Child & Adolescent Psychiatry, Seoul, Republic of Korea,
minsup_shin@hotmail.com
Soo-Churl Cho

Objective: This study was conducted to examine the characteristics of memory function in children with Attention Deficit Hyperactivity Disorder (ADHD), Learning disorder (LD) and ADHD + LD. **Methods:** Thirty-four children (11 ADHD, 5 LD, 9 ADHD + LD, and 8 psychiatric control) were individually assessed with the Korean version of Wechsler Intelligence Scale for Children and the Korean version of Memory Assessment Scale (MAS), and then their performances on those tests were analysed using the non-parametric test (Kruscal-Wallis Test). **Results:** On all memory subtests, the ADHD, the LD and the ADHD + LD group showed lower performances than the control group. The ADHD + LD group showed lowest scores in almost subtests of MAS, suggesting memory dysfunction in children with comorbidity of ADHD and LD. The scores of MAS were positively correlated with the types of memory srategy that children used while being tested. **Conclusion:** The clinical utility of memory test like MAS is discussed in terms of differential diagnosis for ADHD, LD, and ADHD + LD children.

P-019-340   Topic: 84, 95
Impact of Rolandic Spikes on onset, neuropsychology and comorbidity in ADHD

Martin Holtmann, Universität Frankfurt, Kinder- und Jugendpsychiatrie, Frankfurt, Germany, holtmann@em.uni-frankfurt.de
Ulrike Hellmann; Katja Becker; Astrid Matei; Fritz Poustka; Martin Schmidt

Objective: The frequency of Rolandic spikes (benign epileptiform discharges of childhood) in children with Attention-deficit/hyperactivity disorder (ADHD) is significantly higher than expected from epidemiological studies (~6% vs 1–2%). The question arises whether this is simply a co-occurrence of two common childhood disorders or if Rolandic spikes affect the symptomatology in this ADHD subgroup. **Methods:** 16 nonepileptic ADHD outpatients with Rolandic spikes (9.7±2.1 y) and 17 age-matched ADHD children without Rolandic spikes underwent neuropsychological assessment (WISC-III, HSET, STROOP, CPT-AX). In addition, age and global social functioning at admission were assessed retrospectively. **Results:** In the cued continuous performance task (CPT-AX) ADHD children with Rolandic spikes made significantly more commission errors (p=0.045) and tended to exhibit shorter mean hit reaction times (p=0.094). ADHD-children with Rolandic spikes were significantly younger at admission than those without discharges (7.9 vs 9.3 y, p<0.001). The ratio of a comorbid diagnosis of conduct disorder tended to be larger in the ADHD plus Rolandic spikes-group. No significant differences were found between ADHD-patients with and without Rolandic spikes regarding sex, global functioning, intelligence, language function and STROOP test performance. **Conclusion:** ADHD children with Rolandic spikes show increased impulsivity and reduced response inhibition compared to ADHD children without Rolandic spikes. The younger age at admission and the higher rate of comorbid conduct disorder may indicate that Rolandic discharges or underlying, not fully understood mechanisms of epileptogenesis decrease the vulnerability threshold, advance the onset or aggravate the course of ADHD. Whether the occurrence of Rolandic discharges affects the outcome of ADHD needs further research.

P-019-341   Topic: 85, 12
Risperidone in children with Disruptive Behavior Disorders (DBD): A 2-year open-label trial

Magali Reyes-Harde, Johnson & Johnson, Titusville, NJ, USA, mharde@prdus.jnj.com
Jan Croonenberghs; Marielle Eerdekens

Objective: To assess long-term safety and efficacy of risperidone in children with conduct (CD), oppositional defiant (ODD) and disruptive behavior disorder not otherwise specified (DBD-NOS) and below-average IQ. **Methods:** This international, open-label study, an extension to a larger one-year trial (2), followed 48 children, aged 7–15 years, for an additional 12 months treatment with risperidone. Safety was assessed by reported adverse effects, extrapyramidal symptoms, clinical laboratory tests, vital signs, changes in body mass index (BMI), and electrocardiograms. The primary efficacy parameter was the conduct-problem subscale of the Nisonger Child Behavior Rating Form (N-CBRF). **Results:** The mean dose of risperidone was 0.048 mg/kg/day (range 0.01–0.09). N-CBRF scores decreased from a mean of 32.3 (SD 7.1) to a mean of 12.8

(SD 8.51) after two years (p<0.001). Risperidone was generally well tolerated and the incidence of adverse events decreased during the second year of treatment. A modest increase in BMI was observed over the two-year period, which may be mainly attributable to normal growth. **Conclusion:** Risperidone was safe and effective during two years of long-term treatment of children with disruptive behavior disorders.

P-019-342   Topic: 85, 12
Risperidone prevents relapses of Disruptive Behavioral Disorders (DBD) in children and adolescents of average intelligence: A 6-Month trial of Risperidone versus Placebo

Magali Reyes-Harde, Johnson & Johnson, Titusville, NJ, USA, mharde@prdus.jnj.com
Jan Buitelaar; Ilse Augustyns; Marielle Eerdekens

Objective: Risperidone effectively treats Disruptive Behavior Disorders (DBDs) (1,2). This study explored long-term risperidone efficacy in preventing reoccurrence of symptoms in young patients of average intelligence. **Methods:** This international, randomized, double-blind, placebo-controlled relapse prevention study included patients (5–17 years) with DBDs. Patients who responded within 6 weeks to open-label treatment with risperidone and maintained that response for 6 weeks were randomized to 6 months of either risperidone or placebo. Risperidone-treated patients <50 kg received 0.25–0.75 mg/day; and >=50kg received 0.51.5 mg/day. The primary efficacy parameter was time to relapse after switching to double-blind treatment. Secondary parameters included scores on the Clinical Global Impression of Improvement (CGI-I) and the Conduct-problem subscale of the Nisonger Child Behavior Rating Form (N-CBRF). Safety was assessed by reported adverse events, and clinical measures. **Results:** 527 patients (average IQ 92.1±18.06) entered the study with average N-CBRF scores of 35 (±6.74). At 12-weeks, 335 patients entered the 6-month relapse-prevention phase. At 6 months, the Kaplan-Meier relapse estimates were 47.1% (placebo) versus 29.7% (risperidone) (p<0.001). Mean change from baseline on the N-CBRF during the initial 12-week period was 24.8 (±8.0). Mean changes from the start of the double-blind phase at endpoint of the trial were 8.8 (±11.23) and 5.0 (±9.45) (p<0.001) for placebo and risperidone. Risperidone was safe over the complete dosing range. The most common adverse events were upper respiratory tract infection (7.6% vs. 5.5% in risperidone and placebo groups respectively), rhinitis (5.8% vs. 5.5%), pharyngitis (5.8% vs. 2.5%), and headache (4.7% vs. 6.7%). Extrapyramidal symptoms were rare and nobody experienced tardive dyskinesia. **Conclusion:** These data support risperidone for long-term treatment of DBDs and extend prior results to patients with average IQ. This study suggests that pharmacological intervention is important to prevent relapse in this population.

P-019-343   Topic: 84, 59

Attention Deficit Hyperactivity Disorder (ADHD) symptoms and internet addiction in Korean elementary school children

Hee-Jeong Yoo, Gyeongsang Nation. University,
Dept. of Psychiatry, Jinju, Republic of Korea,
neologue@hotmail.com
Ji Hyun Ha; In Hee Cho; Mee Gyeong Kim;
Sook Kyeong Yune; In Kyoon Lyoo

Objective: Internet addiction in children and adolescents is nearly a cultural phenomenon in Korea. Attention deficit/ hyperactivity disorder (ADHD) has been known to be one of the risk factors for the addictive use and abuse of substances in adolescence. Clinical observation has revealed that children with ADHD tend to be indulged in television, video games, and internet while they are reluctant to engage in tasks that require sustained mental efforts. The objective of this study was to evaluate the relationship between ADHD symptoms and internet addiction. **Methods:** Seven hundred twenty two elementary school students (361 boys, 361 girls: mean age: 10.7 ± 1.0 years in boys, 10.8 ± 1.0 years in girls) were recruited. The presence or severity of internet addiction was assessed by the Young's Internet Addiction test (IAT). Parents of children have completed the DuPaul's ADHD rating scale (K-ARS), parents' version. Children with the highest ten percentiles in K-ARS scores have been defined to be ADHD and compared with randomly-selected, age/sex-matched, same number of control subjects. Statistical significances were defined at the 0.05 level, two-tailed. **Results:** 1) One hundred four children (14.4%) met the criteria for a probable internet addiction, which is experiencing occasional or frequent problems because of internet. 2) Degree of inattention and hyperactivity/impulsivity symptoms had significant positive correlations with severity of internet addiction measured by IAT. 3) Internet addiction group had significantly higher degree of ADHD symptoms than control group ($p < 0.05$). 4) ADHD group had significantly higher internet addiction scores compared with the non-ADHD group ($p < 0.05$). **Conclusion:** Significant associations have been found between the level of ADHD symptoms and the severity of internet addiction in children. In addition, current findings suggest that the presence of ADHD symptoms, both in inattention and hyperactivity-impulsivity domains, may be one of the important risk factors for the internet addiction.

P-019-344   Topic: 84, 82

ADHD and language impairment

Bruce Barbro, Logopedics & Phoniatrics, Lund, Sweden

Objective: To investigate the occurrences and types of speech, language and communication problems in a group of children diagnosed as AD/HD and to estimate the relevance of using language ability for identifying clinically meaningful problem dimensions of AD/HD. **Methods:** Subjects: All patients (63 boys and 13 girls) diagnosed with ADHD, who were offered stimulant medication, during the years 2000–2002 at a team, which was part of a general Child and Adolescent Outpatient Clinic. The catchment area consisted of a small university town with surrounding rural areas. A parental questionnaire, The FTF (Five to Fifteen) consisting of 180 items with 8 domains, Motor control, Executive function, Perception, Memory, Language and speech, Learning, Social competence and Emotional/ behavioural problems was analysed regarding items covering speech and language problems. A factor analysis of subdomains revealed 6 factors, Cognition, DAMP, Attention, Impulsivity/Hyperactivity, Dyslexia, Social/Emotonal problems. Aspects of language as well as Socioeconomic status and IQ were analysed in relation to the specific domains as well as the 6 factors. The reults were also compared to a normal control group. **Results:** Two thirds (67%) of the study group were rated as having more language problems than the control group (above the 90th percentile). Problems of communicative skills and language comprehension were more frequently occurring than expressive language problems. However, compared with the control group, the children of the study group seemed to have expressive language problems to a much higher extent (59% > 90th percentile). The language domain had a highly significant correlation with all other domains, except motor development. SES and IQ were not significantly related to the domains and factors except Dyslexia (IQ) and expressive language skill (SES). Pragmatic language problems were related to social/emotional problems. **Conclusion:** A study group of children with ADHD had significantly more language problems than normal controls, mainly in the field of communicative skills and comprehension. Analysis of language in the assessment of ADHD could therefore yield important understanding of the child's problems as well as treatment options.

P-019-345   Topic: 84, 16

Reduction of Attention Deficit Hyperactivity Disorder (ADHD) symptoms with Atomoxetine mediated by cognitive improvement

Jan Buitelaar, University Medical Center,
Psychiatry & Adolescent, Nijmegen, Netherlands,
jb@psy.umcn.nl
Haitao Gao; Douglas Gelowitz

Objective: To examine if atomoxetine improves cognitive functioning in children with attention-deficit/hyperactivity disorder (ADHD) who had impaired Stroop color-word performance, and whether reductions of ADHD symptoms while on atomoxetine might be mediated by improvements in cognitive functioning. **Methods:** Data from 4 long-term atomoxetine clinical studies with Stroop data that focused on children (N = 170) with a cognitive deficit (Stroop color word T-score of 40 or less) at baseline were combined for this analysis. The ADHD RS rated by the parent served as the primary clinical outcome measure. **Results:** Atomoxetine treatment significantly improved age-corrected Stroop color-word and interference T-scores at endpoint compared to baseline (paired t-test, $p < 0.001$). To assess the effect of changes in cognitive function on behavior, multiple regression models were applied with change from baseline in ADHD RS total T-score as the dependent variable, and baseline ADHD RS total T-score and change in Stroop color-word and interference T-score as covariates. A statistically significant relationship was observed between change in ADHD RS Total T-score, baseline ADHD RS Total T-score (slope = –0.70, $p < 0.001$), and change in interference T-score (slope = –0.11, $p = 0.03$), but not for color-word T-score (slope = –0.07, $p = 0.17$). **Conclusion:** Atomoxetine improved cognitive function in children with ADHD who had baseline cognitive deficits. Reductions of ADHD symptoms by atomoxetine may be, in part, mediated by improvement of cognition.

P-019-346 Topic: 84, 26
Attention Deficit Hyperactivity Disorder (ADHD)
prevalence around the world: What are the real sources
of variation in estimates?
Guilherme Polanczyk, Porto Alegre, Brazil,
gvp.ez@terra.com.br

Objective: The aim of this study was to evaluate the impact of country income, origin of the sample, gender, age, source of information, definition of impairment, diagnostic criteria used, and quality of the study design (number of study stages, and attrition coefficient) on the variation of ADHD prevalence estimates across studies. **Methods:** A literature search through PubMed and PsychoInfo (1978 to 2004) was completed to identify studies on ADHD prevalence in different languages. The words prevalence or rate were contrasted against ADHD, ADD, attention-deficit disorder, attention-deficit/hyperactivity disorder, hyperactivity, hyperactive, overactivity, overactive, inattention, inattentive, hyperkinetic disorder, and minimal brain function. After this first screening, abstracts were selected according to the following inclusion criteria: a) sample including children and adolescents (18 years of age or less); b) nonreferred samples (community and school-based); c) diagnoses of attention-deficit/hyperactivity syndromes based on ICD-9, ICD-10, DSM-III, DSM-III-R or DSM-IV. The reference list of each paper was checked. In addition, the reference list of chapters on ADHD from major textbooks of child psychiatry, reviews of the literature that covered ADHD prevalence and major guidelines on the subject were also revised. **Results:** The computerized search identified 6693 abstracts. Although 234 papers were selected for complete reading, only 56 studies fulfilled all inclusion/exclusion criteria. A wide variation at the estimates of ADHD prevalence was found. Age range (highest prevalence in school age children, p=0.01), gender (highest prevalence in males, p<0.001), information source (p<0.001) and diagnostic criteria (highest prevalence with DSM-IV criteria, p<0.01) were the main sources of variation in ADHD prevalence. **Conclusion:** This study documents through an extensive revision of the literature that differences on estimates of ADHD prevalence around the world were mainly determined by methodological differences in the studies. Introduction: The prevalence of Attention-Deficit/Hyperactivity Disorder (ADHD) in children and adolescents vary widely among studies. This variation frequently is attributed to methodological differences in the studies and to peculiarities of the subjects included. These assumptions are well-known but poorly empirically tested.

P-020
Psychosocial and legal issues I

P-020-347 Topic: 51
Abandoned child in Morocco
Zineb Iraqi, CPU Ibn Rushd, Psychiatry, Casablanca,
Morocco, dociraqi@hotmail.com
Nadia Kadri; Driss Moussaoui; Kamal Raddaoui

Objective: Affective deprivation is one main cause of delayed development in abandoned children. The aims of the current study were to investigate the clinical, psychological features of them, and to explore the circumstances of the abandonment. **Methods:** This descriptive study, was conducted in orphanage Center Lalla Meriem, Rabat, Morocco

during the year 2001. 133 children with a mean age of 13±3 months from 0 to 7 years, were investigated. The mean age of abandonment was 2±2 months, a sex ratio male vs female was 4 (85%). The instrument used was, a hetero questionnaire inquiring about socio-demographic aspects, abandonment, clinical and psychological aspects and clinical assessment. **Results:** The main results were, in 52% of cases children were left in streets, and 83% of cases before the age of 3 months. The height-weight development was normal in 43% of cases, 11% had an hypo-trophy with no somatic cause, 11% of the sample had an abnormal anxiety, 18% an abnormal sadness and 50% a delay in language abilities. The number of admission in the center varied across years with a maximum in 1989 and 1992, years of happening of change in laws concerning illegal pregnancies (condemnation of single mothers). The evolution of death had its peak in 1995 (39%) (Infections, and excess on number of children) and then decreased to stabilize to 3%. **Conclusion:** The consequences on the abandonment on the child's health are severe. Therefore early and multidisciplinary interventions are necessary. The legislation constitutes also an important part of the prevention.

P-020-348 Topic: 48
The representation of the parental relationship
in children and adolescents.
Results from a new diagnostic instrument
Karl Titze, Charité-CVK, Kinder- und Jugendpsychiatrie,
Berlin, Germany, karl.titze@charite.de
Susanne Wollenweber; Verena Nell; Andreas Wiefel;
Ulrike Lehmkuhl

Objective: The assessment of the relationship between children and parents is crucial for research, diagnosis, prevention and treatment of psychiatric disorders in childhood and adolescence. However, while existing questionnaires seem to be sufficient for specific research purposes, they are not appropriate for broader clinical use. Therefore, we analyzed theoretical and empirical approaches in assessing the representation of the parental relationship. We constructed a new questionnaire (Parental-Representation-Questionnaire, PRQ). Results from two validation studies are presented. **Methods:** The PRQ consists of 8 scales (36 items) for each parent: "freedom of decision", "emotional burden", "fears/overprotection", "conflict", "hostility/disinterest", "aid for the parents", "punishment", and "support". Study I: 65 children/adolescents with epileptic mothers, 50 controls. Study II: A clinic-referred consecutive sample of 152 patients. Age: 10 to 20 years. **Results:** The dimensional structure was confirmed by factor analyses separately for mother and father. The internal reliability of the 8 scales ranges from 0.64 to 0.91. In study I the PRQ was able to predict in 79% of the cases, whether participants crew up with a chronicle ill or with a control mother. Each PRQ scale correlated significantly with either internalizing or externalizing symptoms or both (YSR, CBCL). In study II we found concordant but moderate correlations with the clinicians diagnosis of abnormal psychosocial situations (Axis 5, Multiaxial Classification System, WHO 1996). Only "conflict" and "freedom of decision" were significantly correlated with increasing age (r=0.18 to 0.24). Adolescent girls reported significant worse relations to both parents in 6 of the 16 scales. **Conclusion:** The present results confirm the PRQ as an economic and discriminating instrument to assess the representation of parent-child relation in childhood and adolescence. The remarkably worse parental representation of adolecent girls may contribute to the understanding of gender differences in psychopathology in adolesecence.

P-020-349   Topic: 47
Parental stress and personality characteristics among hospitalized children

Milica Pejovic-Milovancevic, Institute of Mental Health, Dept. Children & Adolescents, Belgrade, Serbia and Montenegro, mpejovic@eunet.yu
Olivera Aleksic; Smiljka Popovic-Deusic; Biljana Pirgic; Ana Velimirovic

Objective: The objective of following study was to compare personality characteristic of parents whose children were hospitalized at two different clinics one group were parents form department for child and adolescent psychiatry and the other group were parents whose children were hospitalized in a unit for intensive care, University Pediatric Clinic. The group of parents have children who were diagnosed with some developmental disorders for the first time, and the other group were parents whose children were operated because of congential cardiac malformations. **Methods:** Our sample consists of two parental groups; group I were 70 parents of psychiatric children and 70 parents, group II, whose children were treated and operate at Intensive care unit at University Pediatric Clinic. We used the following instruments: Semi structural clinical interview, NEOPIR (Revised NEO Personality Inventory-Costa, McRae, 1992) for personality inventory, PSI (Parental Stress Index) for screening parental stress and SCL-90 (symptom checklist). All data was collected while children were hospitalized at department for the first time. **Results:** Our result show differences among parents in stress reactions and feelings toward their hospitalized children. On the personality test there were no significant differences. Parents from group I significantly differ from group II parents on SCL. There was also evidence of disruptive family dynamics in 45% of analyzed cases in group I. **Conclusion:** Our research showed some very important results concerning parental stress and parental characteristics. Once more the biological dimension and genetic basis of mental disorders, together with the environmental model of understanding mental disorders (such as family dynamics) was demonstrated. We also find a need for parent support groups at Intensive care unit wich aim to reduce parental stress and intensive family therapy for parents at department for developmental disorders treatment.

P-020-350   Topic: 48
Early mother-child dyadic interactions and outcomes of prematurity at 18 months

Margarita Forcada Guex, CHUV Lausanne, Division de Néonatologie, Lausanne, Switzerland, margarita.forcada-guex@chuv.hospvd.ch

Objective: Studies show that premature birth can affect the quality of parent-child interaction. The aim of this study is to explore the relation between interactional characteristics at 6 months and infant's developmental outcomes (symptoms and developmental quotient) at 18 months. We hypothesized that the dyadic quality of interaction could have an impact on the infant's symptoms. **Methods:** Mother-child interaction is explored during a 10-minutes video taped play at 6 months of corrected age, in a population of 47 preterm infants (< 34 weeks), and 25 full term infants and scored with the Care Index. Four significant patterns of dyadic interaction were considered among the preterm population, combining maternal and infant's interactional characteristics: 1) maternal high sensitivity-infant high cooperation (functional preterm dyads); 2) maternal high controlling-infant high compliance; 3) maternal high controlling-infant high difficulty; 4) maternal high unresponsivity-infant high passivity. The infant's symptoms are evaluated at 18 months with the Symptom Check List (SCL), and the psychomotor development by the Griffiths scales. **Results:** Significant differences were found only for the dyadic interactive pattern of mother controlling-infant compliance. At 18 months, these infants present, according to the SCL: more global symptoms than full terms, and more eating disorders than full terms (n=25) and functional preterm's dyads (mother sensitive-infant cooperative; n=13). No differences were found between mother controlling-infant compliance dyads and the other preterm dyads. These infants present a lower DQ than full terms in the personal-social scale, and a lower DQ than full terms as well as functional preterm's dyads in the hearing-speech scale. **Conclusion:** The maternal control is not always associated with infant compliance, but when it is it seems to represent a risk-factor for the infant's development at 18 months. Our results highlight the need of supportive intervention that could promote maternal sensitivity and responsiveness to the infant.

P-020-351   Topic: 48
Grief reaction of adolescents and their mothers after father/husband loss

Basaran Sezer, Uludag University, Child & Adolescent Psychiatry, Bursa, Turkey, yesimtaneli@uludag.edu.tr
Yesim Taneli; Suna Taneli

Objective: This study aimed to assess the grief reaction of adolescents and their mothers after loss of father/husband and to identify risk groups for early intervention. **Methods:** Twenty one adolescents (F: 11, M: 10) and their mothers (n: 21) were enrolled between Jan. 2002–Mar. 2004 in a prospective study of grief. Assessment instruments were: Face-to-face psychiatric interviews and 1) 'Posttraumatic Stress Disorder Reaction Index for Children' (Frederick C, 1992) which we had translated (S.T.) for acute use after the 1999 – 1) Psychosocial Grief Questionnaire of our Department; 2) child (CDI; Kovacs M, 1981) and adult (Zung SDS; Zung W, 1974) depression scales as well as 3) STAI-state/trait (Spielberger CD et al.). SPSS was used for statistical analyses. **Results:** Mean age was 14.3 ± 1.6 years (F: 15;0; M: 13;5 years) for adolescents and 42 ± 5.4 years for mothers. Adolescents' mean scores were Reaction Index: 36.7 ± 13.5; CDI: 14.2 ± 9.2; STAI-state: 38.8 ± 11.7 and STAI-trait: 44.9 ± 10.5. Mothers' mean scores were: Reaction Index: 39.4 ± 14.5; ZungSDS: 61.7 ± 12.7; STAI-state: 45.6 ± 11.2 and STAI-trait: 53.7 ± 8.6. Grief reaction was rated 'severe to very severe' in 38.1% of adolescents and 47.6% of their mothers. A diagnosis of depression (adolescents: 33.3%; mothers: 76.2%), trait anxiety (adolescents: 23.8%; mothers: 61.9%) as well as state anxiety (adolescents: 57.1%; mothers: 95.2%) was common; while mothers seemed to be more affected. Within both groups, the scores of Reaction Index (RI), Depression, STAI-state and STAI-trait correlated significantly ($p < 0.05$ or $p < 0.01$). Adolescents who changed schools after the loss, had significantly higher RI-scores (p < 0.05). Higher RI-scores of adolescents correlated with lower trait anxiety in mothers (p < 0.05) and seemed to correlate with younger mothers (p < 0.09). Higher trait anxiety and higher state anxiety in adolescents both correlated with younger age of adolescents (p < 0.05). **Conclusion:** Assessment of adolescent grief reaction to the loss of their father should include maternal mental health and psychosocial factors.

P-020-352   Topic: 47, 26
Comparison of behavioral problems
of school-aged children in small and large families

Farshid Shamsaei, Hamedan University, Faculty of Nursing, Hamedan, Islamic Republic of Iran, shamsaei68@yahoo.com
Fatemeh Cheraghi

Objective: Children are the largest group of people in the world, and approximately 45% of the Iranian people are below the 15 years old. The health of children is important and first option of public health. Today in the world, mental health and also prevention and treatment of childrens' behavioral problems are very important. This study assessed and compared behavior problems of school aged children in small (one or two children) and large (more than two children) families in Hamedan City. **Methods:** This was a descriptive-cross sectional study. The sample consisted of 320 children school aged in two groups. participants were selected using a stratified random sampling method. Data was gathered with a questionnaire, filled in by the parents. The questionnaire contained two parts: A demographic information (8 items), B-child behavior checklist (CBCL) that consisted 56 items. Statistical analysis was performed by descriptive and inferential statistics and differences in two groups were evaluated with, t-test, Fisher, Chouporof and Cochran tests. **Results:** Outcome showed that adjustment problems of children in large families was higher than those of children in small families, and also, social and school adjustment of children in small families was better than children in large families. **Conclusion:** Family size and factors associated with family sized have an important influence upon adjustment and behavioral problems.

P-020-353   Topic: 47, 29
Parental attitude in families of child psychiatric
and child neurologic out-patients in Turkey

Oytun Hasturk, Uludag University, Child & Adolescent Psychiatry, Bursa, Turkey, yesimtaneli@uludag.edu.tr
Yesim Taneli; Mehmet Okan; Suna Taneli

Objective: This study aimed to assess parental attitudes in families of child psychiatric and child neurologic out-patients. **Methods:** The study group comprised the 120 mothers/fathers of patients who were admitted to the Out-Patient Units of Child & Adolescent Psychiatry (n: 60) and Child Neurology (n: 60) of Uludag University from 10 March 2004 to 20 March 2004 and agreed to take part in the study. Assessment instruments were the PARI (Parental Attitude Research Instrument) and a semi-structured psychosocial questionnaire designed for the study. SPSS was used.

P-020-354   Topic: 48, 42
Does mother's own attachment style affect
her postpartum emotional state and attachment
formation toward her baby?

Naoko Sato, Yamagata Unversity Hospital, Department of Nursing, Yamagata City, Japan, momo@med.id.yamagata-u.ac.jp
Yukiko Morioka; Aya Sato; Arata Oiji

Objective: Past research suggested that postpartum depression affect negatively mother's attachment formation toward her baby. It had been pointed out that mother's own early experience and attachment style may be a risk factor of postpartum depression. This study explored relationship among mothers' attachment style, their postpartum emotional state and attachment formation toward their baby. **Methods:** The subjects of this study were eighty five women in the late pregnancy who gave written informed consent. They were asked to fill out some questionnaires at 8 to 9 months of pregnancy, five days after birth, one month after birth, and three months after birth. Self-rating Depression Scale (SDS; Zung) and Feeling toward Baby Scale (FBS; Hanazawa) were administered four times. Parental Bonding Instrument (PBI; Parker) was administered at 8 to 9 months of pregnancy and Internal Working Model (IWM; Shaver) at one month after birth. Fifty eight subjects responded to all of these questionnaires, so data analysis was given of these 58 subjects. **Results:** The results of Covariance Structure Analysis examining relationship among PBI, IWM and SDS suggested that overprotection score of PBI strongly affected the score of the ambivalent scale of IWM, and the ambivalent scale strongly affected SDS score at one month and three months after birth. The subjects were divided into two groups; the continuously high SDS group (CHS group) and the non CHS group. The CHS group consists of 21 subjects who had scored continuously high (40 points and above) in SDS. The non CHS group consists of the rest of the subjects (n = 37). The score of avoidance scale of FBS was higher in the CHS group than in the non CHS group at one month and three months after birth. **Conclusion:** These results suggested that mother's attachment style affect her postpartum emotional state and attachment formation toward her baby.

P-020-355   Topic: 51, 30
Cognitive neuropsychological profiles
in maltreated children

Francesca Piperno, Rome University, Childhood Neuropsychiatry, Rome, Italy, carla.sogos@uniroma1.it
Eleonora Camillo; Stefania Di Biasi; Daniela Tardiola; Felicia Lauria

Objective: The aim of the study was to investigate whether physical abuse has negative effects on children's cognitive and neuropsychological profiles. We chose to measure the neuropsychological profiles because studies have shown that children who have suffered physical abuse alone or in combination with psychological aggression have lower profiles than control groups of children (Eckenrode et al., 1993; Leiter et al., 1994; Solomon et al., 1999; Kinard, 2001). **Methods:** The cognitive, neuropsychological profiles of 10 maltreated children were assessed and compared with 10 non-abused children with Learning Disorders. All children were between 6–10 years of age. All children were administered the Wechsler Scale of Intelligence Revised (WPPSI-R; WISC-R), that provides Verbal, Performance and Full Scale IQ scores, and specific Tests evaluating reading, writing achievements (Cornoldi et al., 1981; Cornoldi et al. 1991). **Results:** Maltreated children have showed lower cognitive profiles in all areas (verbal, performance) than non-maltreated children. In these children the Learning Disorder affects all areas and is related to the chronically suffered trauma. On the other hand, in the control group there are specific deficits that indicate a Specific Learning Disorders. **Conclusion:** We can say that maltreatment is detrimental to children: maltreatment has negative effects on children's self-esteem and contributes to lowering cognitive, neuropsychological profiles and school achievements. These children are different with respect to the pathogenesis, learning strategies and the clinical evaluation, therefore they need specific and different therapies.

P-020-356   Topic: 47, 86
"Cared Children" and "Thought Children"

Viviana Porcari, University Hospital Palermo,
Child & Adolescent Psychiatry, Palermo, Italy,
viviana.porcari@virgilio.it
Maria Patrizia Salatiello; Sabrina Chifari;
Valentina Dell'Oglio; Militello Rosanna; Carmela Scrò

Objective: The Authors want to demonstrate how a partial change in the incidence and typology of psychopathological disorders of childhood and adolescence has taken place in the last few years. Approximately the 60% of the cases who have come to our attention, at the Institute of Child and Adolescent Psychiatry, University Hospital of Palermo, presents a distortion of their emotional development similar to the one which characterized, years ago, the population of maltreated children coming from poor neighbourhoods. Nowadays instead, this distortion is spreading to the middle and high classes' kids. The Authors try to give a valid interpretation of this phenomenon. **Methods:** The Authors analyse and discuss some of the children who have come to their attention, at the Institute of Child and Adolescent Psychiatry, University Hospital of Palermo. **Results:** The children examined in this study have never been victim of physical maltreatment, they benefit from a material care and their life is fulfilled with planned engagements aimed at an intellectual enrichment. Their emotional life is instead really poor. **Conclusion:** The Authors hypothesize that the emotional decompensation found in the examined child population is correlated with the alteration of the parental role. Children are not present with their emotional needs in their parents' mind. The physiological parents-children asymmetry is turned upside down: nowadays parents more often required to be cared for by their children.

P-020-357   Topic: 51, 57
Sexual trauma and psychosexual developmental problems in male adolescent sexual offenders

Lisette Hart-Kerkhoffs, VU University Medical Center,
Child & Adolescent Psychiatry, Duivendrecht, Netherlands,
liesthart@hotmail.com
A. Ph. van Wijk; L. M. C. Jansen; Robert Vermeiren;
Theodore Doreleijers

Objective: Research on adolescent sex offenders has identified a subgroup of adolescents who display major psychosocial, psychiatric and/or psychosexual problems and who are at risk for repetitive offending, while most adolescent sex offenders do not continue their abusive behaviour. In the present study, it was the intent to gain better insight in

the psychosexual problems of adolescent sexual offenders. **Methods:** Fifty-two male adolescent sexual offenders (mean age 14.5 ± 1.4 years) were studied using a trauma questionnaire and a semi-structured interview regarding psychosexual problems. **Results:** Results indicated that 13.3% experienced sexual trauma themselves. Overall, psychosexual problems were prominent in 32.5%, while 21.9% had committed one or more previous sexual offence. However, no relationship between sexual trauma, psychosexual problems and having committed more than one sexual offence could be established. **Conclusion:** Psychosexual problems and sexual trauma are present in a considerable part of adolescent sexual offenders. Moreover, a considerable part of these adolescents already show persistent sexual offensive behaviour. However, follow-up studies of more extensive groups of male adolescent offenders are needed to establish whether sexual trauma and psychosexual problems are related prospectively.

P-020-358   Topic: 49, 40
Study on the psychological well-being of children from divorced families

Shi Ji Zhang, Beijing Child Health Center,
Dept. of Child Psychiatry, Beijing, China,
shiji-ch-phy@sohu.com

Objective: The rate of divorce from young couple is increasing in China along with the vigorous development of economy. All sections of Chinese people are paying a good deal of attention to the children of divorced parents. The purpose of the study was to investigate the state of psychological well-being of children from divoced families. **Methods:** The Chinese version of the Achenbach's Child Behavior Checklist was used to assess the social competence, emotional and behavioral problems in 50 children from divorced families and 50 children from intact families. **Results:** The results showed that the total social competence scores in children from divorced families was significantly lower then that in children from intact families. The children of divorced parents were found of more anxiety, less feeling of happiness and satisfaction. **Conclusion:** These findings suggested that the emotional and behavioral problems of children from divorced families are related to the post-divorce parent-child relationship and family educating style.

P-020-359   Topic: 51
Assessment of psychiatric juvenile patients, who had become victims of sexual traumas

Heidrun Eichberger, Uni. Clinic of Neuropsychiatry, Vienna,
Austria, heidrun.eichberger@univie.ac.at
Max H. Friedrich

Objective: This examination focuses on the assessment of psychiatric, juvenile patients, who had become victims of sexual trauma. The aim was to find out what impact both their illness and their status as a victim had on the process of judging. **Methods:** A representative sample of the overall population (n = 188) was each given one of the – in total – six different curriculum vitas of a fourteen year old girl and asked to judge on them. In three cases the stimulus person was the victim of rape. In addition, a stable psychotic as well as an acute psychotic disease of the stimulus person were established. Consequently, the results were six test conditions for the design: non victim, acute psychotic stimulus person, stable psychotic stimulus person, victim, acute psychotic victim, stable psychotic victim. **Results:** Victims are granted significantly more trauma, significantly less positive estimation as well as less devaluation. In the acute case of disease trauma is estimated significantly higher, positive estimation turns out to be significantly smaller in both cases of disease as well as devaluation. In all six test conditions, the acute diseased victim gets the highest degree of trauma as well as the smallest degree of positive estimation. **Conclusion:** Ill victims of sexual trauma are estimated less positive.

P-020-360 Topic: 47, 90
Effects of early hospitalization due to prematurity on later separation experiences
Reija Latva, University of Tampere, Dept. of Child Psychiatry, Tampere, Finland, reija.latva@uta.fi
Liisa Lehtonen; Raili Salmelin; Tuula Tamminen

Objective: The aim of the study was to investigate if the early hospitalization of a preterm infant affects separation experiences of the mother five years later. **Methods:** All premature (< 37 weeks and < 2500 g) infants born in Tampere University Hospital 1997–1998 and admitted to the neonatal intensive care unit were included. The neonatal data were collected from the infant's hospital records. A questionnaire developed for this study eliciting parental experiences in separation situations was sent to the families of the prematurely born infants and their gender-matched full-term controls when the children were five years old. The questionnaires were returned by 72% (n = 150/208) of the "preterm" and 45% (n = 119/265) of the control families. Responders and non-responders did not differ by demographic factors. **Results:** Preterm children started day-care older than control group children (median 26 vs 17 months, p < 0.001). The difference remained significant even if the ages were corrected for prematurity. The age when the parents first let the child stay overnight away from home was the same. Mothers' separation experiences between the groups did not differ, but there was a difference within the preterm group. The mothers of smaller and more unstable preterm infants experienced more difficulties when leaving the 5-year-old child in day-care (p = 0.03) or overnight without parents (p = 0.002) than mothers of more stable preterm infants. The difference remained significant even if those preterm children who had developmental difficulties at five years old were removed from the analysis. Maternal perception of the child's separation experience did not differ between the groups or within the preterm group. **Conclusion:** Early hospitalization in the group of small and unstable preterm infants may traumatize the mother in a way which manifests itself in a separation situation still five years later.

P-020-361 Topic: 55
Children of parents suffering from Multiple Sclerosis: Preliminary results
Emmanouel Tsalamanios, University of Athens, Dept. of Child Psychiatry, Athens, Greece, emtsalamanios@hotmail.com
Gerasimos Kolaitis; Elena Paliokosta; Stavroula Diareme; Sofia Anasontzi; Alkis Tsiantis; Irini Limbinaki; John Tsiantis

Objective: This study has been conducted in Greece within the frame of a three year long European project on "Chil-

dren Of Somatically Ill Parents" (COSIP) with the participation of another seven countries (i.e. Austria, Denmark, Germany (coordinator), Great Britain, Finland, Romania and Switzerland). Our hypotheses were that children of M.S. parents will present mental health difficulties: a) in a higher rate than age norms, b) mainly within the internalizing spectrum, and c) in a higher rate if parental depression or/and family dysfunction is/are present. Also M.S. parents are expected to underestimate their children's difficulties compared to children themselves, spouses or/and clinicians **Methods:** Participants are 40 M.S. patients (25–50 years old), their spouses and children (4–18 years old), recruited from Neurology Clinics of general hospitals in Athens. Children's mental health status was examined with CBCL (both parents), YSR (children) and semi-structured interviews for parents and children. Presence of parental depression was examined with BDI, while family functioning was examined with FAD and coping difficulties with F-COPES. One way ANOVA were conducted. **Results:** Preliminary results showed that MS parents presented mental health difficulties in a higher rate than normal.The higher the parents depression, as well as the higher the family dysfunction, the higher the children's mental health problems. Both MS parents and healthy spouses underestimate their children's difficulties compared to children themselves. **Conclusion:** As we had supposed, children and adolescents of somatically ill parents are at risk for developing mental health problems.

P-020-362 Topic: 47, 41
Correlations between family factors and child and adolescent psychiatric disorders
Leontina Dreana-Ianciu, Timisoara, Romania, leo_haragas@yahoo.com
Miriana Vrajitoriu

Objective: To establish the correlations between different family risk factors and the development of psychiatric disorders in children and adolescents. **Methods:** We are studying retrospectively a sample representing all new patients taken into our clinic during 2003. The psychiatric diagnosis is established according to ICD-10. For each patient we looked for the existing family risk factors, concerning family structure, intrafamilial relationships, psychiatric disorders of the other members of the family, professional and economical status. The results are analized statistically. **Results:** After the results' interpretation, we could describe the most frequent pattern of family in which one can find child and adolescent psychiatric disturbances, a "risk family" in our cultural space. We present the degree of association between the main psychiatric diagnosis found and the existence of risk factors in the origin family. **Conclusion:** As found in the psychiatric literature, there is at least an association, if not a causal relation, between family risk factors and psychiatric disorders in children and adolescents.

P-020-363 Topic: 48
Conduct-disordered children's and their mother's attachment representation discrepancies
Laura Lebedeva, University of Latvia, Psychology, Riga, Latvia, laura.l@tvnet.lv

Objective: The aim of this research was to examine if there exists a difference in the degree of similarity or discrepancy between conduct-disordered children's and their mother's attachment representations, and the attachment representations of non-conduct-disordered child-mother dyads. **Methods:** Thirty dyads of conduct-disordered children (ages 7–9 years) and their mothers; and 30 dyads of non-conduct-disordered children (ages 7–9 years) and their mothers were asked to complete a series of Attachment Story Stem-Completions. The narrative representations of each mother-child dyad were analysed in terms of attachment style markers and were compared in regard to structure and content, and the degree of similarity or discrepancy within each dyad was identified. **Results:** The results of the analysis show that there is greater similarity in the structure and content of the narrative attachment representations of the non-conduct-disordered child-mother dyads, than in the case of the conduct-disordered child-mother dyads, where there is greater discrepancy in structure and content. Also, among the conduct-disordered children and their mothers there is a greater percentage of narrative representations which indicate insecure attachment style. **Conclusion:** The practical implication of these findings lies with enabling practitioners to understand better the child-mother relationship in situations of conduct-disordered children. This helps to identify which psychotherapeutic goals and approaches would be best suited in order to facilitate the child-mother relationship and to decrease the conduct-disordered behaviours.

P-020-364   Topic: 50, 24
Developmental characteristics and psychopathology of adopted children in Turkey

Yasemen Taner, Hacettepe Üniversitesi Týp Fak, Cocuk ruh saðlýðý, Ankara, Turkey, taneryasemen@yahoo.com
Betul Bakkaloglu; Füsun Çuhadaroðlu Çetin; Cengiz Ozbesler; Mihriban Erturk

Objective: To find out the developmental characteristics of the adopted children in Turkey and define psychopathological features like internalizing and externalizing problems in such a population. **Methods:** 35 outpatients between ages 2–16 who were adopted were included into the study after taking oral informed consent. Subjects were given Child Behavior Checklist, Wechsler Intelligence Scale or Stanford Binet Intelligence Scale, a questionnaire asking for the developmental stages of children, socioeconomical and demographical characteristics, adoption ways of families. Also attachment styles of the mothers were assesed by the Attachment Styles Questionnaire. In the analysis of the results SPSS 11.0 programme was used. **Results:** The results will be discussed in respect to the attachment style of the mother, the intelligence score, development and the psychopathology of the children.

P-020-365   Topic: 51, 74
Anger and dissociation in relation to experience of abuse across generations in Latvia

Sandra Sebre, University of Latvia, Psychology, Riga, Latvia, sebre@latnet.lv
Laura Lebedeva

Objective: The aim of this study was to examine the levels of anger and dissociation in adolescents and their parents in relation to experienced emotional, physical and sexual abuse in childhood. Anger and dissociation have been found to have mediating effects upon intergenerational transmission of abuse, and these effects were explored as well in the present study. **Methods:** Five hundred sixty five adolescents (ages 11–16) and more than 40% of their mothers and fathers participated in the study. Both adolescents and parents completed the Childhood Trauma Questionnaire, concerning childhood experience of neglect, emotional, physical and sexual abuse. Adolescents completed the Trauma Symptom Checklist for Children, and their parents completed the Trauma Symptom Inventory. In addition, parents reported on their present parenting behaviors, and some of the parents were interviewed in regard to their past and present experience in relation to abuse. **Results:** As expected, results of the study indicate positive correlations between childhood experience of abuse and present ratings of anger and dissociation, and between parents' current parenting behaviors. The mediating effect of anger is particularly apparent in those parents who transmit abusive behaviors intergenerationally. The relationship between anger, dissociation and abuse was found to differ with mothers and fathers. **Conclusion:** In Latvia during the past 5-6 years there has been a marked in increase in awareness of issues of child abuse, and an increase in public discussion of these issues. The identification of anger and dissociation as sequelae of abuse, and also as mediators which perpetuate abuse is important for future national treatment program planning.

P-020-366   Topic: 48
Comparison between maternal rating of emotional state and rater's observation in a prematurity context

Audrey Keller, University Hospital Lausanne, Child & Adolescent Psychiatry, Lausanne, Switzerland, audrey12keller@hotmail.com
Ayala Borghini; Margarita Forcada Guex; Carole Müller Nix; Blaise Pierrehumbert; François Ansermet

Objective: The objective of this study was to examine maternal self-perception of emotions and rater's observations of the mother's emotions in N = 39 mothers with premature infants, and N = 29 mothers with full-term infants. Given the known link between prematurity and maternal post-traumatic stress disorder (PTSD), results will be discussed with a view to clarify whether a premature birth alters the normal mother's awareness of her emotions resulting in lower correlations between self-perception and rater's observation. We will also explore whether such alterations are directly related to the severity of prematurity and/or trauma. **Methods:** The interviews were done when children were 6 and 18 months old (corrected age). Maternal self-perception of emotions was assessed using the R-Interview (Stern et al., 1989) and maternal PTSD was assessed using Perinatal PTSD Questionnaire (PPQ, Quinnell and Hynan, 1999). The raters coded mother's emotions using Working Model of the Child Interview (WMCI, Zeanah et al., 1996). **Results:** The major finding is that in mothers who had signs of PTSD when their child was 18 months old, there was a discrepancy between maternal self-perception of emotions and rater's observations of the mother's emotions. Rater's coded far more negative emotions then these mothers expressed. **Conclusion:** When their child is 18 months old (corrected age), those mothers of premature babies who show signs of PTSD seem to either not report negative emotions, probably because of the guilt that they may feel if they did, or lack the ability to perceive correctly their emotions due to the PTSD they experience.

P-020-367   Topic: 47
Parental estimates of the intelligence of themselves and their children

Rainer Georg Siefen, WKKJPP Marl Sinsen, Haard Klinik, Marl-Sinsen, Germany, rainer_georg.siefen@wkp-lwl.org
Adrian Furnham; Peter Noack; Bruce Kirkcaldy

Objective: Mainly gender related hypotheses concerning self estimates of intelligence were investigated: Do fathers and mothers agree in their rating of general and specific IQ for sons and daughters? Are there significant impacts of age, school track or birth order. **Methods:** The parents of approximately 600 children (average of 11 years of age) in their first year of secondary school education (620 mothers and 533 fathers) in the New German Federal States estimated their general and specific intelligence scores and that of their children. Type of school (general secondary vs. grammar) and gender (boy vs. girl) were used as the independent variables. **Results:** Fathers perceived themselves as more intelligent (analytical IQ). Mothers rated themselves higher in terms of emotional intelligence. Fathers perceived their sons as more intelligent in terms of analytical intelligence and mothers rated their sons higher on practical intelligence. Spatial-numerical IQ data obtained from the children themselves, however, did not differ significantly between boys and girls. There was no gender×school interaction. **Conclusion:** Parental aspirations of school careers and academic achievement of their children are an important part of family counselling in child and adolescent psychiatry. Diagnostic results can be communicated to parents far more successfully if specific influences on parent's estimates of their intelligence and that of their children are taken into account.

P-020-368   Topic: 48, 40
The influence of parent behavior on child distress during voiding cystourethrogram

Sabine Völkl-Kernstock, Medizinische Universität Wien, Inst. für Neuropsychiatrie, Wien, Austria, sabine.voelkl-kernstock@univie.ac.at
Michaela Felber; Stefan Puig; Max H. Friedrich

Objective: Voiding cystourethrogram (VCU) is a common radiological procedure in children, which – due to its invasive nature – is likely to cause considerable distress in children. The purpose of this study was to examine the influence of parent behavior on child distress during the VCU. It was hypothesized that child distress would further be influenced by the child's age and temperament as well as by the parent's VCU-related information and distress. **Methods:** So far, about 30 children 2 to 8 years old diagnosed with urinary tract infection, who had been referred to the University Clinic for Radiology at the General Hospital of Vienna for VCU, were included in the study (outpatients only). Prior to the procedure, the child's behavior and temperament as well as parent VCU-related information were assessed by questionnaires presented to the accompanying parent. During the VCU procedure, parent-child-interaction was audio taped and later transcribed and rated using the 'Child Adult Medical Procedure Interaction Scale - Revised' by Blount et al. (1997), which includes the codes 'child distress behavior', 'child coping be-

havior', 'parent coping promoting behavior' and 'parent distress promoting behavior'. After the procedure, parent's distress during the VCU was assessed. 6–8 days after the VCU procedure, the parent was contacted again in order to assess post-VCU behavioral changes in the child. Data were analysed using SPSS correlation analyses, ANOVA and multiple regression analysis. **Results:** Preliminary results show that parent 'coping promoting behavior' during VCU as well as a higher amount of parental information on the VCU procedure are likely to reduce child distress behavior. **Conclusion:** The results indicate that by providing parents with information on the VCU procedure and by coaching them on how to support their child's coping behavior, children's distress during VCU-procedure can be minimized.

P-020-369   Topic: 48, 35
Brain circuitry and psychology of human parent-infant attachment in the postpartum

James Swain, Yale University, Child Study Center, New Haven, USA, james.swain@yale.edu
James Leckman; Linda Mayes; Ruth Feldman; Robert Constable; Robert Schultz

Objective: We hypothesize a functional overlap in neural circuits mediating obsessive-compulsive disorder (OCD) and human parental attachment, such that: 1. parental preoccupations involving anxious, intrusive, OCD-like thoughts activate striato-thalamo-cortical circuits with baby cry stimuli 2. parental preoccupations involving intrusive, but positive idealizing thoughts and joys activate the ventral striatum, midbrain and hypothalamus by infant visual stimuli 3. parental brain responses to stimuli from their own infants are stronger than from control infants 4. psychometric assessments of parenting correlate with cortisol responses, and brain activity. **Methods:** We are studying parental attachment in two ways, and at two time points (2 weeks and 3 months postpartum): First we are administering interview and self-report versions of the Yale Inventory of Parental Thoughts and Actions, and second, we are performing 3T functional magnetic resonance imaging of the brains of both parents. Brain activation maps are generated while listening to baby stimuli, consisting of cries and pictures of their own and another baby, as well as control stimuli. Salivary cortisol is obtained before and after each scan. **Results:** Preliminary analysis indicates that with baby cry stimuli, activations do overlap with OCD and anxiety circuits, including frontal, cingulate, auditory and visual cortices, as well as midbrain and amygdala. With baby picture stimuli, more visual processing areas are also active. Differences are seen between moms and dads. Brain region-of-interest analysis, and correlation with psychometric constructs including attachment, preoccupation, mood and anxiety will be presented. **Conclusion:** This is the first study to combine neuroimaging of brain regions related to normal attachment (as well as psychopathology) in mothers and fathers with concurrent psychometric and endocrine measures using auditory and visual baby stimuli. Our results fit with human and animal work on affiliative behaviors, and may lead to biological models for protective and vulnerability factors in human family attachments.

P-020-370   Topic: 51, 49
Mental health problems, maltreatment and coping strategies among orphan adolescents

Evgeny Koren, Moscow Research Institute, of Psychiatry, Moscow, Russia, evkoren@yandex.ru

Objective: To investigate relationship between behavioral/emotional symptomatology, the nature and extent of maltreatment experiences and development of dysfunctional coping strategies in a sample orphan adolescents. **Methods:** A study of 67 adolescents aged 12–18 years in orphan rehabilitation center based in the Moscow. Adolescents were surveyed with clinical interview based on criteria ICD-10 and completed the Child Maltreatment Schedule and the Ways of Coping Scale (WAYS). **Results:** Findings revealed different forms abuse and neglect coexisting, high rates of emotional and physical maltreatment. Emotion-focused or avoidant coping strategies was associated with exposure to maltreatment. Dissociation as a coping strategy was particularly linked with sexual abuse where it acts as a mediator of symptoms, such as self-harming behavior. Use of maladaptive coping also predicted emotional difficulties, behavioral problems and may contribute to the development of depressive symptoms in the respondents. **Conclusion:** Coping strategies are an important indicator of psychosocial functioning in orphan adolescents. Identification of coping styles can augment the assessment of at-risk adolescents and child's ability to cope with maladjustment. Emotion-focused strategies, in particular, appear to be widely used by young people from inconsistent and rejecting cultural backgrounds.

P-020-371   Topic: 51, 26
Sexual abuse of children and youth in Thailand: A qualitative study

Umaporn Trangkasombat, Chulalongkorn University, Child & Adolescent Psychiatry, Bangkok, Thailand, familyinthai@yahoo.com

Objective: Sexual abuse in children and youth is a worldwide social and mental health problem. Studies of such phenomenon in the Asian context are limited. The objective of this study was to explore the context of abuse and its psychological and social impacts. **Methods:** The study was qualitative, using the snowball sampling technique and semistructured interview instrument. The sample consisted of 56 girls and 4 boys from the north, south, east and central parts of the country. **Results:** The sample ranged in age from 2 to 18 years. Sixty two percent came from divorced or separated families. Many children were abused by more than one person and 55% of the abusers were family members. The onset of the abuse was mostly in the 12–13 years of age and the duration ranged from one month to more than 3 years. The most frequent psychosocial stressors were family breakdown and poverty. These factors contributed to poor parent-child relationship, lack of supervision and neglect of the children and finally led to abuse. Thirty-two percent of the children were rejected by the families after the disclosure. Due to family rejection and for the safety of the children, 60% were removed to stay at the child protection centers where they later developed adjustment problems. Many physical and mental health problems were found in the sample, for example, HIV infection and suicidal behavior. Despite many negative events most children were optimistic about their future. **Conclusion:** Sexual abuse creates many physi-cal, psychological and social consequences in the lives of the children. Comprehensive rehabilitative and preventive measures that address the overall needs of the children are urgently needed.

P-020-372   Topic: 49, 47
The function of siblings in separating families

Michael Karle, Universität Tübingen, Kinder- und Jugendpsychiatrie, Tübingen, Germany, mlkarle@med.uni-tuebingen.de
Gunther Klosinski

Objective: In the past years research has focused on the impact of divorce for the adjustment of children. There is a controversy about whether siblings are helpful or not in this process. Nevertheless it is accepted as a general rule that siblings should not be separated after separation/divorce of parents. It will be examined if this is considered in expert opinions and which issues are relevant for separating siblings. **Methods:** Retrospective analysis of 124 custody expertises, pertaining to 222 children (mean age 7 years) and a catamnestic survey carried out by a questionnaire (3 1/2 years later) concerning family and child factors. Frequency and significance of different determining factors for the best interest of the child (whishes of the child, the child's interrelationships with parents, continuity of upbringing and living arrangements, fitness of the parents, sibling relationships) are beeing assessed and discussed concerning their relevance. **Results:** Our study confirmed the rule, that siblings should not be separated. In 80.7% of the expert opinions it was recommended, that the siblings should stay together (in 19.3% of the cases a separation was suggested). Decisions to split custody for enhancing the welfare of children were based on various circumstances. The main reasons for split custody are discussed. The most important criteria are the wishes of the children and the sibling relationships. **Conclusion:** The role and function of siblings in separating families is complex and has not been sufficiently considered in literature in the past. Sibling relationship is only one of a variety of criteria. In addition it is important to consider interrelationships with the parents and extrafamilial relation networks and to examine these parameters more differentiated. Furthermore it is not sufficient to explore the sibling relationships without looking at the position of each sibling.

P-020-373   Topic: 55, 32
Maternal hyperthyroidism and mental health of the children

Marina Belianchikova, Reserch Center on, Mental Health, Moscow, Russia, mbelianchikova@mail.ru
Galina Scoblo; Valentin Fadeev

Objective: The aim of the study was to assess the mental health of children from mothers with Graves disease, who suffered from hyperthyroidism during the first trimester of the pregnancy and received oral propylthiouracil from 50 to 100 mg per day. **Methods:** A group of 25 children from mothers with thyroid hyperfunction aged from 5 months to 4 years (14 boys and 11 girls) was studied by the comprehensive mental state examination according to DC: 0–3 (Diagnostic Classification of Mental Health and Developmental Disorders of Infancy and Early Childhood), DDST (Denver Developmental Screening Test), analysis of preperinatal complications. The control group included 25 infants and toddlers of the same age. **Results:** At the time of the birth all infants were clinically euthyroid. 10 mothers rejected the offer to examine their children because they had no problems. The other 15 children did not show any severe psychoneurological disturbances. Regulatory disorder (6), adjustment disorders (2), and disorder of affect (1) were found. The control group did not differ from comparison group concerning the presence of the moderate and mild forms of mental disorders. Children from hyperthyroid mothers showed more relationship disorders (accoding to Axis 2 of DC: 0–3) than the control group. The psychological development of children by DDST was normal in both groups. The analysis of preperinatal complications did not show significant difference between these two groups. **Conclusion:** Our results suggest that children from mothers with thyroid hyperfunction during the first trimester of pregnancy who received oral propylthiouracil had no severe psychoneurological complications or abnormalities in mental development. The relationship between revealed mental disorders, mental health of the mother and relationship disorders in children will be discussed.

P-020-374   Topic: 47, 96
Prematurity, maternal stress and mother-child interactions

Carole Müller Nix, Unité de Développement CHUV, Division de Néonatologie, Lausanne, Switzerland, carole.muller-nix@inst.hospvd.ch
Margarita Forcada Guex; Blaise Pierrehumbert; Lyne Jaunin; Ayala Nicole; Francois Ansermet

Objective: Studies show that premature birth can affect the quality of parent-child interaction, without a clear understanding of the mechanism. The purpose of this longitudinal study is to relate the maternal and infant interactive behaviors with the maternal post-traumatic stressful experience and the infant's perinatal risk factors and to verify their evolution in time. **Methods:** Mother-child interaction is explored during a video typed play, at 6 and 18 months of corrected age, in a population of 47 preterm infants with a gestational age < 34 weeks and 25 full term infants, born in 1998. A gravity score adapted from the Perinatal Risk Inventory, is established, differentiating low and high risk infants. Maternal stress is evaluated with the Perinatal Posttraumatic Stress Disorder Questionnaire, differentiating low and high-stressed mothers. The maternal and infant interactive behaviors are scored with the Care Index. **Results:** At six months mothers of high-risk premature infants, as well as mothers that have suffered posttraumatic stress disorder are less sensitive and more controlling than the full term mothers. Partial correlations show that the PPQ was significant, although the PERI was not. The infant interactional behavior is similar according to these two variables. At 18 months maternal interactional behavior in the preterm dyads shows no more differences with full term dyads. Significant differences appear for infant interactional behavior between groups, only according to the PPQ variable. Interestingly enough, preterm infants showed significantly more compulsive-compliant behaviors with high-stressed mothers and they were more passive with low-stressed mothers. **Conclusion:** The maternal traumatic experience appears to have more influence than the infant's health status on the mother-child interaction. The infant's interactional behavioral characteristics at 18 months, could be understood has a long lasting influence of maternal traumatic experience on the harmonious organization of the dyad.

P-020-375   Topic: 48, 42
Maternal attachment in Japanese women during pregnancy and one month after delivery

Hitoshi Kaneko, Nagoya University, Nagoya, Japan, kaneko@cc.nagoya-u.ac.jp
Shuji Honjo; Tatsuo Ujiie; Satomi Murase; Kenji Nomura; Yasuko Sasaki; Shiori Arai

Objective: The aim of this study was to examine the maternal attachment during pregnancy and after childbirth. **Methods:** The subjects were mothers attending the obstetrics clinic at the Nagoya University Hospital in Japan. One hundred and forty-five pregnant women participated in a longitudinal study. They completed questionnaires at middle pregnancy, and one month after their delivery. The motherÂfs mean age was 30.6 years, ranging from 20 to 41 years. The middle pregnancy questionnaire was composed of the Antenatal Maternal Attachment Scale (AMAS; Honjo, et al., 2003) a scale of anxieties concerning future child rearing, menstrual conditions before pregnancy, and socio-demographic variables. The one month after delivery questionnaire was composed of the Postpartum Maternal Attachment Scale (Nagata, et al., 2000), Self-rating Depression Scale (SDS), and the Edinburgh Postnatal Depression Scale (EPDS). **Results:** A significant moderate correlation was found between AMAS and Postpartum Maternal Attachment Scale ($r = 0.45$, $p < 0.001$). In addition, menstrual tension and anxieties concerning future child rearing showed significant correlations with Postpartum Maternal Attachment Scale, ($r = -0.18$, $p < 0.05$; $r = -0.23$, $p < 0.01$, respectively). The EPDS score was significantly higher among mothers who had had menstrual tension (6.15, S.D. = 5.2) than those who had not had menstrual tension (4.04, S.D. = 5.2). **Conclusion:** These results suggest that the maternal attachment score during pregnancy can predict maternal attachment one month after delivery, and that the menstrual conditions and anxieties concerning future child rearing can also predict maternal attachment one month after delivery.

P-020-376   Topic: 51
Childhood trauma questionnaire-results from a pilot study in young people

Vaska Stancheva-Popkostadinova, South-West University, Medical-Social Sciences, Blagoevgrad, Bulgaria, v_stancheva@abv.bg
Meglena Achkova

Objective: The aim of the study are: to pilot testing the Childhood Trauma Questionnaire in young people in Bulgaria; to reveal the main traumatic experiences in young people during their childhood and to provide some recommendations for prevention programs. **Methods:** Childhood Trauma Questionnaire (53 items version, D. Bernstein, L. Fink, 1993) was selected for the purpose of the study. Double translation and linguistic adaptation was done. The questionnaire was answered by 80 young people, aged 19–23 (high school pupiles and students in helping professions). **Results:** The most prevalent item was emotional neglect. The study group of young people was growing up in a period of severe socio-economic changes (1989–1999). The parents transferred the crisis to the children. Rarely, but there are still existing some inappropriate approaches for discipline on children. **Conclusion:** This study revealed that The Childhood Trauma Questionnaire was socially accepted and might be used for screening of traumatic experiences in childhood, including physical, emotional and sexual abuse, and physical and emotional neglect. Recommendations for prevention programs are made.

P-021
Psychosocial and legal issues II

P-021-377   Topic: 53, 73
Impact of extreme events on the mental health of children

Evgeny Koren, Moscow Research Institute, of Psychiatry, Moscow, Russia, evkoren@yandex.ru

Objective: To establish liability to the influence of extreme events among children victims of local military actions and consequences of terrorism acts and disasters. **Methods:** We have examined 58 child subjects (age 3–17) suffered from armed conflict in Chechenia, victims from terrorism attack in Moscow metro and failure of aquapark according to the clinical interview based on criteria ICD-10 and DSM-IV. **Results:** Different symptoms of PTSD occured in the whole sample of children with prevalence of flash-back type over avoidance type symptoms. High-rate comorbidity with depression, enuresis, tics, hyperactivity disorders and aggressive behaviour are marked. **Conclusion:** Children are a vulnerable group for extreme traumatic events. Variety of symptoms not quite satisfying the requirements of PTSD are marked. It would be important to learn from our experiences to find out a common approach to the problem of diagnostic criteria for PTSD in childhood age.

P-021-378   Topic: 52, 59
The difference of anger expression after violent computer game by adolescents:
Personality characteristics

Young-Sik Lee, Youngsan Hospital, Dept. of Neuropsychiatry, Seoul, Republic of Korea, hawkeyelys@hanmail.net

Objective: It has been well known that violent computer game negatively affect the violence of adolescent. However, some studies proposed the positive effect of violent computer game by catharsis effect. Under the assumption that the different effects of violent computer game were determined by personality character, we performed this experimental study. **Methods:** In 80 male adolescents, Spielberg's STAXI (State-Trait Anger Expression Inventory) was measured before and after exposing violent computer game. We used Warcraft 3 real time simulation game. Subjects' personality character was assessed by MMPI. **Results:** After exposing violent computer game, subjects' Anger-In and Anger-Control subscores were decreased ((p=0.039, p=0.024). However State Anger, Trait Anger, Anger-Out and Anger Expression subscores were not changed. There were different results according to subjects' MMPI subscales. High D scale group (upper 30 percentile) significantly decreased Anger-Out subscale scores (t=−2.196, p=0.033), and high Si scale group also significantly decreased Anger-In subscale scores (t=2.851, p=0.006) after

exposing violent computer game. These phenomenons were reversed in low D scale group and low Si scale group. There was no difference between high and low Pd scale group. **Conclusion:** We found that the violent computer game negatively affect the anger control in adolescents. However, we also support the catharsis theory in some adolescents having depressive and poor social interaction characteristics.

P-021-379   Topic: 52, 41
Self-perception profile of violent adolescents

Emine Kilic, Ankara University, Medical Sch, Child Pscyhiatry, Ankara, Turkey, kilic@dialup.ankara.edu.tr
Gönül Erdogan

This study aims to look for differences in self perception between adolescent boys who are violent in school and who are not. 25 boys from 6th 7th and 8th grades of school who were reported as violent by their teachers were compared to a control group of 25 boys who were rated as not showing violent behavior by their teachers. It is known that children who use violence use this as a way to be accepted by their peers. They have problems forming close relationships and are less liked by their peers. They are mostly lonely children and have an avoidant attachment style. They don't feel secure in close relationships and are mostly pessimistic about their relationships. Self-Perception Profile for adolescents is a scale developed by Harter to tap domain-specific judgements of adolescents about themselves as well as the global perception of one's worth as a person. Studies comparing adolescents who have signs of psychopathology with normals have found that normals rate themselves as better on scholastic competence, job competence, close friendship, and global self-worth. It is hypothesized that adolescents who have a violent attitude will show less self-worth and problems in domains of self, like behavioral conduct and close friendship that are measured by this scale. Differences between violent and non violent adolescents in various domains of self-perception are discussed.

P-021-380   Topic: 54, 45
The psychological condition of refugee children in Hamburg, Germany, and first implications on psychotherapeutic effects

Rami Gaber, Hamburg, Germany, ramigaber@web.de
Areej Qasqas; Martin Aßhauer; Hubertus Adam; Peter Riedesser

Objective: To examine the relation between psychic disorder and exposure to war trauma and the influence of psychotherapy on psychopathology. **Methods:** Patients treated during the last three years and their parents were reinvited in order to obtain an indepth assessment of their psychological status. The sample includes 100 patients aged 8–21 from Afghanistan and the former republic of Yugoslavia. These patients were treated either in the outpatient unit, inpatient unit or in the day hospital of our clinic. The psychological status was assessed with a newly developed set of questionaires for refugee children and their parents. The "Scales for Children afflicted by War and Persecution" (SCWP) measure the following variables: Exposure to War Trauma, Perception of Parental Functioning, PTSD, Depression, Anxiety, Somatization, Coping Strategies and Attitude to Reconciliation. The "Scales for Parents afflicted by War and Persecution" (SPWP) contain among others the CBCL. The number of therapy sessions was assessed with the "Basic Documentation for Child- and Adolescent Psychiatry" (BaDo) at the time of release from the clinic. **Results:** The results are in progress. **Conclusion:** When statistically controlling the degree of exposure to war related experiences, we expect that an improvement of psychopathology is related to the number of therapy sessions.

P-021-381 Topic: 53, 2
Helping war-affected children and youth in Sierra Leone: A qualitative study
Lynne Jones, Cambridge University,
Centre for Family Research, Cambridge, United Kingdom,
lynnemyfanwy@yahoo.co.uk

Objective: To explore the appropriateness of western concepts of CAMHS provision in a war-affected community in Sierra Leone. **Methods:** A mental health needs assessment was conducted 2 years after the war ended. It included: a) 6 focus group discussions with primary and high school children (total 50) exploring: psychosocial concerns; conceptualisations of emotional distress and mental illness; help-seeking behaviours. b) Interviews with key informants including indigenous healers. c) 27 clinical consultations were audited. The results of the focus group discussions, audit and three detailed case histories are presented to demonstrate the issues confronting western service providers in such a setting. **Results:** There is no concept of adolescence. Youth begins at puberty and continues until parents die. The disruption of war means boys in their 20's still attend school. 50% of the boys had been abducted and served in one of the fighting forces. 70% of children had lost one or both parents through abandonment or death. Children identified loss of a parent, memories of frightening events, abuse by foster parents, early marriage, early child bearing, and sexual assault as problems leading to sadness (poil-heart in Creole). Friends or family, not professionals, were the preferred source of support. Western humanitarian agencies were changing this perception. The Creole category "out-of head" encompasses most serious mental disorders recognized by western practitioners. 'Out-of-head' results from witchcraft or evil spirits and requires indigenous treatments. These are ineffective for youth with psychotic illnesses precipitated by a combination of substance abuse, traumatic exposure and organic factors and can cause physical harm. Western help may be

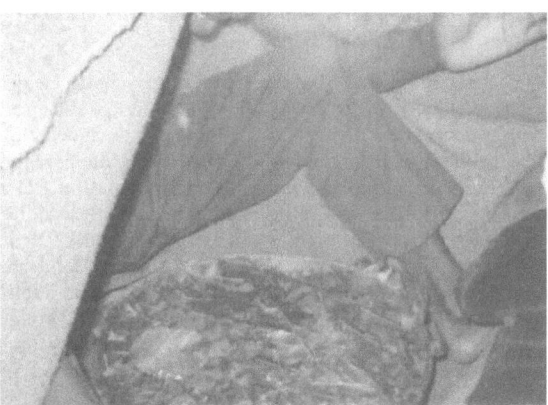

sought after indigenous treatments have failed. **Conclusion:** Western practitioners should rethink their age frameworks for service provision in areas with different constructions of adolescence. The arrival of western mental health services is altering concepts of mental illness and may undermine some effective coping systems while improving damaging ones. A collaborative relationship with indigenous healers is possible and essential.

P-021-382 Topic: 52, 56
Violence among young prisoners
Linda Rachidi, Ibn Rushd University Psychiatr, Psychiatry,
Casablanca, Morocco, rachidili@yahoo.fr
Kawtar Halty; Nadia Kadri; Driss Moussaoui; Omar Battas

Objective: The violence is in increase in all societies, with severe impact particularly in adolescent an his environment. The aim of the present study was to explore the socio-epidemiological and psychiatric profile of young condemned Moroccan for violence. **Methods:** A pilot transsectional study was conducted by residents in psychiatry in jail. Instruments used were: a questionnaire inquiring about sociodemographic characteristics, substance abuse, personal and family history, cause of incarceration, the MINI and overt aggression scale of Yudovsky (OAS). **Results:** 25 adolescents with a mean age of $15 + 3$ years were included. 8.7% of them were illiterate, 73.9% left school at the primary level. The prevalent psychiatric diagnosis were substance abuse (58.3%), a current major depressive episode (41.7%), a psychotic episode (25%), 50% of them had a high score of agressivity (OAS). Family and social environnement was disturbed in 90% of cases. There was a positive association between violence and substance abuse, psychiatric disorders and judicial past-history. **Conclusion:** It is necessary to include the psychological approch in the management of adolescent prisoners

P-021-383 Topic: 53, 52
Early intervention and follow-up of children with acute stress reaction after suicide bombing attacks. Intensiveness of treatment versus prognosis
Agnes Leor, Tel-Aviv Medical Center, Child Psychiatry,
Tel Aviv, Israel, agnesleo@netvision.net.il
Shmuel Tyano; Schaul Shreiber

Objective: Description of acute stress disorder treatment in children and adolescents is rare and controversial in literature. Our objective is to describe the mode and outcome of intensive treatment of ten patients (aged 2.5–17) and their families. **Methods:** 1) Early (at emergency room) and intensive (every day or every other day) intervention. 2) Length of treatment: ten days to three months. 3) No systematization of intervention. 49 The essentials tools of treatment were: holding, support, orientation, cognitive and behavioral advises. Respect the tendency to recall and ventilate, as well as the opposite need. Respect the need for repression 5) Evaluation for need to further intervention. **Results:** 1) In children and adolescents, reaction of parents has great importance in apparition and maintenance of symptoms. 2) Prognosis: 70% full recovery, 20% mild symptoms, 10% PTSD. 3- Correlation of response to treatment with age and with compliance to treatment: The 30% of symptomatic patients at long-term follow-up are all adolescents. The only PTSD patient was with no involvement at all of parents in treatment. **Conclusion:** Early intensive supportive cognitive behavioral intervention, completed by family support is effective in preventing and lowering mental and developmental morbidity including PTSD of children and adolescents after suicide bombing attack.

P-021-384 Topic: 52
Children exposed to domestic violence

Mari Kasahara, National Center for ChildHealt, Psychosocial medicine, Tokyo, Japan, kasahara@kc4.so-net.ne.jp
Nan Hosogane; Kyoto Watanabe; Masaki Kodaira; Makiko Okuyama

Objective: The purpose of this study was to investigate the psychiatric symptoms experienced by children exposed to domestic violence (DV), and the factors which influenced their mental status. **Methods:** The subjects were 16 children (6 boys and 10 girls; mean age 8.1 years old; age range 0–13) who were exposed to DV, and visited the department of child psychiatry of the National Center of Neurology and Psychiatry, or the National Center of Child Health and Development. We investigated mental status of these children, degree of DV, mental status of parents (all mothers) exposed to DV and treatment period. As control, abused children without DV were investigated. **Results:** Children with DV experienced various psychiatric symptoms such as, depressive mood, regulatory disorder, suicidal ideation, PTSD, school refusal, and 5 cases out of 16 also had mild@developmental disorders (e.g. ADHD, Asperger syndrome, mild mental retardation). The result of this study implicated that the severity of psychiatric symptom of children exposed to DV was related with comorbid developmental disorder, and their improvement was influenced by the parental psychosocial level. **Conclusion:** Children exposed to DV show various psychiatric problems, and the involvement of developmental disorders and their mothers' psychosocial problems were implicated.

P-021-385 Topic: 52, 42
Psychopathological consequences of school bullying in Korean middle school students: A prospective study

Young-Shin Kim, UC Berkeley, Child Study Center, Berkeley, CA, USA, kimy02@berkeley.edu
Bennett Leventhal; Yun-Joo Koh; W. Thomas Boyce

Objective: School bullying, the most common type of school violence and peer rejection, is associated with various behavioral, emotional and social problems and can lead to serious psychological sequels. Self-report and peer nomination are the two most widely used instruments to identify students involved with school bullying. This study examines the properties of both self-report and peer nomination in bullying, to compare the differences in psychopathological consequences of experiencing bullying in Korean middle school students, using a 10-month prospective study design. **Methods:** 1666 (out of a possible 1756) 7th and 8th students (94.5% follow-up rate) participated in this prospective study. Study subjects completed the Korean-Peer Nomination Inventory (K-PNI), a Self-report on school bullying, the Korean-Youth Self Report (K-YSR), and a demographic questionnaire. Additionally, parents and teachers of a selected sub-sample (N=330) completed the Korean-Child Behavior Checklist (K-CBCL) and the Korean-Teacher Report Form (K-TRF). Victim, perpetrators and victim-perpetrators (VP) were categorized into 4 groups by self-report and peer nomination: self and peer normal group, peer-only identified bullying, self-only identified bullying, peer and self identified bullying groups. A T-score on the K-YSR, K-CBCL and K-TRF of greater than 65 on the internalizing and externalizing symptoms was considered to be "clinical symptom positive" as suggested by Achenbach. Descriptive statistics, correlational analysis and multivariate logistic regression were performed. **Results:** 1) The correlation between self-report and peer nomination of bullying was minimal. The two victimization scores were significantly correlated, but at a low magnitude (r=0.198). Perpetrator scores were not correlated at all. 2) Higher peer nomination for victimization was significantly correlated with low self-respect (r=−0.254), whereas self-report of bullying was not. 3) With regard to victims, adolescents and parents reported the highest risk of developing new externalizing and internalizing symptoms in self-only identified victims, whereas teachers reported highest risk in peer-only identified victims, 10 months later. 4) In perpetrators, adolescents reported increased risk for externalizing symptoms in all perpetrator groups, whereas parents reported increased risk for internalizing symptoms in self-only identified perpetrators at follow-up. 5) Among the VPs, adolescents reported increased risk for internalizing symptoms in the self-only identified VPs and increased risk for externalizing symptoms in peer-only identified VPs. On the other hand, parents and teachers reported increased risk for externalizing symptoms in self-only identified VPs and peer-only identified VPs, respectively. **Conclusion:** Results from this longitudinal study demonstrate that self-reports and peer nominations regarding school bullying do not converge. As a result, the use of multiple sources of information may be necessary to fully characterize the causes and consequences of school bullying. Additionally, students who considered themselves victims or VPs of bullying, irrespective of the actual occurrence of the bullying, appear to be at the greatest risk for developing psychopathology 10 months after initial identification. This particular group thus warrants careful clinical attention.

P-022
Psychosocial and legal issues III

P-022-386 Topic: 56
Influence of antipsychotic medication on adolescents life quality – pilot study

Vesna Milinkovic, KBC Kragujevac, Klinika za psihijatriju, Kragujevac, Serbia and Montenegro, vesna1972@verat.net
Smiljka Popovic-Deusic; Milica Pejovic-Milovancevic; Olivera Aleksic; Biljana Pirgic

Objective: To examine the impact of antipsychotic medication on subjective quality of life of adolescents after acute psychotic reaction. **Methods:** The research included three groups of patients, previously diagnosed as acute psychotic reaction. First group was on risperidone, second on clozapine, and the third was on convectional antipsychotics. The patient's quality of life was measured by KINDL instrument (child and parent version). **Results:** Conducted investigation proved lower quality of life in treated adolescents compared to healthy population. Clozapine treated patients had higher quality of life than other two groups. **Conclusion:** Higher life quality of clozapine treated patients could be explained with different profile of side effects which are less interfering with normal life style.

P-022-387   Topic: 57

The problem of credibility assessment in people with mental disorders

Sonja Liptai, Universität Tübingen,
Kinder- und Jugendpsychiatrie, Tübingen, Germany,
Marianne.clauss@med.uni-tuebingen.de
Marianne Clauß; Gunther Klosinski

Objective: Systematization of the problematical areas of credibility assessment in people with mental disorders on the three levels of credibility analysis: competence of the witness, failure and quality of testimony. **Methods:** Literature research in the areas of child and adolescent psychiatry, adult psychiatry, psychology and law. Analysis of about 40 reports in which the witnesses had mental malfunction or a history of mental disorder. **Results:** On the level of failure of testimony we mainly found sources of error in personality disorders, especially in histrionic an Borderline personality disorders. Additionally, more unusual sources of error due to mental disorders were shown. On the level of competence of witness most restrictions were found in mental retardation, intellectual disabilities, substance-related disorders, schizophrenia and other psychotic disorders. On the level of quality of testimony possible difficulties were found in several disorders, e.g. in lack of quality in people with history of chronical schizophrenia. **Conclusion:** In literature there has been little discussion and research on this topic. Mental disorders are an important aspect in credibility assessment.

P-022-388   Topic: 61

Production of a concept on sexual self-determination (sexual maturity) in juveniles aged 14 to 16 on the basis of § 182 (2), German Penal Code

Petra Heuer, University Tübingen, Child and Adolescent Psychiatr, Tübingen, Germany,
Marianne.clauss@med.uni-tuebingen.de
Marianne Clauß; Gunther Klosinski

Objective: Attempt of a definition of sexual maturity with criteria for age limitation of sexual self-determination. **Methods:** Literature research from the areas of development psychology, children's and juveniles' psychiatry and law. In addition, there were expert analyses on § 182 (2), German Penal Code. **Results:** Standardised criteria for age limitation of sexual maturity were not found in the literature. There is a requirement for a definition of sexual self-determination, in particular indications of demarcation of sexual immaturity from sexual maturity. **Conclusion:** Criteria of sexual maturity should be researched in further studies.

P-022-389   Topic: 63

Changes in nurse care over child on hospital ward – an educational approach

Maria Danuta Glowacka, Univ. of Medical Sciences,
Dept. of Health Sciences, Poznań, Poland,
ewa.mojs@medscape.com
Ewu Mojs

Objective: Care over child with acute or long term disease brings new demands for nurse care. This is connected with novel social demands, cultural transformation in Poland, progress of technology in medicine and enlargement of parents' awareness concerning social and emotional needs of children. Universities in Poland have long tradition in high education of nurses. Karol Marcinkowski University of medical sciences develops courses in nursing which include: nursing sciences foundation, nursing as individuals and as a profession, nursing professional competencies in management, soft nursing competencies in psychology. **Methods:** The aim of the study was to recognise the expectations toward nurses' work on pediatric ward and to know the profile of nurse working place. 40 nurses and 40 parents of children participated in the study. They fulfilled the questionnaire. **Results:** The results show that the main domain of parents is that nurses should recognise emotional needs of children, their mood and make intervention in this area. Nurses should also have excellent professional skills. The results from the nurse questionnaire show the profile of nurse staff on hospital ward. There are main traits as: ability of making decisions, analytic thinking, social skills, assertiveness, empathy, coping with stress skills. These results show differences in nurse and parent point of view. **Conclusion:** Our academic course in nursing should include demands of working place and parents demands which show the specificity of work with children as well.

P-022-390   Topic: 61

The historical aspects of Stigma attached to children and adolescents with mental illness

Abdul Nasser Kaadan, Aleppo, Syria,
a.kaadan@scs-net.org

Objective: Children with mental illness have traditionally been surrounded by community misunderstanding, fear, and stigma. The aim of this paper is to present details of development of stigma in our society, and a proposal of how could we release an enlightening campaign in our countries, aiming to erase or fight stigma associated with mental diseases, depending on increasing knowledge about mental illness in children. **Methods:** The paper provides an analysis of the historical processes by which stigma has emerged and became associated with these particular disorders. It also explores the process by which these associations have been loosened, identifying distinctive features of stigma that may guide intervention programs; and evaluating changes in the magnitude and character of stigma over time and in response to interventions and social changes. **Results:** Stigma towards children and adolescent with a mental illness has a detrimental effect on their ability to obtain services, their recovery, the type of treatment and support they receive, and their acceptance in the community. The stigma associated with mental illness now is in large part promoted by the media. Improving community attitudes by increasing knowledge and understanding about mental illness, is essential if children with a mental illness are to live in, and contribute to, the community, free from stigma. **Conclusion:** Stigma is one of those social maladies that will probably never be totally eliminated, but there are ways in which it can be diminished. Although, research on stigma has grown dramatically over the past two decades, particularly in the social psychological field in the western countries, I hope that this paper may provoke more studies and researches to be carried out in our region.

P-022-391   Topic: 63, 7
Working with the transference but not in the transference and cognizant of counter-transference: A paediatric perspective

*Samuel Menahem, Monash Medical Centre,
Psychological Peadiatrics, Clayton Melbourne, VC,
Australia, sam.menahem@rch.org.au
Frances Salo-Thompson*

Objective: This reflective paper reviews the importance of the understanding of transference in the day to day practice of the consultant paediatrician, drawing on experience and training over many years. A competent paediatrician learns to take a full history and carry out a complete examination of the infant, child and adolescent. Much, if not most, of the history is taken from the parent(s) or caregiver with some contribution from the older child and adolescent. There is a need to carry out a formulation, arrive at a provisional diagnosis, and impart that information and suggest a plan of management to the parents and child. **Methods:** While there is a need to take into account the important psychological and developmental issues involving the child and their families, in most cases there is little more required from the paediatrician other than that he or she is caring and competent. Even then, especially when the child is ill with the risk of serious sequelae and/or death, the parents may view the paediatrician as omnipotent, an all healing person with powers that he or she does not possess. At times the paediatrician may be caught up in that illusion to the detriment of all concerned with resultant anger and frustration on the part of both parties when the outcome is not as anticipated. In contrast the paediatrician may feel especially vulnerable and impotent to alter the course of an illness, or because of lack of knowledge/skills/resources etc., is unable to achieve a better outcome. That grief may be realistically based but again further compounded by the distressed, needy, dependent parents who may feel inappropriately guilty and neglectful because of what has happened to their sick child. How much more difficult for the paediatrician when he or she has to deal with a child who has become ill because of the parents' wilful or unwitting neglectfulness or injury inflicted by them for whatever reasons. How well can the paediatrician cope with his/her own anger/disgust/despair towards the parents when what is required is a further need for the paediatrician's expertise in understanding and resolving these very difficult situations. How much better is a paediatrician able to cope with the stresses of everyday practice if he or she is aware of the whole basis of transference but guarding against working in the transference, dealing with the here and now, recognising his or her needs and those of the child and the parents, not being seduced to being other than a competent and caring paediatrician. Such a scenario becomes more relevant when the child and adolescent presents to the paediatrician with somatic symptomatology which may have a psychological basis, there being a need to shy away from unconscious interpretation only voiced once the relationship changes to that of a therapist/patient. Behind a transference of negative feelings of anger may be a cluster of feelings of despair, anxiety and shame. Such an awareness may guide the way the paediatrician frames his or her comments and help decide how best to approach the intervention. In this way the paediatrician is working with the knowledge of the transference to ensure the best care of the patient but not in transferences as a therapist might.

Results: Counter-transference, evoked in response to the patient, may have an important defence function although it may seriously interfere with the care being given. Paradoxically, it may have a communicative value, in that being aware of negative feelings even if unable to explain them, helps the paediatrician in his or her work with his child patients. **Conclusion:** Examples from everyday clinical practice will be given to illustrate these points with suggestions as to how paediatricians may improve their area of self knowledge to the benefit of their patients and their own well-being, drawing on personal experience and practice over many years. Training and supervision as a psychoanalytically orientated psychotherapist involved in the treatment of children and adolescents, greatly facilitated this process.

P-022-392   Topic: 58
The survey of environmental health indices of schools in the villages of Mazandaran Province

*Bizhan Shabankhani, Mazandaran University,
of Medical Sciences, Sari, Islamic Republic of Iran,
shabankhani@yahoo.com
Fatemeh Abdollahy*

Objective: It is apparent that schools have an important role on educating and development of schools have always been one of the main focuses of consideration in the societies. The purpose of this study is to survey the health ad environmental conditions in rural schools of Mazandaran Province. **Methods:** This is a descriptive study during which sampling was done from 102 rural schools of Mazandaran for two months. The gathered information was also obtained by the use of questionnaire measurements, at observation. **Results:** Included in the study werer primary schools, secondary schools and high schools. 33.3 percent of the schools are girls school, 30.4 percent are boy's schools and 36.3 percent are coeducational or two shifts of girls and boys. Each class is 3650 square meters on average area. The number of classes in each school is 6 classes on average. The mean of each class is 27.8 square meters and the per capita to be 18 students in each class. 17.6 percent of the schools have less than the minimum per capita of the students in each class. 17.6 percent of the schools have separated drinking fountains and washbasins, also, the angle of incidence of 42 percent of classes is not correct. In addition to this fact that most of the studied factors in this research are not standard (like other researches), the measured variance of these variables are too great. **Conclusion:** This clearly shows that there is no specific planning for production, development and equipment of Mazandaran rural schools.

P-022-393   Topic: 65, 1
The ethical principle of distributive justice: Consequences for the provision of child mental health services

*Christoph Hoeger, Universität Göttingen,
Kinder- und Jugendpsychiatrie, Göttingen, Germany,
choeger@gwdg.de
Aribert Rothenberger*

Objective: To consider the impact of the ethical principle of distributive justice on problems of child mental health (cmh) care allocation **Methods:** 1. Identifying actual problems of child mental health care with respect to scarce resources due to increasing economic constraints in wealthy western societies 2. Reviewing current concepts of distributive justice 3. Considering possible clarifications when this ethical principle is included in the process of problem solving of child mental health care allocation. **Results:** 1. Actual problems are – scarce resources leading to a lack or an unequal distribution of child mental health services – therefore no equal chance for receiving effective treatment – misplacement of young patients due to a lack of agreement concerning diagnostic and therapeutic standards and due to difficulties of defining criteria for need. 2. A meaning of distributive justice which fits the values and traditions of european societies is the 'fair opportunity rule'. It says 'that no persons should be granted social benefits on the basis of undeserved advantageous properties and that no persons should be denied social benefits on the basis of disadvantageous properties' (Beauchamp and Childress). This rule may result in – a right to equal access to health care or – a right to a restricted fundamental health care. The first option seems to become too expensive. Concerning the second option the society is obliged to define what exactly 'fundamental' means. Looking at cmh sevices, the following aspects could be relevant: – Defining needs including the amount of subjective suffering – Setting priorities with respect to severity of the disorder – Equal access to cmh services – Considering not only a just process but a just outcome. **Conclusion:** The inclusion of the ethical principle of distributive justice reveals different options for child psychiatry on the way between economic constraints and just allocation of services.

P-022-394   Topic: 67
Verbal communication of the deaf children at early age
Svetlana Slavnic, University of Belgrade,
Faculty for Special Education, Belgrade,
Serbia and Montenegro, macesicd@yahoo.com
Dragana Macesic-Petrovic

Objective: The purpose of the study was to determine the level and the quality of the verbal communication of the deaf children aged 10-36 months. **Methods:** The study was conducted in the Clinical Center of the Serbia, ORL Institute University of Belgrade, the Department of Rehabilitation of children with hearing problems. The investigated sample includes the 60 children, both sexes, age 10–36 months, with a bilateral hearing impairment of over 90 dB. **Results:** The results of the investigation point up the different degree of complexity in the development at the area of speech and language, which was in this study defined through the following abilities: – color and the intensity of the speech – the ability of articulation – the ability of understanding the speech and language. The preliminary study has shown that voice of investigated sample had normal qualities, the articulation had 1/3 phonemes less than hearing population of the children and the ability of understanding of the speech was delayed – it was at the level of 14-16 months. The ability of verbal production was also delayed – it was at the level of the 10–12 months. **Conclusion:** On the base of the preliminary results we can conclude that an early rehabilitation of the speech and language development in the population of the deaf children is important.

P-022-395   Topic: 59, 96
Computer game playing patterns and relations between computer game addiction and psychopathology in school-age children
Seoung-Hu Lim, Dong-in Hospital, Dept. of Psychiatry,
Kangneung, Republic of Korea, psylim@hanmail.net
Hee-Jung Byun; Seong-Shim Jeong; Sung-Do David Hong;
Jeong-Hwan Park; Ji-Hae Kim

Objective: The object of this study was to examine computer game playing patterns and psychopathologies related to computer game addiction in school-age children. **Methods:** The subjects were 533 elementary school students (4th to 6th grade) in Kangdonggu, Seoul. We evaluated computer playing patterns of all subjects using computer game playing pattern questionnaire, and determined the risk group of computer game addiction by internet game addiction scale score. We evaluated subscale score of K-CBCL of the parents of all subjects, and conducted correlation analysis and logistic regression analysis between computer game addiction and subscale score of K-CBCL. **Results:** Of 488 responders, 10.2% started playing computer game in pre-school age, and 67.2% started at low grade of elementary school. The mean frequency of computer game play per week was 3.66 days. Mean time spent playing computer games per day was 1.89 hours. 'Simply for fun' was the most common reason for playing computer games (40.8%). Male subjects showed statistically significant differences in age of starting computer game, frequency of computer game play per week, reasons for playing computer game and computer game addiction scale scores. There were significant correlations between computer game addiction scale scores and academic performance, somatic symptoms, attention-concentration problems, and internalizing problems on K-CBCL subscales. However, with logistic regression analysis, only attention-concentration problems on K-CBCL subscales showed significant predictability to computer game addiction. **Conclusion:** Upper grade elementary school students experienced computer game playing at a very early age, and spend much time in playing computer games. There were significant correlation and predictability between computer game addiction and attention-concentration problems.

P-022-396   Topic: 57, 47
Adverse childhood experiences and parental bonding in mentally ill offenders
Eduardo Szaniecki, Tavistock Clinic,
Dept. of Child and Family, London, United Kingdom,
eduardo@szaniecki.f2s.com

Objective: 1. To provide information about the type and level of exposure to childhood abuse and neglect. 2. To investigate participants' perception of their parents behaviour and attitudes towards them when they were children. 3. To investigate the association between early adverse experiences and perception of bonding. 4. To obtain data to work out a sample size calculation for the construction of a larger case-control project. **Methods:** Setting: A Regional Medium Secure Unit in London, UK. Subjects: All patients, both male and female (56 recruited). Inclusion criteria: 1. mental disorder as diagnosed by their Medical Responsible Officer 2. offence serious enough to have warranted admission to a medium secure unit 3. compulsorily detained under the British Mental Health Act 1983 4. age between 18-40 5. basic English 6.

Informed consent. Exclusion criteria 7. acutely unwell 8. diagnosis of learning disability. Measures: 1. "Childhood Trauma Questionnaire" (Bernstein et al 1994). The CTQ is a 28-item self-report instrument that retrospectively assesses experiences of abuse and neglect before the age of 18, as well as related aspects of the child-rearing environment. It has been widely used and has high levels internal consistency (Cronbach's alpha: 0.79–0.94), and test-retest reliability over a 2–6 month interval (0.88). 2. "Parental Bonding Inventory" (PBI) (Parker G et al., 1979) is a 25-item self-report instrument designed to assess the attitudes and behaviours of parents during the first 16 years of life as perceived by their children (participant). The measure is split into two dimensional sub-scales: (i) care (from rejection/coldness to warmth/affection) and (ii) protection (allowance of autonomy to overprotection and control). The PBI has been shown to have good internal reliability (0.88 to 0.94). 3. Socio-demographic questionnaire was also used to collect basic background information and corroborate patient's accounts. The patients' notes were used to supplement the information provided by the patients themselves. **Results:** 66.1% response rate. 1. 24.3%–56.8% of the respondents thought they were exposed to some form of abuse and/or neglect of a moderate to extreme degree when they were children/adolescent. 2. 57.1% and 63.3% of the respondents were of the view that they have had distorted bonding with their mothers and fathers, respectively. 3. Amongst respondents who thought they had distorted bonding with their parents the most prevalent style of bonding was "affectionless control" (22.9%–33.3%), whereby the parent presents a high degree of overprotection coupled with low care. 4. 17% of patients who thought their mothers were "affectionless and controlling" also thought that they were emotionally abused to a moderate-extreme degree (Spearman correlation 0.460, approx. sig 0.005). 20% who showed this bonding style thought they were emotionally neglected by their mothers (Spearman correlation 0.575, approx. sig 0.000). 5. 30% of subjects whose fathers were "affectionless and controlling" thought they were emotionally abused moderate-extremely (Spearman 0.627, approx. sig 0.000) as a child or adolescent. 26% of subjects whose fathers had this bonding style thought they suffered emotional neglect to a moderate-extreme degree (Spearman correlation 0.584, approx. sig .001). 23% of subjects thought they were physically abused moderate-extremely (Spearman 0.677, approx. sig 0.000). 6. The majority (54.2%) had no children. Most maintained contact with their families (67.8%) but the vast majority had no live-in partner (88.1%) or no significant relationship (83.1%). 35.6% of this population committed a violent act to family members. 7. 23.7% of the sample presented a history of juvenile conviction and a little more than a quarter (25.5%) had had contact with a Child & Adolescent Mental Health Service. 8. the main diagnosis at CAMHS was Personality Disorder (5.1%), Psychotic disorder and Hyperactivity disorder (3.4% each) **Conclusion:** 1. There was a trend of an association between being a parent who was perceived as "affectionless and controlling" and more likely to be abusive and/or neglectful towards this population when they were children. 2. The figures indicate that these patients' families may well be an important source of contact (and possibly support) with the outside world. This is especially relevant when the history of violence is taken in consideration. 3. Is this finding relevant to understand these aspects of early psychosocial life as potential risk factors in this population? To answer this question it would be ideal to compare the current population (offenders with a psychiatric disorder) with a population of psychiatric patients with no formal for-

ensic history, and/or include a criminal population with no formal psychiatric history. Such a study might give indications of the strength of the association between early parenting, exposure to abuse, and later criminality in this population. This, in turn, may give important clues about early identification, intervention, and prevention. Finally, statistical calculations based on prevalence (30%) for early abuse and neglect in this population estimate that one would have to have 91 patients on each arm to give a CI 95% 6–24.

P-022-398   Topic: 58
Learning disabilities and school situation from a parental perspective

Lise Roll-Pettersson, Stockholm Inst. of Education, Human Development, Stockholm, Sweden, lise.roll-pettersson@lhs.se

Objective: The purpose of this study was to explore perceptions of parents of children with special education needs in Sweden; whether perceptions varied with regard to the child's age, diagnosis or educational placement. **Methods:** Parents of 62 children filled in a 'Parental Perceptions of School support' survey. Mean child age was 15.5. The participants' children had different diagnoses (dyslexia, autism spectrum disorders and mental retardation). 39% of the children were enrolled in the special education programme. A factor analysis on the survey was conducted, internal consistency of the five factors was calculated using Cronbachs alfa which revealed values between 0.69 and 0.91. Group differences regarding diagnosis and in relation to the five factors were investigated using ANOVA. Pearson Product-Moment Correlation was used to obtain an overview of the relation between child's age and the factors. T-tests were conducted to compare group differences (enrolled, not enrolled in the special education programme). **Results:** The findings revealed significant correlations between child's age and parental perceptions. T-tests revealed group differences concerning parental perceptions of their child's school situation, with parents of children enrolled in the special education programme being more satisfied with their relationship to school as well as with teachers' knowledge. Another finding was that parents of children who had a cognitive disability had significantly higher ratings of agreement concerning their collaboration with school than parents of children with dyslexia. **Conclusion:** The findings may reflect a general decrease of quality in Swedish regular education. It is important that policy makers analyse factors within regular education and special education programmes that are well functioning when creating more inclusive schools. The parents of older children with special needs, regardless of diagnosis or placement, want to have more influence on their child's education, be informed of their child's progress, and be contacted before an IEP is written.

P-022-399   Topic: 56
Life quality of children and adolescents in Germany: Results of a representative telephone survey

Patrick Ehnis, Universitätslinikum Marburg, Kinder- und Jugendpsychiatrie, Marburg, Germany, ehnis@med.uni-marburg.de
Maria Trosse; Fritz Mattejat; Helmut Remschmidt

Objective: In order to have a better consideration of the life quality of mentally disordered children and adolescents, the "Inventory of Life Quality in children and adolescents" (ILC) was developed. One of the main intentions of the scientific efforts was the answer to the question, to what extend the quality of life of mentally disordered children and adolescents is affected by their illness. **Methods:** The ILC is a modular questionnaire that consists of a short screening form and a larger, more detailed part. Another option of the ILC is the parallel inquiry of life quality aspects from the child and the parent at the same time. While the child provides information in a self-report manner, the parent rates the same items on an external basis. The goal is to have two sets of information concerning one child which can be compared to determine the differences. In a representative telephone survey 1008 parental interviews and a total of 316 written questionnaires including a parental rating and a self-report of the concerned child were obtained. At the same time data of mentally disordered children and adolescents were assessed in a multi-centre-study which included seven inpatient units as well as seven children and adolescent psychiatrists (practioners). To compare the patient sample with the student sample matched-pairs were formed in order to control for confounding factors. **Results:** Compared to the children in the telephone group the parents of the mentally disordered children and adolescents rated the life quality of their children significantly lower. The most distinct areas with one standard deviance difference were 'emotional health', 'family' and 'overall feeling'. Also differences were found between the parental rating of the inpatients and the outpatients, where the parents of children and adolescents with a inpatient treatment reported a significant lower quality of life. An exception is the area 'school demands and goals'. **Conclusion:** The results document the ability of the ILC to gather relevant information about the life quality of children and adolescents as well as to differ between the mentally disordered and the healthy children. Furthermore the findings show the necessity to include and implement quality of life as a parameter in the everyday treatment of mentally disordered children and adolescents.

P-022-400   Topic: 58, 43
Perception of parental rearing attitudes and school failure during adolescence

Piedade Vaz Rebelo, University of Coimbra, faculty of Sciences, Coimbra, Portugal, pvaz@mat.uc.pt

Objective: This study is centred on the problematic of the school failure during adolescence, which owns specific characteristics, namely in the case of pupils failing at school for the first time during this stage of development. Factors associated with that situation are, for instance, the intellectual inhibition originated by the modifications of the puberty, the depressive problematic or the dynamics of the parents/adolescents relationship. Previous research has shown that the family influence on school failure is developed at different levels, from family socioeconomic status to family psychological variables, such as parental rearing attitudes. In this context, the aim of this study is, then, to contribute for the clarification of the relative influence of parental rearing attitudes on school failure during adolescence, as well as of the characteristics and forms of this relation. **Methods:** The empirical study was carried out in a sample of 2440 portuguese adolescents attending the 9th grade. The analysis is based on the risk concept, which characterizes the factor predicting an unfavourable result, which, in the context of the present study, is the school

failure. Variables representing the perception of parental rearing attitudes (acceptance, control and permissiveness), the family's socio-demographic status (family socioeconomic status, parental education level), the family structure (parents' conjugal situation, birth order, family size, maternal employment) and the subject's personality, IQ and gender were considered. The fact that the variables concerning the perception of the parental rearing attitudes are continuous implied an analysis of its linearity in logit. This analysis allowed the recoded of the parental rearing attitudes variables and enabled a deeply understanding of its relation with school failure. **Results:** Using the logistic regression technique successive models were also constructed, evidencing the importance of maternal employment and control in continued school failure and of acceptance in adolescence school failure. **Conclusion:** The results evidence the importance of relational factors on the school performance of the adolescents.

P-022-401   Topic: 58
The school experience of students with reading and writing disabilities

Eva Heimdahl Mattson, Stockholm Inst. of Education, Dep. of Hum.Dev.&Spec.Ed., Stockholm, Sweden, eva.mattson@lhs.se

Objective: The objective of this work was to study students with specific reading disabilities and their school experience of goals, organization and way of working and relate this to their expressed opinion on possibilities of participation and influence on the process. **Methods:** At the time of the study the 12 students interviewed visited upper level compulsory school or upper secondary school. The questions were semi-structured and had a prospective nature. The interviews were recorded and transcribed and the results were categorized in relation to the issues of the study. **Results:** A main result of the interviews was that it sometimes took up to two or three years before the school reacted on the problems. The parents often had to struggle very hard to get an appropriate education for their child. A frequent solution was remedial teaching in a so called "small group". The students often looked upon this organization as a sort of discrimination and exclusion. Despite this, provided that the teacher was well-educated, they seemed to accept this system as the only way for them to develop their ability in reading and writing. **Conclusion:** Teachers within the regular school system often lacked sufficient knowledge of how to identify and teach students with reading and writing disabilities. This resulted in that the school either neglected the problem and the student was regarded as anybody else, or that he or she was placed in a "small group" with a more or less educated or even non-professional teacher.

P-022-402   Topic: 56, 41
Mental health and quality of life in Brazil: Worse than in Europe?

Giulietta Cucchiaro, State University of Campinas, Brazil, cucchiaro@uol.com.br

Objective: To determine the mental health, quality of life (QOL) and self-esteem of adolescents living in a typical industrialised Brazilian city, and relate these to demographic factors and European findings. **Methods:** 814 adolescents aged 11 to 16 living in two contrasting areas of Campinas,

Brazil were investigated with self and teacher versions of the Strengths and Difficulties Questionnaire (SDQ, Goodman), the Quality of Life Inventory (Mattejat et al.), and the Self-perception Profile for Adolescents (Harter). **Results:** Overall rates: The SDQ algorithm estimated 10% probable cases with any ICD 10 disorder; 6.9% had conduct disorder, 3.1% emotional disorders, and 0.4% hyperkinesis. Area differences: The adolescents living in the outskirts had far lower social, educational and economic status; 57% vs 29% were African-Brazilians. Despite this, there was no difference between areas for the overall prevalence of mental disorder (11.7% vs 8.5%), or in global QOL. However, outskirts adolescents had lower self-esteem (p= 0.02). Sex differences: There was no difference in overall disorder rates or self esteem; boys reported higher global QOL than girls, due to better reported mental health and greater satisfaction with family life. Area differences by sex: Outskirts boys had more conduct disorders (12% vs 6.2%; p=0.04), but girls didn't differ on any disorder. **Conclusion:** The overall rates of disorder in industrialised Brazil are similar to those found in Western Europe, despite mean family incomes being half or less. Within the Brazilian areas, although there were large social disparities, no significant differences were found in the overall rate of psychiatric disorders or global QOL levels. Further analyses showed that the more disadvantaged area did not differ in some important risk factors for disorder, such as divorce rate, and had increased levels of a protective factor, religious observance. The poorest areas, favelas, were not sampled.

P-023
Disorders and other conditions VI

P-023-404   Topic: 72, 14
Obsessive-compulsive Disorder (OCD)
in paediatric patients: Preliminary data of an open
study with Fluvoxamine

Luigi Mazzone, University of Catania, Paediatrics, Catania, Italy, mazzone@unict.it
Diego Mugno; Liliana Ruta; Valentina Genitori D'Arrigo; Mariadonatella Cocuzza; Giada Morales; Domenico Mazzone

Objective: Obsessive-compulsive disorder (OCD) is a frequent and disabling condition that may start at puberty or earlier and is responsive to specific pharmacological and psychotherapy interventions. Aim of our study is to evaluate the efficacy of fluvoxamine monotherapy compared with fluvoxamine associated with cognitive-behavioural therapy (CBT) in children and adolescents with OCD. **Methods:** Twenty patients with OCD, 14 males and 6 females aged 10 to 16 years, were enrolled. Diagnosis was performed according to DSM IV criteria. Informed consent was obtained from their parents. Patients were randomly divided into two groups: the first (10) treated only with fluvoxamine; the second (10) treated with fluvoxamine and CBT. Drug dose ranged 50–200 mg/day. Severity of symptoms was measured with Children's Yale-Brown Obsessive Compulsive Scale (CY-BOCS); Clinical Global Impression-Improvement (CGI-I) was applied to evaluate the individual answer to treatment. Follow-up was performed at 4 months. Chi square was applied for statistical analysis. **Results:** Symptoms had 40% mean reduction on the CY-BOCS in the first group and 47% on CY-BOCS in the second; Clinical Global Impres-

sion-Improvement (CGI-I) revealed a mean moderate improvement relative to a baseline state in both groups. No statistical difference was found. Asthenia and headache were rare side events. **Conclusion:** Our preliminary data show that in children and adolescents with OCD fluvoxamine monotherapy and fluvoxamine with CBT are both effective for improving obsessive-compulsive symptoms at short term follow-up. The different response to treatment could be related to supportive role of CBT.

P-023-405   Topic: 75, 4
Psychosomatic disorders in children and adolescents, revealed in the general practice in the child polyclinic settings

Nataliya Bobrova, Moscow, Russia, baymer@bk.ru

In the child polyclinic settings 140 patients with atypical disorders of digestive system of non-infectious origin were examined (72 boys and 68 girls at age 3–16). The criterions for being atypical were the: 1) discrepancy between the clinical picture and the data of paraclinical studies; 2) atypical changes in the somatic state; 3) atypical response to the somatic treatment. In 126 patients (66 boys and 60 girls) psychiatric disorders were found. The findings of this study indicates that: 1) In most cases (90%) of children and adolescents with atypical gastrointestinal disorders the evident and the masked affective disorders are present. 2) The most common type of depression in general practice is the agitated depression. 4) A very significant (and, perhaps, the most important) factor, contributing to the development of psychosomatic disorders, is the psychic dysontogenesis;. 5) The course of protracted PSD is determined by the number of subsequent stages, namely of transitory psychosomatic reactions, of psychosomatic state and of psychosomatic personality development. 6) Each above mentioned stage is characterized by a definite state of the involuntary nervous system as the one of the links of pathogenesis (including primary and secondary components of psychogenesis and also components of somatogenesis which arrives at the delayed stages of the disease) of PSD in child and adolescents; The arrival of PSD is determined by (along with main affective and disontogenic factors) "personality" factor, residual organic insufficiency of the central nervous system and also by upbringing malpractice. The factors that precipitates the negative course of PSD includes: 1) underestimation of the psychosomatic nature of the disorder, which does not allow the timely pathogeneticdirected intervention to begin; 2) the absence of objective and subjective opportunities to conduct the comprehensive psychotherapeutic intervention, including individual, group and "familial" methods.

P-023-406   Topic: 72, 79
Obsessive-compulsive symptoms in adults with history of rheumatic fever: Sydenham's chorea and type I Diabetes Mellitus – Preliminary results

Fernando Asbahr, Univ. of São Paulo Med. School, Dept. of Psychiatry, São Paulo, Brazil, frasbahr@usp.br
Renato Ramos; André Costa; Roberto Sassi

Objective: To investigate the presence of obsessive-compulsive symptomatology in patients who had rheumatic fever with or without Sydenham's chorea in childhood. **Methods:** The Yale-Brown Obsessive-Compulsive Scale was used to evaluate obsessive-compulsive symptomatology in thirty-

Table 1: Mean Age at Evaluation, Gender, Interval between Beginning of Disease and Evaluation, the Yale-Brown Obsessive-Compulsive Scale Scores of Patients with History of Rheumatic fever and type I Diabetes Mellitus, and the Statistical Results

	RF (n = 38)	DM (n = 19)	
Age	20.55 ± 9.23	20.63 ± 16.69	t = −0.082; df = 55; p = 0.935
Gender	Males = 11 Females = 27	Males = 8 Females = 11	τ^2 = 2.904; p = 0.234
Intenval between the beginning of disease and evaluation	10.06 ± 3.19	8.74 ± 5.38	t = 1.133; df = 52; p = 0.262
Y-BOCS scores – total	6.86 ± 6.79	4.89 ± 5.87	t = 1.080; df = 55; p = 0.285
Y-BOCS scores – obsessions	2.84 ± 3.28	2.42 ± 3.72	t = 0.437; df = 55; p = 0.664
Y-BOC scores – compulsions	3.94 ± 4.32	2.47 ± 3.02	t = 1.329; df = 55; p = 0.189

RF: Rheumatic Fever; DM: type I Diabetes Mellitus; Y-BOCS: Yale-Brown Obsessive-Compulsive Scale

eight adults with history of rheumatic fever (study group: 13 with chorea; 25 without chorea) or Diabetes (control group; N = 19). **Results:** The obsessive-compulsive symptomatology was similar in both groups, although the intensity of the symptoms was not clinically relevant. Separating the study group, though, patients with rheumatic fever without chorea scored higher than patients with chorea in the Yale-Brown Scale. **Conclusion:** In this pilot study, the similar occurrence of obsessions and compulsions in patients with history of RF and DM suggests that the development of this symptomatology, triggered by group-A β-hemolytic streptococcus infections, is restricted to the rheumatic fever acute phase occurred during infancy, and didn't seem to predispose the appearance of these symptoms in adulthood.

P-023-407   Topic: 71, 6
The role of siblings of anxiety disordered children: Symptoms of mental illness and influence on CBT treatment outcome

Maaike Nauta, Accare, Child & Adolescent Psychiatry, Groningen, Netherlands, m.nauta@accare.nl

Objective: The first objective was to describe siblings of children and adolescents with anxiety disorders in terms of symptoms of anxiety symptoms, internalising and externalising behaviour. Second, we wanted to investigate the influence of these symptoms of the siblings on the treatment effectiveness (CBT). The results of this RCT evaluating CBT versus CBT + a cognitive parent training program have been published as Nauta, Scholing, Emmelkamp & Minderaa, 2003. Sibling data were not included in that paper. Since anxiety disorders are known to run in families, we hypothesised siblings to report elevated levels of anxiety symptoms. The level of problem behaviour in a sibling may be a risk factor for treatment failure of CBT for the anxious child. If more children in the family suffer from anxiety, CBT may be less effective for the referred anxious child, especially if the parents are not involved in the treatment program. Sibling's externalising behaviour may also interfere with CBT outcome, since this behaviour may be disruptive for family life. **Methods:** 76 children and adolescents (aged 7–17 years) were referred to general clinical practice for anxiety disorders, were assessed (semi-structured interview (ADIS), child self-report on anxiety symptoms (SCAS), and parent reports on the child's anxi-

ety and internalising symptoms (SCAS-p and CBCL)), and were all treated with CBT. Half of the families received an additional cognitive parent training. Data on child self-reports and parent reports were obtained from 54 siblings in the age of 7–17 years. Diagnostic status (anxiety disorder or not) at post-treatment and at one year follow-up was predicted by the sibling's symptomatology. Further, residual gain scores (RGSs) were computed as a measure for relative treatment gains and RGSs were related to the sibling's symptomatology. **Results:** Siblings of anxiety disordered children reported lower levels of anxiety symptoms than the anxiety disordered child, and were not more anxious than normal controls. Internalising and externalising behaviour or anxiety symptoms of the sibling were not related to CBT outcome for the anxious child. There was no interaction effect with the cognitive parent training program. **Conclusion:** Siblings of anxiety disordered children are not necessarily at risk for anxious symptomatology. Anxiety disordered children benefit from CBT regardless of the anxiety symptoms or internalising and externalising behaviour of their siblings, and a parent training program did not enhance the effectiveness if siblings showed more symptomatology: there seems to be no contra-indication for individual CBT regarding the sibling's symptomatology.

P-023-408   Topic: 73
Children's reactions to stress and trauma

Sonila Tomori, University Hospital Center, Mother Tereza, Tirana, Albania, s_tomorius@yahoo.com
Valbona Alikaj; A. Como

Objective: The study scope was to detect the prevalence of stress and traumatic reactions and other emotional and behavioral disturbances in school age children and adolescents, as well as finding the frequency of violent experiences and other traumatic life events in the latter. **Methods:** Interview with 196 parents using the structured behavioral checklist (SBC-171). The main variables: social background and demographic data, period of migration, type of traumatization, number of traumatic experiences, separation from parents in early childhood, actual context of life conditions, number of anxiety symptoms. Statistical significance is defined at the 95% level (p < 0.05). The frequency of all variables in conformity of the different item's response was reported. Multivariable-adjusted binary logistic regression was used to assess the independent associations between different variables. All statistical analyses were performed using SPSS 10.0 for Windows. **Results:** 71.3% of children had witnessed events of organized violence during the civil-war-like situation in 1997 in Albania, 7% of children had experienced the unexpected death of an unknown in the road within the last year. 28.2% of the families were migrating to the capital within the last 5 years. 23.1% of children were separated for more than 2 years from their parents during the first years of their life due to emigration, 22.5% were showing loss of concentration, 31.8% symptoms of persistent avoidence of stimuli associated with the trauma, 11.8% symptoms of depression. **Conclusion:** Children of school age living in Tirana have experienced severe traumatic experiences. Symptoms of anxiety and depression show that there is a big need for psychological assistance for school age children while the existing system of care for child and adolescent mental health in the country is poor, offering service to only few percentage of children in need.

Table 1. Symptom Dimensions Found after Factor Analysis of 12 Yale-Brown Obsessive-Compulsive Scale Checklist Symptom Categories in 73 Patients with Sydenham Chorea

	Obsessions	Compulsions	Percentage of the Total Variance
Factor 1	Contamination/ Symmetry	Cleaning	19.26
Factor 2	Hoarding	Hoarding/Ordering	13.25
Factor 3		Cechking/Repeating	12.38
Factor 4	Religious	Counting	10.38
Factor 5	Aggressive/Somatic		9.19

P-023-409   Topic: 72, 29
Obsessive-compulsive symptoms among patients with Sydenham chorea

Fernando Asbahr, Univ. of São Paulo Med. School, Dept. of Psychiatry, São Paulo, Brazil, frasbahr@usp.br

Lisa Snider; Marjorie Garvey; Dirce Zanetta; Helio Elkis; Susan Swedo

Objective: The purpose of the present investigation was to document the phenomenology of the obsessive-compulsive symptoms among patients with Sydenham chorea (SC), the neurologic variant of rheumatic fever. Among patients with tic disorders, a distinctive clinical profile of obsessive-compulsive symptomatology has been described, and we hypothesized that the obsessive-compulsive symptoms occurring in association with SC would be similar to those among patients with tic disorders. **Methods:** Seventy-three patients with SC who had obsessive-compulsive symptoms were assessed with the Yale-Brown Obsessive-Compulsive Scale Checklist (Y-BOCS) at the Pediatric Clinics of the University of São Paulo Medical Center (USP) in São Paulo, Brazil (N=45) and at the National Institute of Mental Health (NIMH) in Bethesda, Maryland, USA (N=28). The 12 main symptom categories were factor analyzed using principal components analysis. **Results:** The principal-component analysis yielded a five-factor solution, which accounted for 64.46% of the total variance. Contamination and symmetry obsessions, and cleaning compulsions loaded highly, accounting for 19.26% of the variance, while hoarding obsessions and compulsions and ordering compulsions accounted for an additional 13.25% of the total variance (Table 1). **Conclusion:** The primary symptom factors among the SC sample were different from those reported by patients with Tourette syndrome and tic disorders, but were similar to those previously noted among samples of pediatric patients with primary obsessive-compulsive disorder.

P-023-410   Topic: 72, 45
Phenomenology of Obsessive Compulsive Disorder (OCD) in German and Turkish Patients

Yesim Taneli, Uludag Universitesi Tip Fakult, Cocuk Psikiyatrisi AD, Bursa, Turkey, yesimtaneli@uludag.edu.tr
Suna Taneli; Andreas Warnke; Pinar Vural; Christoph Wewetzer

Objective: The aim of this study was to compare the phenomenology of obsessive compulsive disorder (OCD) in young German and Turkish patients. **Methods:** Y-BOCS subgroups of OCD symptoms were compared in 80 patients (40 each from the Child and Adolescent Psychiatry Departments of Wurzburg University-Germany and Uludag University-Turkey) with an OCD diagnosis (DSM-IV; ICD-10) using SPSS. **Results:** Mean age (German: 13.4 and Turkish: 12.4 years; p>0.05), girl/boy ratio (German: 0.82 and Turkish: 2.08; p>0.05), admission age, age of onset (German: 10.10 and Turkish: 10.6 years), time from onset to admission, time from onset to diagnosis and age at diagnosis did not differ significantly (p>0.05). The German sample comprised more patients with severe OCD. A) In Germany, 90% had obsessions and 100% had compulsions; in Turkey, both ratios were 97% (p>0.05). The most often obsession was contamination (65%) in Germany and aggressive obsessions (62.5%) in Turkey. In both samples, the most often compulsion was cleaning (German: 77.5% and Turkish: 62.5%). B) In Germany, religious obsessions correlated significantly with contamination obsessions and saving obsessions (p<0.05). In Turkey, somatic obsessions correlated significantly with aggressive obsessions and religious obsessions (p<0.05). C) In both samples, compulsions did not relate significantly to eachother. D) In both samples, contamination obsessions related significantly to cleaning compulsions; while obsessions of symmetry related significantly to ordering compulsions. In Germany, an additional significant correlation was 'saving obsessions & hoarding compulsions'. In Turkey, additional correlations were: 'saving obsessions & cleaning compulsion' and 'saving obsessions & repeating compulsion'. **Conclusion:** Our results support the thesis, that culture and/or nationality affect the phenomenology of OCD. This remains to be investigated from a 'nature or nurture' point of view.

P-023-411   Topic: 71
Anxiety Disorders (AN) in a Chinese elementary school pupils

Linyan Su, Mental Health Institute, Dept. of Child Psychiatry, Changsha, China, sulinyan@sina.com
Kai Wang; Yan Zhu

Objective: To understand the prevalence rate of anxiety disorders in Chinese children. **Methods:** 565 pupils of an elementary school in Changsha city completed the 41-item version of the Screen for Child Anxiety Related Emotional Disorders (SCARED). Then the pupils with a total score higher than cut-off point (≥23) of SCARED were interviewed. **Results:** 140 pupils had a total score higher than cut-off point of SCARED (Anx group). The positive rate of screen was 24.78%. In the Anx group, the scores of all CBCL subscales (except social problem and internalizing, externalizing and total problems) were significantly higher than that of the Non-anx group (pupils with a total score lower than cut-off point of SCARED). All scores of Piers-Harris Children's Self-concept Scale were lower than that of the Non-anx group. 32 pupils met the ICD-10 diagnostic criteria of anxiety disorders (15 boys and 17 girls) among 565 pupils (Prevalence rate of anxiety disorders 5.67 %). Among them, separation anxiety disorder is 1.24%, generalized anxiety disorder is 1.95%, phobic anxiety disorder is 1.77% and social anxiety disorder of childhood is 2.48%. **Conclusion:** The anxiety Syndrom was found frequently in elementary school children. Children with anxiety problems have more behavior problems and lower self-concept, they should be screened for appropiate treatment and support.

P-023-412   Topic: 72
The contribution of home family stress to the presentation difference of childhood Obsessive-Compulsive Disorder (OCD) across home and school settings: A preliminary report

Osman Sabuncuoglu, Marmara Un. School of Medicine, Dep. of Child Psychiatry, Istanbul, Turkey, sabuncuoglu@hotmail.com
Meral Berkem

Objective: We have recently described the presentation difference phenomena which is characterized by significant differences in the presentation of obsessive-compulsive disorder at home and school settings. Furthermore, we aimed to find out whether this phenomena is related to the home family stress. **Methods:** 16 schoolchildren who had the diagnosis of OCD were enrolled in the study. CY-BOCS, Clinical Global Impression Scale (CGI) and a questionnaire which consists of items that serve to compare the symptoms across home and school settings were applied. Family stress was rated on a 5-point scale ranging from 1 to 5 which reflected home stressors such as unemployment, parental conflict and care of elderly. Basic informative data was gathered from the file records of the children. **Results:** Of the total number of children, 75% were boys and 25% girls who had a mean age of 12.50 ± 3.2249. The mean obsession and compulsion subscores are 10.4375 ± 4.0161 and 11.0000 ± 3.4641 respectively both summing up a total score of 21.4375 ± 6.4184. CGI scores for both home and school settings are 4.3125 ± 0.9465 ve 2.0000 ± 0.6325 (t: 9.773, Pa 0.0001). The mean home family stress score was $1.875 \pm 1,0878$. Z scores, derived from the CGI and family stress scores, do not suggest any significant correlation. **Conclusion:** Preliminary data does not support any association between home family stress and presentation difference. Although the presentation difference we have noted previously is a significant finding, larger sample is needed to conclude on the contribution of home family stressors to that phenomena.

P-023-413   Topic: 72, 12
Quetiapine monotherapy in adolescents with Obsessive-Compulsive Disorders (OCD)

Viktoryia Krasavina, Municipal Psych Clinic *15, Adolescent psychatry *22, Moscow, Russia, vkrasavina@rambler.ru
Nina Pykhtareva

Objective: The treatment of psychotic disorders in adolescents has some difficulties. So, the choice of the therapeutic strategy must be conditioned not only by clinical effectivity of the drug, pharmakokinetic properties concerning young age. Also it's important to their high side effect sensitivity during the antipsychotic therapy. Quetiapine therapy in adults was shown to have a wide spectrum of the clinical activity. Such treatment causes a reduction of positive and negative symptoms, aggressive behavior and decreases cognitive-perceptual difficulties in patients with schizophrenia. Also, quetiapine has demonstrated efficacy in depressive and anxiety symptoms. Recently we used quetiapine in management of patients with schizophrenia accompanied with affective disorders, obsessive-compulsive disorders (OCD), senesthopathic-hypochondriacal disorders and neurotic symptoms. **Methods:** The quetiapine monotherapy efficacy have been issued in the group of 10

patients with obsessive-compulsive disorders (average age – 16,5 years old). Patients were treated with quetiapine during four weeks. The primary dose were 50 mg/d with following increase up to 300 mg/d. Efficacy was assessed using the Hamilton Rating Scale for anxiety (HAM-A), Clinical Global Impressions scale (CGI). The course of OCD was evaluated by Yale-Brown Obsession-Compulsion (Y-BOCS). **Results:** The four weeks duration quetiapine treatment was demonstrated the 78.1% reduction of anxiety (HAM-A) and 47.2% obsessive-compulsive symptoms (Y-BOCS). Furthermore, the quetiapine treatment has shown high clinical efficacy according CGI scale. The quetiapine safety was confirmed by low frequency of side effects. Only 3 patients demonstrated dizziness that has been ceased by the dose lowering. **Conclusion:** The results of this preliminary trial suggest high clinical efficacy quetiapine monotherapy of obsessive-compulsive disorder patients. However, it's required to increase the amount of the patients in order to test and confirm these observations.

P-023-414   Topic: 73, 51
An evaluation of the psychiatric comorbidity of PTSD in maltreated and ill children

Eleonora Camillo, University of Rome, Childhood Neuropsychiatry, Rome, Italy, carla.sogos@uniroma1.it
Francesca Piperno; Achille Gigliotti; Daniela Tardiola; Bianca Venuti

Objective: The aim of this study was to analyse the comorbidity of PTSD with other psychiatric disorders related to two different patterns of Trauma (Physical abuse and disease) in order to identify clinical clusters with different developmental risk and different therapeutic approaches. **Methods:** Two samples of 10 children (10 physically abused and 10 with chronic diseases), aged between 6 and 9.2 years, were assessed and compared. The subjects were submitted to psychodiagnostic and neuropsychological protocol currently used by our Centre (intelligence scale, projective tests, playing assessment and psychiatric interview with parents). Symptoms were classified following DSM-IV criteria. **Results:** There is a significant association between physical abuse and both Dysthimic and Depressive Disorders NAS. Instead of children with chronic disease have shown the PTSD correlated prevalently with Oppositional and Defiant Disorder and Dystimic Disorder. **Conclusion:** The comorbidity of PTSD is discussed and related to different psychopathological patterns of the two analysed samples: emotional isolation, low self-esteem and overhanging feelings of danger in maltreated children; overhanging fears, need of control, perception of beeing damaged in children with chronic disease.

P-023-415   Topic: 77, 43
Psychological characteristics of eating disorder patients viewed from cosmetic behaviour

Naohiko Tachi, Tamagawa Psychiatric Hospital, Osaka, Japan, n-tachi@msd.biglobe.ne.jp
Naomi Kodoi; Naoko Sakamoto; Michiko Watanabe; Motiko Goto

Objective: Body image distortion is known to be one of main features of eating disorder. It is considered that body image is also strongly related to appearances, which could be modified by cosmetic behavior. Cosmetic behavior is thought to be affected by self image and self consciousness. And it is known that some eating disorder patients make up heavy. In this study, focusing on cosmetic behavior of eating disorder patients, we intend to scrutinize body image distortion of them. **Methods:** We produced cosmetic behavior and body image inquiry test (CBT) and practiced them with eating attitude test (EAT-26) to female collage students as normal control group. We divided this group to high score group and low score group according to the results of EAT-26 and extracted factors. Then, we compared these two groups and group of eating disorder patients. **Results:** There is a remarkable difference in consciousness toward self and body image, and in sensibility of cosmetic behavior between high score group and low score group. High score group is strongly aware of their self and body image, resulting in cosmetic behavior of making display of themselves to others. While, so far as cosmetic behavior is concerned, continuity between high score group and eating disorder patient group us not observed. It is supposed that, for patients, cosmetic behavior is rather performed to cover up. **Conclusion:** From this research, it is demonstrated that eating disorder is not an exaggerated form of dysfunction of eating behavior, and according to CBT, eating disorder patients consists a separate group from EAT high score group. It is supposed that cosmetic behavior of eating disorder patients are not affected by rrelationships to others as observed in normal control.

P-023-416　Topic: 72, 28
Transmission disequilibrium studies pertaining to candidate genes of the Dopaminergic system in children and adolescents with Obsessive-compulsive Disorder (OCD)

Susanne Walitza, Universitätsklinik Würzburg, Kinder- und Jugendpsychiatrie, Würzburg, Germany, walitza@kjp.uni-wuerzburg.de
Christoph Wewetzer; Andreas Warnke; Manfred Gerlach; Frank Geller; J. Reinlein; Nikolaus Barth; F. Hahn; Beate Herpertz-Dahlmann; Christian Fleischhaker; Eberhard Schulz; Helmut Remschmidt; Anke Hinney

Objective: The dopaminergic system was shown to be involved in the etiology of obsessive compulsive disorder (OCD). Here, we screened polymorphisms within the dopamine 4 receptor gene (DRD4) and the catecholamine-O-methyltransferase gene (COMT). For both of these genes positive associations with OCD had previously been reported in adults (Grice et al., 1996, Nicolini et al. 1998, Millet et al. 2003, Karayiourgou et al. 1997; 1999 and Alsobrook 2001). **Methods:** We analysed 50 trios comprising a patient with OCD and both parents. All patients fulfilled the diagnostic DSM-IV criteria for OCD. To confirm the criteria all patients were interviewed with the Y-BOCS and DIPS. For statistical analyses the transmission disequilibrium test (TDT, Spielman et al., 1993) was applied. **Results:** The TDT showed higher transmission of the '7-repeat' allele of the DRD4 48-bp repeat polymorphism ($10\times$ transmitted, $4\times$ not transmitted, one-sided $p=0.054$). There was no evidence for transmission disequilibrium for the alleles of the COMT. **Conclusion:** There is evidence for an involvement of the dopaminergic system in the development of OCD. We found no evidence for an involvement of the COMT SNP in early onset OCD in our study group. However, we detected a higher transmission of the '7-repeat' allele of the DRD4 48-bp repeat in our study group

of children and adolescents with OCD. A similar finding was previously reported in adults with OCD (Grice et al., 1996; Nicolini et al., 1998). Therefore, the '7-repeat' allele of DRD4 or a nearby genetic variation could be a risk factor for development of early onset OCD. Further studies to substantiate the result are warranted.

P-023-417　Topic: 71, 45
A cross-cultural comparison of Brazilian and German disturbed children with anxiety and mood disorders using the Child Behavior Checklist (CBCL)

Henrik Uebel, Universität Göttingen, Kinder- und Jugendpsychiatrie, Göttingen, Germany, huebel@gwdg.de
Tobias Banaschewski; Luis Augusto Rohde; Bjoern Albrecht; Monika Robatzek; Andreas Becker; Aribert Rothenberger

Objective: The aim of this study was to investigate cross-cultural similarities and differences of Brazilian and German children and adolescents with anxiety and mood disorders regarding their psychopathological profile as reported by parents in the Child Behavior Checklist (CBCL). **Methods:** We compared the behavioral and emotional characteristics of a sample of children and adolescents with anxiety and mood disorders from a pediatric psychopharmacology outpatient clinic in Brazil ($N=84$; 23 girls and 61 boys; 8 to 13 years, mean age 10.45 (SD 1.74)) with those of an age and sex matched German sample from an outpatient clinic for child and adolescent psychiatry in Germany ($N=83$; 22 girls and 61 boys; 8 to 13 years, mean age 10.71 (SD 1.74)) as reflected by the subscales of the Children Behavior Checklist (CBCL). A multivariate analysis of variance was computed across the eight subscales of the CBCL. In case of significant differences between Brazilian and German participants additional univariate analyses of variance were calculated. Furthermore receiver operating characteristic (ROC) analyses were carried out to evaluate and compare sensitivity, specificity and positive and negative predictive power of the CBCL at optimum cutoff scores. **Results:** The multivariate analysis revealed significant differences between the two samples. Brazilian parents reported higher levels regarding somatization and anxiety/depression symptoms of their children in the CBCL than those of the German sample. Results of ROC analyses will be reported. **Conclusion:** It has to be clarified by further research if differences in language, culture and the pattern of mental health services or different diagnostic thresholds are responsible for these results.

P-023-418　Topic: 72, 28
Psychopathology in first-degree relatives of OCD children and adolescents

Rosa Calvo, Hospital Mútua de Terrassa, Child and Adolescent Psychiatr, Barcelona, Spain, rcalvoescalona@hotmail.com
Lazaro Luisa

Objective: Few studies have been performed to evaluate the psychopathology in relatives of pediatric OCD and the associations with symptomatology. The purpose of this study is to determine the prevalence of psychiatric disorders in first-degree relatives of children with OCD compared with relatives of controls and to determine whether specific personality characteristics are part of a familial spectrum of OCD. **Methods:** Thirty patients (ages 7–18) with obsessive-compulsive disorder (OCD) and 62 of their first-degree relatives were studied and compared with 30 control probands and a similar number of control relatives. Direct interviews with parents and children were individually performed to asses OCD diagnosis (or indicate the absence of OCD in controls). Instruments used included: Children Yale-Brown Obsessive and Compulsive Scale, CY-BOCS, Structured Clinical Interview for DSM-IV Axis I Disorders (SCID-I), Structured Clinical Interview for DSM-IV Personality Disorders, SCID-II, and Temperament and Character Inventory, Cloninger's TCI to provide a dimensional approach to diagnosis of Personality Disorders (PD). **Results:** The main findings were: 1) early age of onset and severity of OCD were correlated with diagnosis of one or more DSM Axis I disorder in first-degree relatives, 2) The lifetime prevalence of OCD was higher in case compared with control relatives, 3) case relatives had a high prevalence of OCPD. **Conclusion:** Children with earlier age of OCD onset and more severity of symptoms (CY-BOCS) are more likely to have relatives with psychiatric disorders (especially OCD).

P-023-419   Topic: 72, 30
Short term memory and learning ability in adolescents with obsessive compulsive disorder

Nadia Tomassetti, University of Rome, Child & Adolescent Psychiatry, Rome, Italy, n.tomassetti@libero.it
Paola D'Oto; Carlo Di Brina; Francesca Vagnoni; Elvira Rigillo; Lucrezia Cirigliano; Ignazio Ardizzone

Objective: The goal of the present study was to elucidate how a good short term memory capability could provide a significant index of learning ability in obsessive compulsive disorder (OCD) adolescents. **Methods:** Short term memory functions and learning ability was assessed in two adolescents groups: 1) 15 OCD patients, ages 14–17.9 years; 2) 15 healthy subjects peer age and social cultural standard. For the assessment we used two test: Wisconsin Card Sorting Test (WCST) and Test Of Memory And Learning (TOMAL). Especially we focused on Learning to learn score average difference and percent perseverative responses of WCST; on 4 subtests of TOMAL (Word selective reminding, Visual selective reminding, Paired recall, Object recall). **Results:** Statistical data are not available at the moment. Research is in progress yet. However the data available at the moment don't show significant differences between two groups. Moreover data analyses in OCD could yield this trend: a higher percent perseverative responses and negative average difference at Learning to learn score; learning profile subtle higher in relation to expected values in 4 subtest of TOMAL. **Conclusion:** Our data necessitate of further investigations. Nevertheless they allow us to affirm that the OCD adolescents in spite of a diminishing memory confidence don't show an impairment in learning ability.

P-023-420   Topic: 77
Feeding disorders and developmental disorders in early childhood

Anna Costa, Univesity of Rome, Child Adolesc. Neur. Psych., Rome, Italy, costanna1@virgilio.it
Ester Patruno; Anna Fabrizi; Loredana Lucarelli

Objective: Development disorders are typical characterized by neuropsychological dysfunctional patterns. They correspond to different grades of atypical brain development (Gilger and Kaplan 2001 Karmiloff Smith 1998) and are of high psychopathological risk for the affected individuals.

Within theoretical and clinical frame of Infant Research and Development Psychopathology the centrality of interaction between caregiver and child has been proved (Sander 1987; Gianino, Tronick, 1989; Sameroff, Emde, 1989; Stern 1998; Zeanah, 2000). The feeding in early infancy it is an important context of development for the relation between care giver and child where emotional sphere and affect as well sharing of affects promote communication of desires, intentions and needs as well as child's biological rhythms of stabilizations (Stern, 1985; Sander, 1987; Tronick, 1989). The present empiric study is going to proves as following: 1) To valuate with respect of control group, the quality of the relation and individual patterns between care givers and their children in three different clinical groups: – the sample which presents specific childhood language disorder and feeding disorder; – the sample with specific language disorder; – the sample with feeding disorder. 2) To point out the effect of belonging to group variability of the child (DSL, DA. DSL./DA. on the behavior patterns and child emotional functionality). **Methods:** N 30 (couples of care givers and children with DSL, DA, DSL/DA) N 10 (control groups – couples of care giver and children chosen in order by age and sex of the child). Average age of children: 2–7 years (70%) males Average age of care givers: 30 years Tests Feeding Scale (Chatoor) CBCL (Achenbach). **Results:** The most important date to confirm the theoretical hypothesis concerns in the fact that the DSL/DA presents the biggest impact of atypical factors in the feeding scale where compared with children coming from other two clinical groups and the control group.

P-023-421   Topic: 73, 35
Changes in the brain of children and adolescents after traumatic experience:
A review on neuroimaging studies

Uwe Ratz, UKE Hamburg-Eppendorf, Kinder- und Jugendpsychiatrie, Hamburg, Germany, uratz@uke.uni-hamburg.de
Thomas Stegemann; Martin Aßhauer; Hubertus Adam; Peter Riedesser

Objective: Although there have been various studies on neurobiology of PTSD in adults, only little is known about changes in brain structure and function in childhood or adolescence. This review will focus on results from neuroimaging studies in children and adolescents who have experienced severe traumatic incidents. **Methods:** Research was done by means of PTSD-relevant databases (Medline, embase, Psycinfo, Psyndex, PILOTS). Keywords related to PTSD and trauma were combined with neuroimaging techniques in childhood and adolescence. Articles published until January 2004 were included. **Results:** Most of the 12 studies found are based on MRI brain scans, a few studies apply MR spectroscopy and none fMRI to examine anatomical and functional alterations due to PTSD. In most of the examinations smaller intracranial and cerebral volumes are found as well as larger CSF volumes. Duration of traumatic experience correlated negatively and age of onset of trauma positively with brain volume in pediatric PTSD subjects compared to healthy controls. Some studies suggest that brain development is more vulnerable to effects of severe stress in male subjects. A decrease in hippocampal volumes as seen in adult PTSD subjects could not be replicated in pediatric patients. **Conclusion:** Results of reviewed articles provide further evidence to suggest that severe traumatic experiences during childhood and adolescence are associated with alterations in brain structure. In comparison with adults, neuroimaging studies in children and adolescents have to face a number of special ethical and methodological difficulties: e.g. working with child protective services, patients' fear of scanning, age-range and large number of confounding factors that influence brain development. In spite of these limitations, results of anatomical neuroimaging studies have already contributed to a better understanding of the neurobiology of PTSD. Functional investigations, such as fMRI, would be of considerable interest. Especially studies in children are necessary to integrate developmental aspects.

P-023-422   Topic: 72, 28
Obsessive compulsive symptoms in parents of children with OCD and the correlation of OCD symptoms of children and their parents

Pinar Vural, Uludag Universitesi Tip Fakult,
Cocuk Psikiyatrisi AD, Bursa, Turkey,
yesimtaneli@uludag.edu.tr
Suna Taneli; Yesim Taneli

Objective: This study aimed at evaluating the frequency of obsessive compulsive disorder (OCD) and Axis 1 disorders in first and second degree relatives of children and adolescents with OCD. We also aimed to evaluate the relationship of obsessive compulsive symptoms of children and their parents. **Methods:** The study group consisted OCD patients, who were admitted to the Dept. Child & Adolescent Psychiatry at Uludag University in Bursa/Turkey between 1995 and 1999 (40 families). All of the patients (n: 40; f: 27; m: 13) as well as their parents and siblings (first degree relatives; n: 117) were interviewed personally according to DSM-IV diagnostic criteria. Information about second degree relatives (n: 300) was explicitly asked for. OCD Symptoms were assessed according to Y-BOCS subgroups. SPSS was used for statistical analysis. **Results:** Mean age of the patients was 12.4 years. A psychiatric disorder was diagnosed in 80% of the mothers, 69% of the fathers, 18% of the sisters (4/22) and 31.2% of the brothers (5/16). Of first degree relatives, 11% had OCD and 23% showed subclinic OCD. Of the second degree relatives, 4% had OCD and 9.3% showed subclinic OCD. Of first degree relatives, 23% were diagnosed with comorbid depression and 13.6% had comorbid anxiety disorder. Of the children and adolescents with OCD, 62.5% had a comorbid psychiatric disorder (30% depression, 12.5% anxiety, 7.5% ADHD, 5% Tic, 2.5% anorexia, 2.5% enuresis and 2.5% mental retardation). **Conclusion:** Our results show, that comorbidity in children and adolescents with OCD, as well as psychiatric features of first and second degree relatives of these children are similar in Turkey to those reported in other studies.

P-023-423   Topic: 77, 95
Comorbidity of sleep disturbances and behavioral difficulties in school-age children

Ulla Breuer, Universität zu Köln,
Kinder- und Jugendpsychiatrie, Köln, Germany,
ulla.breuer@medizin.uni-koeln.de
Susanne von Widdern; Leonie Fricke; Alexander Mitschke;
Alfred Wiater; Gerd Lehmkuhl

Objective: In childhood and adolescence there exist insufficient and controversial of findings regarding the comorbid occurrence of sleep disturbances and psychiatric disorders, for example with attention deficit hyperactivity disorder (ADHD). Based on this fact, we investigated the prevalence of insomnia, parasomnia, as well as the comorbidity of sleep disturbances and behavioral difficulties in school-age children in a representative sample of school-beginners (Cologne Children's Sleep Study 2002). **Methods:** In the Cologne Children's Sleep Study, parents of the school- beginners (n = 6629) were surveyed, using a checklist for sleep behavior (33 items) and the German Parent Version of Strengths and Difficulties Questionaire – SDQ (Klasen et al. 2000; Woerner et al. 2002). In this study, the response rate was 74%. **Results:** In this sample, we found a two- to three-times elevated risk of hyperactive and emotional problems of children with insomnia or parasomnia with regard to the comorbidity of behavioral difficulties. The greates effect was found in the correlation of daytime sleepiness and emotional problems as reported by the parents. **Conclusion:** These findings indicate a relationship between sleep problems and behavioral problems and underline the necessity for diagnostic clarification of sleep disturbances and intervention programs for behavioral disturbed and sleep disturbed children.

P-023-424   Topic: 73
Treatment for Post-Traumatic Stress Disorders (PTSD) in adolescents

Kyoichi Honda, Matsumura General Hospital,
Child and Adolescent Center, Iwaki, Japan,
k_honda@matsumura-ghp.or.jp

Objective: To examine clinical features of posttraumatic stress disorder(PTSD) in adolescents and develop effective treatment paradigm. **Methods:** We investigated clinical characteristics and prognoses of 9 female patients with PTSD, and studied effective treatment procedure. Our subjects were from 16 to 30 years old (mean age 21 years). Their diagnoses were established according to Hermann's criteria. **Results:** Classification of traumatic episodes consisted of 8 cases with sexual abuse, and 1 case with traffic accident. All subjects in the study were divided into two diagnostic groups, 6 complex PTSD and 3 simple PTSD. Almost of their families were dysfunctional. Clinical symptoms except PTSD were very miscellaneous, such as dissociative disorders including 3 cases of dissociative identity disorder (DID), hallucinations, depressive mood, self-mutilation, and suicide attempt. These subjects were treated with several combinations of psycho-education, expressive or supportive psychotherapy, cognitive therapy, inner child work and milieu therapy. In the 4 cases, their treatment was discontinued or they exchanged hospitals. The relationship between therapist and patients was not stable. **Conclusion:** We regard PTSD as traumatic spectrum disorder from transient simple PTSD to complex PTSD resulting from repeated traumatic exposure for long time. Especially in the complex PTSD, we found serious influence to the personality organization rather than coping behaviors with the traumatic episode. The treatment of PTSD should be administered with several combinations of supportive or expressive psychotherapy and milieu therapy under the safety support system.

P-023-425   Topic: 77, 26
Prevalence of sleep disturbances in school beginners
Leonie Fricke, Universität zu Köln,
Kinder- und Jugendpsychiatrie, Köln, Germany,
leonie.fricke@medizin.uni-koeln.de
Susanne von Widdern; Ulla Breuer; Alexander Mitschke;
Alfred Wiater; Gerd Lehmkuhl

Objective: Diagnostics and therapy of sleep disturbances in adults has been currently recognized as an important health care problem in western countries. Nevertheless epidemiological studies of sleep disturbances in preschool and school-age children are still underrepresented. In the Cologne Children's Sleep Study the sleep behaviour of school beginners was investigated in a representative sample. **Methods:** In cooperation with the public health department the parents of the school beginners were surveyed using a 33-item questionnaire including items related on sleep problems, day time functioning, sleeping environment and sleep hygiene. In total 6629 questionnaires were filled in (response rate: 74%). **Results:** The mean age of the children for whom the questionnaire was completed was 5/6 years old. The sample comprised 48.5% female and 51.5% male individuals. The prevalence of parent-defined insomnia and parasomnia symptoms ranged from 3 to 23%. 18% of the children presented problems falling asleep and/or sleeping all night without awaking. 23% of the parents described that their children wake up frequently in the night. Daytime sleepiness was reported for 4% of the children. The prevalence of parent-reported sleep walking, sleep terror and nightmares was 3%, 4% and 14%. **Conclusion:** The presented data emphasize the importance of sleep disturbances in children. The results may contribute to improve diagnostics and treatment programs for children with sleep problems.

P-023-426   Topic: 73, 45
The presenting symptoms of Post Traumatic Stress Disorder (PTSD) among children in Al-Amiria shelter
Muhmmad Lafta, Al-Rashad Mental, Teaching Hospital,
Baghdad, Iraq, muh1215@yahoo.com

Objective: AL-AMIRIA shelter is one of the common shelters in Baghdad, who had been bombard in Feb. 1991 during the gulf war. The study is aimed to explore the symptom profile of post traumatic stress disorder (PTSD] and any other associated symptoms among Iraqi children. **Methods:** Thirty children, aged from 7–12 y. who were from the survivors or were watching the catastrophe, and met the DSM4 criteria for PTSD, were interviewed twice in 1993 & 1998 respectively. Semi-structured interview and symptom check list of PTSD and stress related neurotic disorder was used. **Results:** All of the patients (100%) had flash backs & ruminations of ideas towards the events. Also avoidance of emotionally charged stimuli was present in all of the group (100%). Night mares 72% ,frequent failure in school 65%, startle reflex 60%, vague abdominal pain 40%, chronic depressive symptoms 27% and nocturnal enuresis 10%, were the main remaining complaints. **Conclusion:** PTSD is a chronic and serious problem, which needs attention and proper management. The avoiding attitude among the children may underestimate the PTSD diagnosis. The associated symptoms of depression or anxiety may overlap the diagnosis of PTSD among children.

P-023-427   Topic: 73, 58
Post-Traumatic Stress Disorder (PTSD), biopsychosocial wellbeing and psychosocial factors in adolescents relocated to a boarding school after the 1999-earthquake in Turkey
Yesim Taneli, Uludag Universitesi Tip Fakult,
Cocuk Psikiyatrisi AD, Bursa, Turkey,
yesimtaneli@uludag.edu.tr
Basaran Sezer; Oytun Hasturk; Secil Oktem Kurultak;
Suna Taneli

Objective: The aim of this study was to evaluate Post-Traumatic Stress Disorder (PTSD), BioPsychoSocial wellbeing and psychosocial factors after a major earthquake, to determine PTSD risk groups and to assess the need for early intervention. **Methods:** In April 2000, eight months after the 1999-Earthquake in Turkey, 27 adolescents (female: 26, male: 1) were assessed, who had been relocated to Bursa because of earthquake damage in their hometowns. Face-to-face psychiatric interviews were conducted in their new boarding school setting, using a semi-structured 'Psychosocial Questionnaire', a 'BioPsychoSocial' (BPS) symptom list (both developed on the basis of the study team's experience with earthquake survivors) and the 'Posttraumatic Stress Disorder Reaction Index for Children' (RI; Frederick C, 1992), which we had translated into Turkish (S.T.) for acute use after the disaster. Nonparametric statistics were applied (SPSS). **Results:** Mean age was $16.7 +/- 0.10$ years (F: 16.6, M: 17.3, $p > 0.05$). All 27 adolescents had 'moderate' to 'very severe' PTSD, the mean Reaction Index score being 49.6 ± 9.9 ('severe PTSD'). Witnessing injury of a loved person increased RI scores (n: 14, $p = 0.094$). RI scores did not (anymore/yet) differ significantly for sex, being without mother/father during the earthquake (n: 7/8), witnessing death of a loved one (n: 13), being burried (n: 2), having physical losses (n: 2), bereavement (n: 19), attending a funeral (n:6) or destruction of the school (n: 13) (all $p > 0.05$). Before-after the earthquake mean number of BPS-symptoms increased significantly; somatic: 1.4–4.1, emotional: 4.3–14.5 and social: 0.15–1.22 (all $p < 0.001$; Wilcoxon). Higher RI scores correlated with more physical, emotional and social symptoms ($p < 0.01$, $p < 0.01$, $p < 0.05$ respectively). **Conclusion:** Eight months after the earthquake, 100% of the adolescents had moderate to severe PTSD and their BioPsychoSocial wellbeing was affected significantly. There is an urgent need for primary/secondary prevention programs, embracing as many individuals as possible affected by a major natural disaster.

P-023-428   Topic: 73
Transgeneration trauma children study
Valbona Alikaj, UHC Mother Tereza, Tirana, Albania,
evag4@yahoo.com
A. Como; S. Tomori; E. Petrela

Objective: The aim was to map the behavioral and emotional difficulties of the children of parents being survivors of imprisonment during the dictatorship of the second part of the last century in Albania. Comparisons with children of parents being survivors of concentration (forced labor)camps were made. **Methods:** 99 imprisoned torture survivors have been randomly selected of a list of 1236 torture survivors drawn by the list of around 43000 former persecuted people available in the ARCT documentation unit, provided by the State Institute for the Political Perse-cuted Individuals (1996). The criteria for selecting the par-ents group: being 18–30 years old in the moment of impri-sonment, being condemned not earlier than 1970, having children under the age of 18 years. A control group of 50 families of parents not being imprisoned but sent to forced labor camps was matched according to childrens age, so-cio-economic status, gender and location. Data gathering: by a team of psychologists previously trained. Instruments used – Parents: General Data Questionnaire, PTSD Diag-nostic Scale, PDS, Family Environment Scale, WHO QoL Bref, PDEQ; Children: STAI, UCLA PTSD Reaction Index. Statistical significance is defined at the 95% level ($p < 0.05$). Multivariable-adjusted binary logistic regression used to assess the independent associations between differ-ent variables. The underlying assumptions of logistic re-gression models were tested with Hoshmer-Lemeshow goodness-of-fit test. All statistical analyses were performed using SPSS 10.0 for Windows. **Results:** 9.98% of the par-ents were diagnosed with the complete picture of PTSD within the study sample, while non from the control group. Partial PTSD was found in 58% of the study sample and in 95% of the control group. Overall QOL score of the imprisoned individuals was 13.13% (concentration camps survivors 36%). Of the 99 child and adolescent partici-pants 23% had at least mild PTSD symptoms (PTSD-RI score $>= 12$); 2% – doubtful PTSD symptoms (PTSD-RI score < 12). 16% met partial diagnostic criteria for PTSD. Of the 50 enrolled participants of the control group 16% met full or partial diagnostic criteria for PTSD. **Conclu-sion:** The children of parents who have survived torture experiences have high level of stress related complaints and high risk in developing the post-traumatic stress dis-order. There is a clear need of focused therapeutic work on this problem group in assisting to overcome the emo-tional and behavioral difficulties.

P-023-429   Topic: 77, 11

An explorative study on the Cologne's treatment program for children with sleep problems

Leonie Fricke, Universität zu Köln,
Kinder- und Jugendpsychiatrie, Köln, Germany,
leonie.fricke@medizin.uni-koeln.de
Ulla Breuer; Susanne von Widdern; Alexander Mitschke;
Alfred Wiater; Gerd Lehmkuhl

Objective: Treatment strategies for sleep problems in chil-dren are only available for the time period of infancy. For example in Germany, several guidelines teach parents how to treat a sleep problem in their child. But we find meth-odological difficulties in psychological treatment strategies concerning children at the age 4 to 13 years. The Cologne Children's Sleep Study pointed out that the prevalence of insomnia and parasomnia symptoms ranged from 3% to 23% in a representative sample of school beginners. The results emphasize the importance of adequate treatment in this age-group. In combination with the described project a psychological group program for parents with children having sleep problems was developed focused mainly on the treatment of insomnia and parasomnia complaints of children. **Methods:** The program was implemented with a small group of parents (4 participants) in order to receive

information on the efficacy of the treatment and also on the necessity of modifying the concept. The children's age was in the mean 7 years. The children of parents attending the group had the following sleep problems: sleep onset delay and night waking, sleep anxiety, sleep walking and nightmares. The parents completed before and after a 3-month interval – in this time the parents were attending on the group program – two questionnaires relating to sleep behaviour, attention and hyperactivity, and as well a questionnaire concerned on the consumer satisfaction re-garding the program. **Results:** Assessed by their parents, the sleep behaviour was improved in all children. More-over the data prove that attention and hyperactivity was reduced in all children. Without any exception the assess-ment of the treatment concept was extremely positive rated. **Conclusion:** Based on these results the program was modified marginally. The conclusion was drawn that the presented group program is a good device treating sleep disturbances in children. The evaluation of the treatment program is in preparation.

P-023-430   Topic: 77

The impact of different information sources for assessing sleep disturbances in school-age children

Susanne von Widdern, Universität zu Köln,
Kinder- und Jugendpsychiatrie, Köln, Germany,
susanne.kraenz@medizin.uni-koeln.de
Ulla Breuer; Leonie Fricke; Alexander Mitschke;
Alfred Wiater; Gerd Lehmkuhl

Objective: In the last few years sleep disorders in child-hood and adolescence are more investigated, especially to assess the comorbidity with cognitive and physical achievements. Most epidemiological studies have consider-ed only parent opinions. The present study assesses the parent-child agreement on sleep problems and connected daytime impairments. **Methods:** Within the Cologne Chil-dren's Sleep Study we investigated the parent and self-re-ported prevalence of sleeping and behavioural parameters in a representative sample of 4587 9–11 year-old primary school students in Cologne in 2002. The assessment in-cludes the parent and self-rated SDQ (Goodman et al. 1997) and a sleep behaviour checklist. **Results:** Sleep-onset problems, night waking, nightmares, difficulty rising on mornings and reduced physical capacity are significant more frequently reported by children than parents (Wil-coxon-statistics: $p < 0.001$). Enuresis, troubled sleep and daytime sleepiness are similar prevalent in parent and self-ratings. Spearman correlations of assessed sleep and fa-tigue problems are in moderate range ($r <= 0.50$) except for enuresis ($r = 0.70$) and difficulty rising on mornings ($r = 0.56$). We found similar correlations between sleep dis-turbances and hyperactive/emotional problems in both child and parent reports, in which the correlations based on self-reports are more pronounced. **Conclusion:** The pre-sent study indicates only a modest agreement of parent and self-reported sleep problems and daytime functioning. Children reported more insomnia problems and night-mares than parents. These findings underline the impor-tance of using multiple information sources to explore children's sleep impairments instead of relying on parent's report only.

Topic Index

A. Care, treatment and prevention

25 Child and mental health issues in the community

26 Epidemiology

84 Attention-deficit/hyperactivity disorders

85 Oppositional defiant and conduct disorders

Author Index

First authors and chairpersons are indicated with bold names. The page number of their appearance in this book is indicated in boldface, too. Page numbers in normal text denote the appearance as co-author.